W0050513

TUMOR INVASION AND METASTASIS

DEVELOPMENTS IN ONCOLOGY 7

Other volumes in this series:

1. F.J. Cleton and J.W.I.M. Simons, eds., Genetic Origins of Tumor Cells
   ISBN 90-247-2272-1
2. J. Aisner and P. Chang, eds., Cancer Treatment Research
   ISBN 90-247-2358-2
3. B.W. Ongerboer de Visser, D.A. Bosch and W.M.H. van Woerkom-Eykenboom, eds., Neuro-Oncology: Clinical and Experimental Aspects
   ISBN 90-247-2421-X
4. K. Hellmann, P. Hilgard and S. Eccles, eds., Metastasis: Clinical and Experimental Aspects
   ISBN 90-247-2424-4
5. H.F. Siegler, ed., Clinical Management of Melanoma
   ISBN 90-247-2584-4
6. P. Correa, ed., Epidemiology of Cancer of the Digestive Tract
   ISBN 90-247-2611-5

Series ISBN: 90-247-2338-8

TUMOR INVASION AND METASTASIS

edited by

L.A. LIOTTA
National Cancer Institute,
Bethesda, Maryland

and

I.R. HART
Frederick Cancer Research Center
Frederick, Maryland

1982

MARTINUS NIJHOFF PUBLISHERS

THE HAGUE / BOSTON / LONDON

Distributors:

for the United States and Canada
Kluwer Boston, Inc.
190 Old Derby Street
Hingham, MA 02043
USA

for all other countries
Kluwer Academic Publishers Group
Distribution Center
P.O.Box 322
3300 AH Dordrecht
The Netherlands

Library of Congress Cataloging in Publication Data CIP

Main entry under title:

Tumor invasion and metastasis.

(Developments in oncology ; v. 7)
1. Metastasis. 2. Cancer cells. 3. Cell interactions.
I. Liotta, L. A. II. Hart, I. R. (Ian R.) III. Series. [DNLM: 1. Neoplasm metastasis.
2. Neoplasm invasiveness. W1 DE998N v. 7 / QZ 202 T9235]
RC269.T85 616.99'407 81-18967
AACR2

ISBN-13: 978-94-009-7513-2 e-ISBN-13: 978-94-009-7511-8
DOI: 10.1007/978-94-009-7511-8

Copyright © 1982 by Martinus Nijhoff Publishers, The Hague.

Softcover reprint of the hardcover 1st edition 1982

All rights reserved. No part of this publication may be reproduced, stored in a retrieval system, or transmitted in any form or by any means, mechanical, photocopying, recording, or otherwise, without the prior written permission of the publishers, Martinus Nijhoff Publishers, P.O. Box 566, 2501 CN The Hague, The Netherlands.

Contents

Preface

The clinical significance of tumor spread has always been appreciated. Yet, in spite of the pioneering work and outstanding contributions of investigators such as D. Coman, H. Green, B. Fisher, S. Wood and I. Zeidman, studies on metastasis rarely achieved the popularity afforded to more esoteric areas of tumor biology. Tumor dissemination, occurring as it does in a responding host and being composed of a series of dynamic interactions, is a highly complex phenomenon. Few investigators were brave enough to attempt to unravel the mechanisms involved.

Paradoxically, this very complexity may have contributed, in part, to the recent upsurge of interest in metastasis research. More and more researchers are becoming fascinated by the complexities of the cellular interactions involved in tumor spread. Accompanying this intellectual stimulation have been technological advances in related fields which allow the derivation of new model systems. The mechanisms of metastatic spread are increasingly amenable to both the reductionist and holistic approaches and it is the purpose of this volume to present many of these model systems while emphasizing the intricacy and complexity of the processes they mimic. We have attempted to emphasize two topics not previously covered in depth in previous books on metastases. These are *in vitro* models of invasion and interactions of tumor cells with connective tissue.

We believe that the present contributions capture some of the excitement and drive that presently pervade this area of tumor biology. Any progress toward the successful achievement of the aims of this book is entirely due to the contributors, whereas any failures may be ascribed to the editors. Constraints of space prevent inclusion of much that is undoubtedly important in metastasis research and the contents of this volume reflect, to a large extent, the personal bias of the editors. This book can do no more than give a hint of the directions in which research into the biology of metastasis is moving. Hopefully, these areas are as of much interest to the reader as they are to the editors.

L.A. Liotta
I.R. Hart

Contributors

BAETSELIER, P. DE, Dienst Algemene Biologie, Vrije Universiteit, Brussels, Belgium.

BARRET, J.C., National Institute of Environmental Health Sciences, P.O. Box 12233, Research Triangle Park, NC 27709, U.S.A.

BARSKY, S.H., Department of Pathology, National Cancer Institute, National Institutes of Health, Bethesda, MD 20205, U.S.A.

BISWAS, C., Developmental Biology Laboratory, Massachusetts General Hospital, 32 Fruit Street, Boston, MA 02114, U.S.A.

CARR, I. and J., Departments of Pathology and Physiology, University of Saskatchewan, Saskatoon, Saskatchewan, S7N 0W0 Canada.

CHU, E.W., Head of Cytopathology, National Cancer Institute, Bldg. 10, Rm. 2A19, 9000 Rockville Pike, Bethesda, MD 20205, U.S.A.

DICKMAN, P., Laboratory of Pathology, National Cancer Institute, Bldg. 10, Rm. 2A27, 9000 Rockville Pike, Bethesda, MD 20205, U.S.A.

FELDMAN, M., The Weizmann Institute of Science, Rehovot, Israel.

FIDLER, I.J., Director, Cancer Metastasis and Treatment Laboratory, Frederick Cancer Research Center, P.O. Box B, Frederick, MD 21701, U.S.A.

FOGEL, M., Institut für Immunologie und Genetik am Deutschen Krebsforschungszentrum, Heidelberg, Federal Republic of Germany.

GARBISA, S., Institute of Histology and General Embryology, University of Padua, Padua, Italy.

GERSHMAN, H., Department of Biochemistry, Case Western Reserve University, School of Medicine, 2119 Abington Road 14263, Cleveland, OH 44106, U.S.A.

GOLDFARB, R.H., Cancer Metastases Research Group, Pfizer Labs, Central Research, Eastern Point Road, Groton, CT 06340, U.S.A.

GORELIK, E., Laboratory of Immunodiagnosis, National Cancer Institute, National Institutes of Health, 9000 Rockville Pike, Bethesda, MD 20205, U.S.A.

HANNA, N., Cancer Metastasis and Treatment Laboratory, National Cancer Institute, Frederick Cancer Research Center, P.O. Box B, Bldg. 539, Frederick, MD 21701, U.S.A.

HART, I.R., Cancer Metastasis and Treatment Laboratory. National Cancer Institute, Frederick Cancer Research Center, P.O. Box B, Bldg. 539, Frederick, MD 21701, U.S.A.

INGBER, D.E., Section of Cell Biology, Yale University, School of Medicine, 333 Cedar Street, P.O. Box 3333, New Haven, CT 06510, U.S.A.

JAMIESON, J.D., Section of Cell Biology, Yale University, School of Medicine, 333 Cedar Street, P.O. Box 3333, New Haven, CT 06510, U.S.A.

JONES, P.A., Children's Hospital of Los Angeles, 4650 Sunset Blvd., Los Angeles, CA 90027, U.S.A.

KATZAV, S., The Weismann Institute of Science, Rehovot, Israel.

KLEINMAN, H.K., National Institute of Dental Research, National Institutes of Health, 9000 Rockville Pike, Bldg. 30, 4th Floor, Bethesda, MD 20205, U.S.A.

KUETTNER, K.E., Chairman, Professor of Orthopedics and Surgery, Department of Orthopedic Surgery, Rush-Presbyterian – St. Luke's Medical Center, 1753 West Congress Parkway, Chicago, IL 60612, U.S.A.

LIOTTA, L.A., Laboratory of Pathophysiology, National Cancer Institute, National Institutes of Health, 9000 Rockville Pike, Bldg. 10, Rm. 5B36, Bethesda, MD 20205, U.S.A.

MAREEL, M.M.K., Academic Hospital, Clinic for Radiotherapy and Nuclear Medicine, Department of Experimental Cancerology, De Pintelaan 135, B-900 Ghent, Belgium.

MARTIN, S.E. Cytopathology Section, Laboratory of Pathology, National Cancer Institute, Bethesda, MD 20205, U.S.A.

MURRAY, J.C., Strangeways Research Laboratory, Wort's Causeway, Cambridge CB1 4RN, England.

NICOLSON, G.L., Department of Tumor Biology (108), University of Texas System Cancer Center, M.D. Anderson Hospital and Tumor Institute, Houston, TX 77030, U.S.A.

PAULI, B.U., Rush Medical College, 1753 West Congress Parkway, Chicago, IL 60612, U.S.A.

POSTE, G., Vice President and Director of Research, Smith, Kline and French Laboratories, 1500 Spring Garden Street, P.O. Box 7929, Philadelphia, PA 19101, U.S.A.

ROSEMAN, J.M., 1399 S.W. First Avenue, Miami, FL 33131, U.S.A.

RUSSO, R.G., Laboratory of Pathophysiology, National Cancer Institute, Bldg. 10, 8-19, National Institutes of Health, Bethesda, MD 20205, U.S.A.

SEGAL, S., The Weizmann Institute of Science, Rehovot, Israel.

SHEELA, S., National Institute of Environmental Health Sciences, P.O. Box 12233, Research Triangle Park, NC 27709, U.S.A.

SIEGAL, G.P., Department of Laboratory Medicine and Pathology, University of Minnesota, Minneapolis, MN 55455, U.S.A.

SUGARBAKER, E.V., 1399 S.W. First Avenue, 200 B, Miami, FL 33131, U.S.A.

TERRANOVA, V.P., National Institute of Dental Research, National Institutes of Health, Bldg. 30, 4th Floor, 9000 Rockville Pike, Bethesda, MD 20205, U.S.A.

THORGEIRSSON, U., Laboratory of Pathophysiology and Pathology, National Cancer Institute, National Institutes of Health, Bethesda, MD 20205, U.S.A.

TRICHE, T.J., Laboratory of Pathology, National Cancer Institute, Bldg. 10, Rm. 2A27, 9000 Rockville Pike, Bethesda, MD 20205, U.S.A.

TRYGGVASON, K., Department of Clinical Chemistry and Medical Biochemistry, University of Oulu, Finland.

VARANI, J., Department of Pathology, University of Michigan, School of Medicine, 1335 E. Catherine Street, Ann Arbor, MI 48109, U.S.A.

WARD, P.A., Department of Pathology, University of Michigan, School of Medicine, 1335 E. Catherine Street, Ann Arbor, MI 48109, U.S.A.

WEINGRAD, D.N., 1399 S.W. First Avenue, Miami, FL. 33131, U.S.A.

WEISS, L., Director of Cancer Research, Roswell Park Memorial Institute, 666 Elm Street, Buffalo, NY 14263, U.S.A.

WOOLLEY D.E., University Department of Medicine, University Hospital of South Manchester, Nell Lane, West Didsbury, Manchester M2O 8LR, England.

1. The role of animal models in the study of experimental metastasis[1]

I.R. HART

1. Introduction

Metastasis is a dynamic process that occurs *in vivo* and, therefore, studies of cancer metastasis must logically include data from *in vivo* experiments and observations. Failure to consider these *in vivo* data can result in the investigation of irrelevant, albeit fascinating, epiphenomena of *in vitro* systems. Identification of the tumor cell or host characteristics that are important for metastatic dissemination can only be made when there are strong correlations between possession of, or alterations in, the observed phenotype and changes in the *in vivo* behavior of that tumor in the appropriate host. All too often investigators have proposed that particular alterations or modifications in cellular properties are responsible for differences in metastatic behavior without first verifying that the cells under investigation were indeed capable of metastasis [1].

Correlations between various cellular properties and metastatic behavior may be obtained by comparing data to historical clinical observations, as is necessary when cells from autochthonous tumors of man or domestic animals are used in *in vitro* assays. However, scientists often use a variety of transplantable tumors in laboratory animals to investigate the process of metastasis. In this chapter, we review some of the salient features of these tumor models and indicate some advantages and limitations.

Stedman's Medical Dictionary [2] defines a model as 'A representation of something, usually idealized and modified to make it conceptually easier to understand.' Although this modification towards simplicity is an obvious advantage, it may, paradoxically, constitute the greatest disadvantage of a model, since simplicity frequently is obtained only at the expense of clinical relevance. More will be said in the following section regarding the advisability of extrapolating from results derived from model systems to produce generalizations of apparent clinical significance. It is sufficient to state at this point that to restrict the use of models to only those that exactly resemble the clinical situation is to impose precisely those con-

[1] Research sponsored by the National Cancer Institute, DHHS, under Contract No. N01-C0-75380 with Litton Bionetics, Inc. The contents of this publication do not necessarily reflect the views or policies of the Department of Health and Human Services, nor does mention of trade names, commercial products, or organizations imply endorsement by the U.S. Government.

L.A. Liotta and I.R. Hart (eds.), Tumor Invasion and Metastasis. ISBN-13: 978-94-009-7513-2.
© 1982 Martinus Nijhoff Publishers, The Hague/Boston/London.

straints that the investigator tried to avoid by resorting to the model in the first place. Metastasis is a complex process, dependent for its final outcome on the results of a variety of interactions between both host defenses and tumor properties [3–5]. Undoubtedly, oversimplification may obscure or negate the subtle interrelationships responsible for tumor spread. Therefore, all these interactions between tumor and host properties must be carefully considered to ensure that an appropriate model is selected for each study. It is readily apparent from the literature that the use of appropriate animal models has been instrumental in elucidating many of the mechanisms of metastasis, and suitable models will continue to play a vital role in future studies.

2. Transplantable versus autochthonous tumor systems

In recent years, considerable debate (frequently of a lively nature) has centered on the adequacy of transplantable tumor systems of rodents as models for human cancer [6–11]. The main concerns have been whether animal models are appropriate for studying the immunology of human cancer, and whether studies using these models overemphasize the clinical relevance of the data. These concerns must be addressed in planning investigations into the nature of metastatis. Hewitt [8, 9, 11] has argued forcibly and eruditely that spontaneous tumors of unknown etiology, which have arisen in strains of rodents with low tumor incidence, may serve as the only true transplantable models of naturally occuring neoplastic disease in man. Certainly, such tumor systems do not display the marked immunogenicity [8] that is so commonly associated with chemically or virally induced neoplasms [12–14]. However, even though spontaneous tumors of rodents may be highly desirable models, other tumor models may be equally valuable, especially with regard to elucidating the mechanisms of tumor cell dissemination. Human tumors may not be highly immunogenic [15–17], but it is possible that the immunogenicity of tumors may have little to do with many of the mechanisms of metastasis [18]. The role of individual cell motility, elaboration and secretion of proteolytic enzymes, and the phenomenon of uncontrolled proliferation are all unlikely to be influenced by tumor immunogenicity. Conversely, the extent and pattern of tumor spread to distant organs may be modified significantly by systemic or local immune reactions, though the degree of modification may be determined by the system studied [18–23]. Such considerations emphasize the inadvisability of making sweeping generalizations about a process as complex as metastasis and the advisability of selecting specific models to answer the specific question under consideration.

There are many naturally occurring neoplasms in domestic animals that, it has been suggested, could serve as excellent models of human cancer [24], even though many of these naturally occuring tumors appear to be virally induced [25–29]. The occurrence of such tumors in outbred animals means that the experimental advantages of multiple isotransplants are unavailable. Nonetheless, the close resemblance of many animal tumors to human tumors suggests they represent an underutilized resource [24, 30]. Unfortunately, many owners of pets, for economic or psychological reasons, do not allow their tumor-bearing animals to be used in experiments. Ironically, treatment for these animals is often based upon protocols initially formulated in human medicine. Naturally occurring animal tumors offer the scientist the opportunity to evaluate aggressive therapeutic modalities on biologically relevant neoplasms before using the regimens on humans. Collaborative programs among medical centers, research institutes and veterinary schools should be instituted to ensure that these tumors are used to their full advantage.

However, for most studies in experimental metastasis, investigators will continue to choose the transplantable tumor model because of its inherent advantages: repeatability of experiments, standardization of procedures, and ease of tumor manipulation. In general, studies using transplantable tumors in inbred strains of mice will be restricted to syngeneic systems, where the genetic compositions of the recipient animals and the tumor are the same. Utilization of only these systems will avoid possible artifacts, mediated by rejection reactions to cell surface transplantation antigens, which can occur in allogeneic systems [31]. Even though it may be possible to study some aspects of metastasis using allogeneic systems [32], it is probably a good policy to limit investigations to syngeneic systems. An exception to this rule, the use of athymic mice for studying the metastatic behavior of allogeneic or xenogeneic tumors, is reviewed elsewhere in this volume (N. Hanna, Chapter 4).

3. Experimental animals

3.1. State of health

Repeatability of results, which is afforded by the use of transplantable tumor systems, can only be obtained when recipient animals are healthy. Tumor colonies should be evaluated routinely for bacterial and viral pathogens, external and internal parasites and histopathological lesions. Since stress can lead to the manifestation of subclinical disease, it is imperative that transported animals become acclimatized before experimental work is initiated. Enhanced activation of host defense mechanisms often follows infection or stress, which may alter the biological behavior of tumors [33, 34]. Improper animal management conditions, such as not providing water, and proper bedding materials or mixing groups of animals which leads to constant fighting, may also profoundly affect experimental results. Every investigator using animals for experimentation should ensure that their experimental animals are properly housed and maintained. The interested reader can consult several publications on this matter [e.g., 35, 36].

3.2. Age

In man, most solid tumors occur in middle-aged or elderly patients. It is generally true that few efforts are made to duplicate this condition in the laboratory where young adult animals are generally the recipients of tumor transplants. There are data which show that the age of recipient animals can have a profound effect upon the course of metastatic disease. The nature of these effects appears to vary according to the tumor system used. Working with Ehrlich ascites tumors and mammary adenocarcinomas, Thompson [37] found that more lung colonies were formed in 71-week-old mice than 15-week-old mice when equal numbers of tumor cells were injected intravenously. Similar results were reported by Yuhas and his colleagues [38, 39] with line 1 carcinoma cells. In contrast, Rockwell [40], who used EMT6 tumors cells injected intravenously into animals of 12–16 weeks and 80–112 weeks of age, found no differences in the number of lung colonies or the incidence or pattern of spontaneous metastases. Interestingly, differences in the latent period of intradermally implanted tumors were apparent between the two groups of mice, as were differences in the number of cells required to effect a 50% take in the subcutaneous site [40]. Because diminution of immunocompetence frequently correlates with senescence [41, 42], it is possible that such variations in biological behavior reflect differences in the immunogenicity of various tumors. However, based on differences in radiation-response curves, indicating an increased incidence of hypoxic cells in tumors established in old animals, Rockwell hypothesized that defects in the tumor vascular bed in older animals could account for this disparate behavior [40]. The age-related development of natural cell-mediated immunity to tumors, and the profound consequences that this mechanism can exert on metastatic spread are covered elsewhere in this volume by Dr. Nabil Hanna (Chapter 3). Age is undoubtedly a factor that must be considered in planning experimental studies of metastasis, and comparisons should be made only between age-matched animals.

3.3 Gender

The behavior of a variety of tumors can be affected significantly by the gender of the host [43, 44]. Similar variations may be observed in many experimental animal tumors, but the model does not invariably mimic its clinical counterpart. This statement can be illustrated by detailing our own experience with one metastasizing murine tumor, the B16 melanoma. In humans, melanomas grow more slowly in women [45] and the prognosis for tumor-bearing females is better than that of tumor-bearing males [46]. These phenomena can be ascribed to the response of the tumor to the differing hormone levels of males and females [47]. Proctor et al. [48] noted a similar pattern in C57BL/6 mice injected with the B16 melanoma. The tumor grew more slowly and produced fewer spontaneous metastases when it was implanted into the hind legs of female, as compared to male, mice [48]. We have confirmed these findings (unpublished observations) but have also noted that sex-determined differences in biological behavior may be influenced by the route of tumor administration. The outcome of injecting male or female mice, of similar ages, with equal numbers of B16 melanoma cells into the lateral tail vein is illustrated in Table 1. In a series of experiments, it was found that female mice developed significantly more ($p < 0.002$) lung nodules than male mice. Castration of the male mice 3 weeks before they were injected with neoplastic cells altered this pattern such that castrated mice developed an increased number of pulmonary tumors compared to the intact or sham-operated controls (Table 1). Indeed, castration resulted in more lung nodules than those that developed in female mice. Obviously, the pulmonary tumor burden, following the intravenous injection of B16 cells, is determined to a considerable extent by the gender of the recipient animal. The influence that is exerted is dependent on the site of tumor implantation since intramuscular growth of the same tumor is enhanced in male animals [48]. Baserga and Kisieleski [49] and Thompson [37] have also reported that the intravenous injection of Ehrlich ascites or mammary adenocarcinoma tumor cells yielded more lung metastases in female mice, indicating that the effect of gender on experimental metastasis is not limited to the B16 melanoma system.

Given the differences in metastatic behavior observed in a single tumor when the health, sex and age of the host animals varied, it is evident that valid comparisons can be made only among age- and sex-matched animals that are housed and maintained under standard conditions.

4. Tumor systems, tumor heterogeneity, and modes of transplantation

An almost bewildering number of different tumor types have been used for experimental studies on metastasis, and it is beyond the scope of this chapter to review all the available models. Each system, despite the frequently fervent claims of its

Table 1. Effect of gender on pulmonary tumor nodule formation produced by B16 melanoma cells injected intravenously into syngeneic mice.

	Median (Range) of Pulmonary Metastases*	
	Male 8-week-old mice	Female 8-week-old mice
Intact animals**	77 (27–300)	142 (94–300)***
Sham castration	66 (45–163)	128 (33–300)
Castration	219 (55–300)***	160 (46–313)

* All mice were injected with 5×10^4 viable melanoma cells i.v. via lateral tail vein. Animals were killed 3 weeks later, and the number of lung nodules was counted.

** 15 mice per group.

*** $p \leq 0.002$ compared to values obtained for intact male animals.

proponents, has its limitations as well as advantages. For example, the B16 melanoma and the Lewis lung carcinoma, which have been used most extensively in metastasis research, are of spontaneous origin but have been propagated *in vivo* and *in vitro* for almost 30 years, or approximately 15 times the average life span of their host, the laboratory mouse. Many spontaneous tumors are capable of metastasizing widely [8], but their capricious occurrence and unpredictable composition marks them unsuitable for some investigations. Chemically induced neoplasms are infrequently metastatic [3, 50–52], and the majority of metastatic rodent tumors metastasize to the lungs, even though the metastatic behavior of their clinical counterpart may be different [52]. Again, it should be stressed that the choice of animal model is dependent upon the nature of the question to be answered.

We have recently described a murine tumor, of spontaneous origin, which selectively metastasizes to the peritoneal viscera [53]. This tumor, known as the M5076, was originally classified as an ovarian carcinoma [54], although functional assays have definitively established that it is of macrophage origin [55]. Regardless of the tissue of origin, this tumor interests us because of the particular patterns of tumor spread it exhibits: it offers a model system with which to study the mechanism of site-specific metastasis [56]. Other efforts to achieve metastatic colonization of particular tissues have often centered on the selection of so-called organ-specific variants from an heterogeneous parent population of tumor cells [57–61]. Such tumor cell diversity allows available models to be adapted and enhanced. Thus, in the example given, site-specific metastasis may be studied either by using a naturally occurring model (e.g. the M5076 tumor) or by using organ-specific variants isolated from a parent tumor by applying specific selection pressure [57–61].

In 1939, Koch [62] showed that the serial transplantation of lymph node metastases led to the derivation of a highly metastatic line. Since that time, numerous studies have shown that many tumors are heterogeneous with regard to the phenotypes of invasion and metastasis [63–70]. Recently, an increasingly popular approach to the determination of the mechanisms of cancer dissemination, and not solely those concerned with site-specific metastasis, has been the comparison of the characteristics of metastatic and nonmetastatic lines derived from the same parental tumor [71–74]. The implications of this diversity have been reviewed extensively elsewhere [4, 75, 76], and Fidler, who has been the leading protagonist in this area of tumor biology, discusses in Chapter 2 of this volume the ramifications of this phenomenon for the selection of the correct therapeutic regimen for metastatic disease.

As far as animal models and their role in experimental metastasis are concerned, there are a number of consequences that result from the existence of tumor cell heterogeneity. Certainly this phenomenon allows an expansion of existing models by permitting the comparison of metastatic and nonmetastatic lines without requiring comparisons between metastatic cells and so-called normal cells.

At the present time, three methods of isolation of tumor cell variants of differing metastatic capacity are available. A large number of clones, each derived from a

Table 2. Experimental metastatic capacity of M5076 clones in syngeneic mice.

Clone	*No. of hepatic tumor nodules: median (range)** Experiment 1	Experiment 2
2	126 (57–209)	198 (78–>300)
3	0 (0–3)	0 (0–2)
4	117 (0–>300)	68 (0–96)
6	8 (0–26)	3 (0–20)
7	155 (36–214)	70 (0–147)

* C57BL/6 × C3H mice (B6C3-F1's) were injected intravenously with 5×10^4 viable M5076 cells in 0.2 ml Hanks' balanced salt solution. Ten mice per group; animals were killed 3 weeks later and hepatic tumor foci were counted under a dissecting microscope.

single cell, may be established *in vitro* and then examined for varying *in vivo* and *in vitro* behavior in an effort to establish positive correlations. An example of this is given in Table 2. Clones of M5076 were established by limiting dilutions into the wells of microtiter dishes such that each cloned line was derived from a single cell. Following identical culture conditions, the clones were harvested, and equal number of cells were injected intravenously into the tail veins of age- and sex-matched syngeneic mice. At a set time, all animals were necropsied, and the grossly evident metastatic foci were counted using a dissecting microscope. As can be seen in Table 2, there are marked differences among the clones with regard to their experimental metastatic capacity. Clones 2, 4, and 7 can be characterized as high metastatic, whereas clones 3 and 6 can be characterized as low metastatic. Having established the relative metastatic behavior of the clones, we could now test them for other differing characteristics, such as enzyme production, resistance or susceptibility to immune lysis, adhesive abilities, etc., which correlate with the biological behavior of these lines. A similar approach has been to select variant lines of different metastatic potential and to compare them with regard to their *in vitro* characteristics; such a procedure is exemplified by the derivation of the B16-F1 and B16-F10 lines selected for lung-colonizing capacity [63]. Alternatively, tumor variants may be selected *in vitro* for specific characteristics, such as motility, detachment from a monolayer or resistance to lymphocyte-mediated lysis, and their *in vivo* behavior may then be assessed [3]. The underlying hope is, of course, that selection will allow the amplification of various characteristics so that the characteristics contributing to biological variation can be identified. This approach, although popular, does not encompass the possibility that cells successful in tumor cell dissemination may not excel in any one of the sequential steps. Rather, what may be required is the ability to complete each step to a limited degree; the search for a single difference between metastatic and nonmetastatic cells then may be doomed to failure by the very nature of the metastatic process.

The diversity of tumor cell populations also presents a challenge in the routine maintenance of tumor cell lines. Morphological studies of tumors have long reported zonal differences. These zonal differences are not restricted to morphology alone, but can encompass antigenicity [77], chemosensitivity [78] and, presumably, the phenotype of malignant behavior. Using a single characteristic as a marker, we have shown recently that the repeated trocar transplantation of tumor fragments can suppress this phenotypic diversity within a very few passages [79]. Choosing the visually striking and grossly evident characteristic of melanin production as our marker, we showed that, within three trocar-mediated passages, the resultant primary tumor could become homogeneous in appearance depending on whether small tumor fragments were derived from the melanotic or amelanotic areas. Transfer of melanotic fragments produced tumors that appeared uniformly black, whereas the passage of fragments derived from amelanotic areas rapidly produced tumors with a uniformly white appearance. In contrast, the passage of cell suspensions derived from the whole primary, heterogeneous tumor maintained the mixed morphology with regard to melanin production [79]. Maintenance of the biological diversity of tumors appears to demand that serial transfers be performed with cell suspensions derived from all zones of the tumor. Although, in the context of this volume, we are primarily concerned with the phenotypes of invasion and metastasis, it appears likely that this principle applies to many phenotypes. Thus, apparently insignificant differences in technical procedures may be partly responsible for differences in findings reported by various laboratories. More important, experimental techniques may artificially limit the diversity and alter the biology of tumor models.

Uniformity in a tumor cell population during *in vivo* passage may not be the consequence of selection by external forces alone. The site of tumor transplantation may have a profound effect not only on the metastatic behavior of a tumor (see below) but also on the eventual composition of the propagated neoplasm. The peritoneal cavity appears to offer solid tumors a milieu of selective pressure that frequently leads to the emergence of more highly metastatic variants from the parent tumor [80–82]. In part, this may be caused by the anatomical compartmentalization of natural host-defense mechanisms [70]. Using the B16 melanoma it has been shown that subcutaneous passage of cells, from either high metastatic (B16-F10) or low metastatic (B16-F1) lines, can maintain stability of these phenotypes over an extended period of time [83]. The subcutaneous site appears then to offer an environment that allows the continued existence of diversity. However, it should be noted that gradients of tumor growth have been described in experimental animals that result in the enhanced growth of tumors in specific anatomical sites [84, 85]. Should such site-determined differences in growth rate lead to the dominance of one subpopulation over another, it is possible that even the apparently nonselective environment of the subcutis might eventually impose uniformity on the cellular composition of the tumor that might not be apparent if other modes of maintenance were used.

5. Tumor implantation, metastatic behavior and quantitation of metastatic burden

The metastatic behavior of transplantable tumors can be altered significantly by the route of tumor cell administration. Several studies on the mechanisms of dissemination have used the direct introduction of tumor cells into a vein as a simplified assay for metastasis [86]. Such a procedure may be criticized because the assay bypasses some of the initial steps associated with metastatic spread. These steps are tumor growth, local invasion and subsequent penetration of venules or lymphatics, and the release of single cells or small emboli into the circulation. Of course, the assay measures the ability of shed cells to survive in the bloodstream, to arrest, to extravasate, and finally, to grow in the organ parenchyma. In many instances the criticism that circumvention of these initial steps renders the intravenous assay too artificial may be invalid. Formation of tumor deposits in host organs requires an almost exactly reversed sequence of events to occur in a distant capillary bed and, presumably, these later processes are accomplished by the same mechanisms that mediated the initial steps. Recently it was shown, using the cloned metastatic cell lines of a UV-induced fibrosarcoma, that good correlations were obtained between the intravenous injection assay and other so-called less artificial assays of spontaneous metastatic capacity [66]. Such correlations, however, do not apply to all tumor systems. We have described the isolation and characterization of an invasive variant from the B16-F10 subline [63] which exhibits enhanced spontaneous metastatic capacity when compared to the parental tumor [87]. However, when injected intravenously, this tumor line formed fewer tumor nodules than equal numbers of the B16-F10 [87]. A recent report on the selection of additional tumor cell variants for enhanced spontaneous metastatic capacity described similar findings [88], namely that cells selected for enhanced spontaneous metastatic capacity did not always perform as well in the intravenous assay as their less spontaneously metastatic counterparts [88]. Although such findings might be explained by any one of a number of mechanisms, such as differential sensitivities to natural killer cell activity [89, 90], the general message remains the same: 'cells selected for a specific aspect and ability in one or many of the steps involved in metastatic spread will not necessarily exhibit enhanced capacities in all other steps.' Consequently, before extrapolations from one assay system to another are made, it is essential that the behavior of the tumor under consideration be tested under a variety of conditions.

As discussed earlier, the site of tumor implantation may determine the growth rate of a tumor [84, 85]. Such differences may reflect variations in blood supply, immune defenses or local environmental conditions [91, 92], and these factors may also regulate metastatic spread, since the site of primary tumor growth may determine the degree of metastasis. For example, the reason that tumors growing in the footpad metastasize to a greater degree than those growing subcutaneously in the flank [71, 89, 93, 94] may not only be related to anatomical considerations such as blood supply, but may also be related to the shedding of tumor cells associated with repeated, minor trauma to the growing neoplasm [95].

Many studies of experimental metastasis measure and compare the final tumor burden in different groups of animals. A common approach to determining metastatic burden, and one extensively used in my laboratory, is the enumeration of tumor colonies on the surface of organs. Such colonies may be easily detected because of color differences between the tumor and the organ parenchyma, as is the case with melanoma foci, or may be artificially delineated by treatment of the organ with agents that heighten the contrast between tumor and tissue [96]. Although these techniques only allow identification of peripheral or surface lesions, they are perfectly adequate when earlier histological studies have shown that surface nodules are representative of the whole tumor burden. A more significant problem is that comparisons between experimental groups based upon numerical counts are only valid when all metastatic foci are uniform in size. Total tumor burden is the determining factor in animal survival, and a few large metastases may contain an equivalent number of tumor cells to ten or twenty times the number of smaller neoplastic foci. Comparisons between groups of animals, where the size of metastatic foci differs, must rely upon other quantitative methods such as organ weights or the incorporation of parenterally administered radioisotopes [97, 99]. As is the case with other aspects of animal models, selection of the correct technique for quantitation of tumor burden depends upon prior knowledge of the biological behavior of the chosen system.

6. Conclusions

There are plethora of animal tumor models available, and the choice of the appropriate model is often as intellectually taxing as deciding which aspect of metastasis is to be investigated. Specific problems can only be resolved when the appropriate model is used and all the inherent limitations of that model are considered. Recognition that all animal models have limitations does not deny the potential value of such systems for the investigation of basic mechanisms. Consideration of the biology of transplantable tumors and metastatic spread must play a central role in the design of experimental protocols. With regard to the limitations of *in vivo* models, it is important to remember that metastasis is a dynamic process which depends for its eventualloutcome on a number of interactions between host and tumor cell. These confrontations cannot be reproduced in an *in vitro* system; they require the environment of a tumor-bearing animal. With these reflections in mind, it seems obvious that good, relevant animal models, correlated with many of the *in vitro* systems described elsewhere in this volume, will be the avenues to broadening our understanding of the biology of cancer metastasis.

References

1. Poste G: The cell surface and metastasis. In: Cancer invasion and metastasis: biologic mechanisms and therapy, Day SB, Laird Myers WP, Stansly P, Garattini S, Lewis MG (eds). New York: Raven Press. 1977, pp 19–47.
2. Stedman's Medical Dictionary. Baltimore: William and Wilkins, 1976.
3. Fidler IJ, Gersten DM, Hart IR: The biology of cancer invasion and metastasis. Adv Cancer Res 28:149–250, 1978.
4. Poste G, Fidler IJ: The pathogenesis of cancer metastasis. Nature 283:139–146, 1980.
5. Hart IR, Fidler IJ: Cancer invasion and metastasis. Quart Rev Biol 55:121–142, 1980.
6. Alexander P: Back to the drawing board – the need for more realistic model systems for immunotherapy. Cancer 40:467–470, 1977.
7. Barlett GL, Kreider JW, Purnell DM: Immunotherapy of cancer in animals: models or muddles? J Natl Cancer Inst 56:207–210, 1976.
8. Hewitt HB, Blake ER, Walder AS: A critique of the evidence for active host defence against cancer, based on personal studies of 27 murine tumors of spontaneous origin. Br J Cancer 33:241–259, 1976.
9. Hewitt HB: The choice of animal tumors for experimental studies of cancer therapy. Adv Cancer Res 27:149–200, 1978.
10. Rapp HJ: Letter to the editor: Appropriateness of animal models for the immunology of human cancer. Cancer Res 39:4285–4286, 1979.
11. Hewitt HB: Answer to the letter to the editor: Appropriateness of animal models for the immunology of human cancer. Cancer Res 39:4286–4287, 1979.
12. Prehn RT, Main J: Immunity to methylcholanthrene -induced sarcomas. J Natl Cancer Inst 18: 769–778, 1957.
13. Embleton MJ, Baldwin RW: Antigenic changes in chemical carcinogenesis. Br Med Bull 36:83–88, 1980.
14. Rapp HJ: Introduction: Animal models of immunotherapy of cancer. Natl Cancer Inst Monogr 39:1–2, 1973.
15. Klein G, Klein E: Rejectability of virus-induced tumors and nonrejectability of spontaneous tumors – a lesson in contrasts. Transplant Proc 9:1095–1104, 1977.
16. Weiss DW: The questionable immunogenicity of certain neoplasms. Cancer Immunol Immunother 2:11–19, 1977.
17. Old LJ: Cancer Immunology: the search for specificity – GHA Clowes Memorial Lecture. Cancer Res 41:361–375, 1981.
18. Tarin D, Price JE: Metastatic colonization potential of primary tumour cells in mice. Br J Cancer 39:710–754, 1979.
19. Kripke ML, Fidler IJ: Enhanced experimental metastasis of ultraviolet light-induced fibrosarcomas in ultraviolet light-irradiated syngeneic mice. Cancer Res 40:625–629, 1980.
20. Fidler IJ, Kripke ML: Tumor cell antigenicity, host immunity and cancer metastasis. Cancer Immunol Immunother 7:201–205, 1980.
21. Fidler IJ, Gersten DM, Kripke ML: Influence of immune status on the metastasis of three murine fibrosarcomas of different immunogenicities. Cancer Res 39:3816–3821, 1979.
22. Fogel M, Gorelik E, Segal S, Feldman M: Differences in cell surface antigens of tumor metastases and those of the local tumor. JNCI 62:585–590, 1979.
23. Weiss L, Glaves D, Waite D: The influence of host immunity on the arrest of circulating cancer cells in tumor-bearing mice. Int J Cancer 18:850–862, 1974.
24. Memoranda: Immunity to cancer: naturally occurring tumors in domestic animals as models for research. Bull WHO 49:205–213, 1973.
25. Burny A, Bex F, Chantrenne H, Clenter Y, Dekagel D, Ghysadael J, Kettmann R, Leclercq M, Leumen J, Mammerick M, Portetelle D: Bovine leukemia virus involvement in enzootic bovine leukosis. Adv Cancer Res 28:251–311, 1978.

26. Payne LN: Pathogenesis of Marek's disease – a review. In: Oncogenesis and herpes viruses, Biggs PM, de-The'G, Payne LN (eds). Lyons: IARC, 1972, pp 21–37.
27. Saveria Campo M, Moar MH, Jarrett WF, Laird HM: A new papilloma virus associated with alimentary cancer in cattle. Nature 286:180–182, 1980.
28. Jarrett WFH, Crawford EM, Martin WB, Davie F: Leukemia in the cat. A virus-like particle associated with leukemia (lymphosarcoma). Nature 202:567–568, 1964.
29. Snyder HW Jr, Hardy WD Jr, Zuckerman EE, Fleissner E: Characterisation of a tumour-specific antigen on the surface of feline lymphosarcoma cells. Nature 275:656–658, 1978.
30. Hart IR, Fidler IJ: Metastatic models. In: The canine as a biomedical research model: immunological, hematological, and oncological aspects, Shifrine M, Wilson FD (eds). Technical Information Center, U.S. Department of Energy, 1980, pp 380–400.
31. Fidler IJ, Gersten DM, Riggs CW: Relationship of host immune status to tumor cell arrest, distribution and survival in experimental metastasis. Cancer 40:23–30, 1977.
32. Carr J, Carr I, Dreher B, Betts K: Lymphatic metastasis: invasion of lymphatic vessels and efflux of tumour cells in the afferent popliteal lymph as seen in the Walker Rat Carcinoma. J Pathol 32:287–305, 1980.
33. Reid LM, Minato N, Gresser I, Holland J, Kadish A, Bloom BR: Influence of anti-mouse interferon serum on the growth and metastasis of tumor cells persistently infected with virus and of human prostatic tumors in athymic nude mice. Proc Natl Acad Sci USA 78:1171–1175, 1981.
34. Fidler IJ, Raz A, Davis TW: The influence of host health and environment on natural cytotoxicity of mouse macrophages. Cancer Immunol Immunother (in press).
35. Guide for the care and use of laboratory animals. Committee on care and use of laboratory animals of the Institute of Laboratory Animal Resources, National Research Council, DHEW Publication, N. (NIH) 78–32, Washington D.C., U.S. Government Printing Office, 1978.
36. Long-term holding of laboratory rodents. A report of the committee on long-term holding of laboratory rodents. ILAR News 19:4–8, 1976.
37. Thompson SC:Effect of age and sex on lung-colony-forming efficiency of injected mouse tumour cells. Br J Cancer 34:566–570, 1976.
38. Yuhas JM, Pazmino NH, Proctor JO, Toya RE: A direct relationship between immune competence and the subcutaneous growth rate of a malignant murine lung tumors. Cancer Res 34:722–728, 1974.
39. Yuhas JM, Ullrich RL: Responsiveness of senescent mice to the antitumor properties of *Corynebacterium parvum*. Cancer Res 36:161–166, 1976.
40. Rockwell S: Effect of host age on the transplantation, growth and radiation response of EMT6 tumors. Cancer Res 41:527–531, 1981.
41. Gatti RA, Good RA: Aging, immunity and malignancy. Geriatrics 25:158–168, 1970.
42. Hollander CF: Animal models for aging and cancer research. J Natl Cancer Inst 51:3–5, 1973.
43. Sugarbaker EV, Ketcham AS: Mechanisms and prevention of cancer dissemination. An overview. Semin Oncol 4:19–32, 1977.
44. Willis RA: The spread of tumors in the human body. London: Butterworth, 1972.
45. White LP: Studies on melanoma. II. Sex and survival in human melanoma. N Eng J Med 260: 789–797, 959.
46. Cochran AJ: Malignant melanoma. A review of 10 years experience in Glasgow Scotland. Cancer 23:1 90–1199, 1973.
47. Paull DE, Seigler HF, Cox ED, McCarty KS Sr, McCarty KS Jr: Factors influencing sex differences in survival for patients with melanoma. Proc Am Assoc Cancer Res 22:646, 1981.
48. Proctor JW, Auclair BG, Stokowski L: Endocrine factors and the growth and spread of B16 melanoma. J Natl Cancer Inst 57:1197–1198, 1976.
49. Baserga R, Kisieleski WE: Increased incidence of tumor metastases in female mice. Science 132: 956–958, 1960.
50. Finlay-Jones JJ, Bartholomaeus WN, Fimmel PJ, Keast D, Stanley NF: Biologic and immunologic studies on a murine model of regional lymph node metastasis. J Natl Cancer Inst 64:1363–1372, 1980.

51. Varani J, Orr W, Ward PA: Hydrolytic enzyme activities, migratory activity, and *in vivo* growth and metastatic potential of recent tumor isolates. Cancer Res 39:2376–2380, 1979.
52. Brattain MG, Strobel-Stevens J, Fine D, Webb M, Sarrif AM: Establishment of mouse colonic carcinoma cell lines with different metastatic properties. Cancer Res 40:2142–2146, 1980.
53. Hart IR, Talmadge JE, Fidler IJ: Metastatic behavior of a murine reticulum cell sarcoma exhibiting organ-specific growth. Cancer Res 41:1281–1287, 1981.
54. Simpson-Herren L, Griswold DP, Dykes DJ: Population kinetics and chemotherapeutic response of transplantable ovarian carcinoma M5076. Proc Am Assoc Cancer Res 20:80, 1979.
55. Talmadge JE, Key M, Hart IR: Characterization of a murine ovarian reticulum cell sarcoma of histiocytic origin. Cancer Res 41:1271–1280, 1981.
56. Hart IR, Fidler IJ: Role of organ selectivity in the determination of metastatic patterns of B16 melanoma. Cancer Res 40:2281–2287, 1980.
57. Brunson KW, Beattie G, Nicolson GL: Selection and altered tumour cell properties of brain-colonizing metastatic melanoma. Nature 272:543–545, 1978.
58. Shearman PJ, Longenecker BM: Selection for virulence and organ-specific metastasis of herpes virus-transformed lymphoma cells. Int J Cancer 25:363–369, 1980.
59. Tao T, Matter A, Vogel K, Burger MM: Liver-colonizing melanoma cells selected from B16 melanoma. Int J Cancer 23:854–857, 1979.
60. Brunson KW, Nicolson GL: Selection of malignant melanoma variant cell lines for ovary colonization. J Supramol Struct 11:517–528, 1979.
61. Brunson KW, Nicolson GL: Selection and biologic properties of malignant variants of a murine lymphosarcoma. J Natl Cancer Inst 61:1499–1503, 1978.
62. Koch RE: Zur Frage der Metastasenbildung bei Impftumoren. Z. Krebsforsch 48:495–507, 1939.
63. Fidler IJ: Selection of successive tumour lines for metastasis. Nature (New Biol) 242:148–149, 1973.
64. Fidler IJ: Tumor heterogeneity and the biology of cancer invasion and metastasis. Cancer Res 38:2651–2660, 1978.
65. Fidler IJ, Kripke ML: Metastasis results from pre-existing variant cells within a malignant tumor. Science 197:893–895, 1977.
66. Kripke ML, Gruys E, Fidler IJ: Metastatic heterogeneity of cells from an ultraviolet light-induced murine fibrosarcoma of recent origin. Cancer Res 38:2962–2967, 1978.
67. Dexter DL, Lowalski HM, Blazar BA, Fligiel A, Nogel R, Heppner GH: Heterogeneity of tumor cells from a single mouse mammary tumor. Cancer Res 38:3179–3186, 1978.
68. Suzuki N, Withers HR, Koehler MW: Heterogeneity and variability of artificial lung colony-forming ability among clones from mouse fibrosarcoma. Cancer Res 38:3349–3351, 1978.
69. Tao TW, Burger MM: Nonmetastasizing variants selected from metastasizing melanoma cells. Nature 270:437–438, 1977.
70. Raz A, Hanna N Fidler IJ: *In vivo* isolation of a metastatic tumor cell variant involving selective and nonadaptive processes. J Natl Cancer Inst 66:183–189, 1981.
71. Hart IR: Selection and characterization of an invasive variant of the B16 melanoma. Am J Pathol 97:587–600, 1979.
72. Varani J, Orr W, Ward PA: Comparison of subpopulations of tumor cells with altered migratory activity, attachment characteristics, enzyme levels and *in vivo* behavior. Eur J Cancer 15:585–591, 1979.
73. Liotta LA, Tryggvason K, Garbisa S, Hart I, Foltz CM, Shafie S: Metastatic potential correlates with enzymatic degradation of basement membrane collagen. Nature 284:67–68, 1980.
74. Wang BS, McLoughlin GA Richie JP, Mannic JA: Correlation of the production of plasminogen activator with tumor metastasis in B16 mouse melanoma cell lines. Cancer Res 40:288–292, 1980.
75. Fidler IJ, Hart IR: The process of cancer metastasis and implications for therapy. In: Principles and practice of oncology. DeVita VT, Hellman S, Rosenberg SA (eds). Philadelphia: JB Lippincott Company (in press).
76. Kerbel RS: Implications of immunological heterogeneity of tumours. Nature 280:358–360, 1979.

77. Prehn RT: Analysis of antigenic heterogeneity within individual 3-methycholanthrene-induced mouse sarcomas. J Natl Cancer Inst 45:1039–1045, 1970.
78. Hakansson L, Trope C: On the presence within tumors of clones that differ in sensitivity to cytostatic drugs. Acta Pathol Microbiol Scand [A] 82:35–40, 1974.
79. Fidler IJ, Hart IR: Biological and experimental consequences of the zonal composition of solid tumors. Cancer Res 41:3266–3267, 1981.
80. Klein E: Gradual transformation of solid into ascites tumors. Evidence favoring the mutation-selection theory. Exp Cell Res 8:188–212, 1955.
81. Klein E: Gradual transformation of solid into ascites tumors. Permanent difference between the original and the transformed sublines. Cancer Res 14:482–485, 1954.
82. Talmadge JE, Starkey JR, Davis WC, Choen A: Introduction of metastatic heterogeneity by short term *in vivo* passage of a cloned transformed cell line. J Supramol Struct 12:227–243, 1979.
83. Poste G, Doll J, Fidler IJ: Interactions between clonal subpopulations affect the stability of the metastatic phenotype in polyclonal populations of B16 melanoma cells. Proc Nat Acad Sci USA (in press).
84. Auerbach R, Morrissey LW, Sidky YA: Gradients in tumour growth. Nature 274:697–699, 1978.
85. Kyriazis AA, Kyrazis AP: Preferential sites of growth of human tumors in nude mice following subcutaneous transplantation. Cancer Res 40:4509–4511, 1980.
86. Fidler IJ: General considerations for studies of experimental cancer metastasis. In: Methods in cancer research. Vol XV, Busch H (ed). New York: Academic Press, 1978, pp 399–439.
87. Poste GH, Doll J, Hart IR, Fidler IJ: *In vitro* selection of murine B16 melanoma variants with enhanced tissue-invasive properties. Cancer Res 40:1636–1644, 1980.
88. Stackpole CW: Distinct lung colonizing and lung-metastasizing cell populations in B16 mouse melanoma. Nature 289:298–300, 1981.
89. Hanna N, Fidler IJ: Role of natural killer cells in the destruction of circulating tumor emboli. JNCI 65:801–809, 1980.
90. Talmadge JE, Meyers KM, Prieur DJ, Starkey JR: Role of NK cells in tumour growth and metastasis in beige mice. Nature 284:622–624, 1980.
91. Bellamy D, Hinsull SM: Influence of lodgement site on the proliferation of metastases of Walker 256 carcinoma in the rat. Br J Cancer 37:81–85, 1978.
92. Reif A: Evidence of organ specificity of defenses against tumors. In: The handbook of cancer immunology. Vol 1, Waters H (ed). New York: Garland STPM Press, 1978, pp. 174–240.
93. Franchi G, Reyers-Degli I, Rosso R, Garattini S: Lymph node metastases after intratibial transplantation of tumours. Int. J Cancer 3:755–760, 1968.
94. VandeVelde CJH, Van Putten LM, Zwaveling A: A new metastasizing mammary carcinoma model in mice: model characteristics and applications. Eur J Cancer 13:555–565, 1977.
95. Liotta LA, Kleinerman J, Saidel GM: Quantitative relationships of intravascular tumor cells, tumor vessels and pulmonary metastases following tumor implantation. Cancer Res 34:997–1004, 1974.
96. Wexler H: Accurate identification of experimental pulmonary metastases. J Natl Cancer Inst 36:641–645, 1966.
97. Giavazzi R, Alessandri G, Spreafico F, Garrattini S, Mantovani A: Metastasizing capacity of tumour cells from spontaneous metastases of transplanted murine tumours. Br J Cancer 42:462–472, 1980.
98. Boeryd B, Ganelius T. Lundin P. Mellgren J: Counting and sizing of tumor metastases in experimental oncology. Int J Cancer 1:497–502, 1966.
99. Baserga R, Kisieleski WE, Halvorsen K: A study on the establishment and growth of tumor metastases with tritiated thymidine. Cancer Res 20:910–917, 1960.

2. Eradication of metastases by tumoricidal macrophages: therapeutic implications*

I.J. FIDLER

1. The biological diversity of metastatic neoplasms

Improved patient care and innovative surgical techniques have led to increasingly effective treatment of primary neoplasms. The principal cause of death from cancer, however, is the growth of metastases. The cure rate for metastasis has not improved as rapidly as that for primary neoplasms. There are several reasons for the failure to treat metastases by direct or adjuvant therapeutic modalities. First, at the time of surgery, metastases may be too small to be detected and already may be disseminated widely throughout the body. Second, even when metastases are discerned, the location of the metastases may limit the effective dose of therapeutic agents that can be delivered to their vicinity. Third, and most important, however, metastases are heterogeneous in their response to therapeutic agents, and metastases may emerge that are resistant to conventional therapy [1–7].

Recent studies suggest that in primary neoplasms there are preexisting subpopulations of cells endowed with special properties that allow them to complete the metastatic process [1, 3, 6]. Moreover, the recognition that malignant neoplasms are populated by cells with diverse biological behavior has prompted investigations into the nature of this diversity and its implications for therapy. Cells obtained from individual animal and human tumors have been shown to be phenotypically diverse with regard to immunogenic and antigenic properties, growth rate, protein production, cell surface receptors, hormone receptors, and response to a variety of cytotoxic drugs [Review 3, 8]. Differences in antigenicity and drug response between cells that populate metastases and those isolated from the localized primary tumor have also been reported [3, 8]. Since metastases could result from the proliferation of different cells which originate from the primary neoplasm [6], it is not surprising that cells obtained from different metastases of the same human patient with breast cancer differ in expression of estrogen receptors [9], and cells collected from various liver metastases produced by human small-cell lung cancer differ with regard to the production of several enzymes [10].

* Research sponsored by the National Cancer Institute, DHHS, under Contract No. N01-C0-75380 with Litton Bionetics, Inc. The contents of this publication do not necessarily reflect the views or policies of the Department of Health and Human Services, nor does mention of trade names, commercial products or organizations imply endorsement by the U.S. Government.

L.A. Liotta and I.R. Hart (eds.), Tumor Invasion and Metastasis. ISBN-13: 978-94-009-7513-2.
© 1982 Martinus Nijhoff Publishers, The Hague/Boston/London.

Several investigators have found differences in drug sensitivity among tumor cell subpopulations of a parent neoplasm. Cells isolated from rat hepatomas [11], methylcholanthrene-induced mouse sarcomas [12], and a mouse mammary tumor [13] have been shown to have different *in vitro* and *in vivo* sensitivities to a variety of cytotoxic agents. These observations are not restricted to experimental tumor systems, because various human neoplasms, such as melanoma [14], colon adenocarcinoma [15], gastric carcinoma [15, 16], ovarian carcinoma [17], breast carcinoma [14], lymphoma [15], and lung adenocarcinomas [18], also have been shown recently to contain various subpopulations of cells with different drug sensitivities.

Immunologic heterogeneity among tumor cells populating a primary neoplasm and between a primary neoplasm and its metastases could also pose serious problems in the treatment of metastases by specific immunotherapy [3, 4, 7, 19–23]. For example, analysis of several AKR mouse lymphomas of recent origin has shown that these tumors are immunologically polyclonal. Immunization of tumor-bearing animals with a representative sample of the tumors was unsuccessful because only the dominant population was rejected. The minor subpopulation(s) of the vaccine did not offer a sufficient immunologic challenge to stimulate the immune response. The rejection of the major clone permitted the other subpopulations to proliferate and become dominant [24]. Thus, both chemotherapy- and/or specific immunotherapy-resistant variants preexisting within the parental tumor population can proliferate unchecked following the destruction of the sensitive populations. Because tumors are not uniform, one successful approach to the therapy of metastases would include a therapeutic agent or modality that circumvents the problem of cellular diversity between primary cancers and their metastases, among various metastatic tumor foci, and against which resistance is less likely to develop.

2. The role of macrophages in the pathogenesis of metastasis: in vitro studies

There is now increasing evidence that stimulation of cells of the reticuloendothelial system (i.e., mononuclear phagocytes) may be effective in the destruction of tumor metastases. Cells of the macrophage-histiocyte series are important in the maintenance of homeostasis. The primary task of phagocytic cells in the body is the phagocytosis and catabolism of effete cells, cellular debris, and serum proteins. Macrophages are involved in the controlled metabolism of lipids [25] and iron [26], host response to injury (inflammation) [27, 28], and defense against microbial invasion [29].

The first indication that macrophages can be tumoricidal came from the work of Granger and Weiser [30] who observed by light microscopy the phagocytosis and digestion of allogeneic neoplastic cells *in vitro* by macrophages from immune animals. Since then, it has been recognized that the activation of cells of the macrophage-histiocyte series to become tumoricidal is an important component in the host defense against neoplasia [5, 19, 20, 28, 31–36].

There are two major ways by which macrophages can be activated *in vivo* to become bactericidal and/or tumoricidal. Frequently, macrophages are activated as a consequence of their interaction with microorganisms and/or their products, such as endotoxins, the bacteria cell wall skeleton and, as shall be discussed below, small components of the bacteria cell wall skeleton such as muramyl dipeptide (MDP) [37–41]. *In vivo* activation of macrophages can also take place after they interact with soluble mediators released by sensitized lymphocytes. The soluble lymphokine responsible for inducing macrophage activation is referred to as macrophage-activating factor (MAF). MAF is able to act across species barriers [31, 35, 36, 41–43], and tumoricidal macrophages activated by MAF induce destruction of a wide range of target tumor cells from a variety of species by a nonimmunological mechanism that requires cell-to-cell contact [33]. Tumoricidal macrophages acquire the ability to recognize and destroy neoplastic cells both *in vitro* and *in vivo*, while leaving nonneoplastic cells unharmed [5, 20, 28, 33–36, 44–46].

The ability of tumoricidal macrophages to discriminate between tumorigenic and normal cells has been studied in a variety of systems, which include syngeneic and allogeneic tumors of mice, syngeneic rat tumors and syngeneic guinea pig tumors [Review 36]. In addition, activated macrophages of one species, such as the mouse, have been shown to discriminate between normal and tumorigenic cells of another species, such as man [33], rat, hamster [36, 44, 45] and dog [47]. The susceptibility of tumor cells to destruction by tumoricidal macrophages is also independent of the *in vivo* biological behavior of the tumor cells, such as invasiveness, metastatic potential, growth rate and resistance to lymphocyte or natural killer (NK) cell-mediated lysis. For example, B16 melanoma variant lines that have a low or high metastatic potential, that have invasive or noninvasive characteristics and that are either susceptible or resistant to syngeneic T-cell-mediated lysis are all lysed *in vitro* by MAF-activated macrophages [36]. Similarly, several cloned cell lines isolated from a C3H mouse fibrosarcoma (UV-2237) induced by ultraviolet radiation (UVR), which vary greatly in their invasive and metastatic potential *in vivo* [48] or immunogenicity, are all susceptible to destruction *in vitro* by tumoricidal macrophages [5].

Recently, we have also examined the tumor target cell's susceptibility to destruction by tumoricidal rat and mouse macrophages by using virus-transformed cell lines in which various elements of the transformed phenotype are temperature dependent. Baby hamster kidney (BHK) cells transformed by the ts3 mutant of polyoma virus, rat embryo 3Y1 cells transformed by a temperature-sensitive A cistron mutant of simian virus 40 (SV40), and the ts-H6-15 temperature-sensitive line of SV40-transformed mouse 3T3 cells were killed *in vitro* by macrophages at both the permissive (33° C) and nonpermissive (39° C) temperatures for expression of the transformed phenotype. 3T3, 3Y1, and BHK cells transformed by wild-type SV40 or polyoma virus were also destroyed by tumoricidal macrophages at both 33 and 39° C, but untransformed 3T3, 3Y1, and BHK cells were not. Thus, transformed cells were killed by macrophages regardless of whether they expressed cell surface LETS protein or Forssman antigens, displayed surface changes that permitted agglutination by low doses of plant lectins, expressed SV40 T antigen, had a low saturation density, or exhibited density-dependent inhibition of DNA synthesis [49].

Taken together, these data indicate that, at least *in vitro*, tumoricidal macrophages discriminate between neoplastic and nonneoplastic cells by a process that is independent of transplantation antigens, species-specific antigens, tumor-specific antigens, cell cycle time, or various phenotypes associated with 'transformation.' Although the exact mechanism(s) by which macrophages do recognize and lyse tumor cells are still unclear, they are probably regulated by a tumor cell characteristic that is linked with the tumorigenic capacity of tumor cells [36].

3. The role of macrophages in the pathogenesis of metastasis: in vivo studies

As stated above, mononuclear cells appear to play a role in determining the outcome of cancer metastasis. Systemic impairment of macrophages by agents such as carrageenan or silica has been associated with an increased incidence of spontaneous [50, 51] and experimental [52] metastasis. There are also several published reports regarding the efficacy of macrophages in the inhibition of metastasis. Syngeneic macrophages activated in culture before intravenous injection reduced the formation of B16 melanoma metastases, and the intravenous injection of nonspecifically activated macrophages prevented the formation of spontaneous fibrosarcoma metastases [53–55]. Activated macrophages also were shown to inhibit the growth of tumors at primary sites [56]. Differences in the cytotoxic activity of macrophages isolated from metastasizing and nonmetastasizing tumors have been reported [57]. Macrophages isolated from a nonmetastasizing sarcoma were cytotoxic *in vitro*. In contrast, macrophages isolated from a weakly immunogenic, metastasizing variant were not [57]. Similar findings have been reported for progressing and regressing mouse sarcomas [58].

In the latter system, however, macrophage-mediated cytotoxicity *in vitro* and the *in vivo* behavior of the tumors from which the macrophages were derived could not always be correlated [59]. In rats, the macrophage content of six carcinogen-induced fibrosarcomas correlated directly with their immunogenicity and inversely with their metastatic potential [60, 61]. It would be convenient to assume that some tumors do not produce metastasis because they contain many macrophages, but this has not been generally the case. We have recently examined the macrophage content of 16 different rodent tumors and failed to demonstrate a correlation between the extent of macrophage infiltration into neoplasms and the tumors' metastatic behavior [62]. We also did not find a correlation between the macrophage content of ultraviolet radiation-induced murine fibrosarcomas growing in normal or immunosuppressed syngeneic mice and the tumors' immunogenic potential. There are several factors that influence the extent of macrophage infiltration into tumors. One of these factors, tumor cell immunogenicity, did not correlate with macrophage content in our study. This observation is in agreement with a study by Evans and Lawler [63], who examined the macrophage content of 33 different methylcholanthrene-induced murine fibrosarcomas and rhabdomyosarcomas and concluded that there was no relationship between macrophage content and the immunogenicity of the tumors. Thus, the role of the mononuclear phagocyte system in metastasis varies for different tumors and does not correlate with tumor cell immunogenicity and/or metastatic properties. In some tumors, a large number of infiltrating macrophages can inhibit metastasis, but the absence of macrophages in a neoplasm will not lead to production of metastasis. For example, a low number of macrophages in benign tumors is unlikely to compensate for their inability to invade host stroma and enter the circulation to produce distant growths. Therefore, neoplasms with low macrophage content may or may not be metastatic, as demonstrated in studies in which nonmetastatic clones isolated from a highly metastatic neoplasm also exhibited low macrophage content when growing subcutaneously [64].

In several experimental systems the presence of progressively growing tumors was accompanied by several alterations in macrophage function, such as enhancement of carbon clearance *in vivo* [65, 66], increased expression of monocyte Fc receptors [67, 68] and suppression of migration or chemotactic response of macrophages from the peritoneal cavity or the site of tumor growth [3, 8, 21–23, 28–31, 67, 69–74]. We recently have investigated whether the presence of progressively growing pulmonary metastases (produced by a syngeneic mammary adenocarcinoma) influenced the number and function of alveolar macrophages (AM) in rats. The functional integrity of AM was determined by their capacity to phagocytose opsonized erythrocytes and by their ability to respond to a variety of activating agents *in vitro*. Moreover, when normal rats and those bearing metastases were injected intravenously with *Nocardia rubra* cell wall skeleton to determine whether the presence of large pulmonary metastases would interfere with AM activation *in situ*, we found that the presence of progressively growing lung metastases did not bring about a decrease in the number of lung macrophages, and the cells harvested from tumor-bearing rats were as phagocytic as the cells obtained from normal rats. Most important was the observation that macrophages harvested from rats with metastases could be rendered tumoricidal against syngeneic tumor target cells in response to activation stimuli *in vitro* and *in vivo* [75]. Such findings have suggested that the presence of a large number of tumor cells in the lung parenchyma does not interfere with macrophage function (in the lung).

4. In vivo activation of macrophages

As discussed above, macrophages can be rendered tumoricidal by a variety of agents, including lymphokines such as MAF released by antigen- and/or mitogen-sensitized lymphocytes. Several recent studies have suggested that, in mice bearing a progressively growing tumor, the interaction between lymphocytes and macrophages does not occur [35, 76]. Lymphocytes from mice bearing large progressive tumors fail to produce MAF when challenged with the specific tumor cells *in vitro*, but are still capable of releasing MAF in response to an unrelated antigen or mitogen [35, 76]. The inability of lymphocytes from tumor-bearing animals to produce lymphokines suggests that an important amplification mechanism may not be functioning in these animals: they may be unable to activate their defense cells for the purpose of destroying tumor cells. Previous studies from our laboratory demonstrated that the lack of tumor cytotoxicity of peritoneal macrophages harvested from mice bearing large syngeneic tumors at a subcutaneous site was not caused by an innate deficiency of the macrophages, but rather by the lack of production of MAF by the autologous lymphocytes [76]. Similarly, macrophages isolated from progressing Moloney virus-induced sarcomas in BALB/c mice were found to be relatively noncytotoxic *in vitro*, whereas those obtained from regressing tumors were cytotoxic [74]. In this experimental system [58], noncytotoxic macrophages could be rendered tumoricidal following incubation with ng/ml quantities of endotoxins. Collectively, these data suggest that macrophages residing in tumor-bearing animals should be able to respond to exogenous activation stimuli to become tumoricidal.

Evidence of the effectiveness of tumoricidal macrophages in controlling cancer metastasis *in vivo* has been obtained from studies in which macrophages activated *in vitro* or *in vivo* were injected intravenously into syngeneic mice bearing pulmonary and lymph node metastases [53–56]. The limitations of this adoptive transfer 'therapeutic modality' are obvious. First, the number of macrophages required for the transfer is very large, and second, the macrophages must be autologous or histocompatible. Because macrophages form tumor-bearing animals can respond to activating stimuli and become tumoricidal, finding a means to activate macrophages *in situ* by delivering activating stimuli (agents) to them becomes desirable. Early attempts to activate macrophages by the systemic administration of lymphokines have not been successful. Although intratumoral inoculation of lymphokine preparations containing MAF has been shown to induce regression of skin tumors and cutaneous metastases [77, 78], the systemic administration of MAF to activate macrophages in distant tumor-bearing tissues has not been feasible. After injection into the circulation, MAF may be inactivated by serum proteins [79], which prevents MAF from being delivered in effective quantities to distant sites. The most serious obstacle to therapeutic activation of macrophages *in situ* by passive immunotherapy with lymphokines could be the finding that macrophages are susceptible to activation for only 3–4 days after their emigration from the circulation into tissues [80]. Moreover, once activated, macrophages are tumoricidal for only 3–4 days, and, with the decay of their tumoricidal properties, they are refractory to reactivation by soluble MAF [79]. Therefore, adoptive immunotherapy with macrophages, although theoretically sound and therapeutically effective in syngeneic animal tumor systems, may be hampered by the difficulty of finding capable immune donors. Passive therapy with systemically injected lymphokines aimed at the *in situ* stimulation of the reticuloendothelial system may be hampered by the inability to achieve therapeutically effective blood levels at the tumor site(s).

5. Activation of tumoricidal properties in macrophages by liposome-encapsulated immunomodulating agents

As stated above, a major pathway for the *in vivo* activation of macrophages involves their interaction with microorganisms and/or their product(s). Because such biologic agents often cause undesirable side effects, such as granuloma formation and allergic reactions [80], it is preferable to activate macrophages *in vivo* with synthetic compounds that are relatively nontoxic, yet possess immunopotentiating activity. N-acetylmuramyl-L-alanyl-D-isolglutamine (muramyl dipeptide, MDP) is the minimal structural unit (mol. wt. 492) with immunopotentiating activity that can replace *Mycobacteria* in Freund's complete adjuvant. MDP is known to influence many macrophage functions including cytotoxic activity [37–40, 46, 81]. It is important to note, however, that therapeutic use of water-soluble synthetic MDP is hindered because, after parenteral administration, this agent is rapidly cleared (<60 min) from the body and excreted in the urine [40].

Recent advances in liposome technology have provided a mechanism for activating macrophages *in situ* with soluble MAF and/or MDP. Liposomes are lipid vesicles composed of one or more lipid bilayers surrounding an internal aqueous space. In the last few years, increasing attention has been given to the potential value of liposomes as carriers of agents used to treat a variety of diseases including cancer [82–85]. At present, liposomes are used to carry agents to cells of the reticuloendothelial system since these cells are responsible for the rapid clearance of particulate material from the circulation. There are several advantages to using liposome-encapsulated materials to activate cells of the macrophage-histiocyte series *in vivo*. Many macrophage-activating agents such as bacterial products (MDP) or lymphokines may be antigenic, and repeated systemic administrations could lead to adverse reactions. Liposomes are nonimmunogenic, and thus elicitation of allergic reactions commonly associated with the systemic administration of other immune adjuvants should be avoided [80].

We have reported that macrophage-activating agents encapsulated within liposomes are far more efficient at activating macrophages *in vitro* than free agents [44–46, 79, 81, 85]. This raised the possibility that liposome-encapsulated agents could be similarly efficient in activating macrophages *in vivo* and thus provide a potential therapeutic modality for enhancing host resistance to metastases. To test this possibility, we gave mice bearing spontaneous metastases intravenous injections of multilamellar vesicle liposomes consisting of phosphatidylserine and phosphatidylcholine (3:7 molar ratio). The liposomes contained entrapped MAF [86] or MDP [87]. C57BL/6 mice were injected in the footpad with 5×10^4 syngeneic

B16-BL6 murine melanoma cells. Four weeks later, when the implants had reached a size of 10–12 mm, the leg bearing the tumor and the popliteal lymph node were amputated. Three days later, animals were injected intravenously with 5 μmol of liposomes containing MAF. Control animals were injected with free MAF or liposomes containing saline but suspended in free MAF. Both test and control groups were treated twice weekly for four weeks. Two weeks after the final treatment, the animals were killed and necropsied. The presence of metastases was determined microscopically, and all suspected lesions were confirmed histologically. Spontaneous pulmonary and lymph node metastases were well established in animals at the time liposome therapy was started; several individual lung metastases were visible macroscopically. Without therapy these tumor foci rapidly developed into lesions exceeding 2–3 mm in diameter. Most mice treated with liposome-encapsulated MAF had no macroscopically or microscopically detectable metastases. Moreover, even in animals with metastasis, the median number of metastases was significantly less than in the other treatment groups [86]. Similar experiments were performed in which liposomes containing MDP were administered systemically. C57BL/6 mice bearing spontaneous lung metastases arising from B16–BL6 melanoma cells were injected intravenously twice a week for four weeks with free MDP (100 μg/mouse), liposomes (5 μmol phospholipid containing 2.5 μg/MDP), or with a similar dose of control liposome preparations. Again, mice were killed two weeks after the eighth and final intravenous injection. Control mice had extensive metastases. In contrast, 74% of mice injected with liposomes containing MDP were free of detectable disease, and, in the few treated animals with lung metastases, the median number of lesions was significantly less than in the other treatment groups. Comparison of the same treatment protocols in survival assays revealed that treatment with liposome-encapsulated MDP produced a highly significant increase in survival relative to control mice or mice injected with free MDP or liposomes containing phosphate-buffered saline suspended in free MDP. In both series of experiments (liposome-MDP and/or liposome-MAF), the regression of lymph node and pulmonary metastases always was associated with the induction of tumoricidal activity in AM. In control studies, in which systemic administration of liposomes containing control substances failed to activate macrophages, tumor regression also failed to occur.

For all these experiments, we used multilamellar vesicles consisting of two natural phospholipids. We chose this particular class of liposomes for our experiments for several reasons. First, studies of body distribution of liposomes of different size and phospholipid composition demonstrated that localization and retention of liposomes in the lung could be achieved with these negatively charged liposomes [85]. Second, toxicity studies in which these liposomes containing MAF were injected intravenously into mice (10 μmol phospholipid) or beagle dogs (5–60 mg phospholipid/kg) failed to reveal any adverse reactions in recipient animals even after repeated injections [88]. Finally, the intravenous injection of these liposomes has been shown to activate murine AM to become tumoricidal [87].

Our results indicate that the multiple intravenous injections of MLV liposomes containing macrophage-activating agents such as MAF or MDP, but not free agents, eradicated spontaneous pulmonary and lymph node metastases (arising from B16–BL6 melanoma or K–1735 melanoma primary tumors resected before therapy) in mice. In mice bearing the B16–BL6 tumor, the tumor burden in lung and lymph node metastases at the start of therapy was great (perhaps in excess of 10^7 cells). Yet, 70% of mice treated with liposome-encapsulated MDP survived for 190 days after tumors were implanted into the footpad. In this tumor system, the median life span of mice inoculated with as few as 10 viable cells has been shown to be 40–50 days [89, 90]. Therefore, the tumor burden in surviving mice must have been reduced to fewer than 10 viable cells, because the mice survived longer than required to be classified as disease free.

The optimal conditions for systemic therapy with liposome-encapsulated immunomodulators, and the efficacy of this modality alone, or in combination, in treating large metastatic tumor burdens has not been defined. Although the initial results reported here are encouraging, it is unlikely that this therapeutic approach could serve as the sole treatment for advanced metastatic disease. As with many other antitumor therapies, optimal application of these modalities will probably require their use in combination with other antitumor agents. Potential therapeutic regimens designed to stimulate host immunity must be used in combination with other treatments such as chemotherapy, in order to first reduce the 'bulk' tumor burden to a sufficiently low level at which activated macrophages can kill the surviving or drug-insensitive tumor cells.

6. Conclusions

These findings suggest that amplification of host defense systems by liposome-encapsulated immunomodulators can be a useful addition to the therapy of metastatic disease. Activated macrophages appear to be able to recognize and destroy neoplastic cells without regard to their phenotypic diversity, and macrophage-mediated cytotoxicity appears to be devoid of the problem of cellular resistance to killing which is routinely encountered in efforts to destroy tumor cells by cytotoxic drugs. However, even if the activated macrophage were consistently effective in circumventing the problem of tumor cell heterogeneity, macrophage-mediated destruction of large tumor burdens may not be feasible. In many neoplastic lesions, the number of macrophages is too low to destroy all tumor cells, even under conditions of optimal macrophage activation and expression of cytotoxic activity. Thus, it seems likely that the potential application of liposome-encapsulated macrophage-activating agents will not be the destruction of massive tumor burdens but rather the destruction of micrometastases and the residual tumor cell burden that remain after elimination of the majority of tumor cells by other means such as chemotherapy.

References

1. Fidler IJ, Gersten DM, Hart IR: The biology of cancer invasion and metastasis. Adv Cancer Res 28:149–250, 1978.
2. Sugarbaker EV: Cancer metastasis: a product of tumor-host interactions. Curr Probl Cancer 7:3–59, 1979.
3. Poste G, Fidler IJ: The pathogenesis of cancer metastasis. Nature 283:139–146, 1979.
4. Fidler IJ: Tumor heterogeneity and the biology of cancer invasion and metastasis. Cancer Res 37:2481–2486, 1978.
5. Fidler IJ, Cifone MA: Properties of metastatic and nonmetastatic cloned subpopulations of an ultraviolet light-induced murine fibrosarcoma of recent origin. Am J Pathol 97:633–648, 1979.
6. Fidler IJ, Kripke ML: Metastasis results from preexisting variant cells within a malignant tumor. Science 197:893–895, 1977.
7. Fidler IJ, Kripke ML: Biological variability within murine neoplasms. Antibiot Chemother 28: 123–129, 1980.
8. Hart IR, Fidler IJ: The implications of tumor heterogeneity for studies on the biology and therapy of cancer metastasis. Biochem Biophys Acta 651:37–50, 1981.
9. Brennan MJ, Donegan WL, Appleby DE: The variability of estrogen receptors in metastatic breast cancer. Am J Surg 137:260–262, 1979.
10. Baylin SB, Weisburger WR, Eggleston JC, Mendelsohn G, Beaven MA, Abeloff MD, Ettinger DS: Variable content of histamine, L-dopa decarboxylase and calcitonin in small-cell carcinoma of the lung. Biologic and clinical implications. N Engl J Med 299:105–110, 1978.
11. Barranco SC, Haenelt BR, Gee EL: Differential sensitivities of five rat hepatoma cell lines to anticancer drugs. Cancer Res 38:656–660, 1978.
12. Hakansson L, Trope C: On the presence within tumors of clones that differ in sensitivity to cytostatic drugs. Acta Pathol Microbiol Scand [A] 82:35–40, 1974.
13. Heppner GH, Dexter DL, DeNucci T, Miller FR, Calabresi P: Heterogeneity in drug sensitivity among tumor cell subpopulations of a single mammary tumor. Cancer Res 38:3758–3763, 1978.
14. Lotan R: Different susceptibilities of human melanoma and breast carcinoma cell lines to retinoic acid-induced growth inhibition. Cancer Res 39:1014–1019, 1979.
15. Trope, C: Different susceptibilities of tumor cell subpopulations to cytotoxic agents. In: Design of models for testing cancer therapeutic agents, Fidler IJ, White RJ (eds). New York: Van Nostrand, 1982.
16. Trope C, Hakansson L, Dencker H: Heterogeneity of human adenocarcinomas of the colon and the stomach as regards sensitivity to cytostatic drugs. Neoplasma (Bratislava) 22:423–430, 1975.
17. Trope C, Aspegren K, Kullander S, Astedt B: Heterogeneous response of disseminated human ovarian cancers to cytostasis *in vitro*. Acta Obstet Gynecol Scand 58:543–546, 1979.
18. Baylin SB: Clonal selection and heterogeneity of human solid neoplasms. In: Design of models for testing cancer therapeutic agents, Fidler IJ, White RJ (eds). New York: Van Nostrand, 1982.
19. Fidler IJ, Kripke ML: Tumor cell antigenicity, host immunity and cancer metastasis. Cancer Immunol Immunother 7:201–205, 1980.
20. Kerbel RS: Implications of immunological heterogeneity of tumours. Nature 280:358–360, 1979.
21. Killion JJ, Kollmorgen GM: Isolation of immunogenic tumor cells by cell-affinity chromatography. Nature 259:674–676, 1976.
22. Prehn RT: Analysis of antigenic heterogeneity within individual 3-methylcholanthrene-induced mouse sarcomas. J Natl Cancer Inst 45:1039–1045, 1970.
23. Heppner GH: The challenge of tumor heterogeneity. In: Commentaries on research in breast disease, Bulbrook RD, Taylor DJ (eds). New York: Alan R. Liss. 1979.
24. Olsson L, Ebbesen P: Natural polyclonality of spontaneous AKR leukemia and its consequence for so-called specific immunotherapy. JNCI 62:623–627, 1979.
25. Day AJ: The macrophage system, lipid metabolism and atherosclerosis. J Atherosclerosis Res 4:117–131, 1964.

26. MacDonald RA, MacSween RNM, Pechet GS: Iron metabolism by reticuloendothelial cells *in vitro*. Physical and chemical conditions, lipotrope deficiency, and acute inflammation. Lab Inves 21: 236–241, 1969.
27. Tompkins EH: Reaction of the reticuloendothelial cells to subcutaneous injections of cholesterol. Arch Pathol 42:299–302, 1946.
28. Hibbs JB, Jr, Lambert LH, Jr, Remington JS: Control of carcinogenesis: a possible role for the activated macrophage. Science 177:998–1000, 1972.
29. Mackaness GB: The influence of immunologically committed lymphoid cells on macrophage activity *in vivo*. J Exp Med 129:973–982, 1969.
30. Granger GA, Weiser RS: Homograft target cells: specific destruction in vitro by contact interaction with immune macrophages. Science 145:1427–1429, 1964.
31. Churchill WH, Jr, Piessens WF, Sulis CA, David JR: Macrophages activated as suspension cultures with lymphocyte mediators devoid of antigen become cytotoxic for tumor cells. J Immunol 115: 781–790, 1975.
32. Evans R, Alexander P: Role of macrophages in tumor immunity. I. Cooperation between macrophages and lymphoid cells in syngeneic tumor immunity. Immunology 23:615–620, 1972.
33. Hibbs JB, Jr: Discrimination between neoplastic and non-neoplastic cells *in vitro* by activated macrophages. J Natl Cancer Inst 53:1487–1492, 1974.
34. Kaplan AM, Morahan PS, Regelson W: Induction of macrophage-mediated tumor-cell cytotoxicity by pyran copolymer. J Natl Cancer Inst 52:1919–1927, 1974.
35. Fidler IJ: Activation *in vitro* of mouse macrophages by syngeneic, allogeneic, or xenogeneic lymphocyte supernatants. J Natl Cancer Inst 55:1159–1163, 1975.
36. Fidler IJ: Recognition and destruction of target cells by tumoricidal macrophages. Isr J Med 14:177–191, 1978.
37. Lederer E: Synthetic immunostimulants derived from the bacteriol cell wall. J Med Chem 23:819–825, 1980.
38. Chedid L, Carelli L, Audibert F: Recent developments concerning muramyl dipeptide, a synthetic immunoregulating molecule. J Reticuloendothel Soc 26:631–641, 1979.
39. Matter A: The effects of muramyl dipeptide (MDP) in cell-mediated immunity. A comparison between *in vitro* and *in vivo* systems. Cancer Immunol Immunother 6:201–210, 1979.
40. Parant M, Parant F, Chedid L, Yapo A, Petit JF, Lederer E: Fate of the synthetic immunoadjuvant, muramyl dipeptide (14C-labelled) in the mouse. Int J Immunopharmacol 1:35–41, 1979.
41. David JR: Macrophage activation by lymphocyte mediators. Fed Proc 34:1730–1736, 1975.
42. Fidler IJ, Darnell JH, Budmen MB: Tumoricidal properties of mouse macrophages activated with mediators from rat lymphocytes stimulated with concanavalin A. Cancer Res 36:3608–3615, 1976.
43. Fidler IJ, Raz A: The induction of tumoricidal capacities in mouse and rat macrophages by lymphokines. In: Lymphokine reports, Pick E (ed). New York: Academic Press, 1981.
44. Poste G, Kirsh R, Fogler W, Fidler IJ: Activation of tumoricidal properties in mouse macrophages by lymphokines encapsulated in liposomes. Cancer Res 39:881–892, 1979.
45. Sone S, Poste G, Fidler IJ: Rat alveolar macrophages are susceptible to free and liposome-encapsulated lymphokines. J Immunol 124:2197–2202, 1980.
46. Sone S, Fidler IJ: *In vitro* activation of tumoricidal properties in rat alveolar macrophages by synthetic muramyl dipeptide encapsulated in liposomes. Cell Immunol 57:42–50, 1981.
47. Hart IR, Fidler IJ: The colLection, purificaton and characterization of canine peripheral blood monocytes. J Reticuloendothel Soc 26:121–133, 1979.
48. Kripke ML, Gruys E, Fidler IJ: Metastatic heterogeneity of cells from an ultraviolet light-induced murine fibrosarcoma of recent origin. Cancer Res 38:2962–2967, 1978.
49. Fider IJ, Roblin RO, Poste G: *In vitro* tumoricidal activity of macrophages against virus-transformed lines with temperature-dependent transformed phenotypic characteristics. Cell Immunol38: 131–146, 1978.

50. Sadler TE, Jones PDE, Castro JE: The effects of altered phagocytic activity on growth of primary and metastatic tumour. In: The macrophage and cancer, James K, McBride B, Stuart A (eds). Edinburgh: Econoprint, 1977, pp 155–163.
51. Jones PDE, Castro JE: Immunological mechanisms in metastatic spread and the anti-metastatic effects of *C. parvum*. Br J Cancer 35:519, 1977.
52. Mantovani A, Giavazzi R, Polentarutti N, Spreafico F, Gavattini S: Divergent effects of macrophage toxins on growth of primary tumors and lung metastases in mice. Int J Cancer 25:617, 1980.
53. Fidler IJ: Inhibition of pulmonary metastasis by intravenous injection of specifically activated macrophages. Cancer Res 34:1074–1078, 1974.
54. Liotta LA, Gattozzi C, Kleinerman J, Saidel G: Reduction of tumor cell entry into vessels by BCG-activated macrophages. Br J Cancer 36:639–641, 1977.
55. Fidler IJ, Fogler WE, Connor J: The rationale for the treatment of established experimental micrometastases with the injection of tumoricidal macrophages. In: Immunobiology and immunotherapy of cancer, Terry WD, Yamamura Y (eds). New York: Elsevier, 1979, pp 361–375.
56. Den Otter W, Dullens Hub FJ, Van Lovern H, Pels E: Anti-tumor effects of macrophages injected into animals: a review. In: The macrophage and cancer, James K, McBride B, Stuart A (eds). Edinburgh: Econoprint, 1977, pp 119–141.
57. Mantovani A: Effects on *in vitro* tumor growth of murine macrophages isolated from sarcoma lines differing in immunogenicity and metastasizing capacity. Int J Cancer 22:741–747, 1978.
58. Russell SW, McIntosh AT: Macrophages isolated from regressing Moloney sarcomas are more cytotoxic than those recovered from progressing sarcomas. Nature 268:69–71, 1977.
59. Evans R: Tumor macrophages in host immunity to malignancies. In: The macrophage in neoplasia, Fink MA (ed). New York: Academic Press, 1976, pp 27–42.
60. Eccles SA: Macrophages and cancer. In: Immunological aspects of cancer, Castro JE (ed). Lancaster, England: MTP Press, 1978, pp 123–154.
61. Eccles SA, Alexander P: Macrophage content of tumors in relationship to metastatic spread. Nature 250:667–669, 1974.
62. Talmadge JE, Key M, Fidler IJ: Macrophage content of metastatic and nonmetastatic rodent neoplasms. J Immunol 126:2245–2248. 1981.
63. Evans R, Lawler EM: Macrophage content and immunogenicity of C57BL/6J and BALB/cByJ methylcholanthrene-induced sarcomas. Int J Cancer 26:831–835, 1980.
64. Kerbel RS, Twiddy RR: Host cell analysis of a rapidly metastasizing mouse tumor and derived low metastatic variant lines. In: Contemporary topics in immunology, Witz IP, Hanna MG, Jr (eds). New York: Plenum Press, 1980, pp 239–254.
65. Blamey RW, Crosby DL, Baker JM: Reticuloendothelial activity during the growth of rat sarcomas. Cancer Res 29:335–337, 1969.
66. Old LJ, Clarke DA, Benacerraf B, Goldsmith M: The reticuloendothelial system and the neoplastic process. Science 88:264–280, 1960.
67. Rhodes J: Altered expression of human monocyte Fc receptors in malignant disease. Nature 265:253–255, 1977.
68. Rhodes J: Resistance of tumor cells to macrophages. Cancer Immunol Immunother 7:211–215, 1980.
69. Bernstein ID, Zbar B, Rapp HJ: Impaired inflammatory response in tumor-bearing guinea pigs. J Natl Cancer Inst 49:1641–1647, 1972.
70. Eccles SA, Alexander P: Sequestration of macrophages in growing tumors and its effect on the immunological capacity of the host. Br J Cancer 30:42–49, 1974.
71. Meltzer MS, Stevenson MM: Macrophage function in tumor-bearing mice: tumoricidal and chemotactic response of macrophages activated by infection with Mycobacterium bovis, strain BCG. J Immunol 118:2176–2181, 1977.

72. Meltzer MS, Stevenson MM: Macrophage function in tumor-bearing mice: dissociation of phagocytic and chemotactic responsiveness. Cell Immunol 35:99–111, 1978.
73. Normann SJ, Sorkin E: Cell-specific defect in monocyte function during tumor growth. J Natl Cancer Inst 57:135–140, 1976.
74. Snyderman R, Pike MC, Blaylock BL, Weinstein P: Effect of neoplasms on inflammation: depression of macrophage accumulation after tumor implantation. J Immunol 116:585–589, 1976.
75. Sone S, Fidler IJ: Activation of rat alveolar macrophages to the tumoricidal state in the presence of progressively growing pulmonary metastases. Cancer Res 41:2401–2406, 1981.
76. Kripke ML, Budmen HB, Fidler IJ: Production of specific macrophageactivating factor by lymphocytes from tumor-bearing mice. Cell Immunol 30:341–352, 1977.
77. Papermaster BW, Holtermann OA, Rosner D, Klein E, Dao T, Djerassi I: Regressions produced in breast cancer lesions by a lymphokine fraction from a human lymphoid cell line. Res Commun Chem Pathol Pharmacol 8:413–428, 1974.
78. Salvin SB, Youngner JS, Nishio J, Neta R: Tumor suppression by a lymphokine released into the circulation of mice with delayed hypersensitivity. J Natl Cancer Inst 55:1233–1236, 1975.
79. Poste G, Kirsh R: Rapid decay of tumoricidal activity and loss of responsiveness to lymphokines in inflammatory macrophage. Cancer Res 39:2582–2590, 1979.
80. Allison AC: Model of action of immunological adjuvants. J Reticuloendothel Soc 26:619–630, 1979.
81. Sone S, Fidler IJ: Synergistic activation by lymphokines and muramyl dipeptide of tumoricidal properties in rat alveolar macrophages. J Immunol 125:2454–2460, 1980.
82. Poste G, Papahadjopoulos D: Lipid vesicles as a carrier for introducing materials into culture cells: influence of vesicle lipid composition on mechanism(s) of vesicle incorporation into cells. Proc Natl Acad Sci USA 73:1603–1607, 1976.
83. Kimelberg HK, Mayhew EG: Properties and biological effects of liposomes and their uses in pharmacology and toxicology. CRC Crit Rev Toxicol 9:25–44, 1978.
84. Allison AC, Gregoriadis G: Liposomes as immunological adjuvants. Nature 252:252–254, 1974.
85. Fidler IJ, Raz A, Fogler WE, Kirsh R, Bugelski P, Poste G: The design of liposomes to improve delivery of macrophage-augmenting agents to alveolar macrophages. Cancer Res 40:4460–4466, 1980.
86. Fidler IJ: Therapy of spontaneous metastases by intravenous injection of liposomes containing lymphokines. Science 208:1469–1471, 1980.
87. Fidler IJ, Sone S, Fogler WE, Barnes ZL: Eradication of spontaneous metastases and activation of alveolar macrophages by intravenous injection of liposomes containing muramyl dipeptide. Proc Natl Acad Sci USA 78:1680–1684, 1981.
88. Hart IR, Fogler WE, Poste G, Fidler IJ: Toxicity studies of liposome-encapsulated immunomodulators administered intravenously into dogs and mice. Cancer Immunol Immunother 10:
157–166, 1981.
89. Griswold DP, Jr: Consideration of the subcutaneously implanted B16 melanoma as a screening model for potential anticancer agents. Cancer Chemother Rep 3:315–323, 1972.
90. Schabel FM, Jr, Griswold DR, Jr, Corbett TH, Lloyd HH: Quantitative evaluation of anticancer agent activity in experimental animals. Pharmacol Ther [A] 1:411–435, 1977.

3. The role of natural killer (NK) cells in the control of tumor metastasis*

N. HANNA

1. Introduction

Elucidation of the host defense mechanisms that control tumor dissemination is essential for the design of successful approaches for the prevention and therapy of tumor metastasis. It has been demonstrated that immunity against tumor-specific antigens [1, 2] and generalized nonspecific stimulation of the immune response [3, 4] may inhibit metastasis formation. In contrast, immunosuppression enhances metastatic spread of immunogenic tumors [5, 6]. Host responses mediated by T lymphocytes [6], macrophages [7, 8] and NK cells [9] participate in host resistance against tumor metastasis. Considering the nature of the metastatic process [10–12], such effector mechanisms could prove effective in controlling lymphatic and hematogenous spread of tumor cells, although they might exert only a limited effect against the primary tumor. For example, once tumor cells enter the circulation, in the form of single cells or small clumps [13], they are confronted with highly destructive immune and nonimmune host defense mechanisms that might not exist within the primary tumor mass. Indeed, the majority of tumor cells that enter the circulation are destroyed and only a small fraction survive and develop into secondary tumor foci in the organ parenchyma [14]. Little is known about the mechanisms responsible for the rapid destruction of most circulating tumor cells. In this chapter, the *in vivo* role of NK cells in the destruction of circulating tumor cells and the inhibition of hematogenous tumor metastasis will be discussed. The applicability of NK cell activation by biological response modifiers to the prevention and therapy of tumor metastasis will be evaluated.

2. The NK cell system

The cellular characteristics, target cell specificity, and possible *in vivo* significance of NK cells have been the focus of several recent reviews [15–17]. Although NK cells

* Research sponsored by the National Cancer Institute Contract No. N01-C0-75380 with Litton Bionetics, Inc. The contents of this publication do not necessarily reflect the views or policies of the Department of Health and Human Services, nor does mention of trade names, commercial products, or organizations imply endorsement by the U.S. Government.

L.A. Liotta and I.R. Hart (eds.), Tumor Invasion and Metastasis. ISBN-13: 978-94-009-7513-2.
© 1982 Martinus Nijhoff Publishers, The Hague/Boston/London.

represent a heterogeneous population of cells, most findings indicate that murine NK cells are distinct from macrophages, B cells and mature T cells [15–17]. They express specific antigens (NK1, Qa-5, GM-1) and, therefore, could be killed by treatment with specific antibodies and complement [18–21]. In addition, NK cells express low concentrations of Fc receptors and Thy 1.2 antigens [16]. NK cells have a characteristic organ distribution: their activity is highest in peripheral blood and then in descending order spleen, lymph nodes and bone marrow and absent in the thymus [22, 23]. In mice, the expression of NK cell activity is controlled genetically and is strain- and age-dependent [15, 22, 23]. It is very low in mice younger than 3 weeks of age, peaks at 6 to 10 weeks, then declines gradually. Of the many factors that may be involved in the regulation of NK cell activity, interferon seems to play a central role. Interferon and interferon inducers were shown to activate NK cells following *in vivo* administration or incubation with normal lymphoid cells *in vitro* [24, 25]. The activation process is rapid and transient. Recent studies indicate that interferon influences the maturation of pre-NK cells that develop into highly active and functional effector NK cells [26]. It is noteworthy that mature NK cells produce interferon during their interaction with tumor target cells. This could be an important mechanism for activation and recruitment of NK cells *in situ*.

Studies on the target cell specificity of NK cells have revealed that, in addition to being tumoricidal, NK cells are cytotoxic *in vitro* to a variety of target cells including virus-infected normal or transformed cells, immature thymocytes and bone marrow stem cells [16, 27, 28]. In general, lymphoid and myeloid tumor cells are more sensitive to NK cell-mediated cytotoxicity than cells of solid tumors. However, a high degree of killing against fibrosarcomas and melanomas could be demonstrated following prolonged (18–24 h) incubation of effector and target cells *in vitro* [29, 30]. Under these *in vitro* conditions, however, another naturally cytotoxic (NC) cell, which is distinct from NK cells, may be active in killing of non-lymphoma tumor cells [31, 32].

3. Role of NK cells in resistance against transplantable tumors in vivo

Evidence that NK cells may play a role in resistance to transplantable lymphoma cells is based primarily on the correlation between the levels of NK cell activity of the host as measured *in vitro* and resistance against tumor growth *in vivo*. Nude mice exhibit high NK cell activity and strong resistance against syngeneic, allogeneic and xenogeneic lymphoma cells (see chapter on nude mice). Warner et al. [33] found that the growth rate of most lymphoma cells transplanted into syngeneic nude mice was much slower than that observed in syngeneic normal or heterozygous littermates. However, only lymphoid tumor cells that are sensitive to killing by spleen cells from nude mice *in vitro* showed reduced growth rate *in vivo*. Similarly, Minato et al. [34] found that xenogeneic cell lines infected with RNA viruses, unlike their tumorigenic parent cell lines, failed to form tumors when transplanted into nude mice. The virus-infected cell lines, but not the uninfected cells, were sensitive to NK cell-mediated cytotoxicity *in vitro*. Moreover, a virus-infected cell variant that escaped rejection *in vivo* was resistant to killing by NK cells *in vitro*. Haller et al. [35] reported that *in vivo* resistance against the growth of the NK-sensitive YAC lymphoma is positively correlated with the levels of NK cell activity of the hosts measured by *in vitro* assays. Thus, lethally irradiated F1 hybrid mice reconstituted with histocompatible bone marrow derived from high NK responders resisted the YAC-1 lymphoma cells more effectively than mice reconstituted with bone marrow from low NK responder donors. Reisenfeld et al. [36] expanded these studies and investigated the *in vivo* behavior of two lymphomas that differ in their susceptibility to killing by NK cells *in vitro*. They have demonstrated that recipients with high NK cell activity exhibited marked resistance against the growth of the NK-sensitive lymphoma and only marginal inhibition of the NK-resistant lymphoma.

Direct evidence that NK cells may prevent tumor growth *in vivo* was obtained by Kasai et al. [37] who, using specific anti-Ly5 serum, demonstrated that $Ly5^+$ NK cells positively selected from nonimmune spleen cells prevented the local growth of lymphomas in a Winn-type assay *in vivo*.

The possible role of NK cells in the inhibition of growth of transplantable nonlymphoma tumors was suggested by the findings that the growth rate of Lewis lung carcinoma (3LL) in F1 hybrid mice that exhibit high NK cell activity was slower than that observed in syngeneic recipient mice [38]. Similarly, Talmadge et al. [39] have demonstrated that NK-sensitive B16 melanoma cultured cells injected into beige mice, known to be deficient in NK cell activity, exhibited shorter induction time, and faster growth rate than those observed in normal syngeneic mice. Karre et al. [40] also have demonstrated that virally or chemically induced leukemias administered in small doses develop faster and at higher frequency in beige mice than in normal syngeneic mice. In these studies it was suggested that beige mice lack a rapidly acting defense mechanism that is involved in the early destructive events after tumor inoculation. On the other hand, Salomon et al. [41] observed no differences in the time of appearance or frequency of tumors in normal or beige mice injected with 3-methylcholanthrene. Furthermore, the rate of 3LL tumor growth was the same in both types of recipients. In this study, however, no data were provided regarding the sensitivity of the tumor cells to NK cell-mediated killing *in vitro*.

Recently, we have compared the time of appearance and growth rate of the NK-sensitive UV-2237 fibrosarcoma to those of the NK-resistant variant cell line UV-2237 NK-5 [29] following transplantation to normal syngeneic mice. We have found that the latent period preceding the growth of the parent UV-2237 tumor was significantly longer than that of the NK-resistant cell line. However, the slopes of the growth curves of both tumors were very similar. Studies on the fate and survival of transplanted radiolabelled tumor cells *in vivo* revealed that, 24–48 h following inoculation into the footpad of syngeneic recipient mice, 60% of the injected NK-resistant tumor cells were alive as compared to only 25% of the NK-sensitive UV-

2237 parent tumor cells. Therefore, it appears that NK cells may be involved in the early destruction of implanted tumor cells, whereas they exert little or no effect on the growth rate at later stages of tumor establishment and progression.

4. Role of NK cells in the control of tumor metastasis

The outcome of the metastatic process is determined by the interaction of tumor cells with various host factors [6]. Once tumor cells enter the circulation, they interact with host cells such as lymphocytes [6] and platelets [42]. In a quantitative analysis of metastasis, it was found that only a small fraction of tumor cells that enter the circulation can survive and develop into tumor colonies in organ parenchyma [14]. Little is known about the exact mechanisms that lead to the destruction of most circulating tumor emboli. The following studies indicate that NK cells play a major role in the destruction of tumor cells that enter the circulation and thus inhibit hematogenous metastatic spread. To establish a correlation between the levels of NK cell activity and the incidence of tumor metastasis, we studied metastasis in hosts that naturally exhibit low (3-week-old mice or adult beige mice) or high (nude mice) NK cell activity and in hosts whose NK cell activity was suppressed or enhanced by treatment with cyclophosphamide (Cy) or interferon inducers, respectively.

A single dose of Cy (120 or 240 mg/kg) administered four days before intravenous tumor injection enhanced pulmonary and extrapulmonary tumor metastasis [9; Table 1]. The enhancement of metastasis by Cy was not related to tumor immunogenicity or sensitivity to killing by immune T lymphocytes. Treatment with Cy enhanced experimental metastasis of all metastatic tumors tested, regardless of whether they metastasized at low or high frequencies in adult normal mice. That the enhancement of tumor metastasis was caused by the depletion of host effector immune cells by Cy was evident from lymphoid reconstitution experiments. These studies have indicated that adoptive transfer of normal spleen cells to Cy-treated recipient mice 24 h before intravenous tumor injection reversed the Cy-induced enhancement of experimental metastasis. The timing of spleen cell transfer was crucial, since lymphoid cells were effective only when inoculated before, but not after, tumor cells. These observations suggested that the host effector cells responsible for abrogating the Cy effect are active during a short period (12–24 h) following intravenous tumor cell injection and that their target is probably the circulating tumor cell [9]. Fractionation studies have indicated that the reactive cells in the reconstitution experiments are non-T, non-B, non-macrophage, Cy-sensitive and share the organ distribution and age dependency described for NK cells. Furthermore, it has been shown that Cy treatment inhibits NK cell activity [43] and that the peak of metastasis enhancement by Cy and its decline [44] corresponds with the kinetics of inactivation and recovery of NK cells following a single dose of the drug [45]. The involvement of NK cells in the present system may also explain the equally

Table 1. Number of pulmonary metastases following i.v. injection of melanoma cells into normal and Cy-treated C57BL/6 mice.

Cy-treatment dose (mg/kg)	Number of injected B16 cells/mouse	Average number of pulmonary tumor colonies	Extrapulmonary metastases
0	20000	29 ± 8	2/10 pleural
120	20000	62 ± 26	3/10 pleural
240	20000	149 ± 30	4/10 pleural; 4/10 lymph nodes; 6/11 liver; 1/11 kidney
0	40000	40 ± 6	None
120	40000	96 ± 33	3/10 pleural; 2/10 liver; 2/10 lymph nodes
240	40000	364 ± 57	8/10 pleural; 6/10 lymph nodes; 7/10 liver; 2/10 kidney; 3/10 mesentery; 1/10 stomach

protective effect of lymphoid reconstitution for all metastatic tumors regardless of their immunogenicity or susceptibility to killing by immune T lymphocytes. The most definitive evidence that NK cells are the effectors in this system was provided by recent experiments in which specific anti-NK antibodies were utilized to deplete NK cells from the lymphoid cell preparation before transfer to Cy-treated recipients [46]. Thus, we have shown that selective depletion of NK cells by treatment with anti-NK-1.2 antibodies and complement abolished the ability of normal spleen cells to override the Cy-induced enhancement of metastasis (Table 2).

4.1. Tumor metastasis in mice treated with β-estradiol

Recent reports have indicated that treatment of mice with β-estradiol leads to a marked depression of NK cell activity which cannot be boosted by the administration of interferon inducers [47, 48]. We have demonstrated that the depressed NK activity against UV-2237 and B16 melanoma tumors *in vitro* is associated with a marked enhancement of experimental pulmonary metastasis of both tumors in β-estradiol-treated syngeneic mice.

Moreover, the intraperitoneal injection of poly I:C or *C. parvum* failed to boost NK cell activity or inhibit metastasis formation in β-estradiol-treated mice. This is in

Table 2. Effect of lymphoid reconstitution on Cy-induced enhancement of experimental pulmonary metastasis.

Treatment of recipient mice	Median number (range) of lung tumor colonies
None, control	16 (2–27)
Cy	186 (123–300)
Cy-reconstituted with spleen cells:	
unfractionated	35 (8–52)
nylon wool nonadherent	18 (5–36)
treated with anti-θ + C	46 (22–78)
treated with anti-NK − 1.2 + C	168 (98–300)

Cy (200 mg/kg) was administered intraperitioneally 4 days before tumor cell injection. Lymphoid cells were injected intravenously 24 h before tumor cell inoculation. Mice were killed 21 days after intravenous injection of 10^5 UV-2237 fibrosarcoma tumor cells, and pulmonary metastases were counted.

sharp contrast to their antimetastatic effect when administered to normal mice. In these experiments, treatment with β-estradiol did not inhibit interferon production or interfere with the *in vivo* activation of alveolar or peritoneal macrophages following the injection of poly I:C or *C. parvum*. Therefore, β-estradiol-treated mice may be used to achieve selective activation of non-NK-effector cells and thus, evaluate their role in the prevention and/or therapy of tumor metastasis.

4.2. Experimental tumor metastasis in 3- and 6-week-old syngeneic mice

The *in vivo* expression of NK cell activity is age dependent [15]. Only low levels of cytotoxicity against UV-2237 fibrosarcoma and B16 melanoma target cells could be demonstrated with spleen effector cells from normal 3-week-old mice. On the other hand, lymphoid cells obtained from mice 6–10 weeks old exhibited significant levels of cytotoxicity *in vitro*. However, NK cell activity in 3-week-old mice could be boosted readily by the administration of bacterial adjuvants and/or interferon inducers (Figure 1). Injection of metastatic tumor cells into 3-week-old syngeneic mice produced larger numbers of lung tumor colonies (10- to 100-fold) than those observed in 8-week-old mice [9]. Activation of NK cells in 3-week-old mice by the intraperitoneal administration of poly I:C or *C. parvum* 24 h prior to tumor challenge reduced the incidence of metastasis to levels observed in adult 8-week-old mice. These agents were effective only when given before, but not after, tumor cell injection. This period coincides with the presence of tumor cells in the circulation and before extravasation into the organ parenchyma occurs. Similarly, an inverse correlation between the levels of NK cell activity exhibited by 3- and 8-week-old mice and the incidence of experimental tumor metastasis was observed in athymic nude mice (see chapter on nude mice).

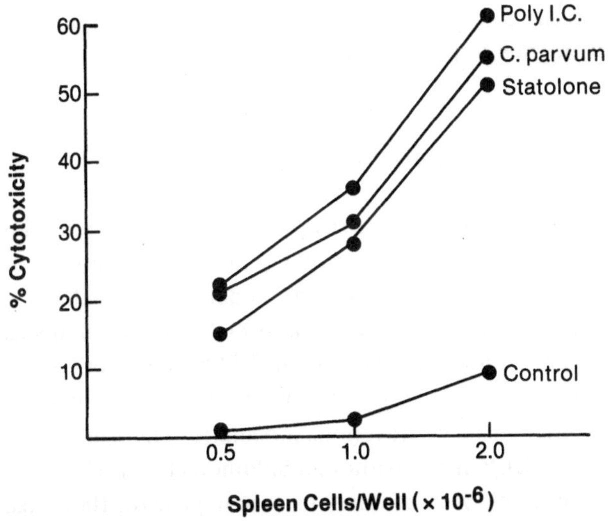

Figure 1. Enhancement of NK cell-mediated cytotoxicity by poly I:C, *C. parvum* and statolone injected into 3-week-old C3H⁻ mice 24 h before testing *in vitro*. Percent killing was determined after a 24 h incubation of spleen effector cells with ^{3}H-proline-labeled UV-2237 fibrosarcoma target cells.

Although enhancement of experimental metastasis was observed in both 3-week-old mice and Cy-treated adult mice, NK activation by poly I:C or *C. parvum* inhibited metastases formation in 3-week-old but not in Cy-treated mice, unless normal lymphocytes were also supplied to the drug-treated mice [9]. These data indicate that NK cells are present but not yet activated (pre-NK) in young normal mice, whereas they are depleted in Cy-treated mice. These results are relevant to the application of combined immuno- and chemotherapeutic drugs in cancer treatment, which may result in antagonism rather than synergism. For example, by depleting or inactivating the effector cells involved in host defense against tumor metastasis, chemotherapeutic drugs may enhance metastasis formation, especially by tumor cell variants that are resistant to the drug and also interfere with the antimetastatic effect of biological response modifiers. In the aforementioned studies, the adoptive transfer of normal syngeneic lymphoid cell preparations (spleen or bone-marrow cells) after drug treatment and before the application of the immunomodulators proved to be beneficial in reconstituting the antimetastatic response of the recipient mice [9].

The high incidence of pulmonary metastasis in 3-week-old mice and Cy-treated mice was not caused by a more efficient trapping of tumor cells in the capillary bed of the lungs, since the initial arrest of radiolabeled tumor cells did not differ from that observed in normal adult mice. However, the survival of the arrested tumor cells during the first 24 h after intravenous tumor cell injection was higher in mice with low NK cell activity (3-week-old mice and Cy-treated mice). Likewise, Riccardi et al. [49] have demonstrated a close correlation between the levels of NK cell activity and the ability of normal mice to eliminate lymphoma cells during the first 4 h following intravenous inoculation.

4.3. Enhanced tumor metastasis in beige mice

Recently, the beige mutant of the C57BL/6 mouse was shown to exhibit low levels of NK cell activity *in vitro* [50]. The macrophage and T cell functions, however, appear to be normal [51]. Therefore, this animal model may provide a valuable tool for evaluating the *in vivo* role of NK cells in natural defense mechanisms against tumor growth and dissemination. Talmadge et al. [39] have demonstrated that NK-sensitive B16 melanoma cells metastasized more readily and at a higher frequency (following subcutaneous or intravenous inoculation) in beige mice than in heterozygous normal C57BL/6 mice. Although Salomon et al. [41] were unable to detect differences in the rates of subcutaneous tumor growth, they observed a higher incidence of pulmonary tumor metastasis in beige mice than in normal syngeneic controls. We have shown that more lung tumor colonies developed in beige mice given intravenous injections of B16-F10 and B16-F1 melanoma cell lines than in age-matched C57BL/6 recipients [29]. These findings provide further evidence that NK cells are effective in host defense against circulating tumor cells and can prevent the hematogenous tumor spread and subsequent establishment of distant organ metastasis.

4.4. The relationship between the expression of metastatic potential of tumor cells in vivo and resistance to NK cell-mediated cytotoxicity in vitro

Many tumors are heterogeneous and contain subpopulations of cells that differ in their immunogenicity [52], metastatic potential [53] and perhaps also in their resistance to killing by immune and natural cytotoxic cells. In a recent report, Gorelick et al. [38] have suggested that cells obtained from a metastasis of 3LL carcinoma are more resistant to NK cell-mediated lysis *in vitro* than cells from the local primary tumor.

Since we have demonstrated that NK cels play a major role in the destruction of circulating tumor cells and the inhibition of hematogenous metastatic spread, we examined 1) whether the metastatic potential of *in vivo* isolated tumor variants or *in vitro* cloned cell populations correlated with resistance or susceptibility to killing by NK cells, 2) whether the *in vivo* selection of highly metastatic cell variants is associated with selection for resistance to NK cell-mediated lysis, and 3) whether *in vitro* selection for tumor cells resistant to NK cell-mediated cytotoxicity is associated with the emergence of cells that are highly metastatic *in vivo*.

In the B16 melanoma system, the F10 (high lung colonization), F1 and F10^{Lr} (low lung colonization) cell lines exhibited similar but modest degrees of sensitivity to killing by normal or poly I:C-activated NK cells, irrespective of whether they have high or low metastatic potential [29]. This result correlated with the *in vivo* increase in the incidence of metastasis by all three B16 tumor variants when injected into recipients with low levels of NK cell activity, such as beige mice or 3-week-old syngeneic recipients.

In the K-1735 melanoma system, cell lines established from different individual lung metastatic nodules invariably exhibited high lung colonization potential. Nonetheless, their sensitivity to killing by NK cells varied significantly. Similar results were obtained with *in vitro* cloned cell populations of the K-1735 tumor in which NK resistance did not always segregate with high metastatic potential [29].

The UV-2237 fibrosarcoma produces few metastases in the normal syngeneic $C3H^-$ mouse and is highly sensitive to NK cell-mediated lysis *in vitro*. Here also, four highly metastatic cell lines established *in vivo* from spontaneous pulmonary metastases and five cloned lines selected *in vitro* were as sensitive to NK cell-mediated lysis as the parent UV-2237 cell line, regardless of their metastatic behavior *in vivo* [29].

In order to determine the relationship between target cell susceptibility to NK cell-mediated lysis *in vitro* and expression of metastatic potential *in vivo*, we studied the metastatic behavior of NK-resistant and NK-sensitive tumor cells following injection into hosts with high or low levels of NK cell activity. Therefore, we selected tumor cells *in vitro* that are resistant to NK-cell-mediated cytotoxicity [29]. The UV-2237 fibrosarcoma was incubated with nylon-wool-nonadherent spleen cells obtained from normal 8- to 10-week-old syngeneic $C3H^-$ mice. Surviving cells were allowed to proliferate and were reincubated six times with NK cells. The cells surviving each cycle of NK cell treatment were designated as NK-1, NK-2 and so on. Control cultures included UV-2237 parent cells incubated six times with spleen cells obtained from 3-week-old syngeneic mice that have low NK cell activity. A

Table 3. Relationship between susceptibility to NK cell-mediated cytotoxicity *in vitro* and metastatic behavior *in vivo*.

Tumor cell lines	% Cytotoxicity	Median number (range) of lung tumor colonies
UV-2237 parent	53	22 (7–31)
NK-1	45	15 (2–28)
NK-2	31	12 (3–22)
NK-3	38	28 (8–42)
NK-5	15	119 (67–182)
NK-6	10	130 (76–231)
C1-C6	48–62	8–26 (2–43)

Percent cytotoxicity was measured after 24 h incubation of normal spleen cells (1×10^6 cells/well) with ^{3}H-proline-labeled tumor target cells (1×10^4 cells/well). Number of lung colonies was measured 3 weeks following the intravenous injection of 10^5 tumor cells into 8-week-old syngeneic $C3H^-$ mice.

marked and consistent resistance to NK cell-mediated lysis was exhibited by the NK-5 and NK-6 cell lines (Table 3). The control tumor cells treated with spleen cells devoid of NK cell activity did not display any trend toward increased resistance to NK cell-mediated lysis.

To determine whether selection of tumor cells resistant to NK cell-mediated lysis *in vitro* is associated with enhanced metastasis formation *in vivo*, the UV-2237, NK-1 to NK-6 and C1 to C6 cell lines were injected intravenously into adult 8- to 10-week-old syngeneic $C3H^-$ recipients. Only the NK-resistant cell lines (NK-5 and NK-6) produced significantly more pulmonary metastases than the UV-2237 parent, NK-1 to NK-3, and C1 to C6 cell lines. Moreover, only the NK-resistant cell lines (NK-5 and NK-6) produced large numbers of lung tumor colonies in adult nude mice that exhibit high levels of NK cell activity and increased resistance to metastasis development [29]. These results indicate that NK-resistant tumor cell lines, isolated under defined selective conditions *in vitro* from the predominantly NK-sensitive UV-2237 parent tumor, express high metastatic potential when injected into recipients that exhibit either low or high NK cell cytotoxicity. Collectively, the selective process of metastasis *in vivo* need not be associated with parallel selection for resistance to NK cell-mediated lysis. Resistance to NK cell-mediated cytotoxicity, however, can enhance the expression of metastatic potential of tumor cells. Thus, metastases may be populated by NK-resistant or NK-sensitive tumor cells that escaped NK cell-mediated killing. Therefore, the levels and state of activation of NK cells in tumor-bearing hosts may influence the outcome of metastasis to distant organs.

Even though NK cells seem to be effective primarily during the early stages of metastasis development and even though malignant neoplasms may have already spread by the time of diagnosis, activation of NK cells has clinical relevance. For example, it has been reported that during diagnostic and/or surgical procedures, tumor cells may be released from the primary neoplasm and eventually develop into metastatic foci in distant organs. Perhaps, the activation of NK cells shortly before and after such manipulation will destroy the newly released circulating tumor cells and thus prevent additional metastatic growths. For this reason, elucidation of the mechanisms that regulate the activation and suppression of NK cells will help achieve and maintain the high levels of NK cell activity required for the control of hematogenous spread of tumor cells.

References

1. Hanna MG: Active specific immunotherapy of residual micrometastases: a comparison of post-operative treatment with BCG-tumor cell vaccine to preoperative intratumoral BCG injection. In: Immunobiology and immunotherapy of cancer, Terry WD and Yamamura Y (eds). New York: Elsevier North Holland, 1979, pp 331–350.
2. Fidler IJ, Gersten DM, Riggs C: Relationship of host immune status to tumor cell arrest, distribution and survival in experimental metastasis. Cancer 40:46–55, 1977.

3. Bomford R, Olivotto M: The mechanism of inhibition by Corynebacterium parvum of the growth of lung nodules from intravenously injected tumor cells. Int J Cancer 14:226–235, 1974.
4. Jones PDE, Castro JE: Immunological mechanisms in metastatic spread and the antimetastatic effects of C. parvum. Br J Cancer 35:519–527, 1977.
5. Fidler IJ, Kripke ML: Tumor cell antigenicity, host immunity and cancer metastasis. Cancer Immunol Immunother 7:201–205, 1980.
6. Fidler IJ, Gersten DM, Kripke ML: Influence of immune status on the metastasis of three murine fibrosarcomas of different immunogenicities. Cancer Res 39:3816–3821, 1979.
7. Fidler IJ: Therapy of spontaneous metastases by intravenous injection of liposomes containing lymphokines. Science 208:1469–1471, 1980.
8. Poste G, Fidler IJ: The pathogenesis of cancer metastasis. Nature 283:139–146, 1980.
9. Hanna N, Fidler IJ: The role of natural killer cells in the destruction of circulating tumor emboli. JNCI 65:801–809, 1980.
10. Fidler IJ, Gersten DM, Hart IR: The biology of cancer invasion and metastasis. Adv Cancer Res 28:149–250, 1978.
11. Sugarbaker EV, Ketcham AS: Mechanism and prevention of cancer dissemination: an overview. Semin Oncol 4:19–32, 1977.
12. Weiss L: A pathobiologic overview of metastasis. Semin Oncol 4:5–17, 1977.
13. Liotta LA, Kleinerman J, Saidel GM: Quantitative relationships of intravascular tumor cells, tumor vessels and pulmonary metastases following tumor implantation. Cancer Res 34:997–1004, 1974.
14. Fidler IJ: Metastasis: quantitative analysis of distribution and fate of tumor emboli labeled with ^{125}I-5-Iodo-2′-deoxyuridine. J Natl Cancer Inst 45:733–782, 1970.
15. Kiessling R, Wigzell H: An analysis of the murine NK cells as to the structure, function, and biological relevance. Immunol Rev 44:165–208, 1979.
16. Herberman RB, Djeu JR, Kay HD, Ortaldo JR, Riccardi C, Bonnard GD, Holden HT, Fagnani R, Santoni A, Pucetti P: Natural killer cells: characteristics and regulation of activity. Immunol Rev 44:43, 1979.
17. Herberman RB, Holden HR: Natural cell-mediated immunity. Adv Cancer Res 27:305–377, 1978.
18. Glimcher L, Shen FW, Cantor H: Identification of a cell-surface antigen selectively expressed on the natural killer cell. J Exp Med 145:1–9, 1977.
19. Burton RC: Alloantisera selectively reactive with NK cells: characterization and use in defining NK cell classes. In: Natural cell-mediated immunity to tumors, Herberman RB (ed). New York: Academic Press, pp 19–36.
20. Koo GC, Jacobson JB, Hammerling GJ, Hammerling U: Antigenic profile of murine natural killer cells. J Immunol 125:1003–1006, 1980.
21. Young WW, Hakomori SI, Durdik JM, Henney CS: Identification of ganglio-N-tetraosylceramide as a new surface marker for murine natural killer (NK) cells. J Immunol 124:199–201, 1980.
22. Herberman RB, Ninn ME, Laurin DH: Natural cytotoxic reactivity of mouse lymphoid cells against syngeneic and allogeneic tumors. I. Distribution of reactivity and specificity. Int J Cancer 16:216–229, 1975.
23. Keissling, R, Klein E, Wigzell H: Natural killer cells in the mouse. a. Cytotoxic cells with specificity for mouse Moloney leukemia cells. Specificity and distribution according to genotype. Eur J Immunol 5:112–117, 1975.
24. Gidlund M, Orn A, Wigzell H, Senik A, Gresser I: Enhanced NK cell activity in mice infected with interferon and interferon inducers. Nature 273:750–761, 1978.
25. Djeu JY, Heinbaugh JA, Holden HT, Herberman RB: Augmentation of mouse natural killer cell activity by interferon inducers. J Immunol 122:175–181, 1979.
26. Minato N, Reid L, Cantor H, Lengyel P, Bloom B: Mode of regulation of natural killer cell activity by interferon. J Exp Med 152:124–137, 1980.
27. Nunn ME, Herberman RB, Holden HT: Natural cell-mediated cytotoxicity in mice against non-lymphoid tumors and some normal cells. Int J Cancer 20:381–387, 1977.

28. Hansson M, Kiessling R, Andersson B, Karre K, Roder J: NK cell-sensitive T-cell subpopulation in thymus: inverse correlation to host NK activity. Nature 278:174–176, 1979.
29. Hanna N, Fidler IJ: Relationship between metastatic potential and resistance to NK cell-mediated cytotoxicity in three murine tumor systems JNCI 66:1183–1190, 1981.
30. Hanna N: Expression of metastatic potential of tumor cells in young nude mice is correlated with low levels of natural killer cell-mediated cytotoxicity. Int J Cancer 26:675, 1980.
31. Stutman O, Paige CJ, Figarella EF: Natural cytotoxic cells against solid tumors in mice. I. Strain and age distribution and target cell susceptibility. J Immunol 121:1819–1826, 1978.
32. Paige CJ, Figarella EF, Cuttito MJ, Cahan A, Stutman O: Natural cytotoxic cells against solid tumors in mice. II. Some characteristics of the effector cells against solid tumors in mice. J Immunol 121:1827–1835, 1978.
33. Warner NL, Woodruff MFA, Burton RC: Inhibition of the growth of lymphoid tumours in syngeneic athymic (nude) mice. Int J Cancer 20:146–155, 1977.
34. Minato N, Bloom BR, Jones C, Holland J, Reid LM: Mechanism of rejection of virus persistently infected tumor cells by athymic nude mice. J Exp Med 149:1117–1133, 1979.
35. Haller O, Hansson M, Kiessling R, Wigzell H: Role of non-conventional natural killer cell in resistance against syngeneic tumour cells *in vivo*. Nature 270:609–611, 1977.
36. Riesenfeld I, Orn A, Gidlund M, Axberg I, Alm GU, Wigzell H: Positive correlation between *in vitro* NK activity and *in vivo* resistance towards AKR lymphoma cells. Int J Cancer 25:399–403, 1980.
37. Kasai M, Leclerc JC, McVay-Boudreau L, Shen FW, Cantor H: Direct evidence that natural killer cells in nonimmune spleen cell populations prevent tumor growth *in vivo*. J Exp Med 149:1260–1264, 1979.
38. Gorelick E, Fogel M, Feldman M, Segal S: Differences in resistance of metastatic tumor cells and cells from local tumor growth to cytotoxicity of natural killer cells. JNCI 63:1397–1404, 1979.
39. Talmadge JE, Meyers KM, Prieur DJ, Starkey JR: Role of NK cells in tumor growth and metastasis in beige mice. Nature 284:622–624, 1980.
40. Karre K, Lein GO, Kiessling R, Klein G, Roder JC: Low natural *in vivo* resistance to syngeneic leukemias in natural killer-deficient mice. Nature 284:624–626, 1980.
41. Salomon JC, Creau-Goldberg N, Lynch NR: Cancer induction by methylcholanthrene and metastatic spread of transplantable tumor in Chediak Higashi (beige) mice. Cancer Immunol Immunother 8:67–70, 1980.
42. Gasic GJ, Gasic TB, Galanti N, Johnson T, Murphy S: Platelet-tumor cell interaction in mice. The role of platelets in the spread of malignant disease. Int J Cancer 11:704–718, 1973.
43. Djeu JY, Heinbaugh JA, Vieira WD, Holden HT, Herberman RB: The effect of immunopharmacological agents on mouse natural cell-mediated cytotoxicity and on its augmentation by poly I.C. Immunopharmacology 1:231–244, 1979.
44. Steel GG, Adams K: Enhancement by cytotoxic agents of artificial pulmonary metastasis. Br J Cancer 36:653–658, 1977.
45. Mantovani A, Luini W, Peri G, Vechi A, Spreafico F: Effect of chemotherapeutic agents on natural cell-mediated cytotoxicity in mice. JNCI 61:1255–1261, 1978.
46. Hanna N, Burton RC: Definitive evidence that natural killer (NK) cells inhibit tumor metastasis *in vivo*. J Immunol 127:1754–1758, 1981.
47. Seaman WE, Blackman MA, Gindhart TD, Roubinia JR, Loeb JM, Talal N: β-estradiol reduces natural killer cells in mice. J Immunol 121:2193–2198, 1978.
48. Seaman WE, Merigan TC, Talal N: Natural killing in estrogen-treated mice responds poorly to poly I:C despite normal stimulation of circulating interferon. J Immunol 123:2903–2905, 1979.
49. Riccardi C, Puccetti P, Santoni A, Herberman RB: Rapid *in vivo* assay of mouse natural killer cell activity. JNCI 63:1041–1045, 1979.
50. Roder J, Duwe A: The beige mutation in the mouse selectively impairs natural killer cell function. Nature 278:451–453, 1979.

51. Roder JC, Lohmann-Matthes ML, Domzig W, Wigzell H: The beige mutation in the mouse. II. Selectivity of the natural killer (NK) cell defect. J Immunol 123:2174–2181, 1979.
52. Killion JJ, Kollmorgen GM: Isolation of immunogenic tumor cells by cell-affinity chromatography. Nature 259:674–676, 1976.
53. Fidler IJ, Kripke ML: Metastasis results from preexisting variant cells within a malignant tumor. Science 197:893–895, 1977.

4. Metastasis of xenogeneic and allogeneic tumors in nude mice*

N. HANNA

1. Introduction

Understanding the pathogenesis of cancer metastasis is fundamental to the design of successful therapeutic modalities for treatment of disseminated cancer. Metastasis development is determined by both host factors and intrinsic properties of the tumor cells [1]. To establish metastases, tumor cells must invade the surrounding local tissue and eventually penetrate into blood vessels and/or the lymphatic system. In the circulation, they must survive the potentially lethal interaction with host defense mechanisms, be arrested in the capillary bed of distant organs, extravasate into organ parenchyma, vascularize, and proliferate to form distinct foci of metastatic tumor growth [2–4]. Interruption of the sequence at any of these steps can inhibit metastasis formation. It is, therefore, not surprising that modification of either host factors or tumor cell properties influences the outcome of tumor dissemination and the establishment of distant organ metastases [5–8]. Host immune mechanisms (specific and nonspecific; natural and acquired) can intervene at different stages of the metastatic process and, thereby, inhibit the development of visible clinical metastases [9–11]. Studies using animals with selective immune deficiencies have contributed considerably to the elucidation of the host factors involved in tumor metastasis [10, 12–14]. Such animal models also have potential for studies of effective therapy of metastasis. Unfortunately, studies of metastases of human malignant neoplasms have been hampered by a lack of adequate *in vivo* models. The discovery of the athymic T-cell-deficient nude mouse and its successful use for heterotransplantation of normal and malignant tissuès provided a highly desirable *in vivo* model for studying the biology of human tumors [15–17]. In this chapter, I will review briefly the applicability of the nude mouse model to studies of tumor growth and metastasis and discuss the possible role of T-cell-independent natural cell-mediated immunity in the resistance of nude mice to tumor dissemination. Also, I will describe our recent findings that young nude mice with low levels of natural cell-mediated immunity could serve as a sensitive model for assessing the

* Research sponsored by the National Cancer Institute Contract No. NO1-C0-75380 with Litton Bionetics, Inc. The contents of this publication do not necessarily reflect the views or policies of the Department of Health and Human Services, nor does mention of trade names, commercial products, or organizations imply endorsement by the U.S. Government.

L.A. Liotta and I.R. Hart (eds.), Tumor Invasion and Metastasis. ISBN-13: 978-94-009-7513-2.
© 1982 Martinus Nijhoff Publishers, The Hague/Boston/London.

metastatic potential of allogeneic and xenogeneic tumors and perhaps for isolating highly metastatic cell subpopulations to be used for testing the activity of anti-metastatic agents.

2. Growth of allogeneic and xenogeneic tumors in nude mice

Since the initial observation by Rygaard and Povlsen [18] that xenogeneic human tumors could grow in athymic nude mice, intensive efforts have been made to use this *in vivo* model for studies of the cellular characteristics and metastatic potential of xenogeneic human tumors [16, 17] and for evaluation of tumorigenicity of transformed cells of various origins [19, 20].

Progressive growth of xenogeneic tumors transplanted into nude mice is dependent on host- and tumor-related properties, such as the origin and type of tumor, the route of inoculation, and the age, strain and state of health of the recipient mice. Studies with human tumors have found that melanomas, carcinomas of soft tissues and sarcomas can be transplanted successfully into nude mice [21–23]. In contrast, carcinomas of the breast [24, 25], stomach [26], and prostate [26] are more difficult to establish. To successfully grow lymphomas and leukemias in nude mice, the recipient host must be immunosuppressed and/or the tumor must be injected intracranially [27].

Of the 48 carcinomas implanted into nude mice by Shimosato et al. [23], lung tumors were transplanted most easily (10 of 21), followed by gastric (2 of 14) and breast (1 of 13) carcinomas. Other investigators have reported a similarly modest rate of success (12 to 15%) with human mammary carcinomas implanted in female nude mice [28, 29]. In contrast, the percentage of successful 'takes' of human malignant melanomas transplanted into nude mice is impressive (70 to 80%) [30, 31].

The *in vivo* tumorigenic and malignant properties of cultured tumor cell lines transplanted to nude mice have been studied extensively [21, 32, 33]. Giovanella et al. [21] made the observation that, although surgically excised fresh human tumors could grow progressively in nude mice, cultured tumor cell lines expressed malignant properties of invasiveness and metastasis more readily.

In addition to tumor cell properties, host-related factors influence the growth of tumor xenografts in nude mice. Kameya et al. [34] reported that the percentage of human choriocarcinomas successfully grown in specific pathogen-free (SPF) nude mice was markedly higher than that observed in animals housed in conventional facilities (95% versus 35%, respectively). Kyriazis et al. [35] reported that, unlike SPF mice, nude mice infected with mouse hepatitis virus exhibit greater resistance to transplanted xenogeneic human neoplasms. Our own experience with a limited number of human melanoma cell lines and surgically excised colon carcinoma tumors indicates that the percentage of successful transplantations and the growth rate of these tumors were higher in BALB/c nude mice than in age-matched

NIH/Swiss nude recipients. Tumors grew faster in mice (of a particular strain) housed in barrier or isolator facilities than in those housed in conventional facilities.

3. Host resistance to tumor growth

Although the athymic nude mouse lacks functionally mature T lymphocytes, it should not be considered totally immunodeficient. Nude mice show an almost normal response to T-cell-independent antigens [36] and have high titers of natural antibodies that react with tumor cells [37]. Tumoricidal macrophages can be isolated from untreated nude mice [38, 39] and their activity can be enhanced following *in vivo* stimulation with bacterial adjuvants [39]. Moreover, nude mice exhibit consistently high natural killer (NK) cell activity [40]. All three T-cell-independent effector mechanisms could play a significant role in host-tumor interaction and contribute to natural resistance of nude mice against xenogeneic human neoplasms. Strong evidence of the *in vivo* role of such defense mechanisms in limiting tumor growth is provided by the observation that further immunosuppression of nude mice or the use of newborn recipients increases the rate of successful transplantation, the growth rate and, occasionally, the invasiveness and metastatic spread of implanted xenogeneic human tumors [30, 41, 44]. For example, Watanabe et al. [44] reported that lymphoid cell lines were accepted in 38.5% of irradiated mice and 100% of splenectomized and irradiated mice as opposed to 0% of untreated mice. However, transplantation of fresh leukemia and lymphoma cells into pretreated mice was successful in only 29% of the 24 cases studied. This limited success could be attributed to a radioresistant defense mechanism operating against lymphoma cells that express Hh antigens [45]. A recent report by Minato et al. [46] demonstrated that xenogeneic cell lines known to be highly tumorigenic in the nude mouse were rejected when persistently infected with a variety of RNA viruses. Unlike the parent cell lines, the virus-infected cells were susceptible to NK-cell-mediated cytotoxicity *in vitro*. Similarly, Warner et al. [47] described a close correlation between the sensitivity of lymphoma cells to killing by NK cells *in vitro* and a reduced growth rate in syngeneic nude mice.

4. Tumor invasion and metastasis in nude mice

The usefulness of the nude mouse for studies of cancer metastasis has been limited because malignant allogeneic and xenogeneic neoplasms rarely metastasize following transplantation into nude mice [18, 48, 49]. The expression of metastatic potential of tumor cells in nude mice is dependent on the tumor system, transplantation protocols, and on the natural defense mechanisms of the host. Such variables may account for the apparently conflicting results reported from different laboratories [18, 50, 51]. Giovanella et al. [21, 50] detected lymph node and lung metastases following subcutaneous (s.c.) inoculation of human melanoma cultured cell lines into nude mice. On the other hand, Povlsen [31], using several different tumors including human malignant melanomas, was unable to detect any metastases. Sharkey and Fogh [33] observed lymph node and lung metastases in only 1.3% of nude mice injected with 10^6 malignant tumor cells. In this study, breast tumor cell lines metastasized more frequently than other tumor types, whereas none of the sarcoma lines metastasized. Similarly, an extremely low incidence of metastasis was reported by Shimosato et al. [23], who detected lymph node metastases of a hepatocellular carcinoma in one of 91 surgically excised human tumors transplanted into nude mice. Microscopic pulmonary metastases were observed by Zamecnik and Long [52] in four of 36 nude mice with progressively growing s.c. tumors derived from Hodgkin's lymphoma cultured cell lines. Hata et al. [53] reported that human neuroblastomas that are transplanted into nude mice metastasize to the lymph nodes, ovaries and cerebrum. The pattern of organ distribution of metastases in nude mice was similar to that seen in the donor. Another study, by Maguire et al. [54], showed that xenogeneic human, dog and guinea pig tumors that were successfully transplanted into nude mice did not metastasize. However, when a highly aggressive methylcholanthrene (MCA)-induced reticulum cell sarcoma from a Syrian hamster was implanted s.c. into nude mice, local invasion and both hematogenous and lymphatic tumor spread were observed. Wiltrout et al. [55] found that allogeneic murine MCA-induced sarcomas implanted into BALB/c nude mice metastasize successfully. In this tumor system, the kinetics and organ distribution pattern of the metastases in nude mice were identical to those observed in the syngeneic host.

The site of tumor implantation in nude mice seems to influence the growth rate, invasiveness and metastatic behavior of the tumor cells. Kyriazis et al. [56] transplanted human tumor cell lines derived from carcinoma of the larynx and the colon into s.c. or intraperitoneal (i.p.) sites of BALB/c nude mice. Only tumor cells administered i.p. invaded the intra-abdominal organs and metastasized in 60% of the mice to mediastinal lymph nodes and lungs. Takahashi et al. [57] reported similar results with adenocarcinoma cells administered i.p. into nude mice.

Although the use of antilymphocyte serum-treated and x-irradiated immunosuppressed nude mice increases the percentage of successful transplants of human tumors [41, 43, 44], a study of 10 malignant lymphoblastoid cell lines showed no gross or histologic evidence for local or distant metastases [43]. On the other hand, Sordat et al. [30] reported that human solid tumors and/or established lymphoid and myeloid cell lines injected into newborn, but not adult, nude mice exhibited pronounced local invasiveness and frequent dissemination to the lungs and kidneys. Similar results were obtained with the K-562 myeloid cell line injected s.c. or intravenously (i.v.) into newborn nude mice [42]. The resistance of T-cell-deficient mice to tumor growth and metastasis was considered as evidence in support of the immunostimulation theory of tumor growth [58]. However, the relatively enhanced susceptibility of immunosuppressed or newborn nude mice to tumor growth and metastasis strongly suggests that an active T-cell-independent defense mechanism is responsible for the poor tumor growth and the low incidence of tumor metastasis in nude mice.

5. Resistance of nude mice to tumor metastasis

The rarity of metastasis, despite the local growth of malignant tumors, can be attributed to host defense mechanisms that are more effective in destroying small numbers of circulating tumor cells than in inhibiting the growth of the local tumor. For example, unlike the cells within a solid tumor, the progenitors of metastasis circulate as single cells or small clumps and are, therefore, highly vulnerable to the destructive effects of immune and nonimmune host defense mechanisms. Moreover, in the blood, which is a primary route for tumor dissemination, tumor cells are exposed to highly destructive forces that may not be present in the primary tumor mass. Fidler et al. [59] and Skov et al. [60] observed that i.v. injection of metastatic murine tumor cells into adult nude mice resulted in a lower incidence of lung tumor colonies as compared with age-matched syngeneic mice. This does not seem to be a unique feature of experimental tumor metastasis, since Lozzio et al. [61] reported that leukemia cells could be detected in the blood of tumor-bearing nude mice in the absence of detectable metastases. Thus, the presence of tumor cells in the circulation is necessary, but certainly not sufficient, to produce metastases [1]. It is well established that most tumor cells that enter the circulation do not survive to establish metastases [62–64]. An understanding of the host defense mechanisms that participate in the destruction of circulating tumor emboli will be important in establishing highly sensitive animal models that exhibit low resistance against metastatic spread of neoplastic cells.

5.1. Role of NK cells in the control of hematogenous tumor dissemination

Recent reports from our laboratory [10, 65] and others [66] strongly suggest that NK cells are involved in the early destruction of circulating tumor cells. We have demonstrated an inverse correlation between the levels of NK cell activity and the incidence of experimental metastases, i.e. the incidence of tumor metastases was higher in recipients that exhibited low NK cell levels and was lower in hosts with high NK cell activity [10, 13, 65]. For example, the *in vivo* depletion of NK cells by pretreatment of syngeneic mice with cyclophosphamide (Cy) resulted in enhancement of pulmonary and extrapulmonary metastases. Similarly, a high incidence of metastasis was observed in 3-week-old syngeneic mice [10] and the beige mutant (bg^J/bg^J) of C57BL/6 mice [14, 67]. Both recipients exhibited low levels of NK cells which correlated with the increased tumor cell survival in the circulation. Activation of NK cells in young syngeneic mice by the administration of interferon-inducing

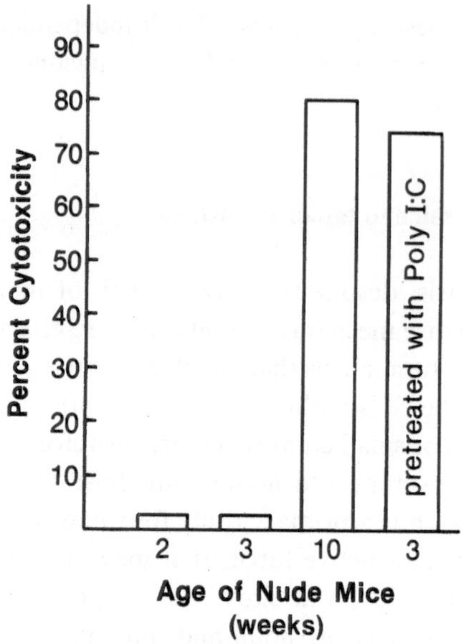

Figure 1. Natural cell-mediated cytotoxicity of spleen cells obtained from 2-, 3- and 10-week-old nude mice and its enhancement by treatment with poly I:C. Pretreated 3-week-old nude mice received an i.p. injection of 50μg of poly I:C 18 hours before the *in vitro* assay. ^{3}H-proline-labelled UV-2237 fibrosarcoma cells served as targets in a 24-hour *in vitro* assay.

agents such as poly I:C and statolone markedly inhibited tumor metastasis. These drugs were effective when administered 24 hours before (but not after) tumor cell inoculation. This indicates that the activated effector cells were functional (during a short period) following tumor cell injection, and that their target is probably the circulating tumor cell (see chapter 3).

6. The expression of the metastatic potential of allogeneic and xenogeneic tumors in young nude mice with low levels of NK cell activity

The finding that a higher incidence of tumor metastases in 3-week-old syngeneic mice correlates with low NK cell activity initiated a search for a similar correlation between age dependence of NK cell expression and the incidence of allogeneic and xenogeneic tumor metastases in nude mice.

The natural cell-mediated cytotoxicity of spleen cells obtained from 2- to 3-week old and 6- to 10-week-old nude mice was assessed *in vitro* against NK-sensitive fibrosarcoma target cells. The results of such experiments clearly show that only low levels of NK cell activity could be detected in spleens from 2- or 3-week-old donors. In contrast, mice older than 6 weeks of age consistently exhibited high NK cell activity [13, 40]. However, the low NK cell cytotoxicity observed in young mice could be boosted readily by interferon inducers and bacterial adjuvants injected 1–3 days before the *in vitro* tests (Figure 1).

The i.v. injection of metastatic allogeneic murine melanomas and fibrosarcomas and xenogeneic chemically induced rat adenocarcinomas into 3-week-old, but not 6- to 8-week-old, nude mice resulted in the formation of many lung tumor colonies (Table 1). Although all tumors grew s.c., only metastatic neoplasms formed pulmonary metastatic foci following i.v. inoculation. The successful metastasis of allogeneic and xenogeneic tumors in young nude mice correlated with the low levels of NK cells detected in the recipient mice. The *in vivo* activation of NK cells by the injection of interferon inducers shortly before tumor inoculation rendered the 3-week-old nude mice resistant to metastases development [13, 65]. Kinetic analysis of tumor cell arrest and survival indicated that the higher frequency of tumor metastases in the lungs of young nude mice is not due to increased initial tumor cell arrest in the capillary bed, but rather to increased survival of the arrested tumor cells during the first 24 hours after tumor cell injection [65].

Although i.v. injection of tumor cells bypasses the initial steps of detachment from the primary tumor and invasion of blood vessels, all subsequent barriers in the metastatic process must be overcome before metastases can be established [3, 4]. Moreover, extravasation of arrested tumor cells probably occurs by mechanisms similar to those that mediate invasion. A good correlation between the ability of

Table 1. Experimental pulmonary metastasis of murine tumor cells in syngeneic hosts and in 3- and 6-week-old nude mice.

Strain	Tumor	Cell dose	Recipients		
			6-week-old syngeneic mice	3-week-old nude mice	6-week-old nude mice
C3H	UV-2237 parent	10^5	25 (15–78)	68 (38–115)	0
	Clone 38	10^5	1 (0–6)	2 (0–14)	0
	Clone 46	10^5	5 (0–16)	96 (55–178)	1 (0–3)
	Clone 25	10^5	35 (17–92)	89 (42–141)	0 (0–2)
	UV-2237-M_1	10^5	145 (85–278)	238 (110–300)	0 (0–4)
	UV-2237-M_2	10^5	178 (110–300)	all >300	2 (0–6)
	UV-1591	5×10^5	0	0 (0–1)	0
	UV-1316	5×10^5	0	0	0
	K-1735 parent	10^5	55 (17–98)	165 (75–300)	0
	Clone 16	10^5	0 (0–2)	0 (0–7)	0
	Clone 13	10^5	0 (0–2)	27 (3–68)	0
	Clone 2	10^5	108 (81–210)	156 (65–233)	0
C57BL/6	B16-F1	5×10^4	6 (0–18)	28 (3–55)	0
	B16-F10	5×10^4	62 (21–95)	98 (35–300)	2 (0–4)
	B16-F10^{Lr}	5×10^4	2 (0–3)	11 (1–28)	0

tumor cells to produce metastases following i.v. (experimental) and s.c. (spontaneous) implantation has been reported for two murine tumor systems [68, 69]. These findings indicate that the development of experimental metastases following i.v. injection of tumor cells is a valid assay for the metastatic potential of malignant neoplasms.

The applicability and validity of using young nude mice for ascertaining the metastatic potential of tumor cells are supported by the fact that the metastatic patterns of allogeneic and xenogeneic rat tumors were strikingly similar when injected into syngeneic hosts and young nude mice. All metastatic neoplasms, irrespective of their antigenicity or sensitivity to killing by immune T lymphocytes or NK cells, produced lung tumor colonies in young nude mice, whereas non-metastatic tumors did not (Table 1). Moreover, the quantitative differences in ability to form experimental metastases among tumor cell lines and clones observed in syngeneic hosts were maintained in the young nude recipients. In experimental tumor systems, the inability of highly immunogenic tumors to metastasize in normal immunocompetent syngeneic hosts could be attributed either to their immunogenicity or to their inability to complete the metastatic process. The use of immunosuppressed syngeneic hosts or young nude mice allows investigators to distinguish between these possibilities.

Because of the close correlation between high levels of NK cells and resistance to experimental tumor metastasis, it is evident that the genetic and perhaps environmental factors that influence NK cell activity also affect the sensitivity of the nude mouse to metastasis development. Our recent findings demonstrate that nude mice with a BALB/c background exhibit lower NK cell activity and higher incidence of metastasis of allogeneic and xenogeneic human tumors than age-matched NIH/Swiss nude mice. Moreover, with a given strain of nude mice, the housing conditions influenced both NK cell activity and the incidence of tumor metastasis. Thus, nude mice raised under pathogen-free conditions in barrier or isolator facilities were always superior to age-matched littermates housed under conventional conditions in supporting metastatic growth. High interferon levels induced by viral infections with mouse hepatitis virus, for example, activate NK cells and thus render young nude mice highly resistant to metastasis formation. As discussed in chapter 3, C57BL/6 and C3H mice treated with Cy or β-estradiol exhibit low NK cell activity and a higher incidence of experimental metastases. Similarly, adult nude mice treated with Cy show a marked increase in the frequency of lung tumor colonies produced after i.v. injection of B16-F10 melanoma tumor cells. Nude mice treated with β-estradiol for a period of 8–10 weeks exhibit low NK cell activity and a high incidence of experimental metastases as compared to untreated age-matched controls. However, both treatments rendered nude mice susceptible to viral and bacterial infections that could be responsible for early death. This imposes a serious limitation for applying such procedures to long-term studies and perhaps requires that the mice be housed under gnotobiotic conditions. These findings imply, however, that successful metastasis in young 3-week-old nude mice is not unique, and experimental depletion of NK cells renders adult 8-to 12-week-old nude mice quite susceptible to metastasis formation. Such results support the belief that NK cells are indeed responsible to a great extent for the resistance of nude mice to tumor dissemination. Moreover, we have demonstrated that metastatic tumor cells selected *in vitro* for resistance to NK-cell-mediated killing metastasize readily in both 3- and 6-week-old nude mice [67]. The expression of significant NK cell activity at 4 to 5 weeks of age, accompanied by marked resistance to experimental tumor metastasis, renders the 3-week-old nude mouse inadequate for studying spontaneous metastasis of tumors growing at a s.c. site. By the time the implanted tumor reaches a critical size, the already highly active NK cells will destroy tumor cells released from the primary tumor into the circulation.

7. The use of young nude mice for isolation of highly metastatic tumor cells

Recent studies have provided ample evidence that malignant primary neoplasms are heterogeneous and contain subpopulations of cells that differ in immunogenicity, antigenicity, enzyme activity, radiosensitivity, drug susceptibility and metastatic potential [70, 71]. Since metastases originate from specialized subpopulations of cells that preexist within the primary tumor [2, 70, 71], methods were designed for the isolation and identification of tumor cells capable of invasion and metastasis. The possibility that cells with high metastatic potential can be isolated from a heterogeneous primary neoplasm by an *in vivo* selection procedure was first demonstrated by Koch [72], who isolated a highly metastatic cell line of Ehrlich carcinoma by serially transplanting lymph node metastases. By using similar approaches, several investigators have demonstrated that tumor cells isolated from metastatic lesions during successive passages *in vivo* exhibited greater metastatic potential than cells of the original parental tumor [73–76]. The isolation of tumor cell subpopulations with high metastatic potential has great clinical implications for the testing of potential antimetastatic agents. Differences in the response of primary and metastatic lesions to therapeutic agents is well documented in clinical practice [77–79]. Recently, it has been pointed out that most methods used to define drug sensitivity of experimental animal tumors are based on the belief that transplantable tumors are homogeneous and, therefore, these methods may produce misleading results. Assays that rely primarily on partial regression of the primary tumor may be inadequate for predicting the antimetastatic activity of therapeutic agents. Therefore, metastatic cell subpopulations selected from the primary neoplasms may prove beneficial for screening agents for the treatment of tumor metastases.

The successful metastasis of allogeneic and xenogeneic tumors in young nude mice offers a unique opportunity to use the nude mouse as a means to select and isolate highly metastatic tumor cells from heterogeneous xenogeneic neoplasms. Evidence supporting the validity of this *in vivo* model is provided by our recent observation that tumor cells isolated from lung nodules of young nude mice injected with allogeneic or xenogeneic rat tumors are highly metastatic when reinjected into either young nude recipients or the syngeneic hosts. By the same method, we were able to select from a human melanoma cell line (A-375) several cell subpopulations that following i.v. injection into young nude mice produced 20 to 50 times more lung colonies than the parent cell line. Tumor cells grown at a s.c. site maintain the metastatic phenotype of the injected cells. The selection for high metastatic potential was observed only when pulmonary metastatic foci were harvested. These results strongly indicate that the enhanced metastatic potential observed in tumor cells isolated from lung metastases is a result of a highly selective process and not a mere adaptation to growth in the nude mouse.

In summary, young nude mice may be useful for ascertaining the metastatic potential of surgically excised human primary neoplasms and for selecting metastatic tumor cell subpopulations. Pulmonary metastases (and not s.c. tumor growths) established from highly metastatic cell variants in nude mice could be used for assessing the antimetastatic activity of therapeutic agents.

References

1. Fidler IJ, Gersten DM, Hart IR: The biology of cancer invasion and metastasis. Adv Cancer Res 28:149–250, 1978.
2. Fidler IJ, Kripke ML: Metastasis results from preexisting variant cells within a malignant tumor. Science 197:893–895, 1977.
3. Sugarbaker EV, Ketcham AS: Mechanisms and prevention of cancer dissemination. An overview. Semin Oncol 4:19–32, 1977.
4. Weiss L: A pathobiologic overview of metastasis. Semin Oncol 4:5–17, 1977.
5. Fidler IJ, Gersten DM, Riggs C: Relationship of host immune status to tumor cell arrest, distribution and survival in experimental metastasis. Cancer 40:46–55, 1977.
6. Brown JM: A study of the mechanism by which anticoagulation with warfarin inhibits blood-borne metastases. Cancer Res 33:1217–1224, 1973.
7. Bomford R, Olivotto M: The mechanism of inhibition by *Corynebacterium parvum* of the growth of lung nodules from intravenously injected tumor cells. Int J Cancer 14:226–235, 1974.
8. Van Putten LM, Kram LK, Van Dierendonck HH, Smink T, Fuzy M: Enhancement by drugs of metastatic lung nodule formation after intravenous tumour cell injection. Int J Cancer 15:588-595, 1975.
9. Fidler IJ, Kripke ML: Tumor cell antigenicity, host immunity and cancer metastasis. Cancer Immunol Immunother 7:201–205, 1980.
10. Hanna N, Fidler IJ: The role of natural killer cells in the destruction of circulating tumor emboli. JNCI 65:801–809, 1980.
11. Poste G, Kirch R, Fogler WE, Fidler IJ: Activation of tumoricidal properties in mouse macrophages by lymphokines encapsulated in liposomes. Cancer Res 39:881–892, 1979.
12. Hart IR, Fidler IJ: Cancer invasion and metastases. Quart Rev Biol 55:121–142, 1980.
13. Hanna N, Fidler IJ: Expression of metastatic potential of allogeneic and xenogeneic neoplasms in young nude mice. Cancer Res 41:438–444, 1981.
14. Talmadge JE, Meyers KM, Prieur DJ, Starkey JR: Role of NK cells in tumor growth and metastasis in beige mice. Nature 284:622–624, 1980.
15. Kindred B: Nude mice in immunobiology. Prog Allergy 26:137–238, 1979.

16. Fogh J, Giovanella BC: The nude mouse in experimental and clinical research. New York: Academic Press, 1978.
17. Nomura T, Ohsawa N, Tamaoki N, Fujiwara K: Proceedings of the second international workshop on nude mice. Tokyo: University of Tokyo Press, 1977.
18. Rygaard J, Povlsen CO: Heterotransplantation of human malignant tumor to nude mice. Acta Pathol Microbiol Scand [A] 77:758–760, 1969.
19. Stiles CD, Desmond W, Chuman LM, Sato G, Saier MH, Jr: Relationship of cell growth behavior *in vitro* to tumorigenicity in athymic nude mice. Cancer Res 36:3300–3305, 1976.
20. Shin S, Freedman VH: Neoplastic growth of animal cells in nude mice. In: Proceedings of the second international workshop on nude mice, Nomura T, Ohsawa N, Tamaoki N, Fujiwara K (eds). Tokyo: University of Tokyo Press, 1977, pp 337–349.
21. Giovanella BC, Stehlin JS, Williams LJ, Jr: Heterotransplantation of human malignant tumors in 'nude' thymusless mice. II. Malignant tumors induced by injection of cell cultures derived from human solid tumors. J Natl Cancer Inst 52:921–927, 1974.
22. Povlsen CO, Rygaard J: Heterotransplantation of adenocarcinomas of the colon and rectum in the mouse mutant nude. A study of nine consecutive transplantations. Acta Pathol Microbiol Scand [A] 79:159–169, 1971.
23. Shimosato Y, Kameya T, Nagai K, Hirohaski S, Koide TM, Hayashi H, Nomura T: Transplantation of human tumors in nude mice. J Natl Cancer Inst 56:1251–1260, 1976.
24. Kuga N, Yoshida K, Seido T, Oboshi S, Koide T, Shimosato Y, Nomura T: Heterotransplantation of cultured human cancer cells and human cancer tissues into nude mice. Gann 66:547–560, 1975.
25. Outzen HC, Custer RP: Growth of human normal and neoplastic mammary tissues in the cleared mammary fat pad of the nude mouse. J Natl Cancer Inst 55:1461–1463, 1975.
26. Reid LC, Shin SI: Transplantation of heterologous endocrine tumor cells in nude mice. In: The nude mouse in experimental and clinical research, Fogh J, Giovanella B (eds). New York: Academic Press, 1978, pp 313–351.
27. Epstein AL, Herman MM, Kim H, Dorfman RF, Kaplan HS: Biology of the human malignant lymphomas III. Intracranial heterotransplantation in the nude, athymic mouse. Cancer 37:2158–2176, 1976.
28. Sebesteny A, Taylor-Papadimitriu J, Ceriani R, Millis R, Schmitt C, Trevan D: Primary human breast carcinomas transplantable in the nude mouse. JNCI 63:1331–1333, 1979.
29. Rae-Venter B, Reid LM: Growth of human breast carcinomas in nude mice and subsequent establishment in tissue culture. Cancer Res 40:95–100, 1980.
30. Sordat B, Merenda C, Carrel S: Invasive growth and dissemination of human solid tumors and malignant cell lines grafted subcutaneously to newborn nude mice. In: Proceedings of the second international workshop on nude mice, Nomura T, Ohsawa N, Tamaoki N, Fujiwara K (eds). Tokyo: University of Tokyo Press, 1977, pp 313–326.
31. Povlsen CO: Heterotransplantation of human malignant melanomas to the mouse mutant nude. Acta Pathol Microbiol Scand [A] 84:9–14, 1976.
32. Fogh J, Fogh JM, Orfeo T: One hundred and twenty-seven cultured human tumor cell lines producing tumors in nude mice. J Natl Cancer Inst 59:221–226, 1977.
33. Sharkey FE, Fogh J: Metastasis of human tumors in athymic nude mice. Int J Cancer 24:733–738, 1979.
34. Kameya T, Shimosato Y, Tumuraya M, Ohsawa N, Nomura T: Human gastric choriocarcinoma serially transplanted in nude mice. J Natl Cancer Inst 56:325–329, 1976.
35. Kyriazis A, DiPersio L, Michael JG, Pesce AJ: Influence of the mouse hepatitis virus (NHV) infection on the growth of human tumors in the athymic mouse. Int J Cancer 23:402–409, 1979.
36. Manning JK, Reed ND, Jutila JW: Antibody response to *Escherichia coli* lipopolysaccharide and type III pneumococcal polysacchaaride by congenitally thymusless (nude) mice. J Immunol 108: 1470, 1972.
37. Martin WJ, Martin SE: Naturally occurring cytotoxic anti-tumor antibodies in sera of congenitally

athymic (nude) mice. Nature 249:564–565, 1974.

38. Meltzer MS: Tumoricidal responses *in vitro* of peritoneal macrophages from conventionally housed and germ-free nude mice. Cell Immunol 22:176–181, 1976.
39. Johnson WJ, Balish E: Macrophage function in germ-free, athymic (nu/nu), and conventional-flora (nu/+) mice. J Reticuloendothel Soc 28:55–66, 1980.
40. Herberman RB, Ninn ME, Laurin DH: Natural cytotoxic reactivity of mouse lymphoid cells against syngeneic and allogeneic tumors. I. Distribution of reactivity and specificity. Int J Cancer 16: 216–229, 1975.
41. Gershwin ME, Ikeda RM, Erickson K, Owens R: Enhancement of heterotransplanted human tumor graft survival in nude mice treated with antilymphocytic serum and in congenitally athymic-asplenic (lasat) mice. JNCI 63:295–298, 1980.
42. Lozzio BB, Machodo EA, Lair SV, Lozzio CB: Reproducible metastatic growth of K-562 human myelogenous leukemia cells in nude mice. JNCI 63:295–298, 1980.
43. Ohsugi Y, Gershwin ME, Ownes RB, Nelson-Rees WA: Tumorigenicity of human malignant lymphoblasts: comparative study with unmanipulated nude mice, antilymphocyte serum-treated nude mice, and x-irradiated nude mice. JNCI 65:715–718, 1980.
44. Watanabe S, Shimosato Y, Juroki M, Sato Y, Nakajima T: Transplantability of human lymphoid cell line, lymphoma, and leukemia in splenectomized and/or irradiated nude mice. Cancer Res 40:2588–2595, 1980.
45. Bonmassar E, Campanile F, Houchens D, Crino L, Goldin A: Impaired growth of a radiation-induced lymphoma in intact or lethally irradiated allogeneic athymic (nude) mice. Transplantation 20:343–346, 1975.
46. Minato N, Bloom BR, Jones C, Holland J, Reid LM: Mechanism of rejection of virus persistently infected tumor cells by athymic nude mice. J Exp Med 149:1117–1133, 1979.
47. Warner NL, Woodruff MFA, Burton RC: Inhibition of the growth of lymphoid tumors in syngeneic athymic (nude) mice. Int J Cancer 20:146–155, 1977.
48. Gershwin ME, Ikeda RM, Kawakami TG, Ownes RB: Immunobiology of heterotransplanted human tumors in nude mice. J Natl Cancer Inst 58:1455–1461, 1977.
49. Povlsen CI, Fialkow PJ, Klein E, Klein G, Rygaard J, Wiener F: Growth and antigenic properties of a biopsy-derived Burkitt's lymphoma in thymusless (nude) mice. Int J Cancer 11:30–39, 1973.
50. Giovanella BC, Yim SO, Morgan AC, Stehlin JS, Williams LJ: Metastases of human melanomas transplanted in 'nude' mice. J Natl Cancer Inst 50:1051–1053, 1973.
51. Giovanella BC, Yim SO, Stehlin JS et al.: Development of invasive tumors in the 'nude' mouse after injection of cultured human melanoma cells. J Natl Cancer Inst 18:1531–1533, 1972.
52. Zamecnik PC, Long JC: Growth of cultured cells from patients with Hodgkin's disease and transplantation into nude mice. Proc Natl Acad Sci USA 74:754–758, 1977.
53. Hata J, Ueyama Y, Tamaoki N, Furukawa T, Morita K: Human neuroblastoma serially transplanted in nude mice and metastases. Cancer 42:468–473, 1978.
54. Maguire H, Outzen HC, Custer P, Prehn RT: Invasion and metastasis of xenogeneic tumor in nude mice. J Natl Cancer Inst 57:439–442, 1976.
55. Wiltrout RH, Frost P, Morrison MK, Kerbel RS: Immune-mediated arrest and reversal of established visceral metastases in athymic mice. Cancer Res 39:4034–4041, 1979.
56. Kyriazis AP, DiPersio L, Michael GJ, Pesce AJ, Stinnett JD: Growth patterns and metastatic behavior of human tumors growing in athymic mice. Cancer Res 38:3186–3190, 1978.
57. Takahashi S, Konishi Y, Nakatani K, Inui S, Kojima K, Shiratori T: Conversion of a poorly differentiated human adenocarcinoma to ascites form with invasion and metastasis in nude mice: brief communication. J Natl Cancer Inst 60:925–929, 1978.
58. Prehn RT, Lappe M: An immunostimulation theory of tumor development. Transplant Rev 7:26–51, 1971.
59. Fidler IJ, Caines S, Dolan Z: Survival of hematogenously disseminated allogeneic tumor cells in athymic nude mice. Transplantation 22:208–212, 1976.

60. Skov CB, Holland JM, Perkins EH: Development of fewer tumor colonies in lungs of athymic nude mice after intravenous injection of tumor cells. J Natl Cancer Inst 56:193–195, 1976.
61. Lozzio BB, Lozzio CB, Machado EA: Human myelogenous (Ph^1 +) leukemia cell line: transplantation into athymic mice. J Natl Cancer Inst 56:627–629, 1978.
62. Fidler IJ: General considerations for studies of experimental cancer metastasis. In: Methods in cancer research, Bush H (ed). New York: Academic Press, 1978, pp 399–439.
63. Liotta LA, Kleinerman J, Saidel GM: Quantitative relationships of intravascular tumor cells, tumor vessels and pulmonary metastases following tumor implantation. Cancer Res 34:997–1004, 1974.
64. Fidler IJ: The relationship of embolic homogeneity, number, size and viability to the incidence of experimental metastasis. Eur J Cancer 9:223–227, 1973.
65. Hanna N: Expression of metastatic potential of tumor cells in young nude mice is correlated with low levels of natural killer cell-mediated cytotoxicity. Int J Cancer 26:675–680, 1980.
66. Riccardi C, Puccetti P, Santoni A, Herberman RB: Rapid *in vivo* assay of mouse natural killer cell activity. JNCI 63:1041–1045, 1979.
67. Hanna N, Fidler IJ: Relationship between metastatic potential and resistance to NK cell-mediated cytotoxicity in three murine tumor systems. JNCI 66:1183–1190, 1981.
68. Kripke ML, Gruys E, Fidler IJ: Metastatic heterogeneity of cells from an ultraviolet light-induced murine fibrosarcoma of recent origin. Cancer Res 38:2962–2967, 1978.
69. Wang BS, McLoughlin GA, Richie JP, Mannick JA: Correlation of the production of plasminogen activator with tumor metastasis in B16 melanoma cell lines. Cancer Res 40:288–292, 1980.
70. Poste G, Fidler IJ: The pathogenesis of cancer metastasis. Nature 283:139–146, 1980.
71. Fidler IJ: Tumor heterogeneity and the biology of cancer invasion and metastasis. Cancer Res 38:2651–2660, 1978.
72. Koch FE: Zur Frage der Metastasenbildung bei Impftumoren. Z Krebsforsch 48:495, 1939.
73. Fidler IJ: Selection of successive tumor lines for metastasis. Nature 242:148–149, 1973.
74. Suzuki N, Withers HR, Koehler MW: Heterogeneity and variability of artificial lung colony-forming ability among clones from mouse fibrosarcoma. J Natl Cancer Inst 60:179–183, 1978.
75. Brunson KW, Nicolson GL: Selection and biologic properties of malignant variants of a murine lymphosarcoma. JNCI 61:1499-1503, 1978.
76. Fogel M, Gorelik E, Segal S, Feldman M: Differences in cell surface antigens of tumor metastases and those of the local tumor. JNCI 62:585–588, 1979.
77. Fugmann RA, Anderson JC, Stolfi RL, Martin DS: Comparison of adjuvant chemotherapeutic activity against primary and metastatic spontaneous murine tumors. Cancer Res 37:496–500, 1977.
78. Schabel FM, Jr: Concepts for systemic treatment of micrometastases. Cancer 35:15–24, 1975.
79. Trope C: Different sensitivity to cytostatic drugs of primary tumor and metastasis of the Lewis carcinoma. Neoplasma 22:171–180, 1975.

5. Cell surface properties of metastatic tumor cells

G.L. NICOLSON

1. Surface properties of metastatic tumor cells

Since the interaction of tumor cells with their environment is mediated by cell surface constituents, this structure is thought to play one of the most important roles in metastasis. Modifications in cell surface properties have been described in detail and compared in particular, between transformed cells and their untransformed counterparts. In these systems modifications at the cell surface have generally correlated with neoplastic transformation (see reviews by Hynes [1], Nicolson [2] and Roblin et al. [3]); however, few of these changes are probably relevant to metastasis [2, 4]. Using the animal model systems described elsewhere in this volume (Chapter 1), it has been possible to examine in detail cell surface properties and their potential involvement in metastasis.

1.1. Cell surface involvement in metastasis

Two major lines of evidence have been used to demonstrate the involvement of cell surface membranes in certain aspects of metastasis, particularly blood-borne implantation. The first is that enzymatic modification of cell surface components modifies malignant cell arrest in the microcirculation without modifying cell viability. Hagmar and Norrby [5] utilized trypsin and trypsin-EDTA treatment to modify the cell surface properties of B16 melanoma cells and found that these treatments could change the degree and location of experimental metastasis. Using lymphosarcoma and Walker carcinoma cells Sinha and Goldenberg [6] noted that neuraminidase treatment shifted experimental metastatic colonization from lung to liver. Fidler [7] also used trypsin to modify the surfaces of B16 melanoma cells. At various times during the treatment cells were washed, checked for viability and injected i.v. into syngeneic mice. Without affecting cell vaibility or plating efficiency *in vitro* prolonged trypsin treatment dramatically and significantly reduced the average number of pulmonary tumor colonies [7].

The second line of evidence for the involvement of cell surfaces in metastasis comes from the transfer of portions of the plasma membrane from highly metastatic B16 melanoma cells to B16 cells of low metastatic potential [8]. To transfer cell membrane components we took advantage of the fact that B16 melanoma cells shed

L.A. Liotta and I.R. Hart (eds.), Tumor Invasion and Metastasis. ISBN-13: 978-94-009-7513-2.
© 1982 Martinus Nijhoff Publishers, The Hague/Boston/London.

spontaneously closed plasma membrane vesicle *in vivo* as well as *in vitro*. These vesicles can be harvested, purified and subsequently fused with plasma membranes of homologous or heterologous cells to introduce plasma membrane components into the surface membranes of other cells. When vesicles from the high metastatic subline B16-F10 were fused into the cell surface of the low metastatic subline B16-F1, the ability of the F10 vesicle-modified B16-F1 cells to localize in lung and form experimental metastases was increased significantly. An important control for this experiment was to prove that the transferred components were actually integrated into plasma membranes of the recipient cells. In order to demonstrate this a B16 subline resistant to T-cell-mediated cytotoxicity was rendered sensitive by fusion of plasma membranes obtained from T-cell-sensitive B16 sublines. In this case the vesicle-modified B16 cells were sensitive to the cytotoxic action of T-cells, but the vesicle-induced changes were transient and correlated with the natural turnover of cell membrane components [8].

1.2. Cell surface biophysical parameters and metastasis

Biophysical parameters of the cell surface such as surface charge density have been proposed as determinants of metastastic properties. Earlier studies employing cell electrophoresis indicated that tumor cells have a higher net negative charge compared to their normal cell counterparts [9] and in turn cells of higher metastatic potential have higher net negative charge compared to cells of low metastatic potential [10]. However, after a careful analysis of the data correlating net negative surface charge with malignancy or relative metastatic potential in different tumor systems, Weiss [11] concluded that there was no obvious relationship between surface charge and malignancy.

Cell surface biophysical properties have been utilized to separate malignant cell subpopulations from heterogeneous parental tumor cell lines. Grdina et al. [12] found that low density fibrosarcoma cells could be separated on linear density gradients of Reografin-60, and these low density cells were more metastatic in experimental lung colonization assays compared to high density cells from the same tumor. Similarly, Baniyash et al. [13] showed that cells from the low metastatic B16-F1 subline had a higher mean density profile in colloidal silica isopyknic density gradients compared to the more metastatic subline B16-F10. Using the original, unselected B16 tumor, these authors demonstrated broad distribution profiles indicative of cell density heterogeneity. When B16 cells from various densities were injected into mice, the lower density cells formed more experimental lung metastases. Miner et al. [14] utilized both cell surface charge and hydrophobic partitioning characteristics to separate subpopulations of RAW117 lymphosarcoma cells by countercurrent distribution in a dextran-poly(ethylene glycol) phase system having an electrostatic potential difference between the phases. Both low and high metastatic RAW117 sublines were heterogeneous with respect to cell surface properties as shown by their broad countercurrent distribution curves, but the mean partition coefficient of the highly metastatic RAW117-H10 subline was always greater than that of the low metastatic parental line (Figure 1). An examination of metastatic potentials of parental lymphosarcoma cells obtained from different parts of the countercurrent extraction train confirmed that the highly metastatic subpopulations resided at positions of higher mean partitioning. In this case cells obtained from countercurrent distribution cavities to the right (higher partitioning) were always more malignant and colonized liver with greater efficiencies (Figure 1) [14].

1.3. Cell surface proteins and glycoproteins on metastatic cells

Differences between cell surface glycoproteins on sublines of low or high metastatic potential have been detected by the use of lectins [for a discussion on lectins see ref. 15]. Quantitative lectin binding to B16 melanoma sublines of differing metastatic potential has shown that some low metastatic sublines bind less ^{125}I-concanavalin A (such as the lymphocyte-resistant subline B16-F10^{Lr-6}), while the highly metastastic subline B16-F10 was found to have fewer wheat germ agglutinin- and soy bean agglutinin-binding sites [16]. Alternatively, quantitative labeling with ^{125}I-*Ricinus communis* agglutinin failed to show a numerical difference in receptors for this lectin on various B16 melanoma sublines [4] unless the cells were first treated with neuraminidase [17]. Differences in the binding of ^{125}I-labeled lectins have also been documented in the RAW117 metastatic system. The most dramatic difference found was the sequential loss of concanavalin A receptors with increasing malignancy and metastatic potential [18]. Reading et al. [19] have examined a number of cell lines and clones selected *in vivo* for enhanced metastasis or *in vitro* for loss of adherence to immobilized-lectins for any relationship between malignancy and lectin binding in the RAW117 system.In almost every cell line and clone examined there was a correlation between the loss of concanavalin A-binding sites and metastatic potential, while there was no correlation between the number of wheat germ agglutinin-binding sites and malignancy. Similarly, Tao and Burger [20] selected subline of B16 melanoma for their resistance to wheat germ agglutinin cytotoxicity, and this same group [21] found that a wheat germ agglutinin-resistant clone of a B16 subline had alterations in the major wheat germ agglutinin-binding cell surface glycoproteins. Using cell clones obtained from an hepatocarcinoma cell line, Talmadge et al. [22] found that metastatic potential correlated with the number of concanavalin A-binding sites but did not correlate with a number of other *in vitro* parameters such as cell growth rates, saturation densities, cell shedding and adhesion characteristics, plasminogen activator production and pro-coagulant activities.

The lectin-binding components involved in metastatic cell interactions have in some cases been analyzed by the binding of radioactive lectins to the solubilized, separated cellular glycoproteins on SDS-polyacrylamide slab gels. Although differ-

RAW117-P Cavity No.	RAW117-P Liver Tumor Colonies Formed (5×10^3 Cells i.v.)
Load	0,0,0,0,0,0,0,10,12,200
0-3	0,0,0,0,0,0,0,0,0,50
8-11	0,0,0,0,0,0,0,0,200,200
24-27	0,0,0,0,0,0,0,0,100,200
32-35	0,0,0,0,0,0,0,50,200,200
40-43	0,0,0,0,0,50,100,200,200,200
44-47	30,200,200,200,200,200,200,200,200,200,200
48-51	0,0,0,0,0,0,0,200,200

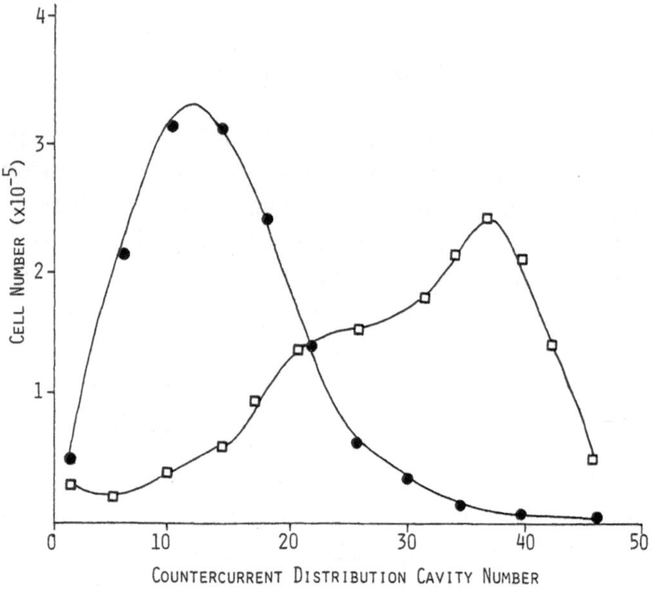

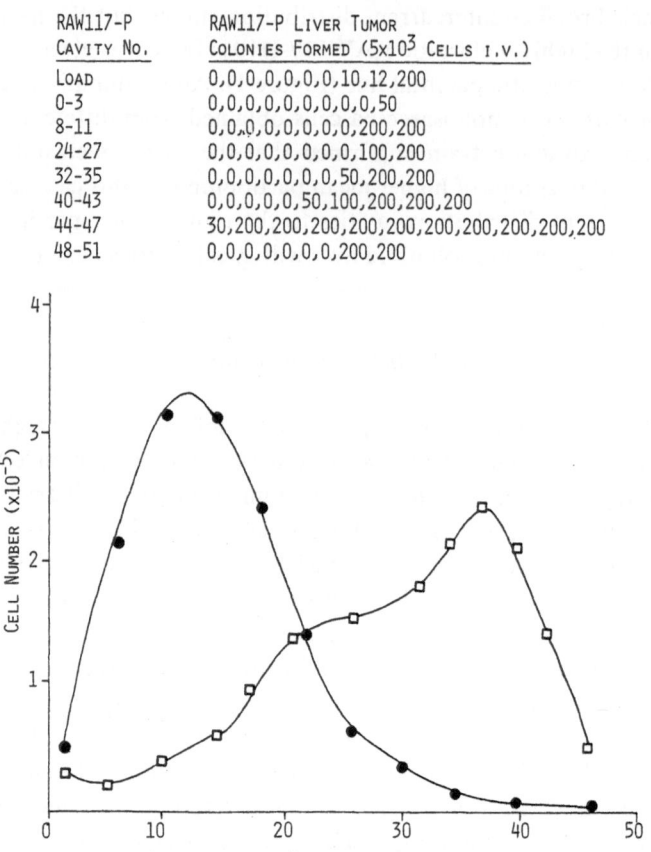

Figure 1. Subfractionation of RAW117 lymphosarcoma cells of varying metastatic potentials by countercurrent distribution in a dextran-poly(ethylene glycol) aqueous phase system. Fifty transfers were carried out at 4° C, and data presented as the number of cells found in different cavities along the extraction train as described by Miner et al. [14]. Cells were pooled (four cavity fractions each), washed and injected (5×10^3 viable cells) intravenously into BALB/c mice. Experimental liver metastases were determined after 23 days.

ences are often not found using this technique [e.g., see refs. 4, 16] lectin-binding glycoprotein alterations have been found which sometimes correlate well with the potential to metastasize. Irimura et al. [17] used ^{125}I-labeled *Ricinus communis* agglutinin to detect differences on tunicamycin-treated B16 melanoma sublines. Tunicamycin treatment inhibited experimental metastasis and resulted in loss of high molecular weight sialogalactoproteins. The reappearance of these sialogalactoproteins correlated with the reappearance of metastatic properties after drug removal [17]. Finne et al. [21] utilized ^{125}I-labeled wheat germ agglutinin to detect modifications in wheat germ agglutinin-selected low metastatic sublines and found that the lectin-resistant sublines had lost malignancy and wheat germ agglutinin-binding sites.

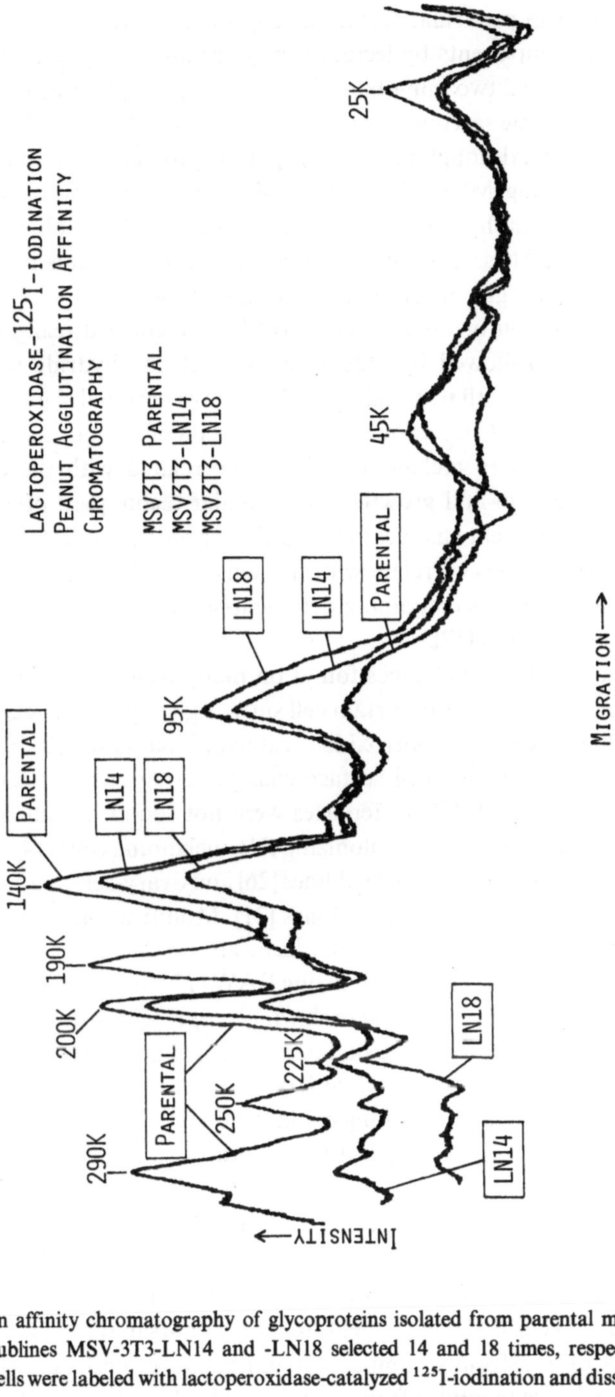

Figure 2. Lectin affinity chromatography of glycoproteins isolated from parental murine MSV-3T3 sarcoma and sublines MSV-3T3-LN14 and -LN18 selected 14 and 18 times, respectively, for lung colonization. Cells were labeled with lactoperoxidase-catalyzed ^{125}I-iodination and dissolved in Trixton X-100. The detergent extracts were applied to a peanut agglutinin affinity column, and the column was eluted with 100 mM D-galactose. The eluates were then electrophoresed, and autoradiograms were prepared and scanned with a densitometer to identify labeled proteins as described [24].

Modifications in particular surface glycoproteins have been detected after isolation of these components by lectin affinity chromatography [23]. For example, Nicolson [24] utilized two immobilized galactose-specific lectins to isolate galactoproteins from murine sarcoma virus-transformed fibroblastic sublines selected for lung colonization. Although most of the galactoproteins were similar on low and high lung colonizing MSV-3T3 sublines, distinct changes were seen after lectin affinity chromatography and SDS-polyacrylamide gel electrophoresis autoradiography (Figure 2). These data indicate the usefulness of lectins in identifying and isolating cell surface glycoproteins on metastatic tumor cells.

Galactoproteins on metastatic cells have been identified using oxidation with galactose oxidase followed by reduction with ^{3}H-borohydride with or without pretreatment of cells with neuraminidase to remove terminal sialic acid. Using this procedure Raz et al. [16] have found that expression of a major sialogalactoprotein on lung-colonizing B16 melanoma sublines correlated with the degree of lung implantation, survival and growth. Using similar techniques, other workers [25] have also found different changes in sialogalactoproteins on B16 melanoma glycoproteins. These findings correlate with those using ^{125}I-labeled galactose-specific lectins to stain SDS gels containing detergent-solubilized, neuraminidase-treated B16 melanoma sublines [17].

One of the generalized changes found on many transformed compared to untransformed cells is the loss of certain cell surface glycoproteins identifiable by cell surface labeling utilizing lactoperoxidase-catalyzed iodination [1–3]. Not all metastatic systems show distinct cell surface changes using lactoperoxidase-catalyzed iodination techniques. While differences were not found in iodinatable proteins exposed on the surfaces of lung-colonizing B16 melanoma cells [14, 16], differences have been found on brain-selected sublines [26] and ovary-selected sublines [27] and on wheat germ agglutinin-resistant clones [21]. Modifications in lactoperoxidase-catalyzed iodinatable surface proteins have also been seen in other metastatic systems. Highly metastatic liver-colonizing RAW117 lymphosarcoma sublines progressively lost exposure of a 70 000 mol. wt. glycoprotein with *in vivo* selection for enhanced liver colonization, while simultaneously gaining exposure in a component of 135 000 mol. wt. [18, 19]. Alterations have also been noted on virus-transformed 3T3 cell sublines of high and low lung colonization potential [24, 28] and mammary adenocarcinoma clones differing in their abilitk to spontaneously metastasize to lymph nodes and lungs [29].

Cell surface glycopeptide fragments removed from tumor cells by trypsinization and rendered free of oligopeptides by pronase treatment have been studied on metastatic tumor cells. These experiments originate from studies on untransformed and transformed cell surface glycopeptides (see reviews in refs. [30, 31]. The results from a variety of transformed compared to untransformed cell systems indicate that trypsin-released glycopeptides from transformed cells (of approx. 4 000 mol. wt.) are of higher apparent molecular weight when chromatographed on Sephadex G-50 columns. Possible alterations of cell surface peptides and their relationship to the malignant proces was assessed by metabolically labeling B16 lines of low and high metastatic potential with ^{14}C- and ^{3}H-sugars, respectively. Mild trypsinization removed cell surface glycopeptides which were further digested by pronase and examined as described above [137]. Co-chromatography of peptides from low and high lung-colonizing sublines of B16 melanoma revealed few if any differences [4, 32].

One of the more interesting cell surface changes after transformation is the loss or decrease in exposure of cell surface fibronectin [1–3]. It has been proposed [33, 34] that cell surface expression of fibronectin, a glycoprotein involved in adhesion [35] which is found on many types of connective and epithelial cells [36, 37], correlates with malignancy. Smith et al. [38] examined several human tumor-derived cell lines for the presence of fibronectin and found this glycoprotein expressed on cell lines obtained from primary mammary carcinomas but not on cell lines from metastatic carcinomas. On the other hand, Neri et al. [39] did not find a good correlation between fibronectin expression *in vivo* or *in vitro* and the potential of rat mammary adenocarcinoma cell lines and clones to metastasize spontaneously from mammary sites to lung. Although the cell lines obtained from secondary sites generally expressed less fibronectin compared to cell lines from primary sites, there was no absolute relationship between loss of fibronectin and ability to metastasize [39].

1.4. Glycolipids on metastatic cells

Modifications in the chemical composition of membrane glycolipids have been found in various transformed cells when compared to their untransformed counterparts. The most common changes found are simplification of the glycosphingolipid patterns [40, 41]. However, these changes are not always found on transformed or tumor cells.

The glycolipids of various metastatic sublines have been examined by cell extraction and thin layer chromatography. In the case of the B16 melanoma system, which has a relatively low content of glycolipids compared to transformed fibroblastic cell lines, a very simple ganglioside pattern was found. The most prominent components were the sialoganglioside G_{M1} [Cer-Glc-Gal-(NANA)] found in large amounts in all B16 melanoma cells along with minor amounts of G_{M2} [Cer-Glc-Gal-(NANA)-GalNAc] and G_{M1} [Cer-Glc-Gal-(NANA)-GalNAc-Gal]. The most distinctive change in glycolipid pattern found in selected B16 cells was an increase in G_{M3} and a reduction in the ganglioside GD_{1a} [Cer-Glc-Gal-(NANA)-Gal-NAc-Gal-(NANA)] in lung-colonizing sublines of high metastatic potential [4, 16, 25]. Yogeeswaran and Stein [42] have examined the glycosphingolipids on several metastatic variant sublines of virus-transformed 3T3 lines. They found differences between various sublines depending on cell growth characteristics, state of transformation, type of transforming virus and metastatic potential. In the latter case only the enhanced external labeling of G_{M2} by glactose oxidase-$NaB^{3}H_{4}$ correlated with lung metastasis potential [42].

1.5. Enzymatic properties of metastatic cells

Enzymatic analysis of malignant animal and human tumor tissues has revealed higher levels of degradative enzymes compared to surrounding normal tissues or benign lesion [43–46]. It has been proposed that these enzymes, mainly proteases, degrade tissue extracellular matrix and aid in the infiltration of host tissue stroma by malignant cells (see chapters by Liotta, Wooley, Kuettner). However, the release of degradative enzymes does not always correlate with local invasion [47–49].

One of the more dramatic changes occuring after neoplastic transformation is an increase in released and cell surface-bound degradative enzymes. For example, the production of high levels of proteolytic enzymes is thought to be an important property of transformed cells [50–52]. When tumor tissue has been homogenized and assayed, the homogenates generally contain higher levels of protease activities compared to normal tissues [45, 46, 53, 54]. In studies where tumor tissue was compared to surrounding host tissue it is difficult to distinguish between tumor-associated enzymatic activities and host cell enzymes released from immunocytes, inflammatory cells or even endothelial cells within the tumor. High levels of neutral protease, aminopeptidase, and collagenase activities have been found at the peripheries of invasive tumors and in the fluid from tumor necrotic regions [46, 54–59], although there are exceptions to these reports [47, 48].

The proteolytic enzymes associated with neoplastic cells are present in both secreted and cell surface-bound forms which could be important in tissue invasion. Their cell surface location was shown by Tökés et al. [60] using protease substrates covalently attached to latex beads. By allowing the bead-immobilized substrates to make contact with cells or be in close proximity to the cells but not make contact, cell surface-associated and secreted proteases could be measured, and these were both found to be higher in the neoplastic cells. There have been few studies on the proteases associated with invasive or metastatic cell systems. Bosmann et al. [61] studied the proteolytic enzymes of B16 melanoma sublines of low and high lung-colonizing potential and found higher levels of trypsin-like enzymes in the more metastatic B16 sublines, but only when the cells were replated at low cell densities in culture. Using the same system Liotta et al. [62] found that the more metastatic B16 sublines produce higher levels of collagenase active against type IV collagen of basement membranes.

One of the groups of enzymes which has attracted wide attention due to its possible role in tissue matrix destruction and tumor invasion is the collagenases. Dresden et al. [45] examined a variety of human neoplasms for their abilities to produce collagenases and found that most tumors produce high levels of collagenase activities while some did not, and normal tissues rarely produced the enzyme. Collagenolytic activities in squamous cell carcinoma [46] and malignant melanoma [54] were dramatically higher in concentration in tumor regions compared to surrounding normal tissue. When Strauch [43] examined benign and malignant tumors for collagenases, he found that the malignant tumors possessed high levels of these enzymes, and the enzymatic activities in tissue slices recovered from invasive tumor regions were higher than non-invasive regions or surrounding normal tissues. However, as mentioned above, these experiments could be criticized on the grounds that infiltrating host immunocytes, endothelial cells, etc. as well as degenerating tumor cells may contribute significant amounts of the detected activities [63]. High collagenase activities have been found in cell cultures of highly metastatic tumor cells [62, 64], and these activities correlate with metastatic potential [62]. Liotta et al. [65] have partially purified a collagenase from the media of cultured metastatic PMT sarcoma cells, and they have found that this metaloenzyme requires proteolytic cleavage for activation, is very active against type IV collagen substrates, but fails to significantly degrade other collagens or glycoproteins such as fibronectin.

Transformed cells are known to release a serine protease called plasminogen activator which converts serum plasminogen to plasmin [66–68]. Plasminogen activator secretion by transformed cells is generally higher than corresponding untransformed or normal cells [62, 68–71]. Production of plasminogen activator does not always correlate with neoplastic transformation [70, 72, 74] and is not restricted to transformed cell lines; many normal tissue are known to be high in plasminogen activator levels [70, 73]. The possible role of plasminogen activator in tumor spread and metastasis is uncertain, and in some studies there was no difference in plasminogen activator production between low and high metastatic sublines [75], although recent reports indicate highly metastatic cells release higher levels of plasminogen activator [76, 77]. Talmadge et al. [22] found no obvious relationship between plasminogen activator production and metastatic potential in rat hepatocarcinoma sublines of different metastatic potential. The relationship between plasminogen activator production and invasion is unclear, in part because the formation and dissolution of a fibrin deposit around tumor cells, for example after blood-borne arrest, may either enhance or inhibit malignant cell survival at a secondary site or its ability to undergo secondary invasion.

A variety of oligosaccharide degrading enzymes or glycosidases have been found in transformed and malignant cells. Bosmann and Hall [53] found higher levels of β-galactosidase, a-mannosidase and neuraminidase in malignant breast and colon tissue homogenates compared to surrounding normal tissue. Although they were not able to rule out filtrating normal host leukocytes and histiocytes, their results are thought to represent tumor cell release of stromal degrading enzymes. Bosmann et al. [61] found that a high metastatic B16 subline produced significantly glycosidases such as β-galactosidase, α-fucosidase, N-acetyl-β-galactosaminidase and N-acetyl- β-glucosaminidase, although these differences were only found at low cell densities *in vitro*.

Another class of oligosaccharide-modifying enzymes found at normal and tumor cell surfaces are the glycosyltransferases. Human breast colonic tumor tissue homogenates were found have higher sialyltransferase activities toward endogenous and exogenous glycoproteins compared to homogenates to of non-malignant tissue [53], although in other systems such as untransformed transformed cells *in vitro* the neoplastic cell sialytransferases show reduced activities [78]. Chatterjee and Kin [79, 80] have found a relationship between glycosyltransferases and metastasis in spontaneously metastasizing rat mammary carcinomas. Sialyltransferase [79] was low, while galactosyltransferase [79, 80] and fucosyltransferase [81] activities were higher in metastasizing tumor homogenates. When the serum from tumor-bearing animals was analyzed for glycosyltransferase activites, the rats with highly metastatic subcutaneously (s.c.) growing tumors had significantly increased serum levels of sialyl- and galactosyltransferases [80]. Cappel et al. [82] have used the serum levels of galactosyltransferase as a marker for metastatic disease in mice bearing Lewis lung carcinoma metastases and have found that tumor burden after chemotherapy correlates with serum enzyme levels.

More recent techniques in studying the enzymes associated with invasion and metastasis have utilized physiologically relevant substrates such as basement membrane [83, 84] or extracellular matrix produced by smooth muscle [85] or endothelial [86, 87] cells. Liotta et al. [83] found that metastatic murine T241 cells collected from venous drainage were able to solubilize basement membrane components and a collagen substrate at faster rates than tumor cells isolated from primary growth sites, and Jones and DeClerk [85] noted that human HT1080 fibrosarcoma cells express elastinolytic, collagenolytic and fibrinolytic (plasminogen activator-mediated) activities which solubilized smooth muscle basal lamina. Using metabolically-labelled endothelial cell basal lamina Kramer et al. [88] found that metastatic B16 melanoma cells solubilize matrix fibronectin in a serum plasmin-independent process and release sulfated glycosaminoglycans, particularly a unique heparin sulfate-containing glycosylaminoglycan of about one-third the size of the glycosylaminoglycans released during normal endothelial cel basal lamina turnover.

1.6. Adhesive properties of metastatic cells

The adhesion characteristics of malignant cells are thought to be relevant to their state of aggregation and distribution *in vivo*. Although little is known concerning the actual surface structures involved in cell adhesion, Oppenheimer [89, 90] has shown that cell adhesion requires the utilization of saccharide precursors which are synthesized into cell surface complex carbohydrates, and Chipowsky et al. [91] have found that cell adhesion is mediated via cell surface carbohydrates. This was shown by the binding of cells to various sugars covalently linked to Sephadex beads [91] or to sugar-derivatized gels [92, 93].

The role of adhesion in determining metastatic properties of malignant cells was studied by Coman [94] who proposed, on the basis of his experiments on the mechanical forces required to detach or separate malignant and normal cells, that malignant cells are less self (homotypic)-adhesive than their normal counterparts. Many investigators have felt that malignant cells should have reduced homotypic adhesive properties to aid in the release of cells from the primary tumor site. However, most experiments designed to test this hypothesis have utilized assays which measure cell attachment as opposed to cell detachment. For example, Criborn et al. [95] used an aspiration technique to remove tumor biopsies and found that aspirates from carcinomas contained more free cells than similar aspirates from benign epithelial tumors. Using assays for measuring homotypic and heterotypic adhesive attachment of untransformed and transformed cells Dorsey and Roth [96] and Wright et al. [97] found that transformed cells have higher adhesive attachment rates to a variety of homotypic or heterotypic cell substrates. However, these properties were not always found with transformed, tumorigenic cell lines. Some of these experiments must be criticized on the grounds that trypsin was used to harvest cells, a procedure which could result in cell surface proteolytic modification [98]. In studies where the homotypic rates of adhesion have been measured *in vitro* using tumor cells of varying metastatic potentials, the more metastatic cells were always found to have higher rates of homotypic attachment [75, 99–101]. In fact, it is well known that cell adhesion leading to multi-cell aggregates allows much better implantation in the microcirculation [102, 103].

Cell detachment from the primary site is of obvious importance in metastasis. Weiss [104] has stressed the concept that cell detachment is a different phenomena from cell attachment. Coman [94, 105] labeled these two properties 'adhesiveness' and 'stickiness' to differentiate between detachment of tumor cells from each other and attachment of tumor cells to different cells and tissues. The latter was expected to be important for blood-borne arrest, whereas the former was thought to be essential for escape from the primary tumor mass. In general, neoplastic cells are more easily separated from a solid tumor mass than are normal cells from corresponding tissues. The role of lysozomal enzymes in the cell release process has been considered elsewhere [106, 107]. Using an assay based upon the transfer of tumor cells between cell aggregates in one chamber across a nylon meshwork to cell aggregates in another chamber Umbright and Erbe [108] found that tumor cells detach, pass through the nylon mesh and attach to fibroblast aggregates much more readily than normal cells suggesting that both detachment and attachment or homotypic and heterotypic adhesive phenomenon are altered in tumor cells.

During transport in the blood malignant cells undergo cellular interactions with other circulating host cells, solubile blood components and the vascular endothelium. Heterotypic cell adhesion of malignant cells with platelets [109–112] are known to be important in blood-borne implantation. For example, it has been shown that experimental metastasis can be reduced by inducing thrombocytopenia in animals, as well as administration of anti-platelet agents [113–115]. Platelet aggregation activities have been found in a variety of tumor cell lines [109, 111, 112, 116, 117], in isolated cell membrane vesicles from tumor and transformed cells [117, 118]. Hara et al. [119] have partially characterized the platelet-aggregating activity of tumor cells, and they have found it to be composed of protein, lipid and carbohydrate components. All of these components appear to be required for platelet

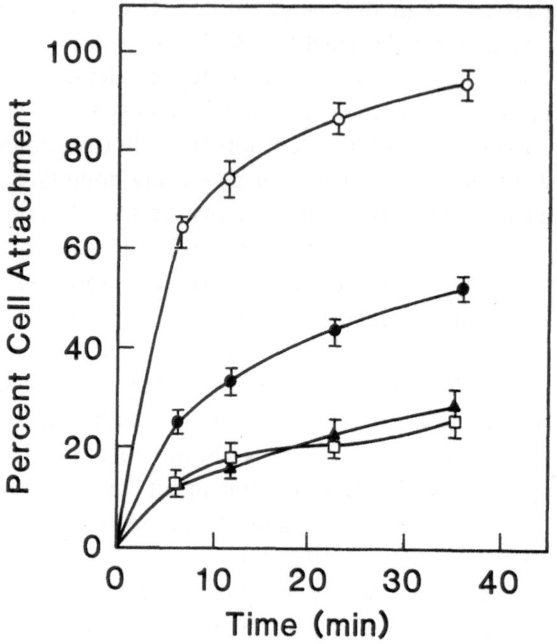

Figure 3. Kinetics of adhesion of B16 melanoma sublines to endothelial cells or their basal lamina. ▲—▲ B16-F1 melanoma cell attachment to CBE endothelial cell monolayer; □—□, B16-F1 melanoma cell attachment to murine brain endothelial cell monolayer; •—•, B16-B14B (brain-selected) melanoma cell attachment to murine brain endothelial cell monolayer; ○—○, B16-F1 melanoma cell attachment to CBE basal lamina [131].

aggregation. Metastatic cells also aggregate with host lymphocytes. Fidler found that metastatic B16-F10 cells adhere to host lymphocytes at higher rates than B16-F1 cells of lower metastatic potential. Using sequential selection procedures based on lymphocyte killing of B16 melanoma cells Fidler et al. [123] was able to obtain after six *in vitro* selections sublines that were no longer susceptible to lymphocyte-mediated cytotoxicity; the lymphocyte-resistant sublines no longer bound lymphocytes to the same degree [121] and formed significantly fewer experimental lung metastases *in vivo* [121, 123].

One of the most important events in blood-borne metastasis is implanation in the microcirculation. The fact that malignant cells can enter the blood does not necessarily indicate that arrest and metastatic colonization will follow [124–127]. Stable attachment or adhesion to the capillary endothelium is necessary to prevent detachment and recirculation, and the larger the circulating tumor cell emboli the greater the chance for successful arrest [102, 103]. Adhesion of malignant cells to host organ cells has been used to demonstrate a role for specific cell adhesion in determining specificity of organ arrest and metastasis. Nicolson and Winkelhake [100, 128] used B16 melanoma sublines and measured their abilities to heterotypically adhere to suspended organ cells. They found that the sublines selected for

A

B

C

D

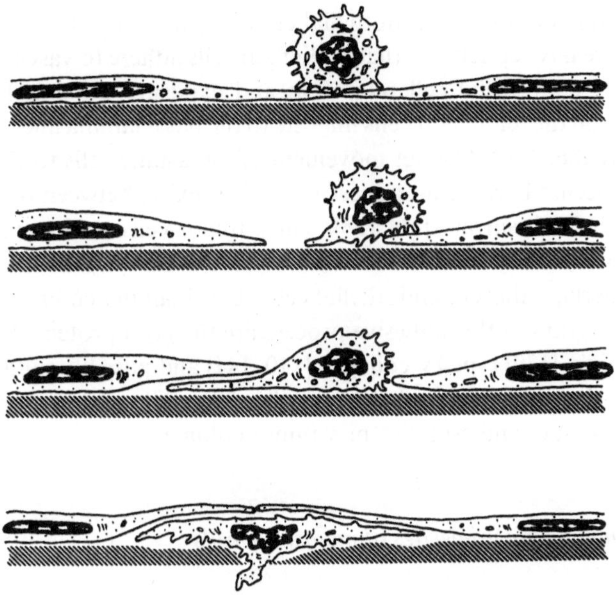

Figure 4. Sequence of events during metastatic cell attachment and invasion of vascular endothelial cell monolayers and their basal lamina. A, tumor cell attachment to endothelial cells; B, endothelial cell retraction; C, tumor cell invasion and underlapping of adjacent endothelial cells; D, destruction of endothelial basal lamina and reformation of endothelial intercellular junctions [131].

enhanced lung colonization and metastasis adhere at much faster rates to lung cells than to cells obtained from other organs not involved in metastasis [75, 100, 128]. Similarly, Phondke et al. [129] found that leukemia cells that colonize spleen but not lung adhere to isolated spleen cells but fail to adhere to suspended lung cells, and Schirrmacher et al. [130] have found that liver colonizing lymphoma variants adhere to hepatocytes in relation to their metastatic properties. Since these interactions normally take place at the level of the vascular endothelium, adhesion experiments should take this into account by using endothelial cells. By establishing endothelial cells from brain and using B16 melanoma sublines selected for enhanced lung or brain implantation the relationship between target organ endothelial cells and organ-selected B16 melanoma subpopulations has been explored further [131]. Brain-selected B16 melanoma cells adhered at faster rates to brain endothelial cell monolayers compared to lung-selected melanoma cells (Figure 3). During and after tumor cell adhesion to the vascular endothelium the deposition of fibrin occurs in many tumor systems [110, 132–134]. The formation of a fibrin thrombus or coating around arrested malignant cells is thought to be related to their thomboplastic properties [135, 136] which in turn are important in blood-borne tumor cell arrest.

Once tumor cell arrest has occurred, the malignant cells must escape the vascular compartment by invading the underlying basement membrane or basal lamina. We have examined the sequence of events in this process using malignant cell binding to monolayers of vascular endothelial cells (Figure 4) [86–88, 131, 137]. From these studies we have concluded that malignant cells adhere to vascular endothelial cells, stimulate endothelial cell retraction and exposure of underlying basal lamina, whereupon the malignant cells migrate to the basal lamina and adhere firmly to this structure [86, 138]. The net movement of metastatic cells to the endothelial basal lamina occurs because an adhesive gradient exists between this structure and the endothelial cell surface [86, 138]. Thus, tumor cells tend to migrate to the basal lamina where they adhere more strongly and eventually the malignant cells spread and underlap adjacent endothelial cells. Basal lamina components that are probably important in this adhesive process are the glycoproteins fibronectin [86, 138] and laminin [139] type IV collagen [140, 141] and possibly sulfated-proteoglycans. Once the basal lamina has been solubilized [83–87] malignant cells can enter extravascular tissues and establish new tumor colonies.

1.7. Immunologic properties of metastatic cells

When cells obtained from highly malignant tumors or from metastases have been compared to their parental or primary tumor counterparts, they frequently possess differing antigenicities and immunogenicities (see Fidler, Chapter 2). In immunologically competent hosts it is thought that immuno-selection may occur at the level of the primary or secondary tumor, resulting in the eventual emergence of tumor cell subpopulations which lack strong antigens that could lead to their recognition and destruction. Evidence for this type of selection has come from experiments where the selected, highly malignant cells have been shown to display reduced antigen levels or to have antigen deletions on their cell surfaces. When Sugarbaker and Cohen [142] examined spontaneous lung metastases from a murine fribrosarcoma for transplantation antigens, they found that several metastases that were tested had lost or expressed lowered amounts of these antigens when assayed by subcutaneous transplantation into tumor-immunized mice. Kim et al. [143] found less ruthenium red staining and antibody binding to metastasizing rat mammary carcinoma cells compared to non-metastastizing carcinomas and suggested that the relatively non-metastatic carcinoma lines had greater amounts of cell surface acidic glycocalyx and cell surface antigens. These authors also found that the highly metastatic carcinomas released more cell surface-derived material which was detected in the blood of tumor-bearing animals. Although both classes of carcinomas possessed and released some of the same common surface antigens, the nonmetastatic carcinomas had, in addition, other cell surface-bound antigens that were immunologically related to the common antigen. Kim and his collaborators proposed that the soluble antigens released from the metastasizing carcinoma interfered with host anti-tumor immune responses. Reading et al. [19] have analyzed a number of *in vivo*- and *in vitro*-selected murine RAW117 lymphosarcoma cell lines (and clones derived from these cell lines) for their metastatic properties and cell

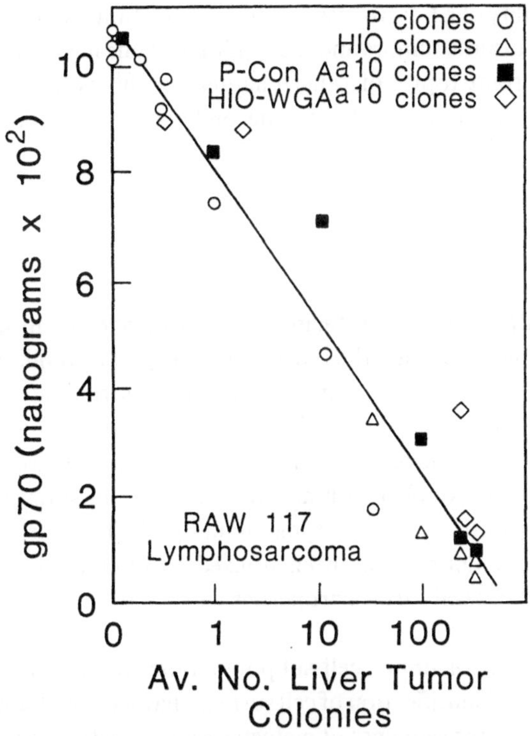

Figure 5. Relationship of murine RAW117 lymphosarcoma liver metastasis to content of RNA tumor virus envelope glycoprotein gp70. Cell clones obtained from the parental line (P clones), ten-times liver-selected subline (H10 clones), parental line selected ten times for lack of adherence to immobilized-concanavalin A (P-Con A^{a10} clones) and ten-times liver-selected subline that was additionally selected ten times for lack of adherence to immobilized-wheat germ agglutinin (H10-WGA^{a10} clones) were analyzed for gp70 by competition radioimmune assay according to Reading et al. [19].

surface antigen content. They found that the amounts of viral antigens such as the RNA tumor virus envelope glycoprotein gp70 determined by competition radioimmune assays correlated well with the metastatic potential to colonize liver (Figure 5). In this system successful metastasis apparently required escape from host immune surveillance which occurred via antigen deletion on the highly metastatic lymphosarcoma cells [18, 19]; however, in other metastatic systems such as B16 melanoma there was no relationship between metastasis and viral antigens such as gp70 [124]. Shearman and Longenecker [144] have found an increase in antigen content correlating with metastasis to liver in the chicken. These authors utilized a Marek's disease virus-transformed chick lymphoma to investigate antigenic changes on metastasizing cells, and found a cell surface antigen detectable with monoclonal antibody that increased in amounts concomitant with the ability of the lymphoma cells to metastasize to and colonize liver [144]. Thus, there is no simple relationship between the display of cell surface antigens, immunogenecities and metastasis. The ability of a host to respond to or to be stimulated to respond against primary and/or metastatic tumors and the type of immune mechanism(s) used in the response are important topics of other chapters in this volume, and the reader should consult these chapters for discussions on host anti-tumor immune response systems.

2. Final comments

Two of the most difficult problems facing researchers involved in studying tumors cell properties and metastasis are the inherent phenotypic instabilities of malignant cells and the continual *in vovo* selection pressures that discriminate against portions of the tumor cell populations. These characteristics of the malignant cell and its environment lead to tumor progession in the host where the incessant emergence of new tumor cell variants coupled with natural selection pressures generate tumors that are undergoing continuous phenotypic change [145]. The heterogeneous nature of malignant cell populations has been utilized to obtain subpopulations with differing metastatic and cell surface properties which have been discussed here and elsewhere.

Careful comparisons of tumor cell subpopulations varying in their metastatic potentials has allowed identification of cell surface characteristics important to each event occurring during the sequence of metastasis and could eventually lead to their biochemical elucidation. However, malignant cell subpopulations are often unstable, even in the absence of host selective pressures [29, 124, 144, 150 and Table 4], and this fact has made it more difficult to distinguish cell surface properties that are important to the metastatic sequence. Most of the research in this area has utilized cell populations that have been expanded by long term growth *in vitro* or have been obtained from tumors contaminated with dead or dying cells and containing unknown numbers of normal host cells. Although frequent assays of metastatic potential performed in parallel with biochemical and immunological experiments have eliminated some of the problems associated with phenotypic divergence of tumor cell properties during growth *in vivo* or *in vitro*, this has not been practical when using malignant human cells. Strict ultilization of short-term tissue culture may or may not exclude some of the problems of phenotypic instability. Finally it should be mentioned that in some systems growth *in vivo* can lead to even more rapid phenotypic divergence than that found in tissue culture [150] so the stringent growth of a tumor cell population *in vivo* does not necessarily remove problems associated with phenotype instability. Phenotypic instability (due to genotypic instability?) and the rapid generation of tumor cells with altered properties could be the unique characteristics that are common to all highly malignant tumor cell populations.

Acknowledgments

I wish to thank Adele Brodginski and Shirley Nunnally for assistance in the preparation of this chapter. Support has been provided by USPHS National Cancer Institute grants 1RO1-CA-28844, 2RO1-CA-28867 and 2RO1-CA-29571 and the Kleberg Foundation.

References

1. Hynes RO: Cell surface proteins and malignant transformation. Biochim Biophys Acta 458:3–107, 1976.
2. Nicolson GL: Transmembrane control of the receptors on normal and tumor cells. II. Surface changes associated with transformation and malignancy. Biochim Biophys Acta 458:1–72, 1976.
3. Roblin R, Chou I-N, Black PH: Proteolytic enzymes, cell surface changes and viral transformation. Adv Cancer Res 22:203–259, 1975.
4. Nicolson GL, Birdwell CR, Brunson KW, Robbins JC, Beattle G, Fidler IJ: Cell interactions in the metastatic process: some cell surface properties associated with successful blood-borne tumor spread. In: Cell and tissue interactions, Lash J, Burger MM (eds). New York: Raven Press, 1977, pp 225–241.
5. Hagmar B, Norrby K: Influence of cultivation, trypsinization and aggregation on the transplantability of melanoma B16 cells. Int J Cancer 11:663–675, 1973.
6. Sinha BK, Goldenberg GJ: The effect of trypsin and neuraminidase on the circulation and organ distribution of tumor cells. Cancer 34:1956–1961, 1974.
7. Fidler IJ: General considerations for studies of experimental cancer metastasis. Meth Cancer Res 15:399–439, 1978.
8. Poste G, Nicolson GL: Arrest and metastasis of blood-borne tumor cells are modified by fusion of plasma membrane vesicles from highly metastatic cells. Proc Natl Acad Sci USA 77:399–403, 1980.
9. Weiss L, Subject JR, Poste G: Some electrical properties of the peripheries of murine 3T3 cells with respect to viral transformation and reversion. Int J Cancer 16:914–921, 1975.
10. Klein G, Klein E: Conversion of solid neoplasms into ascites tumors. Ann NY Acad Sci 63:640–661, 1956.
11. Weiss L: Membrane dynamics and the metastasis of cancer. Cell Biophys 1:331–343, 1979.
12. Grdina DJ, Hittelman WM, White RA, Meistrich ML: Relevance of density, size and DNA content of tumour cells to the lung colony assay. Br J Cancer 36:659–669, 1977.
13. Baniyash M, Netanel T, Witz IP: Differences in cell density associated with differences in lung colonizing ability of B16 melanoma cells. Cancer Res 41:433–437, 1981.
14. Miner KM, Walter H, Nicolson GL: Subfractionation of malignant variants of metastatic murine lymphosarcoma cells by countercurrent distribution in two-polymer aqueous phases. Biochemistry 20:6244–6250, 1981.
15. Nicolson GL: The interactions of lectins with animal cell surfaces. Int Rev Cytol 39:89–190, 1974.
16. Raz A, McLellan WL, Hart IR, Bucana CD, Hoyer LC, Sela BA, Dragsten P, Fidler IJ: Cell surface properties of B16 melanoma variants with differing metastatic potential. Cancer Res 40:1645–1651, 1980.
17. Irimura T, Gonzalez R, Nicolson GL: Effects of tunicamycin on B16 metastatic melanoma cell surface glycoproteins and blood-borne arrest and survival properties. Cancer Res 41:3411–3418, 1981.
18. Nicolson GL, Reading CL, Brunson KW: Blood-borne tumor metastasis: some properties of selected tumor cell variants of differing malignancies. In: Tumor progression, Crispen RG (ed). Amsterdam: Elsevier North-Holland, 1980, pp 31–48.

19. Reading CL, Brunson KW, Torrianni M, Nicolson GL: Malignancies of metastatic murine lymphosarcoma cell lines and clones correlate with decreased cell surface display of RNA tumor virus envelope glycoprotein gp70. Proc Natl Acad Sci USA 77:5943–5947, 1980.
20. Tao T-W, Burger MM: Non-metastasising variants selected from metastasising melanoma cells. Nature 270:437–438, 1977.
21. Finne J, Tao T-W, Burger MM: Carbohydrate changes in glycoproteins of a poorly metastasizing wheat germ agglutinin-resistant melanoma clone. Cancer Res 40:2580–2587, 1980.
22. Talmadge JE, Starkey JR, Stanford DR: *In vitro* characteristics of metastatic variant subclones of restricted genetic origin. J Supramol Struct 15:139–151, 1981.
23. Lotan R, Nicolson GL: Purification of cell membrane glycoproteins by lectin affinity chromatography. Biochim Biophys Acta 549:329–376, 1979.
24. Nicolson GL: Cell surface proteins and glycoproteins of metastatic murine melanomas and sarcomas. In: Biological markers in neoplasia: basic and applied aspects, Ruddon RW (ed). New York: North-Holland Publishing Co., 1978, pp 227–239.
25. Yogeeswaran G, Stein SB, Sebastian H: Altered cell surface organization of gangliosides and sialylglycoproteins of mouse metastatic melanoma variant lines selected *in vivo* for enhanced lung implantation. Cancer Res 38:1336–1344, 1978.
26. Brunson KW, Beattie G, Nicolson GL: Selection and altered tumour cell properties of brain-colonising metastatic melanoma. Nature 272:543–545, 1978.
27. Brunson KW, Nicolson GL: Selection of malignant melanoma variant cell lines for ovary colonization. J Supramol Struct 11:517–528, 1979.
28. Yogeeswaran G, Stein BS, Sebastian H: Characterization of tumorigenic and metastatic properties of murine sarcoma virus-transformed non-producer BALB/373 cell lines. J Natl Cancer Inst 64:951–957, 1980.
29. Neri A, Nicolson GL: Phenotypic drift of metastatic and cell surface properties of mammary adenocarcinoma cell clones during growth *in vitro*. Int J Cancer 28:731–738, 1981.
30. Warren L, Fuhrer JP, Buck CA: Surface glycoproteins of cells before and after transformation by oncogenic viruses. Fed Proc 32:80–85, 1973.
31. Glick MC, Rabinowitz Z, Sachs L: Surface membrane blycopeptides correlated with tumorigenesis. Biochemistry 12:4864–4869, 1973.
32. Warren L, Ziedman I, Buck CA: The surface glycoproteins of a mouse melanoma growing in culture and as a solid tumor *in vivo*. Cancer Res 35:2186–2190, 1975.
33. Chen LB, Burridge K, Murray A, Walsh ML, Copple CD, Bushnell A, McDougall JK, Gallimore PH: Modulation of cell surface glycocalyx: studies on large, external transformation-sensitive protein. Ann NY Acad Sci 312:366–381, 1978.
34. Chen LB, Summerhayes I, Hsieh P, Gallimore PH: Possible role of fibronectin in malignancy. J Supramol Struct 12:139–150, 1979.
35. Yamada KM, Olden K: Fibronectins: adhesive glycoproteins of cell surface and blood. Nature 275:179–184, 1978.
36. Stenman S, Vaheri A: Distribution of a major connective tissue protein, fibronectin, in normal human tissues. J Exp Med 147:1054–1064, 1978.
37. Wartiovaara J, Leivo I, Vaheri A: Expression of the cell surface-associated glycoprotein, fibronectin, in the early mouse embryo. Develop Biol 69:247–257, 1979.
38. Smith HS, Riggs JL, Mosesson MW: Production of fibronectin by human epithelial cell lines. Cancer Res 39:4138–4144, 1979.
39. Neri A, Ruoslahti E, Nicolson GL: The distribution of fibronectin on clonal cell lines of a rat mammary adenocarcinoma growing *in vitro* and *in vivo* at primary and metastatic sites. Cancer Res 41:5082–5095, 1981.
40. Brady RO, Fishman PH: Biosynthesis of glycolipids in virus-transformed cells. Biochim Biophys Acta 355:121–148, 1974.
41. Hakomori S-I: Structure and organization of cell surface glycolipids dependency on cell growth

and malignant transformation. Biochim Biophys Acta 417:55–89, 1975.

42. Yogeeswaran G, Stein BS: Glycosphingolipids of metastatid variants of RNA virus-transformed nonproducer Balb/3T3 cell lines: altered metabolism and cell surface exposure. J Natl Cancer Inst 65:967–973, 1980.
43. Strauch L: The role of collagenases in tumor invasion. In: Tissue interactions in carcinogenesis, Tarin D (ed). New York: Academic Press, 1972, pp 399–434.
44. Sylvén B, Snellman O, Sträuli P: Immunofluorescent studies on the occurrence of cathepsin B1 at tumor cell surfaces. Virchows Arch B Cell Path 17:97–112, 1974.
45. Dresden MH, Heilman SA, Schmidt JD: Collagenlytic enzymes in human neoplasms. Cancer Res 32:993–996, 1972.
46. Hashimoto K, Yamanishi Y, Maeyens E, Dabbous MK, Kanzaki T: Collagenolytic activities of squamous cell carcinoma of the skin. Cancer Res 33:2790–2801, 1973.
47. Sträuli P, Weiss L.: Cell locomotion and tumor penetration. Eur J Cançer 13:1–12, 1977.
48. Carr I, Mc Ginty F, Norris P: The fine structure of neoplastic invasion: invasion of liver, skeletal muscle and lymphatic vessels by the Rd/3 tumour. J Pathol 118:91–99, 1976.
49. Mareel M, De Bruyne G, De Ridder L: Invasion of malignant cell into ^{51}Cr-labeled host tissue in organotypical culture. Oncology 34:6–9, 1977.
50. Schnebli HP: A protease-like activity associated with malignant cells. Schweiz Med Wochenschr 102:1194–1197, 1972.
51. Bosmann HB: Elevated glycosidases and proteolytic enzymes in cells transformed by RNA tumor virus. Biochim Biophys Acta 264:339–343, 1972.
52. Bosmann HB, Lockwood T, Morgan HR: Surface biochemical changes accompanying primary infection with Rous sarcoma virus, II. Proteolytic and glycosidase activity and sublethal autolysis. Exp Cell Res 83:25–30, 1974b.
53. Bosmann HB, Hall TC: Enzyme activity in invasive tumors of human breast and colon. Proc Natl Acad Sci USA 71:1833–1837, 1974.
54. Yamanishi Y, Maeyens E, Dbbous MK, Ohyama H, Hashimoto K: Collagenolytic activity in malignant melanoma: physiochemical studies. Cancer Res 33:2507–2512, 1973.
55. Koono M, Ushijima K, Hayashi H: Studies on the mechanisms of invasion in cancer. III. Purification of a neutral protease of rat ascites hepatoma cell associated with production of chemotactic factor for cancer cells. Int J Cancer 13:105–115, 1974.
56. Sylvén B, Bois-Svensson I: On the chemical pathology of interstitial fluid. I. Proteolytic activities in transplanted mouse tumors. Cancer Res. 25:438–468, 1965.
57. Sylvén B, Malmgren H: The histological distribution of proteinase and peptidase activity in solid tumor transplants. Acta Radiol (suppl) 154:1–24, 1957.
58. Poole AR, Tiltman KJ, Recklies AD, Stocker TAM: Differences in secretion of the proteinase cathepsin B at the edge of human breast carcinomas and fibroadenomas. Nature 273:545–547, 1978.
59. Zimmerberg J, Greengard O, Knox WE: Peptidyl proline hydroxylase in adult, developing, and neoplastic rat tissues. Cancer Res 35:1009–1014, 1975.
60. Tökés ZA, Sorgente N, Okigaki T: Proteolysis associated with norman, carcinogen-treated and transformed rat liver epithelial cells. Prog Clin Biol Res 615–624, 1977.
61. Bosmann HB, Bieber GF, Brown AE, Case KR, Gersten DM, Kimmerer TW, Lione A: Biochemical parameters correlated with tumour cell implantation. Nature 246:487–489, 1973.
62. Liotta LA, Tryggvason S, Garbisa S, Hart I, Foltz CM, Shafie S: Metastatic propensity correlates with tumor cell degradation of basement membrane collagen. Nature 284:67–68, 1980.
63. Weiss L: The cell periphery metastasis and other contact phenomenon. Amsterdam: North Holland Publishing Co., 1967, pp 289–338.
64. Liotta LA, Abe S, Robey PG, Martin GR: Preferential digestion of basement membrane collagen by an enzyme derived from a metastatic murine tumor. Proc Natl Acad Sci USA 76:2268–2276, 1979.

of a neutral protease which cleaves type IV collagen. Biochemistry 20:100–104, 1981.

66. Unkeless JC, Dan K, Kellerman GM, Reich E: Fibrinolysis associated with oncogenic transformation. Partial purification and characterization of the cell factor, a plasminogen activator. J Biol Chem 249:4295–4305, 1974.
67. Christman JK, Acs G: Purification and characterization of a cellular fibrinolytic factor associated with oncogenic transformation: the plasminogen activator from SV40-transformed hamster cells. Biochem Biophys Acta 340:339–347, 1974.
68. Ossowski L, Unkeless JC, Tobia A, Quigley JP, Rifkin DB, Reich E: An enzymatic function associated with transformation of fibroblasts by oncogenic viruses. II. Mammalian fibroblast cultures transformed by DNA and RNA tumor viruses. J Exp Med 137:113–126, 1973.
69. Goldberg AR: Increase protease levels in transformed cells: a casein overlay assay for the detection of plasminogen activator production. Cell 2:95–102, 1974.
70. Rifkin DB, Loeb JN, Moore G, Reich E: Properties of plasminogen activators formed by neoplastic human cell cultures. J Exp Med 139:1317–1328, 1974.
71. Chen LB, Buchanan JM: Plasminogen-independent fibrinolysis by proteases produced by transformed chick embryo fibroblasts. Proc Natl Acad Sci USA 72:1132–1136, 1975.
72. Unkeless JC, Gordon S, Reich E: Secretion of plasminogen activator by stimulated macrophages. J Exp Med 139:84–850, 1974.
73. Mott DM, Fabisch PH, Sani BP, Sorof S: Lack of correlation between fibrinolysis and the transformed state of cultured mammalian cells. Biochem Biophys Res Commun 61:621–627, 1974.
74. Tökés ZA, Sorgente N: Cell surface-associated and released proteolytic activity of bovine aorta endothelia cell. Biochem Biophys Res Commun 73:965–971, 1976.
75. Nicolson GL, Winkelhake JL, Nussey AC: An approach to studying the cellular properties associated with metastasis: some *in vitro* properties of tumor variants selected *in vivo* for enhanced metastasis. In: Fundamental aspects of metastasis, L Weiss (ed). Amsterdam: North-Holland Publishing Co., 1976, pp 291–303.
76. Wang BS, McLoughlin GA, Richie JP, Mannick JA: Correlation of the production of plasminogen activator with tumor metastasis in B16 melanoma cell lines. Cancer Res 40:288–292, 1980.
77. Ossowski L, Reich E: Experimental model for quantitative study of metastasis. Cancer Res 40:2300-2309, 1980.
78. Grimes WJ: Glycosyl transferase and sialic acid levels of normal and transformed cells. Biochemistry 12:990–996, 1973.
79. Chatterjee SK, Kim U: Galactosyltransferase activity in metastasizing and non-metastasizing rat mammary carcinomas and its probable relationship with tumor cell surface antigen shedding. J Natl Cancer Inst 58:273–280, 1977.
80. Chatterjee SK: Glycosyltransferases in metastasizing and non-metastasizing rat mammary tumors and the release of these enzymes in the host sera. Eur J Cancer 15:1351–1356, 1979.
81. Chatterjee SK, Kim U: Fucosyltransferase activity in metastasizing and non-metastasizing rat mammary carcinomas. J Natl Cancer Inst 61:151–162, 1978.
82. Capel ID, Jenner M, Pinnock MH, Dorrell HM, Payne DC, Williams DC: Correlation between tumour size, metastatic spread and galactosyl transferase activity in cyclophosphamide-treated mice bearing the Lewis lung carcinoma. Oncology 36:242–244, 1979.
83. Liotta LA, Kleinerman J, Catanzaro P, Rynbrandt D: Degradation of basement membrane by murine tumor cells. J Natl Cancer Inst 58:1427–1431, 1977.
84. Garbisa S, Kniska K, Tryggvason K, Foltz C, Liotta LA: Quantitation of basement membrane collagen degradation by living tumor cells *in vitro*. Cancer Lett 9:359–366, 1980.
85. Jones PA, DeClerck YA: Destruction of extracellular matrices containing glycoproteins, elastin, and collagen by metastatic human tumor cells. Cancer Res 40:3222–3227, 1980.
86. Kramer RH, Gonzalez R, Nicolson GL: Metastatic tumor cells adhere preferentially to the extracellular matrix underlying vascular endothelial cells. Int J Cancer 26:639–645, 1980.

87. Kramer RH, Nicolson GL: Invasion of vascular endothelial cell monolayers and underlying matrix by metastatic human cancer cells. In: International cell biology, Schweiger S (ed). Heidelberg: Springer-Verlag, 1981, pp 794–799.
88. Kramer RH, Vogel K, Nicolson GL: Solubilization and degradation of subendothelial matrix glycoproteins and proteoglycans by metastatic tumor cells. J Biol Chem 257:2678–2686, 1982.
89. Oppenheimer SB, Utilization of L-glutamine in intercellular adhesion: ascites tumor and embryonic cells. Exp Cell Res 77:175–182, 1973.
90. Oppenheimer SB: Functional involvement of specific carbohydrate in teratoma cell adhesion factor. Exp Cell Res 92:122–126, 1975.
91. Chipowsky S, Lee YC, Roseman S: Adhesion of cultured fibroblasts to insoluble analogues of cell-surface carbohydrates. Proc Natl Acad Sci USA 70:2309–2312, 1973.
92. Weigel PH, Schmell E, Lee YC, Roseman S: Specific adhesion of rat hepatocytes to β-galactosides linked to polyacrylamide gels. J Biol Chem 253:330–333, 1978.
93. Weigel PH, Schnarr RL, Kuhlenschmidt MS, Schmell E, Lee RT, Lee YC, Roseman S: Adhesion of hepatocytes to immobilized sugars. A threshold phenomenon. J Biol Chem 254:10830–10838, 1979.
94. Coman DR: Decreased mutual adhesiveness, a property of cells from squamous cell carcinomas. Cancer Res 4:625–629, 1944.
95. Cribon CO, Franzen S, Unsgaard B, Zajieck J: Studies on the effect of aspiration biopsy on the viability of aspirated cells. I. Registration of pressure differences during aspiration. Scand J Haemetol 1:272–279, 1974.
96. Dorsey JK, Roth S: Adhesive specificity in normal and transformed mouse fibroblasts. Develop Biol 33:249–256, 1973.
97. Wright TC, Ukena TE, Campbell R, Karnovsky MJ: Rates of aggregation, loss of anchorage dependence, and tumorigenicity of cultured cells. Proc Nat Acad Sci USA 74:258–262, 1977.
98. Weiss L: Studies on cellular adhesion in tissue culture. V. Some effects of enzymes on cell detachment. Exp Cell Res 30:509–520, 1963.
99. Winkelhake JL, Nicolson GL: Determination of adhesive properties of variant metastatic melanoma cells to BALB/3T3 cells and their virus-transformed derivatives by a monolayer attachment assay. J Natl Cancer Inst 56:285–291, 1976.
100. Nicolson GL, Winkelhake JL: Organ specificity of blood-borne tumour metastasis determined by cell adhesion? Nature 255:230–232, 1975.
101. Nicolson GL: Cell and tissue interactions leading to malignant tumor spread (metastasis). Amer Zool 18:77–86, 1978.
102. Fidler IJ: The relationship of embolic homogeneity, number, size and viability to the incidence of experimental metastasis. Eur J Cancer 9:223–227, 1973.
103. Liotta LA, Kleinerman J, Saidel GM: The significance of hematogenous tumor cell clumps in the metastatic process. Cancer Res 36:889–894, 1976.
104. Weiss L: Biophysical aspects of the metastatic cascade. In: Fundamental aspects of metastasis, Weiss L (ed). Amsterdam: North-Holland Publishing Co., 1976, pp 51–70.
105. Coman DR: Adhesiveness and stickiness: two independent properties of the cell surface. Cancer Res 21:1436–1438, 1961.
106. Poste G: Sublethal autolysis. Modification of the cell periphery by lysosomal enzymes. Exp Cell Res 67:116–125, 1971.
107. Poste G, and Weiss L: Some consideration on cell surface alterations in malignancy. In: Fundamental aspects of metastasis, Weiss L (ed). Amsterdam: North-Holland Publishing Co., 1976, pp 25–47, 1976.
108 Umbreit JN, Erbe RW: Transfer of tumor cells between cell aggregates as a model for adhesive changes in metastasis. Cancer Res 39:2001–2005, 1979.
109. Gasic CJ, Gasic TB, Galanti N, Johnson T, Murphy S: Platelet-tumor cell interaction in mice. The role of platelets in the spread of malignant disease. Int J Cancer 11:704–718, 1973.

110. Warren BA: Environment of the blood-borne tumor embolus adherent to vessel wall. J Med 4:150–177, 1973.
111. Hilgard P: The role of blood platelets in experimental metastases. Br J Cancer 28:429–435, 1973.
112. Gasic CJ, Koch PAG, Hsu B, Gasic TB, Niewiarowski S: Thrombogenic activity of mouse and human tumors: effect on platelets, coagulation, and fibrinolysis, and possible significance for metastases. Z Krebsforsch 86:263–277, 1976.
113. Gasic GJ, Gasic TB, Murphy S: Antimetastatic effects of aspirin. Lancet ii:932–933, 1972.
114. Fisher B, Fisher ER: Experimental studies of factors which influence hepatic metastases. VIII. Effect of anticoagulants. Surgery 50:240–247, 1961.
115. Gespar H: Inhibition of cancer cell stickiness by anticoagulants, fibrinolytic drugs and pyrimido-pyrimidine derivatives. Hematol Rev 3:1–51, 1972.
116. Chew EC, Wallace AC: Demonstration of fibrin in early stages of experimental metastasis. Cancer Res 36:1904–1909, 1976.
117. Pearlstein E, Salk PL, Yogeeswaran G, Karpatkin S: Correlation between spontaneous metastatic potential, platelet-aggregating activity of cell surface extracts, and cell surface sialylation in 10 metastatic-variant derivatives of rat renal sarcoma cell line. Proc Natl Acad Sci USA 77:4336–4339, 1980.
118. Gasic GJ, Boettiger D, Catalfamo JL, Gasic TB, Stewart GJ: Aggregation of platelets and cell membrane vesiculation by rat cells transformed *in vitro* by Rous sarcoma virus. Cancer Res 38:2950–2955, 1978.
119. Hara Y, Steiner M, Baldini MG: Characterization of the platelet-aggregating activity of tumor cells. Cancer Res 40:1217–1221, 1980.
120. Fidler IJ: Biological behavior of malignant melanoma cells correlated to their survival *in vivo*. Cancer Res 35:218–224, 1975.
121. Fidler IJ, Bucana C: Mechanism of tumor cell resistance to lysis by syngeneic lymphocytes. Cancer Res 37:3945–3956, 1977.
122. Fidler IJ, Nicolson GL: Tumor cell and host properties affecting the implantation and survival of blood-borne metastatic variants of B16 melanoma. Isr J Med Sci 14:38–50, 1978.
123. Fidler IJ, Gersten DM, Budmen MB: Characterization *in vivo* and *in vitro* of tumor cells selected for resistance to syngeneic lymphocyte-mediated cytotoxicity. Cancer Res 36:3160–3165, 1976.
124. Fidler IJ, Nicolson GL: The immunobiology of experimental metastatic melanoma. Cancer Biol Rev 2:171–234, 1981.
125. Fidler IJ: tumor heterogeneity and the biology of cancer invasion and metastasis. Cancer Res 38:2651–2660, 1978.
126. Salsbury AJ: The significance of the circulating cancer cell. Cancer Treat Rev 2:55–72, 1975.
127. Fisher ER, Fisher B: Circulating cancer cells and metastasis. Int J Radiat Oncol Biol Phys 1:87–91, 1976.
128. Nicolson GL, Robbins JC, Winkelhake JL: Tumor cell surface and metastasis: dynamic changes in neoplastic membrane structure and their relationship to tumor spread. In: Cellular membrane and tumor cell behavior, Walborg EF (ed). Baltimore: Williams and Wilkins, 1975, pp 81–127.
129. Phondke GP, Madyastha KR, Madyastha PR, Barth RF: Relationship between Concanvalin A-induced agglutin-ability of murine leukemia cells and their propensity to form heterotypic aggregates with syngeneic lymphoid cells. J Natl Cancer Inst 66:643–647, 1981.
130. Schirrmacher V, Cheinsong-PoPov R, Arheiter H: Hepatocyte-tumour cell interaction *in vivo*. I. Conditions for rosette formation and inhibition by anti-H2 antibody. J Exp Med 151:984–989, 1980.
131. Nicolson GL: Metastatic tumor cell attachment and invasion assay utilizing vascular endothelial cell monolayers. J Histochem Cytochem 30:214–220, 1982.
132. Chew EC, Josephson RL, Wallace AC: Morphologic aspects of the arrest of circulating cancer cells. In: Fundamental aspects of metastasis, Weiss L (ed). Amsterdam: North-Holland Publishing Co., 1976, pp 121–150.

133. Baserga R, Saffiotti U: Experimental studies on histogenesis of blood-borne metastases. Arch Pathol 59:26–34, 1955.
134. Wood Jr S: Mechanisms of establishment of tumor metastasis. Pathobiol Ann 1:281–308, 1971.
135. Day ED, Planinisek JA, Pressman D: Localization *in vivo* of radioiodinated anti-rat fibrin antibodies and radioiodinated rat fibrinogen in the Murphy rat lymphosarcoma and in other transplantable rat tumors. J Natl Cancer Inst 22:413–426, 1969.
136. Mootse G, Agostino D, Cliffton EE: Alterations in fibrinogen, plasminogen and inhibitors of plasmin with the growth of V2 carcinoma in rabbits. J Natl Cancer Inst 35:567–572, 1965.
137. Kramer RH, Nicolson GL: Interactions of tumor cells with vascular endothelial cell monolayers: A model for metastatic invasion. Proc Natl Acad Sci USA 76:5704–5709, 1979.
138. Nicolson GL, Irimura T, Gonzales R, Rouslahti E: The role of fibronectin in adhesion of metastatic melanoma cells to endothelial cells and their basal lamina. Exp Cell Res 135:461–465, 1981.
139. Terranova VP, Rohrback DH, Martin GR: Role of laminin in the attachment of PAM212 (epithelial) cells to basement membrane collagen. Cell 22:719–726, 1980.
140. Murray CJ, Liotta LA, Rennard SI, Martin GR: Adhesion characteristics of murine metastatic and non-metastatic tumor cells *in vitro*. Cancer Res 40:347–351, 1980.
141. Liotta LA, Tryggvason K, Garbisa S, Robey PG, Murrey JC: Interaction of metastatic tumor cells with basement membrane collagen. In: Metastatic tumor growth, Grundmann C (ed). New York: Verlag, 1980, pp 21–30.
142. Sugarbaker EV, Cohen AM: Altered antigenicity in spontaneous pulmonary metastases from an antigenic murine sarcoma. Surgery 72:155–164, 1972.
143. Kim V, Baumler A, Carruthers C, Bielat K: Immunological escape mechanism in spontaneously metastasing mammary tumors. Proc Natl Acad Sci USA 72:1012–1016, 1975.
144. Shearman PJ, Longenecker BM: Clonal variation and functional correlation of organ-specific metastasis and an organ-specific metastasis-associated antigen. Int J Cancer 27:387–395, 1981.
145. Nowell PC: The clonal evolution of tumor cell populations. Science 194:23–28, 1976.
146. Miner KM, Lotan R, Nicolson GL: Metastatic and melanogenic properties of *in vivo*-selected B16 melanoma sublines and their clonal derivatives. In: Phenotypic expression in pigment cells, Seiji M (ed). Tokyo: Univ. Tokyo Press, 1981, pp 529–532.
147. Chambers AF, Hill RP, Ling V: Tumor heterogeneity and stability of the metastatic phenotype of mouse KHT sarcoma cells. Cancer Res 41:1368–1372, 1981.
148. Kerbel RS: Immunologic studies of membrane mutants of a highly metastatic murine tumor. Am J Pathol 97:609–622, 1979.
149. Olsson L, Ebbesen P: Natural polyclonality of spontaneous AKR leukemia and its consequences for so-called specific immunotherapy. J Natl Cancer Inst 62:623–627, 1979.
150. Chow DA, Greenberg AH: The generation of tumor heterogeneity *in vivo*. Int J Cancer 25:261–265, 1980.

6. Metastatic inefficiency

L. WEISS

1. Introduction

Any operational definition of metastatic efficiency must surely focus on the capacity of a cancer to generate clinically overt metastases during the lifetime of its host. The latter qualification will appear less curious to experimentalists than clinicians, since the former have the opportunity to make bioassays on apparently normal organs for metastatic cancer cells in fresh hosts, and thus achieve a sensitivity of detection which may have little clinical relevance.

As the major underlying causes of cancer-related deaths in patients are metastasis and recurrence, it may at first sight appear paradoxical to even consider the metastatic process as inefficient. However, when the primary causes of death in patients with non-leukemic cancers are examined (Table 1), it can be seen that the majority of deaths were not due to overwhelming metastatic 'burdens' in either the host or individual vital organs. Small metastases at anatomically strategic sites can, for example, result in bronchiolar or ureteric obstructions, leading to potentially lethal infections or renal failure. Thus, in the sense used here, the ultimate death of patients with metastases is not evidence that, at the level of cancer cells, metastasis is an efficient process, and in the present context, it should be noted that even an inefficient process will achieve measurable success, if repeated often enough.

For an individual cancer cell, the metastatic process consists of a number of 'all-or-none' sequential steps as outlined simplistically in Figure 1. At the level of individual cells, survival through each step and progression to the next is mandatory for metastasis formation, and failure to survive or progress leads to total metastatic inefficiency. At the level of whole cancers, when many malignant cells are likely to

Table 1. Some primary causes of death in patients with non-leukemic cancer.

Infection	41.6%
Vital organ 'failure'	19.2%
Hemorrhage	8.8%
Thromboembolism	12.2%
Emaciation and/or electrolyte imbalance	7.7%

Based on studies on a total of 1479 patients made by Klastersky et al. [1], Inagaki et al. [2] and Ambrus et al. [3].

L.A. Liotta and I.R. Hart (eds.), Tumor Invasion and Metastasis. ISBN-13: 978-94-009-7513-2.
© 1982 Martinus Nijhoff Publishers, The Hague/Boston/London.

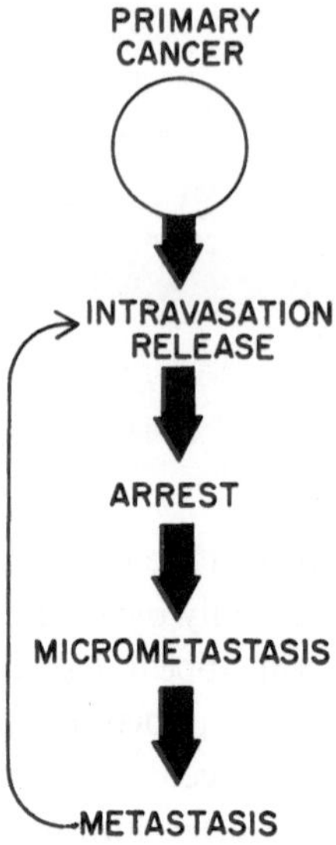

Figure 1. Simplistic outline of metastasis.

be involved on many separate occasions in the initiation of metastasis, it seems improbable in general, that one particular step could constitute a unique or complete block to the metastatic process. However, partial blocks, by determining the proportions of cancer cells progressing from one step to the next, are likely to constitute rate-regulating processes bearing on metastatic efficiency. In this chapter, some of these processes will be examined in detail.

Actuarial survival, following confirmed total removal of primary cancers, leads to some basis for comparison of their metastatic efficiencies within a given time-frame. For such comparisons to be valid in reflecting their respective natural histories, cancers should be at the same stage, and should have been subject to local treatment only, otherwise the comparisons are biased, by differentials in ease of diagnosis and response to therapy. If staging is inaccurate at the time of local therapy, then false impressions of relative metastatic efficiency will be generated. A good example of this comes from comparing the effects of local therapy on Stage I, Group I endometrial carcinoma with Stage I ovarian carcinoma. Following local therapy of operable (Group I) Stage I endometrial cancer which is limited to the fundus uteri, the actuarial survival rates in one series were 94.5% and 92.6% at 5 and 10 years, respectively [4]. In contrast, the mean 5-year survival rate of patients with Stage IA ovarian carcinoma, which is limited to one ovary, is approximately 60% following total hysterectomy and bilateral salpingo-oophorectomy, with or without local radiation. Although at first sight, these data suggest Stage I ovarian cancer is more metastatic than Stage I endometrial cancer, this is not the case. Data reviewed by Piver et al. [5] and Castaldo et al. [6] show that of those women with *presumed* Stage I ovarian cancer, metastases were present in the pelvic lymph-nodes in approximately 8%, in the aortic nodes in 13%, in the diaphragm in 11% and in the omentum in 3%. In addition, 33% had free malignant cells in the peritoneal cavity. Thus, in these data, Stage I ovarian cancers had metastasized more than Stage I endometrial cancers at the time of diagnosis, and cannot determine whether the ovarian cancers were diagnosed comparatively later and/or metastasized earlier; direct comparison of metastatic efficiencies between the two types of cancer is therefore not possible.

2. Evidence that metastasis in people is an inefficient process

It must be emphasized that over 270 types of human cancer are recognizable on morphologic grounds, which implies potential differences in biologic behavior. Coupled with this are many well-known associations between metastasis, differentiation and loss of differentiation. Therefore, any generalizations on metastasis without regard to the nature of the primary cancer must be treated with skepticism.

The routes of metastasis are via blood and lymphatic channels and through natural body cavities. Except for those cancers, often sarcomas, having direct access to vascular clefts which are not lined by vascular endothelium, and cancers such as ovarian carcinomas having direct assess to body cavities, some sort of invasive phase is a prerequisite to the disseminative phase of metastasis. The basal cell carcinoma provides an obvious example of invasive efficiency coupled with inefficiency in subsequent steps of the metastatic process. These cancers which account for approximately 70% of all skin cancers, occur almost exclusively on hair-bearing skin and, if untreated, may invade the tissues causing a great deal of destruction. In spite of this, metastasis from these tumors is rare; Costanza et al. [7] found only 90 cases in the world literature, and according to Farmer and Helwig's [8] study of 17 cases of metastatic basal cell carcinoma, metastatic lesions generally have a basosquamous or adenoid pattern. In spite of their obvious capacity to invade, and the occurrence of presumptive hematogenous metastases, it is virtually unknown to find intravascular cancer cells close to non-metastasizing tumors. The stromal relations of basal cell carcinomas have been stressed by many authors in terms of tumor survival and more recently as some sort of invasion-inhibiting pseudoencapsule. However, since most basal cell carcinomas appear to have invasive potential, it seems a more reasonable and testable speculation that different enzymes are required for general stromal invasion than for lysis of basement membranes, and that the non-metastatic cancers lack the enzymes necessary for penetration of basement membranes, and hence intravasation.

Another indication that invasiveness per se is not synonymous with metastasis is provided by data on microinvasive carcinoma (MC) of the cervix uteri. Although the diagnosis of MC (Stage 1A) is often vague and controversial, Lohe [9] has attempted to give a 3-dimensional definition of this entity as a carcinoma of maximum length and width of 10 mm, with a maximum depth of up to 5 mm.

Assuming a unicentric origin, to achieve a maximum volume of $0.5\,cm^3$, an MC would have gone through approximately 28 doublings and would contain more than 10^8 cells. In spite of this large cancer cell reservoir, a definite pattern of stromal invasion and a frequency of 'capillary-like' space invasion in excess of 40% of cases [10], the incidence of pelvic lymph-node metastases is less than 1% in Lohe's [11] series. The fact that the pattern of stromal invasion, whether finger-like or the more advanced confluent type, does not correlate with invasion of the 'capillary-like' lymphatic spaces, and that invasion of these spaces is very seldom associated with metastasis [12], is indicative of a considerable degree of metastatic inefficiency.

There have been many attempts to correlate the presence of cancer cells in the blood-stream with metastasis, although many of the studies reported over the period of 1950 to 1965 are suspect, because degenerate non-cancer cells and megakarocytes were incorrectly reported as malignant cells [13]. It has been recognized for many years that the presence of circulating cancer cells is not synonymous with metastasis [14] because on morphologic evidence, many if not most cells, are somehow killed in the circulation [15] within tumor emboli [16, 17, 18]. At present there are no human data relating input of cancer cells into the blood-stream with the numbers of metastases subsequently developing, and without these data numerical estimates of metastatic efficiency cannot be made. However, cancer cells have unequivocally been detected in the blood albeit in low numbers, in specimens of only a few mm^3 volume, and by extrapolation, 1 cancer cell/mm^3 of blood is equivalent to approximately 5×10^6 cells in the blood of a 70 kg man at any one time. At autopsy, the numbers of *overt* metastases detected are orders of magnitude less than this calculated number of circulating cancer cells. Thus, with overt metastasis as the end-point, metastatic efficiency is very low indeed, even without allowance for continuous input of cancer cells into the circulation.

3. Experimental approaches

Although a qualitative impression of metastatic inefficiency is gained from human data, more quantitative estimates may be obtained from experiments made on rodents. In using experimental data, it must be remembered that many animal tumors are immunogenic in their hosts whereas human tumors are not; that although in people, cancer is a disease of later life, the life-span of a laboratory mouse under normal conditions is approximately 2 years, yet most experiments are made with 'young adult' 6- to 8-week-old animals; that a 5 g tumor in a 22 g mouse corresponds to a 16 kg tumor in a 70 kg man and that in many, if not most experiments, an animal is abruptly exposed to initiation of a 'primary' cancer by thousands of cells as distinct from a uni- or paucicentric origin in people, or intravenous injections made in volumes of fluid which may be artifactually large compared with the animals' blood volume [19, 20]. Some of these qualifications and others on the use of animal models are critically reviewed by Hewitt [21, 22].

4. Circulating cancer cells

By the use of an isolation technique in which tumors are implanted into an ovarian site in the rat where effluent blood is confined to the ovarian vein, Butler and Gullino [23] evaluated cell shedding from the MTW9 mammary carcinomas into the circulation; some 3 to 4 $\times$ 10^6 cells/24 h/g of primary tumor were shed. Liotta and his colleagues [24], using the T241 fibrosarcoma in mice, showed that as tumors grew, progressively more cancer cells were shed into the circulation. On the fifth post-implantation day 1.4 $\times$ 10^3 cells were released per 24 h; on day 10, 3 $\times$ 10^4 and on day 15, 1.5 $\times$ 10^5 cells. These two sets of data indicate that very large numbers of cancer cells are released into the blood during the natural history of metastasis, and metastases occur some orders of magnitude less frequently than expected if every circulating cancer cell formed one metastasis.

It is well known that circulating cancer cells may be present as both single cells and multicellular clusters; it has also been demonstrated that circulating clusters have a greater chance of generating tumors than single cells [25, 26]. This greater efficiency on the part of the clusters appears in part due to their earlier arrest by impaction in small vessels and partly to the protection of the innermost cells by those at the periphery. Regardless of mechanism, the question arises of whether inefficiency in this phase of metastasis can be explained in terms of proportions of 'efficient' clusters and 'inefficient' single cells. In this respect, the data of Liotta et al. [27] on T241 fibrosarcoma in C57B1 mice are illuminating.

Intravenous injection of 10^3 cells in clumps containing 6 to 7 cells produced 10 times as many pulmonary tumors as 10^3 single cancer cells, and doubling in cluster size doubled the number of tumors. In this system, approximately 65% of the cancer cells were released from the fibrosarcomas as single cells and the remainder were in clusters containing 2 to 3 (20%), 4 to 5 (5%), 6 to 7 (2%) or 8 (5%) or more cancer cells. Some 1.5 $\times$ 10^5 cancer cells were released from these tumors into the circulation each 24 h [24]; therefore if metastases were formed exclusively by cell clusters arrested in the lungs, and if the metastatic process in these animals had 100% efficiency, we might expect very approximately 5 $\times$ 10^4 metastases to be generated per day. In point of fact, a mean of only 17 macroscopic pulmonary metastases developed by the 19th day following tumor implantation. In another study, Liotta et al. [27] showed that following the intravenous injection of 10^3 cancer cells in clusters of 6 to 7 cells, a mean of only 1.75 'metastases' developed by 12 days after injection. Thus, 140 clusters generated 1.75 pulmonary transplants, corresponding to an overall efficiency of less than 1%, this value corresponds to a calculated efficiency of approximately 0.01% following injections of 10^3 single cells. Therefore, although these factors are major considerations in discussions of metastatic inefficiency, they are not the only ones.

5. Metastatic subpopulations

Another possibility to account for metastatic inefficiency is the suggestion that metastases arise exclusively from small, pre-existing subpopulations of cancer cells having a highly metastatic genotype, as distinct from randomly surviving cells released from the primary tumor [28].

The complex problem of subpopulations will not be discussed in depth, since the topic has recently been critically reviewed elsewhere [29]; however, a few salient points can be made within the present context. While there is no doubt that cancer cells in any population exhibit a great deal of heterogeneity, a major problem lies in relating this heterogeneity to naturally occurring metastasis, within the time-frame of the host's life-time. Fidler and his colleagues have cloned cells *in vitro* from B16 melanomas [30] and UV-2237 fibrosarcomas [31] and have unquestionably demonstrated that following intravenous injection into mice, cells grown from some clones produce more or less pulmonary transplants than others.

If metastatic inefficiency is to be explained in terms of metastatic subpopulations, then these subpopulations must represent a minority of the total cancer cell population; however, the experimental evidence does not really support this view. Thus, of 17 B16 sublines described by Fidler [30], nine given rise to more pulmonary tumor colonies following intravenous injection than the parent line, and two of these produce more than 10 times the number of colonies, and in the case of the parental UV-2237 fibrosarcoma and its cloned subpopulations, the incidence of spontaneous metastases was as high or higher with 13 of 17 tumorigenic clones to the UV-2237 fibrosarcoma than in the parent line [32]. Kerbel [33] obtained clones of the anaplastic MDAY-D2 murine cancer, using similar techniques to those of Fidler, and reported that only three of 20 clones examined were less metastatic than the parental line on the basis of the tabulated 'gross' metastatic profiles, but these were unstable *in vitro* and reverted to the metastatic behavior of the parent. This instability *in vitro* may be the key to interpretative problems with these clones. On the one hand, if it is argued that cloning procedures are highly selective for metastatic subpopulations and therefore do not give representative pictures of cancer cell populations, then quantitative inferences cannot be drawn on the importance of pre-existing metastatic subpopulations in spontaneous metastasis. On the other hand, if the cloning procedures do give representative population samples, then metastatic inefficiency cannot be explained in terms of minor, pre-existing metastatic subpopulations, because the data indicate that the majority of cancer cells present in the sampled populations have high metastatic potential.

6. Circulatory trauma

It is generally accepted that cancer cells are damaged in transit from their site of intravasation to their site of arrest, and although some of the causes of circulatory trauma have been identified for some cancers, knowledge of the process is far from complete. Humoral factors possibly contributing to the death of circulating cancer cells include non-immunologic agents and antibodies; the latter are expected to be more important in immunogenic animal tumors than in people. It is often impossible to discriminate between ill-defined immunologic and non-immunologic phenomena in much of the literature [34].

Mechanical trauma is also important in causing death of circulating cancer cells, and the work of Sato and Suzuki [35] emphasizes the cytotoxic effects of the repetitive squeezing of cancer cells through small blood-vessels. Using rat ascites hepatoma cells, these workers demonstrated that 98% of AH100B cells were killed by one pulmonary passage compared with AH66F cells, of which 8% were killed. The former cells were much more resistant to mechanical deformation than the latter. Resistance to deformation is in part dependent on the density of sialic acids in the cell periphery [36] and in some types of cancer cells the surface density of sialic acid approximately doubles around mitotic peak-phase [37, 38]. Thus, it is possible that at this time the resistance to deformation increase, and that circulating cancer cells in this phase of the mitotic cycle are more susceptible to being literally squeezed to death than similar cells in other phases. In addition, changes in cell deformability can follow exposure to proteolytic enzymes and other agents [39]. Thus, in the present context, the existence of transient inefficient metastatic 'compartments' within cancer cell populations should also be considered in addition to relatively fixed genotypic properties.

7. Cancer cell retention

It is a common observation that the majority of cancer cells injected into the tail-veins of rodents are present in the lungs, temporarily attached to the vascular endothelium, for some minutes after injection. However, within a few minutes, detectable numbers of cells begin to be released and, after 24 h, few cells remain. Studies such as these measure cell retention, which is the result of arrest and release. Thus, as metastases can arise only from retained cells, and as the circulation is a hostile environment for released cells, a low metastatic efficiency could be generated by inhibition of arrest and/or promotion of release. It must be emphasized that cell arrest and release are basically different phenomena, that release is not physically the exact reverse of the arrest process and that different experimental techniques must be used to study these two phenomena [40].

8. Cell arrest

Both cancer cells and the vascular endothelium carry a net negative surface charge, and it is therefore inescapable that contact between them should tend to be pre-

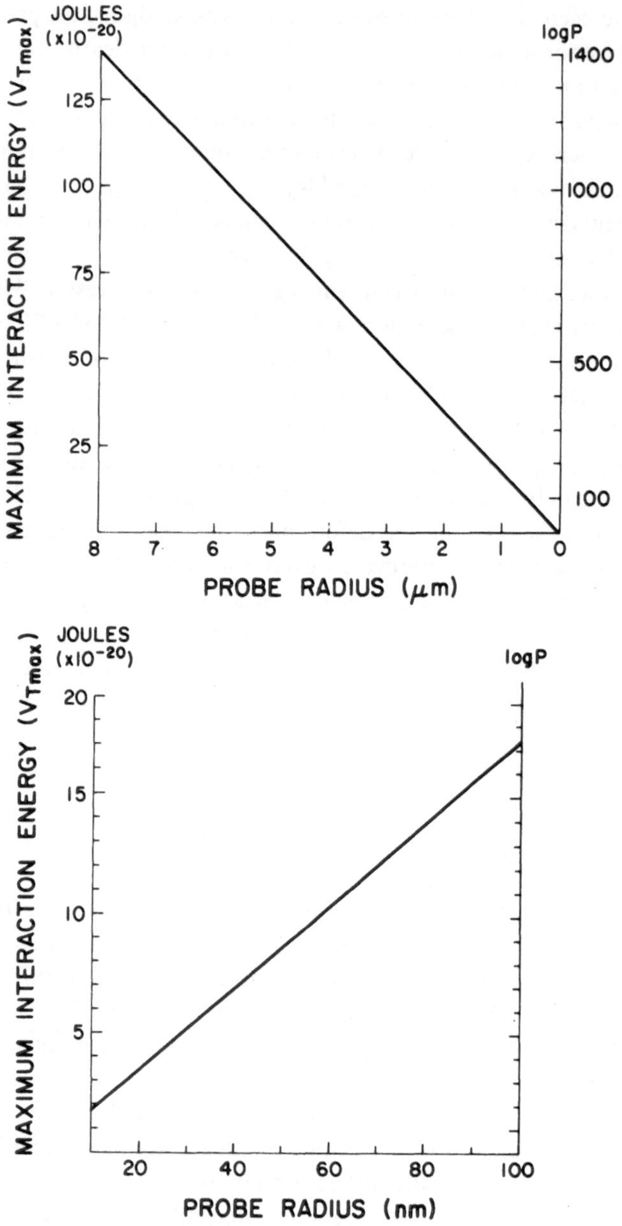

Figure 2. Maximum interaction energies between 'flat' vascular endothelium and cancer cell 'probes' of radii in the range (a) 0 to 8 μm, and (b) to 100 nm.

vented by their mutual electrostatic repulsion. By the use of previously published procedures [41, 42], the magnitudes of these contact-inhibiting, potential energy barriers may be calculated. The chances (p) of contact-making collisions between cancer cells and the vascular endothelium mediated by thermal (Browman) agitation may be estimated from a knowledge of the maximum (total) potential energy barrier (V_{Tmax}) by:

$$p = \exp. (V_{Tmax}/kt) \qquad [43]$$

where k is Boltzmann's constant and T is absolute temperature.

The computations of average maximum total potential energy barriers (V_{Tmax}) shown in Figures 2a and b indicate that as the radii of projections from circulating cancer cells and/or the vascular endothelium decrease, the potential energy barriers between them are expected to decrease. The figures also graphically illustrate that as this barrier to contact diminishes, the chances of collisions between the two surfaces are expected to increase. However, the probabilities are so small that such collisions involving whole cells would indeed be rare events even with repetition. As shown in Figure 2a, in the defined energy situation, in only one out of 10^{1650} attempts is it expected that contact will be established between all of the opposing surfaces of 10 μm radius cancer cells and a flat vascular endothelium. The chances of collisions are further reduced by the boundary 'layers' present at vessel walls, due to velocity profiles across viscous plasma. The chances of collisions would be increased considerably if contact were to be made between regions of cell surfaces carrying less than average charge density, by means of low radius of curvature macromolecular 'hairs' or 'glues.' Thus, as shown in Figure 2b, collisions are expected to occur between a 10 nm probe and the vascular endothelium in one attempt out of 100. Fibronectin may be considered as such a binding agent, and the low levels of fibronectin reported at the peripheries of some cancer cells makes it interesting to speculate that this operational fibronectin-deficiency either inhibits their adhesion to the vascular endothelium altogether, or alternatively results in such an unstable attachment that cancer cells held at the vascular endothelium are easily detached from it by the shear forces generated by the circulating blood, which are greater in the larger vessels. However, as fibronectin bridges between malignant cells and an arrest site could be provided by platelets, endothelial cells, by circulating fibronectin or possibly cold-insoluble globulins, the failure of circulating cancer cells to utilize these sources could indicate a relative deficiency in their fibronectin-receptors as a consequence of deficient synthesis, 'masking' or enzymatic degradation of fibronectin. These various considerations indicate that the energetic barriers hindering contact between cancer cells and vessel walls, dictate that if contact is made at all it must be made initially by structures which are ultimately mechanically weak, leading to relatively frequent release of the arrested cells. This may well be a key to metastatic inefficiency and is deserving of more intensive study.

9. Cell release

Cancer cells introduced into the venous circulation are temporarily arrested in the first organ encountered, and are then gradually released into the circulation. One

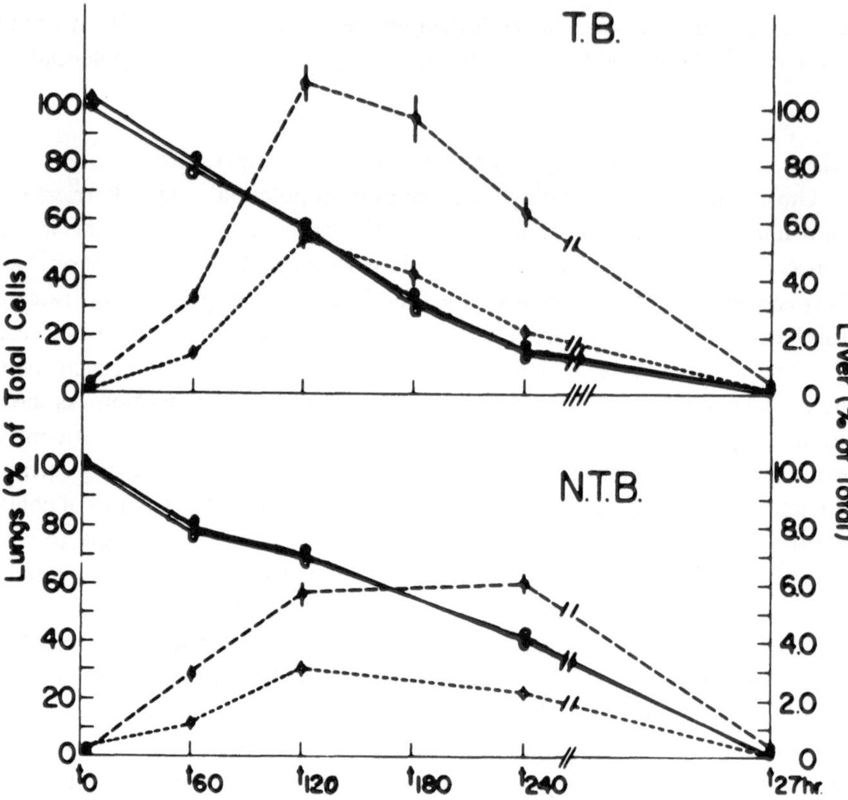

Figure 3. Following tail-vein injections of radio-labeled 4 × 10^6 W-256 cells into tumor-bearing (T.B.) or non-tumor-bearing (N.T.B.) rats, the lungs and livers were removed at the times (minutes) shown on the abscissa and γ-counted, before (lungs, — • —; livers --- • ---) and after (lungs — o —; livers, --- o ---) alcohol extraction, which removes radioactivity not associated with intact cells. The counts are expressed as percentages of the original injected dose as shown on the ordinates. Standard errors are shown for the livers and for the lungs at t_5 (Weiss [45]).

possible consequence of 'first organ encounters' is that cancer cells are processed so that they die before or shortly after arrival in a second organ. This possibility was investigated in a series of experiments [45] in which the lung-to-liver traffic of [^{125}I]dUrd-labelled Walker-256 cancer cells was examined in rats following tail-vein injections where, after 27 h, few cells remained in the lungs. Throughout the experiment, only 2% of the cells in the lungs were non-viable, compared with approximately half of those in the liver (Figure 3); these viability estimates correlated with higher (10:1) incidence of lung transplants over liver transplants following tail-vein injections of unlabelled cancer cells, and with the common observation that natural, extrapulmonary metastases are uncommon in animals carrying this tumor. Direct injections of cancer cells into the liver indicated that the reduced viability of lung-derived cells in this site was not due to an inherently hostile hepatic environment. Injections into and sampling from, other sites indicate that only small proportions of cells were killed on their way to the lungs, during their arrest in the pulmonary capillaries and arterioles, or between the left ventricle, aorta, hepatic artery and liver. By a process of elimination, it was concluded that significant trauma resulting in cancer cell death occurs during the events culminating in their release from temporary arrest sites at the pulmonary vascular endothelium. As the lungs are commonly the first organ encountered by circulating tumor cells, it was suggested that in this host/tumor system at least, the low viability of cells released from the lungs contributes to metastatic inefficiency.

Some clue to the mechanisms of cell release comes from *in vitro* experiments in which cell detachment was shown to be enhanced by agents activating lysosomes including non-cytotoxic antisera [46] and endotoxin [47]; this enhancement was abrogated by the lysosomal stabilizer hydrocortisone. *In vivo* experiments are more difficult to interpret since bacterial endotoxins affect a number of key homeostatic mechanisms including activation of coagulation and complement systems and enhancement of fibrinolysis and stimulation of the secretory and phagocytic activities of reticuloendothelial cells; in addition, glucocorticoids also have wide-ranging pharmacologic effects, many of which counteract those of endotoxin. Nonetheless, it is of considerable interest that on the one hand, Glaves [48] has shown that endotoxin-induced stimulation of the reticuloendothelial system (RES) markedly increases the release of previously arrested cancer cells from the lungs of tumor-bearing mice, resulting in the decreased incidence of lung tumors. On the other hand, Fidler and Lieber [49] and Glaves and Weiss [50] have shown that glucocorticoids alone decrease the release of arrested cancer from the lungs, and increase the incidence of lung tumors. Glaves and Weiss [50] have also demonstrated that in mice treated with both endotoxin and triamcinolone acetonide, after the arrest of intravenously injected B16 melanoma, nullified the endotoxin-induced, increased release of cancer cells from the lungs.

If the hypothesis is correct that proteinases play a key role in promoting the release of arrested cells from the vascular endothelium thereby contributing to

Table 2. Effects of aprotinin on metastasis from Lewis lung tumors and on retention of LL cells following I.V.I. [51].

	Aprotinin = treated	Controls
Mean numbers (± S.E. (no. of obs.)) of lung metastases from s.c. tumors after 21 days	69.2 ± 4.4 [29]3	43.9 ± 3.4 [29]
% Retention of I.V.I. of radio-labeled cells after 6 h in lungs of tumor-bearing mice	17.0 ± 2.5 [14]**	7.6 ± 1.1 [14]

* $p < 0.001$.
** $0.01 > p > 0.001$.

metastatic inefficiency, then appropriate antiproteinases should have an opposite effect. Experiments made by Turner and Weiss [51] on the effects of the antiproteinase aprotinin, on mice bearing subcutaneous Lewis lung tumors which are summarized in Table 2, show that compared with appropriate controls, mice receiving intraperitoneal injections of 5000 KIU aprotinin on 14 consecutive days following tumor implantation developed significantly more lung metastases by 21 days. In addition, in mice receiving intravenous injections of radiolabeled cells, a single intravenous injection of 5000 KIU aprotinin significantly increased the numbers of cells retained in both the lungs and liver when measurements were made 6 h later.

The roles of fibrinogenesis and fibrinolysis in this phase of metastasis are complex; the literature which is often confusing and contradictory has been critically reviewed elsewhere [52]. Although the initial arrest of cancer cells at the vascular endothelium of mice was unaffected by agents inhibiting thrombin production, platelet release reactions and fibrin formation [Table 3; 53], the temporary deposition of fibrin arround arrested emboli tends to both stabilize their adhesion and retard their release [54]. The fibrin cocoon investing such emboli also appears to provide protection for the cancer cells from humoral agents. In contrast to fibrinogenesis, fibrinolysis may be regarded as a component of host-defense, which contributes to metastatic inefficiency by abrogation of the generally cancer-cell protective effects of fibrinogenesis. By virtue of their own plasminogen activators, in addition to their host's contribution to fibrinolysis, cancer cells may thus contribute to their own destruction. Therefore, although it is fashionable to regard all attributes of cancer cells as contributing positively to expressions of their malignancy, this view is probably naive.

By acting as sources of proteolytic enzymes, cancer cells themselves, vascular endothelial cells and RES cells can promote the release of arrested cancer cells; this may be an example of a host defense mechanism of vascular- 'purging'. Since both macrophages and polymorphs can induce contact-mediated destruction of cancer cells, and macrophage-induced cytolysis may be enhanced by endotoxins [55] and depressed by glucocorticoids [56], the RES appears to be responsible for the concomitant release and destruction of arrested cancer cells.

Table 3. Effects of anticoagulants on lung localization in mice of ^{125}IdUrd-labeled tumor cells one hour after injection [53].

	TA3 carcinoma percent dose		Gardner lymphosarcoma percent dose	
	Treated	Control	Treated	Control
Aspirin	98.5 ± 2.3	98.4 ± 2.1	44.3 ± 6.2	38.9 ± 0.5
Heparin	87.2 ± 4.4	92.0 ± 1.5	69.9 ± 4.1	64.8 ± 3.6
Warfarin	93.4 ± 1.7	96.0 ± 2.0	62.1 ± 4.4	66.8 ± 2.4

10 to 14 animals for each observation.

10. Micrometastases

A proportion of cells retained in the microvasculature grow into micrometastases which may progress into metastases. Although the factors influencing the development or non-development of micrometastases are not well understood, this has the potential to be the terminal limiting factor in metastatic inefficiency.

It is not entirely satisfactory to discriminate between covert micrometastases and overt metastases exclusively on the basis of size, since with improvement of diagnostic techniques lesions which would have been labeled as covert a few years ago can now be visualized. A more operational definition of micrometastases is that of lesions obtaining their nutrition by diffusion, rather than by their own blood supply. The importance of vascularization in controlling tumor proliferation was elegantly demonstrated by experiments in which tumor fragments were implanted in the vitreous humor of experimental animals [57]. The tumors grew very slowly for some weeks as non-vascularized cell aggregates, which eventually made contact with the retinal blood-vessels, became vascularized, and then grew rapidly. Thus, in the present context, factors promoting vascularization (the tumor angiogenic factors, TAF) are expected to contribute to the conversion of micrometastases to metastases, while those factors inhibiting TAF and hence the conversion, contribute to metastatic inefficiency.

In purely descriptive terms, a refractory micrometastasis can be said to be in the *dormant* state. It is usually impossible to distinguish between cells arrested in the so-called Go state, or in the pseudodormant state where cell loss matches cell proliferation. In either case, activation of these micrometastases from their dormant state poses a constant therapeutic problem.

Although the effects of TAF can be abrogated *in vitro* by xenogeneic antiserum [58] or by the direct action of somewhat ill-defined extracts of cartilage [59], at present there is no direct evidence for the *in vivo* activity of antiangiogenesis factors, unless the occurrence of dormant tumors themselves is unwarrantably interpreted exclusively in terms of angiogenesis.

In tumor-bearing animals, removal of their primary cancers and immunosuppression sometimes results in the abrupt manifestation of metastases, leading to the suggestion that immunologic interactions contribute to the maintenance of dormancy [60]. If it is assumed that the establishment of micrometastases occurs early in the history of cancer, while any immune response is still partially effective, then it is not unreasonable to suggest that further growth of these lesions can occur in the immunodepressed host, particularly if the cancer cells in the micrometastases contain much less tumor-associated antigen than those in the primary cancer [61]. However, if the argument is accepted that immune response to human cancer is negligible, then the results of these experiments with immunogenic tumors are irrelevant to humans.

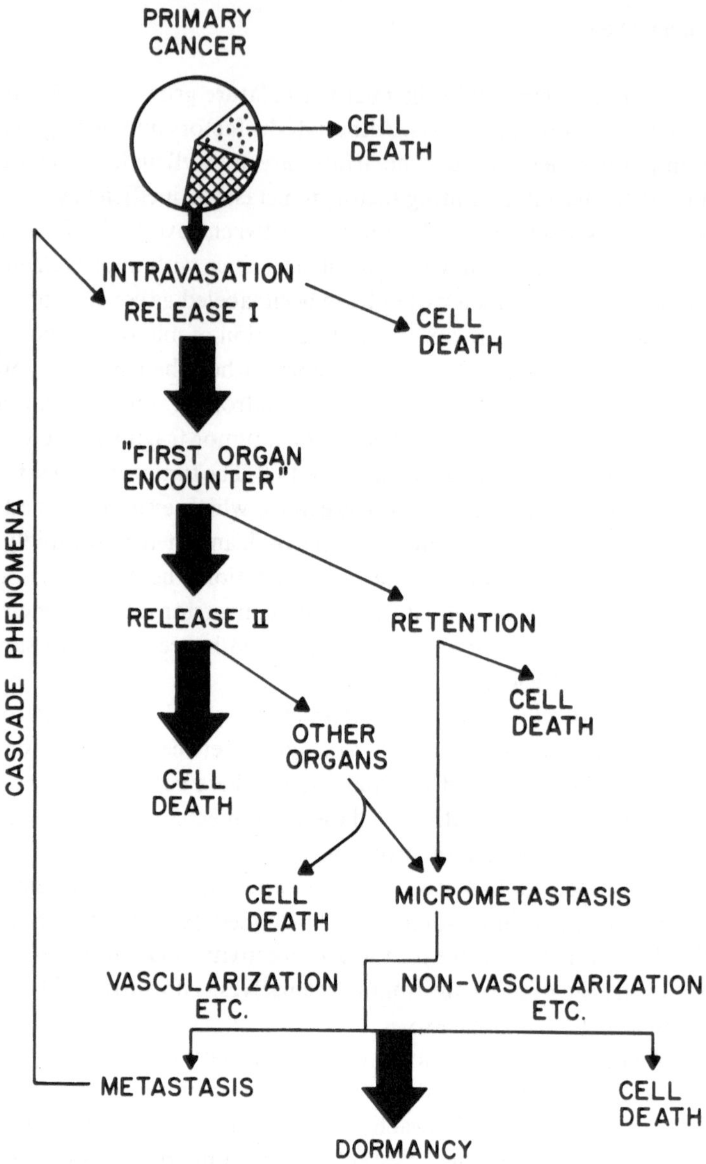

Figure 4. Metastatic inefficiency. The main pathways in metastasis lead to death or dormancy in cancer cells. (From Weiss [52], with permission.)

11. Metastatic patterns

In considering the distribution of metastases from cancer of the breast, Paget in 1889 [62] was the first to write in English on questions posed earlier by Langenbeck, Billroth and Fuchs, namely: 'What is it that decides what organs shall suffer in a case of disseminated cancer? ... When a plant goes to seed, its seeds are carried in all directions; but they can only live and grow on congenial soil.' In terms of metastatic inefficiency, the focus on the 'seed and soil' theory is on the nature of uncongenial soil!

A non-exclusive alternative to the 'seed and soil' hypothesis is the hemodynamic or mechanical hypothesis, which states that the frequency of metastases in organs is determined by their arterial blood-supply since this determines the dose of cancer cells delivered [63]. By the use of recent physiologic data on organ arterial blood-flow derived from non-invasive measurements, correlations significant to the 4 to 8% levels were obtained between organ blood-flow per gram and metastatic frequency in eight organs from primary carcinomas of the esophagus, pancreas, colon and rectum. However, in nine of ten primary cancers with initial venous drainage into the superior or inferior vena cava, no correlations were obtained. Thus, regardless of explanation, for some primary cancers with an appropriate transit history, metastatic inefficiency after retention is apparently similar for some gastrointestinal cancer cells in a number of different organs, since the frequency of the development of overt metastases in them correlates with the dose of cancer cells delivered in the arterial blood [64].

12. Conclusions

If the criterion for success of the metastatic process is reasonably considered to be the development of overt metastases, then in terms of the total numbers of involved cancer cells, it is indeed an inefficient process. Thus, Figure 1 may be redrawn to indicate metastatic inefficiency in a proportional flow-chart for the majority of cancer cells involved in each step of the process, whereas as shown in Figure 4, each of these designated steps terminates in cell death or dormancy.

References

1. Klastersky J, Daneau D, Verhest A: Causes of death in patients with cancer. Eur J Cancer 8:149–154, 1972.
2. Inagaki J, Rodriquez V, Bodey GP: Causes of death in cancer patients. Cancer 33:568–573, 1974.
3. Ambrus JL, Ambrus CM, Mink IB, Pickren JW: Causes of death in cancer patients. J Med 6:61–64, 1975.
4. Piver MS, Yazigi R, Blumenson L, Tsukada Y: A prospective trial comparing hysterectomy, hysterectomy plus vaginal radium, and uterine radium plus hysterectomy in stage I endometrial carcinoma. Obstet Gynecol 54:85–89, 1979.
5. Piver MS, Barlow JJ, Lele SB: Incidence of subclinical metastasis in stage I and II ovarian carcinoma. Obstet Gynecol 52:100–104, 1978.
6. Castaldo TW, Petrilli ES, Ballon SC, Berman ML: Lymph-node metastases from epithelial carcinoma of the ovary. In: Lymphatic system metastasis, Weiss L, Gilbert HA, Ballon SC (eds). Boston: G.K. Hall and Co., 1980, pp 383–389.

7. Costanza ME, Dayal Y, Binder S, Nathanson L: Metastatic basal cell carcinoma. Cancer 34:230–235, 1974.
8. Farmer ER, Helwig EB: Metastatic basal cell carcinoma: a clinicopathologic study of seventeen cases. Cancer 46:748–757, 1980.
9. Lohe KJ: Early squamous cell carcinoma of the uterine cervix. I. Definition and histology. Gynecol Oncol 6:10–30, 1978.
10. Sedlis A, Sall S, Tsukada Y, Park R, Mangan C, Shingleton H, Blessing JA: Microinvasive carcinoma of the uterine cervix: a clinical-pathologic study. Am J Obstet Gynecol 133:64–74, 1979.
11. Lohe KJ: Early squamous cell carcinoma of the uterine cervix. III. Frequency of lymph node netastases. Gynecol Oncol 6:51–59, 1978.
12. Roche WD, Norris HJ: Microinvasive carcinoma of the cervix. Cancer 36:180–186, 1975.
13. Cole WH, Roberts SS, Webb RS, Strehl FW, Oates GD: Dissemination of cancer with special emphasis on vascular spread and implantation. Ann Surg 161:753–768, 1965.
14. Goldmann EE: Anatomische Untersuchungen über die verbreitungsweise bösartiger Geschwülste. Beitr z klin Chir (Tübingen) 18:595–612, 1897.
15. Iwasaki T: Histological and experimental observations on the destruction of tumour cells in the blood vessels. J Pathol Bacteriol 20:85–105, 1915.
16. Schmidt MB: Die Verbreitungswege der Karzinome und die Beziehung generalisierter Sarkome zu den leukämischen Neubildungen. Jena: G. Fischer, 1903.
17. Takahashi M: An experimental study of metastasis. J Pathol Bacteriol 20:1–13, 1915.
18. Saphir O: The fate of carcinoma emboli in the lung. Am J Pathol 23:245–254, 1947.
19. Weiss L, Glaves D: Arrest patterns of circulating lymphosarcoma cell in tumour-bearing mice as modified by previously injected cell suspensions. Br J Cancer 37:363–368, 1978.
20. Weiss L, Holmes J, Crispe IN: The effects of a prior injection of Walker cancer cells in the rat on the lung-retention pattern of a second dose. Br J Cancer 40:483–488, 1979.
21. Hewitt HB: Projecting from animal experiments to clinical cancer. In: Fundamental aspects of metastasis, Weiss L (ed). Amsterdam: N. Holland/American Elsevier, 1976, pp 343–358.
22. Hewitt HB: The choice of animal tumors for experimental studies of cancer therapy. Adv Cancer Res 27:149–200, 1978.
23. Butler TP, Gullino PM: Quantitation of cell shedding into efferent blood of mammary adenocarcinoma. Cancer Res 35:512–516, 1975.
24. Liotta LA, Kleinerman J, Saidel GM: Quantitative relationships of intravascular tumor cells, tumor vessels, and pulmonary metastases following tumor implantation. Cancer Res 34:997–1004, 1974.
25. Watanabe S: Metastasizability of tumor cells. Cancer 7:215, 1954.
26. Fidler IJ: The relationship of embolic homogeneity, number, size and viability to the incidence of experimental metastasis. Eur J Cancer 9:223–227, 1973.
27. Liotta LA, Kleinerman J, Saidel GM: The significance of hematogenous tumor cell clumps in the metastatic process. Cancer Res 36:889–894, 1976.
28. Fidler IJ, Kripke ML: Metastasis results from pre-existing variant cells within a malignant tumor. Science 197:893–895, 1977.
29. Weiss L: Metastasis: Differences between cancer cells in primary and secondary tumors. Pathobiol Annu 10:51–58, 1980.
30. Fidler IJ: The heterogeneity of metastatic neoplasms. In: Pulmonary metastasis, Weiss L, Gilbert HA (eds). Boston: G.K. Hall, 1978, pp 43–61.
31. Kripke ML, Gruys E, Fidler IJ: Metastatic keterogeneity of cells from an ultraviolet light-induced murine fibrosarcoma of recent origin. Cancer Res 38:2962–2967, 1978.
32. Fidler IJ: Cifone MA: Properties of metastatic and nonmetastatic cloned subpopulations of an ultraviolet-light-induced murine fibrosarcoma of recent origin. Am J Pathol 97:633–648, 1979.
33. Kerbel RS: Immunologic studies of membrane mutants of a highly metastatic murine tumor. Am J Pathol 97:609–622, 1979.
34. Weiss L: Factors leading to the arrest of cancer cells in the lungs. In: Pulmonary metastasis, Weiss L,

Gilbert HA (eds). Boston: G.K. Hall, 1978, pp 5–25.

35. Sato H, Suzuki M: Deformability and viability of tumor cells by transcapillary passage, with reference to organ affinity in metastasis in cancer. In: Fundamental aspects of metastasis, Weiss L (ed). Amsterdam: North-Holland, 1976, pp 311–317.
36. Weiss L: Studies on cell deformability. I. Effect of surface charge. J Cell Biol 26:735–739, 1965.
37. Mayhew E: Cellular electrophoretic mobility and the mitotic cycle. J Gen Physiol 49:717–725, 1966.
38. Glick MC, Gerner EW, Warren L: Changes in the carbohydrate content of the KB cell during the growth cycle. J Cell Physiol 77:1–6, 1971.
39. Weiss L: Cell deformability: some general considerations. In: Fundamental aspects of metastasis, Weiss L (ed). Amsterdam: North-Holland, 1976, pp 305–310.
40. Weiss L: The cell periphery, metastasis and other contact phenomena. Amsterdam: North-Holland, 1967.
41. Weiss L: Biophysical aspects of initial cell interactions with solid surfaces. Fed Proc 30:1649–1657, 1971.
42. Weiss L, Harlos JP: Cell contact phenomena and their implication in cell communication. In: Intercellular communication, DeMello WC (ed). New York: Plenum Press, 1977, pp 33–59.
43. Verwey EJW and Overbeck JTG: Theory of the stability of lyophobic colloids. Amsterdam: Elsevier, 1948, p 164 et seq.
44. Weiss L, Nir S, Harlos JP, Subjeck JR: Long-distance interactions between Ehrlich ascites tumour cells. J Theor Biol 51:439–454, 1975.
45. Weiss L: Cancer cell traffic from the lungs to the liver: an example of metastatic inefficiency. Int J Cancer 25:385–392, 1980.
46. Weiss L: Studies on cell adhesion in tissue-culture. VIII. Some effects of antisera on cell detachment. Exp Cell Res 37:540–551, 1965.
47. Neiders ME, Weiss L: The effects of endotoxin on cell detachment in vitro. Arch Oral -Biol 18:499–504, 1973.
48. Glaves D: Metastasis: reticuloendothelial system and organ retention of disseminated malignant cells. Int J Cancer 26:115–122, 1980.
49. Fidler IJ, Lieber S: Quantitative analysis of the mechanism of glucocorticoid enhancement of experimental metastasis. Res Commun Chem Pathol Pharmacol 4:607–613, 1972.
50. Glaves D, Weiss L: Metastasis and the reticuloendothelial system. II. Effect of triamcinolone acetonide on organ retention of malignant cells in endotoxin-treated mice. Int J Cancer 27:475–479, 1981.
51. Turner GA, Weiss L: An analysis of aprotinin-induced enhancement of metastasis of Lewis lung tumors in mice. Cancer Res 41:2576–2580, 1981.
52. Weiss L: Metastatic inefficiency. In: Liver metastasis, Weiss L, Gilbert HA (eds). Boston: G.K. Hall, 1982, pp 126–157.
53. Glaves D, Weiss L: Initial tumor cell arrest in animals of defined coagulative status. Int J Cancer 21:741–746, 1978.
54. Chew EC, Josephson RL, Wallace AC: Morphologic aspects of the arrest of circulating cancer cells. In: Fundamental aspects of metastasis, Weiss L (ed). Amsterdam: North-Holland, 1976, pp 121–150.
55. Ruco LP, Meltzer MS: Macrophage activation for tumor cytotoxicity. Tumoricidal activity by macrophages from C3H/HeJ mice requires at least two activation stimuli. Cell Immunol 41:35–51, 1978.
56. Gallily R, Eliahy H: Mechanism and specificity of macrophage mediated cytotoxicity. Cell Immunol 25:245–255, 1976.
57. Brem H, Folkman J: Inhibition of tumor angiogenesis mediated by cartilage. J Exp Med 141:427–439, 1975.
58. Phillips PJ, Kumar S: Tumour angiogenesis factor (TAF) and its neutralisation by xenogenic antiserum. Int J Cancer 23:82–89, 1979.

59. Kuettner K and Pauli BU: Resistance of cartilage to invasion. In: Bone metastasis, Weiss L, Gilbert HA (eds). Boston: G.K. Hall, 1981, pp 131–167.
60. Alexander P: Dormant metastases which manifest on immunosuppression and the role of macrophages in tumours. In: Fundamental aspects of metastasis, Weiss L (ed). New York: American Elsevier Publ. Co., 1976, pp 227–239.
61. Wheelock EF, Goldstein LT, Weinhold KJ, Carney WP, Marx PA: The tumor dormant state. In: Cancer invasion and metastasis: biologic mechanisms and therapy, Day SB, et al. (eds). New York: Raven Press, 1977, pp 105–116.
62. Paget S: The distribution of secondary growth in cancer of the breast. Lancet i:571–573, 1889.
63. Ewing J: Metastasis. In: Neoplastic diseases, Saunders WB. Philadelphia, 1928, 3rd Ed.
64. Weiss L, Haydock K, Pickren JW, Lane WW: Organ vascularity and metastatic frequency. Am J Pathol 101:101–113, 1980.

7. Tumor cell chemotaxis

J. VARANI and P.A. WARD

1. Introduction

Recent evidence from several laboratories has clearly demonstrated that neoplastic cells (as well as normal, non-leukocytic cells such as fibroblasts) are capable of responding to chemotactic factors *in vitro*. In many respects the responses of these cells are similar to the responses of polymorphonuclear leukocytes (PMN). It has been postulated that the mechanism accounting for the localization of tumor cells at metastatic foci *in vivo* is similar to the process by which leukocytes localize at sites of inflammatory responses. In this chapter we will review some of the more recent findings in the field of tumor cell chemotaxis. Particular emphasis will be placed on describing similarities between chemotactic responses of tumor cells and leukocytes – in so far as this may allow for inferences about the tumor cell response. Finally, we will present evidence that suggests tumor cell chemotactic factors influence the biological behavior of tumor cells *in vivo*.

2. Responses of tumor cells to chemotactic factors

2.1. *Sources of chemotactic factors for tumor cells*

2.1.1. Tumor tissue. Several factors have been discovered in the past decade which are capable of inducing directed (or chemotactic) motility of tumor cells *in vitro*. The first factor to be identified was discovered by Hayashi and his coworkers in 1970 [1, 2]. The factor was obtained from extracts of solid tumor tissue. After purification, the chemotactic factor behaved as a protein with a molecular weight of approximately 70 000 dalton. Subsequent work suggested that the purified material contained at least two distinct chemotactic factors – one that was identical to the originally-defined factor and a second small molecular weight (14 000 dalton), non-protein factor. A number of different tumor cells derived from rats, mice and humans responded to these factors although PMNs did not.

2.1.2. The fifth complement component. A second chemotactic factor for tumor cells was discovered by Romualdez and Ward [3, 4]. The fifth component of complement (C5) – a major source of chemotactic peptides for leukocytes – was identified as the

L.A. Liotta and I.R. Hart (eds.), Tumor Invasion and Metastasis. ISBN-13: 978-94-009-7513-2.
© 1982 Martinus Nijhoff Publishers, The Hague/Boston/London.

source of this tumor cell chemotactic factor. The tumor cell chemotactic factor could be obtained by protease treatment of zymosan-activated normal human serum or by proteolysis of purified C5 or C5a, the latter being isolated from human serum. The chemotactic factor could also be generated from the serum of several different species of animals including rats, mice and rabbits. It could be generated in the serum from rabbits deficient in the sixth complement component but not from the serum of C5-deficient (B10.D2, OSN) mice. Nor could the chemotactic factor be generated from purified preparations of the third complement component (C3) [3–7].

Several studies have shown that the tumor cell chemotactic factor is chemically related to, and may be derived from, the C5-derived chemotactic factor for leukocytes. Both leukocyte chemotactic factor-rich fractions of zymosan-activated serum and purified C5a (the major C5-derived leukocyte chemotactic factor) serve as suitable substrates for the generation of the tumor cell chemotactic factor. Limited proteolytic digestion of either substrate results in generation of the tumor cell chemotactic factor. As digestion proceeds, chemotactic activity for tumor cells is generated in parallel with the loss of leukocyte chemotactic activity. Excessive proteolysis results in degradation of generated chemotactic activity. Based on gel-filtration data, the peptide with chemotactic activity for tumor cells appears to have a molecular weight of approximately 6000 dalton. This would suggest that the tumor cell chemotactic peptide consists of approximately one-half of the C5a molecule [4–6]. The tumor cell chemotactic peptide stimulates a half-maximal response in the Boyden Chamber assay in appropriate tumor cells at doses as low as 10^{-12} M(6), making the peptide one of the most biologically active peptides derived from the complement system.

2.1.3. Bone resorption factor. A third chemotactic factor for tumor cells has been identified in the supernatant fluids from cultures of resorbed bone [8]. Culture fluids from fetal rodent long bones induced to undergo resorption with a number of agents (parathyroid hormone, prostaglandin E_1 or the culture supernatant fluid from Walker carcinosarcoma cells) acquire high levels of the chemotactic activity for tumor cells. The concentration of activity in the supernatant fluids is independent of the mediator of bone resorption but is directly related to the extent of resorption. The bone-derived chemotactic factor has not been highly purified or identified. It is, however, heat labile and has an apparent molecular weight of 6000 dalton based on gel filtration studies [9]. This factor seems to be unrelated to the chemotactic factor derived form C5 since none of this activity can be suppressed with antibody to C5.

2.1.4. Synthetic tripeptides. It has recently been shown that the synthetic tripeptide, N-formyl-methionyl-leucyl-phenylalanine (f-met-leu-phe), a peptide with chemotactic activity for PMNs also has chemotactic activity for several tumor cell types [10, 11]. In further studies it has been found that certain other di-, tri- and tetrapeptides containing the same amino acids lack chemotactic activity when tested with the tumor cells that respond to f-met-leu-phe.

In summary, several factors have been identified that induce the directed migration of tumor cells as defined *in vitro* by the Boyden Chamber assay. The factors that are chemotactic for tumor cells bear no apparent functional relationship to one another. Furthermore, there is no direct relationship between chemotactic activity for tumor cells and chemotactic activity for leukocytes. In the case of the synthetic tripeptide, f-met-leu-phe, the same peptide is chemotactic for PMNs [12] and for tumor cells. The C5-derived tumor cell chemotactic peptide on the other hand is not chemotactic for leukocytes but is similar to, and probably derived from, the C5-related leukocyte chemotactic factor [4–6]. Supernatant fluids from cultures of resorbed bone, which have tumor cell chemotactic activity also contain a chemotactic activity for human monocytes but not for PMNs [13]. Finally, the tumor cell chemotactic factor isolated from tumor tissue extracts has no effect on PMNs.

It is essential to keep in mind that just as the various types of leukocytes do not all respond to the same chemotactic factors, neither do all tumor cell types respond to each of the currently-known tumor cell chemotactic factors. It would seem essential, in fact, for there to be some selectivity if responsiveness has any biological importance *in vivo*.

2.2. *In vitro response of tumor cells to chemotactic factors*

Tumor cells respond to chemotactic factors by demonstrating directed migration in the Boyden Chamber assay. Indeed, responsiveness in this assay is the functional definition of chemotaxis. Using the Walker 256 carcinosarcoma cells it has been shown that the chemotactic response is dose dependent, falls off at concentrations of chemotactic factor that are above the optimal dose and fits the typical Zigmond-Hirsch checkerboard pattern [5], i.e., the cells demonstrate increased motility in the presence of the chemotactic factor regardless of whether or not there is a gradient present but the maximum response is seen in the presence of a gradient. Several other tumor cell types including those of rodent and human origin also respond in the Boyden chamber assay [2, 3, 5, 14, 15]. In addition, normal non-leukocytic cells such as fibroblasts have also been shown capable of responding to chemotactic factors in the Boyden chamber assay [16, 18].

With regard to the mechanism of tumor cell response to chemotactic factors, this appears to be similar to the response observed with human or rabbit PMNs. Using leukocytes it has been shown that directed migration in response to chemotactic factors is only one of several functional responses of the cells. Additional, parallel responses of leukocytes to chemotactic stimuli include an increase in cell-substrate adhesiveness and cell-cell aggregation [19–21], release of lysozomal enzymes [22], cell swelling [20, 21] and the generation of oxygen-free radicals [23]. It has been proposed that these functional responses are important parts of the leukocyte response to inflammatory stimuli. Particularly with regard to cell-cell aggregation and cell-substrate adhesiveness, these responses may contribute to the ability of the cells to localize at sites of inflammation.

Until recently, very little was known about the response of tumor cells to chemotactic factors. Recent work, however, has shown that some of the same responses that occur in leukocytes also occur in tumor cells when they come in contact with chemotactic factors. For example, tumor cells undergo a temporary change in cell size [10, 11] during chemotactic factor stimulation. The temporary alteration in cell size can be measured using a particle counter with a mean cell volume analyzer. When the Walker 256 carcinosarcoma cells are examined in this way the average cell volume increases by approximately 20%. The response is rapid (the maximum change is observed between 0–2 min) and is readily reversible. Tumor cell types other than the Walker carcinosarcoma cells that respond in the Boyden Chamber assay also demonstrate cell volume changes upon contact with the chemotactic peptide [11]. The swelling response in the tumor cells appears to be qualitatively and quantitatively similar to that described by O'Flaherty et al. [21, 24, 25] who described changes in leukocyte volume following exposure to chemotactic stimuli.

A major difference between the response of leukocytes and tumor cells is that the cell swelling response in leukocytes is accompanied by the formation of cell-cell aggregates [21, 24, 25] while it appears that cell-cell aggregation of tumor cells does not occur as a consequence of chemotactic factor stimulation [10, 11]. Although no evidence for the formation of tumor cell aggregates can be found using methods which are satisfactory for identifying aggregate formation in leukocytes, the formation of short-lived tumor cell aggregates cannot be ruled out. The formation of leukocyte aggregates in response to chemotactic factors *in vitro* is possibly related to the mechanism accounting for the neutropenia observed in animals treated with chemotactic factors *in vivo* [21]. The neutropenia is accompanied by a temporary localization of the leukocytes in the vascular bed of the lungs. It would be interesting if similar observations could be made with tumor cells.

Although no evidence exists to suggest that tumor cell aggregation occurs, it has recently been discovered that chemotactic factor-treated tumor cells do show increased adherence to foreign surfaces [27]. This has been demonstrated using the nylon fiber assay described by MacGregor et al. [28]. In this assay, treated or untreated tumor cells are added to prewashed columns of nylon fibers and allowed to adhere for 1–3 min. Following this the nonadherent cells are washed through and counted. Table 1 summarizes the known responses of tumor cells to chemotactic factors.

Because it is easy to see how increased adhesiveness, if it occurs *in vivo*, could influence tumor cell localization, our laboratory is making a major effort to characterize this response. We have found in studies to date that a number of cell types adhere to the nylon fibers in the absence of chemotactic factors. These include chemotactically responsive cells such as the Walker carcinosarcoma cells and the murine fibrosarcoma cells as well as the chemotactically nonresponsive normal fibroblasts. Since the Walker cells grow as ascites cells in rats or in suspension in culture while the fibroblasts and fibrosarcoma cells grow as substrate-attached monolayers, there appears to be no relationship between adherence in the nylon

Table 1. Responses of tumor cells to chemotactic factors.

Response	How demonstrated	Characteristics	References
Chemotaxis	Boyden chamber assay	Up to 50% increase in the number of cell migrating into 12 micropore diameter nitrocellulose filters	3–5
Cell swelling	Particle counter assay	Reversible drop in cell count (45%) accompanied by an increase in mean cell volume (20%). No evidence of 2 and 3 cell aggregates	10, 11
Adherence	Nylon fiber assay	Increased adherence to nylon fibers of up to 50%.	26

fiber assay and the attachment to and growth as monolayers on plastic or glass.

The conditions under which the cells are assayed greatly affects the results. In the presence of serum-free Hanks' balanced salt solution (or serum-free culture medium) the percentage of adhering cells is normally between 15 and 25%. When a chemotactic factor is added to a suspension of responsive cells, the number of adhering cells increases to 40–45%. Nonresponsive cells do not show this increase. In the presence of a small amount of serum (0.1–1.0%) the number of cells that will adhere in the absence of chemotactic factor falls nearly to zero. However, when a chemotactic factor is added to a suspension of responsive cells in the presence of serum, 15–20% of the cells adhere. In terms of absolute numbers of adhering cells, this value is just about the same as that obtained in the absence of serum.

Chemotactic factor-induced adherence to nylon fibers depends on the proper ionic milieu. When Ca^{++} and Mg^{++} are omitted from the suspending medium, the percentage of cells specifically adhering in response to the chemotactic factor decreases by about half. The addition of EDTA or EGTA (a Ca^{++} specific chelator) to Ca^{++} and Mg^{++}-free medium causes the number of adhering cells to fall nearly to zero. The findings suggest that Ca^{++} and Mg^{++} are required for optimal chemotactic factor-induced adherence but that traces of the ions may be sufficient.

These results are in generally good agreement with the results of similar studies in which leukocytes were used. It has been reported that optimal responsiveness to chemotactic factors in the Boyden Chamber assay and in the nylon fiber adherence assay require the presence of both Ca^{++} and Mg^{++} [28–34]. More work will need to be done before it can be determined how closely leukocytes and tumor cells compare in their requirements for divalent cations.

Certain inhibitors have been examined for effects on the adherence response. These include 2-deoxyglucose, which interferes with glucose metabolism; cychloheximide, a protein synthesis inhibitor; colchicine, a microtubule disrupting agent and cytochalasin B, an agent which interferes with microfilaments. When 10^{-3} M 2-

deoxyglucose was added to the suspending medium (Hanks' balanced salt solution without glucose), chemotactic factor-induced adherence was almost completely inhibited. The dramatic effect is similar to what we have reported previously in the Boyden Chamber and cell swelling assays with the tumor cells [10, 11]. In contrast, cychloheximide did not inhibit the adherence response. Both colchicine and cytochalasin B inhibited the adherence response at high concentrations (10^{-5} M) but had no effect or slightly potentiated the response at lower doses.

The demonstration that chemotactic factors can increase the adhesiveness of responding cells may be a significant finding since several recent studies in other model systems suggest a correlation between high adhesiveness and malignancy. With the high and low metastatic variants of the B16 melanoma tumor isolated by Fidler [35], a correlation has been found between metastatic capability (after intravenous injection of the cells) and ability of the cells to adhere to normal lymphoid cells from syngeneic animals, to lung tissue cells from syngeneic animals and to monolayers of unrelated tumor cells [36–39]. The cells with high metastatic behavior adhered more rapidly and to a greater extent to each of the other cell types than did the low metastatic cells. When injected intravenously, a greater proportion of the cells with high metastatic behavior were found to remain localized in the lungs of the recipient animals, subsequently forming a greater number of tumors in these animals.

In a separate study it has been shown that treatment of tumor cells with agents such as colchicine and cytochalasin B reduces both their ability to adhere to substrates *in vitro* and their ability to localize and form tumors in the lungs of syngeneic mice after intravenous injection [40].

In studies carried out by Hart [41], Briles and Kornfeld [42] and Varani et al. [43–47] correlations have been found between malignancy and adhesiveness as indicated by resistance of cells to removal from surfaces of plastic dishes. The cells used by Briles and Kornfeld were selected on the basis of resistance to EDTA-induced release from plastic dishes. Subsequently, the more resistant cells were found to form more lung tumors after intravenous injection than were the less resistant cells [42]. Hart, on the other hand, selected cells on the basis of altered invasive and metastatic capacity and subsequently showed that the cells with high invasive and metastatic capacity were the most resistant to removal from plastic dishes with trypsin [41].

In studies carried out by Varani et al. [15, 43–47] a subpopulation of murine fibrosarcoma cells was isolated from an uncloned parent culture by repeated passage in medium supplemented with human serum. Several clones of cells were eventually isolated in this way. When compared to the parent population or to clones of cells obtained from tumors induced in syngeneic mice following injection of the parent cells, the human serum adapted cells were found to be much less malignant. They formed many fewer tumors after injection of 1×10^5 cells into the footpad (20% vs 100%) than did the parent or high malignant cells and did not spontaneously metastasize in striking contrast to the parent and high malignant

Table 2. Correlation between adhesiveness and malignancy.

Parameter	Findings	References
Aggregate formation between normal lymphoid cells and tumor cells.	Direct correlation between rate and extent of aggregate formation *in vitro* and cell localization in lungs after intravenous injection.	36
Aggregate formation between normal lung tissue cells and tumor cells; attachment to monolayers of unrelated tumor cells.	Direct correlation between rate and extent of aggregate formation and rate and extent of monolayer attachment with cell localization and tumor formation in the lungs after intravenous injection.	37–39
Attachment of tumor cells to monolayers of bovine endothelial cells.	Direct correlation between inhibition of adherence induced by colchicine and cytochalasin B and inhibition of cell localization and tumor formation in the lungs after intravenous injection.	40
EDTA-mediated detachment of tumor cells from plastic dishes.	Inverse correlation between sensitivity to EDTA-mediated detachment and lung tumor formation after intravenous injection.	42
Trypsin-mediated detachment of tumor cells from plastic dishes.	Inverse correlation between sensitivity to trypsin-mediated detachment and lung tumor formation after intravenous injection.	41
Trypsin-mediated detachment of tumor cells from plastic dishes, protein-coated dishes and monolayers of endothelial cells.	Inverse correlation between sensitivity to trypsin-mediated detachment and cell localization and tumor formation in the lungs after intravenous injection. Also, inverse correlation with primary tumor formation and spontaneous metastasis after intra-footpad injection.	45–47
Adherence of tumor cells to nylon fibers.	Direct correlation between increased adherence to nylon fibers and increased numbers of tumors in peritoneal mesenteries induced by chemotactic factors.	27

cells. A number of differences distinguish the high and low malignant cell types. Among them is the difference in sensitivity to trypsin-mediated detachment from culture dishes or from monolayers of endothelial cells. All of the low malignant clones are much more sensitive to detachment than the high malignant clones. The difference in sensitivity to trypsin-mediated detachment is accompanied by a difference in motility. The more sensitive cells are less motile [43, 44, 46]. Recent evidence indicates that they also do not respond to chemotactic factors [15].

These recent studies in no way contradict the classical observations made by Coman and others [48–50] suggesting that a low degree of cohesiveness allows tumor cells to separate from primary tumors. Both the initial separation and the secondary reattachment must occur. The recent studies correlating high adhesiveness with successful reattachment implies that the secondary reattachment step is a critical point in the metastatic sequence of events and that its successful occurrence is not a foregone conclusion. A summary of recent reports showing a correlation between high adhesiveness and high malignant potential is shown in Table 2.

Taken together, these recent studies imply that cellular adhesiveness contributes to a number of biological outcomes including primary and metastatic tumor formation. This is not surprising, since, once tumor cells are released from a primary tumor, they must become localized at secondary sites during the process of metastases. In the transplantable tumor models commonly used, single-cell suspensions of cells are injected into syngeneic animals – either into localized sites or intravascularly. In either case, the situation is analogous to what occurs in a spontaneously-developing tumor after the cells have been separated from the primary tumor.

3. Chemotaxis and metastasis

Although a large amount of data now confirms the ability of tumor cells to respond to chemotactic factors *in vitro*, there still is some question about the significance of the response relative to the metastatic process. A large amount of effort is being directed, therefore, to obtaining information which might answer this question. Two approaches are being taken. One involves obtaining data correlating chemotactic responsiveness with metastatic potential; the second involves altering the *in vivo* behavior of tumor cells with chemotactic factors.

With regard to the first approach, recent studies in our laboratory have shown a correlation between chemotactic responsiveness to the C5-derived tumor chemotactic peptide and metastatic capability of the responding cells. Several tumor cell types including the Walker 256 carcinosarcoma cells, a rat tumor which tends to spread from lymphnode to lymphnode after injection into the thigh, and a murine fibrosarcoma tumor which first appears as pulmonary metastasis (without evidence of lymphnode involvement) respond to the peptide. In contrast, normal fibroblasts from rats and mice do not respond *in vitro* to this chemotactic factor [15, 27].

Although the normal fibroblasts do not respond to the C5-derived factor, these cells (unpublished observation) as well as human fibroblasts [16–18, 51, 52] have been shown capable of responding to other factors.

The strongest evidence correlating chemotactic responsiveness with metastatic activity derives from studies in which the fibrosarcoma cells with high and low malignant potential have been used [43, 44]. The high malignant cells, which metastasize freely from footpad tumors and which form pulmonary tumors in the lungs of a high proportion of animals after intravenous injection, respond to the C5 chemotactic peptide while the cells with low malignant potential, which do not spontaneously metastasize, fail to respond to chemotactic stimulation [15].

Although the indirect studies provide suggestive evidence that chemotactic responsiveness contributes to metastatic activity, more direct evidence is needed. This requires the ability to manipulate tumor cell localization and growth *in vivo* with chemotactic factors. Evidence that this, in fact, can be done was presented by Hayashi et al. [1, 53]. In their studies, chemotactically-responsive tumor cells were injected intrarterially into rats while the chemotactic factors were injected intradermally. The chemotactic factor used in these studies was the tissue derived factor initially described by them [1, 2]. The skin sites were excised at intervals of 6, 12 and 24 h and at 3, 5, 7 and 11 days following intradermal injection. Within 24 h after injection a number of tumor cells were seen, apparently sticking to the endothelium of the venules. Some of the cells were seen emigrating through the walls of the vessels. By 72 h, the number of extravascular tumor cells had increased and some mitotic figures could be seen. At periods of longer than 3 days, the tumors showed widespread invasion of the underlying connective tissue and muscle.

In animals not injected with tumor cells the intradermal injection of the chemotactic factor produced a mild edematous change with localization of a few PMNs. When permeability-increasing factors or leukocyte chemotactic factors were injected they produced edema and PMN accumulation, respectively but neither induced the localization of tumor cells.

These studies provide direct evidence that the localization of tumors can be manipulated *in vivo* through the use of chemotactic factors. They do not address the question of the mechanism. It is often construed that the term chemotaxis, because it refers to the phenomenon of directed migration *in vitro*, implies the localization of cells *in vivo* by a similar mechanism-involving active, directed motility. While this may certainly be a part of it, it is likely that some of the other responses (i.e., adhesiveness) to chemotactic factors are also involved. O'Flaherty et al. [26] observed that the infusion of preformed leukocyte chemotactic factors into rabbits or the activation of intrinsic chemotactic factors caused a rapid, reversible neutropenia that was accompanied by the accumulation of PMNs in the pulmonary capillaries. This rapid response could hardly be due to active motility on the part of the leukocytes, particularly since the chemotactic factor was already systemically distributed. On the other hand, the aggregation or hyperadherence responses could readily account for this activity. Likewise with the tumor cells, increased adherence of the tumor cells to endothelial cells could contribute to the initial localization of the tumor cells. Once localized, the ability of the cells to directionally migrate toward the focus of chemotactic factor production could contribute to their becoming extravascular.

One question which has yet to be adequately answered concerns the mechanism by which active, tumor cell chemotactic factors are generated *in vivo*. If chemotaxis is a factor in the *in vivo* localization of tumor cells, what event(s) triggers the system? A mechanism has been proposed by Koono et al. [54, 55] to explain the generation of the tumor tissue-derived chemotactic factor. According to the proposed mechanism, the active factor is generated by the action of a tumor cell neutral protease acting on an unidentified tissue protein. The tumor protease is thought to be specifically released from the tumor cells by the action of a specific releasing factor. The system provides for specificity since the releasing factor does not release the neutral protease activity from normal cells.

A similar mechanism could account for the generation of an active, tumor cell chemotactic factor from C5. It has been shown that the tumor cells, themselves, can cleave intact C5 to produce a factor with chemotactic activity for the tumor cells [3, 4]. Furthermore, a number of normal tissues [4] also have the ability to produce the active factor. How these cells are triggered to begin the cascade is not known at present. Another mechanism which could account for the generation of chemotactic activity for tumor cells involves the host's inflammatory cells. It has been shown that the major neutral proteases (elastase and cathepsin G) of human PMNs can both split whole C5 to produce the tumor cell chemotactic peptide [7]. Since these enzymes are released at sites of inflammation this could explain the propensity of certain tumors to metastasize to sites of inflammation [56–63].

With regard to the chemotactic factor for tumor cells obtained from resorbed bone, this factor could readily be produced *in vivo* since bone is continually undergoing breakdown and rebuilding – both in normal and abnormal conditions. Although it is difficult to speculate on the relevance of the synthetic tripeptide, f-met-leu-phe, to *in vivo* metastases, it could be argued that this represents a common sequence of amino acids which is likely to be present *in vivo*. The same argument is used with leukocytes. Definitive answeres to these questions await additional work.

4. Future work

Much progress has been made in recent years in demonstrating that tumor cells and other non-leukocytic cells are capable of demonstrating chemotactic behavior *in vitro*. Although the response has not been studied nearly as extensively in these cells as in leukocytes, recent studies indicate that, at least in many respects, the response is similar to that observed in leukocytes. This would suggest that the underlying biological basis is similar for leukocytes and for tumor cells. It would also suggest which avenues of research are likely to be profitable. For example, much work remains to be done with regard to identifying and characterizing the physiological responses that occur in these cells upon interaction with chemotactic factors. Those responses known to occur in leukocytes should be examined in the tumor cells. Likewise, attempts to understand the events that occur at the membrane level as tumor cells interact with chemotactic factors should also take into account the findings made in the study of leukocytes. Studies are currently in progress in several of these areas. While very little is known directly about what occurs at the molecular level when tumor cells and chemotactic factors interact, Postlethwaite et al. [51] provide strong evidence that the interaction between normal fibroblasts and the collagen peptide chemotactic factor is a receptor-mediated event. Future work with the tumor cells will, hopefully, produce similar findings.

Although the study of tumor cell chemotaxis can benefit much from using the leukocytes as a model, the tumor cell systems provide opportunities to obtain basic biological data which would be extremely difficult to obtain with leukocytes. Unlike leukocytes, tumor cells are not end-stage cells programmed for an early death. Thus, with these cells, studies can be done and the cells retrieved for analysis. As has already been accomplished with the high and low malignant fibrosarcoma cells [15], variants derived from a common parent but with differing chemotactic responses might be isolated. These variants could then be invaluable in delineating the basis for the chemotactic response.

Finally more direct evidence to substantiate the relevance of the chemotactic response to the process of metastasis should be obtained. Although the studies which need to be done in order to obtain this information will be difficult to do, they should be attempted. If it can be shown that the response to chemotactic factors does influence the behavior of tumor cells *in vivo*, not only will this be a major advance in study of cancer metastasis but it will also broaden considerably the implications of chemotaxis in general.

Acknowledgment

The authors would like to acknowledge the support of NIH grants CA 29550 and CA 29551.

References

1. Hayashi H, Yoshida K, Ozaki T, Ushijima K: Chemotactic factor associated with invasion of cancer cells. Nature 226:174–175, 1970.
2. Yoshida K, Ozaki T, Ushijima K, Hayashi H: Studies on the mechanism of invasion in cancer. I. Isolation and purification of a factor chemotactic for cancer cells. Int J Cancer 6:123–132, 1970.
3. Romualdez AG, Ward PA: A unique complement-derived chemotactic factor for tumor cells. Proc Nat Acad Sci USA 72:4128–4132, 1975.
4. Romualdez AG, Ward PA, Torikata T: Relationship between the C5 peptides chemotactic for leukoctyes and tumor cells. J Immunol 117:1762–1766, 1975.

5. Orr W, Varani J, Ward PA: Characteristics of the chemotactic response of neoplastic cells to a factor derived from the fifth component of complement. Am J Pathol 93:405–422, 1978.
6. Orr W, Phan S, Varani J, Ward PA, Kreutzer DL, Webster RO, Henson PM: Chemotactic factor for tumor cells derived from the C5a fragment of complement component 5. Proc Nat Acad Sci USA 76:1986–1989, 1979.
7. Orr FW, Varani J, Kreutzer DL, Senior RM, Ward PA: Digestion of the fifth component of complement by leukocyte enzymes: sequential generation of chemotactic activities for leukocytes and for tumor cells. Am J Pathol 94:75–84, 1979.
8. Orr W, Varani J, Gondek MD, Ward PA, Mundy GR: Chemotactic responses of tumor cells to products of resorbing bone. Science 203:176–179, 1979.
9. Orr FW, Varani J, Gondek MD, Ward PA, Mundy GR: Partial characterization of a bone-derived chemotactic factor for tumor cells. Am J Pathol 99:43–52, 1980.
10. Wass JA, Varani J, Ward PA: Size increase induced in Walker ascites cells by chemotactic factors. Cancer Lett 9:313–318, 1980.
11. Wass JA, Varani J, Piontek GE, Goff D, Ward PA: Characteristics of the chemotactic factor-mediated cell swelling response of tumor cells. J Nat Cancer Inst (in press).
12. Showell HJ, Freer RJ, Zigmond SN, Shiffmann E, Aswanikunar I, Corcoran B, Becker EL: The structure-activity relations of synthetic peptides as chemotactic factors and inducers of lysozomal enzyme secretion for neutrophils. J Exp Med 143:1454–1469, 1968.
13. Mundy GR, Varani J, Orr W, Gondek MD, Ward PA: Resorbing bone is chemotactic for monocytes. Nature 275:132–135, 1978.
14. Remualdez AG, Ward PA: Further studies on the C5-derived chemotactic factor for tumor cells. In: Membranes and neoplasia: new approaches and strategies, progress in clinical and biological research Vol. 9, Marchesi VT (ed). New York: Alan R. Liss, 1976, pp 65–71.
15. Jain N, Orr W, Delikatny J, Varani J, Ward PA: Chemotactic responsiveness of high and low malignant fibrosarcoma clones. Am J Pathol (in press).
16. Postlethwaite AE, Snyderman R, Kang AH: The chemotactic attraction of human fibroblasts to a lymphocyte-derived factor. J Exp Med 144:1188–1203, 1976.
17. Postlethwaite AE, Seyer JM, Kang AH: Chemotactic attraction of human fibroblasts to type I, II, and III collagen and collagen-derived peptides. Proc Nat Acad Sci USA 75:871–875, 1978.
18. Postlethwaite AE, Snyderman R, Kang AH: Generation of fibroblast chemotactic factor in serum by activation of complement. J Clin Invest 64:1379–1385, 1979.
19. Hoover RL, Riggs RT, Karnovsky MJ: The adhesive interaction between polymorphonuclear leukocytes and endothelial cells *in vitro*. Cell 14:423–428, 1978.
20. O'Flaherty JT, Kreutzer DL, Ward PA: The influence of chemotactic factors on neutrophil adhesiveness. Inflammation 3:37–48, 1978.
21. O'Flaherty JT, Kreutzer DL, Ward PA: Neutrophil aggregation and swelling induced by chemotactic agents. J Immunol 119:232–239, 1977.
22. Kreutzer DL, O'Flaherty JT, Orr W, Showell HJ, Ward PA, Becker EL: Quantitative comparisons of various biological responses of neutrophils to different active and inactive chemotactic factors. Immunopharamacology 1:39–47, 1978.
23. Becker EL, Sigman M, Oliver JM: Superoxide production induced in rabbit polymorphonuclear leukocytes by synthetic chemotactic peptides and A23187: the nature of the receptor and the requirement for Ca^{2+}. Am J Pathol 95:81–97, 1979.
24. O'Flaherty JT, Kreutzer DL, Ward PA: Chemotactic factors influences on the aggregation, swelling and foreign surface adhesiveness of human leukocytes. Am J Pathol 90:537–550, 1978.
25. O'Flaherty JT, Ward PA: Leukocyte aggregation induced by chemotactic factors. Inflammation 3:177–194, 1978.
26. O'Flaherty JT, Showell HJ, Ward PA: Neutropenia induced by systemic infusion of chemotactic factors. J Immunol 118:1586–1589, 1977.
27. Varani J, Wass J, Piontek G, Ward PA: Chemotactic factor-induced adherence of tumor cells. Cell Biol Inter Reports 5:525–530, 1981.

28. MacGregor R, Spagnuolo P, Lentnek A: Inhibition of granulocyte adherence by ethanol, prednisone and aspirin measured with an assay system. N Eng J Med 291:642–646, 1974.
29. Becker EL, Showell HJ: The effects of Ca^{2+} and Mg^{2+} on the chemotactic responsiveness and spontaneous motility of rabbit polymorphonuclear leukocytes. Z Imm unit acts for sch 143:466–476, 1972.
30. Gallin JI, Rosenthal AS: The regulatory role of divalent cations in human granulocyte chemotaxis. J Cell Biol 62:594–609, 1974.
31. Wilkenson PC: Leukocyte locomotion and chemotaxis: the influence of divalent cations and cation ionophores. Exp Cell Res 93:420–426, 1976.
32. Estensen RD, Reusch ME, Epstein ML, Hill HR: Role of Ca^{2+} and Mg^{2+} in some human neutrophil functions as indicated by ionophore A23187. Infect Immun 13:146–151, 1976.
33. Kvarstein B: Effects of proteins and inorganic ions on the adhesiveness of human leukocytes to glass beads. Scand J Clin Lab Invest 24:41–48, 1969.
34. Bryant RE, Sutcliffe MC: A method for quantitation of human leukocyte adhesion to glass. Proc Soc Exp Biol Med 141:196–202, 1972.
35. Fidler IJ: Selection of successive tumor lines for metastasis Nature (New Biol) 242:148–149, 1973.
36. Fidler IJ: Biological behavior of malignant melanona cells correlated to their survival *in vivo*. Cancer Res 35:218–224, 1975.
37. Fidler IJ, Nicholson GL: Tumor cell and host properties affecting the implantation and survival of blood-borne metastatic variants of B16 melanoma. Isr J Med Sci 14:38–50, 1978.
38. Nicolson GL, Winkelhake JL: Organ specificity of blood-borne tumor metastases determined by cell adhesion. Nature 255:230–232, 1975.
39. Winkelhake JL, Nicolson GL: Determination of adhesive properties of variant metastatic melanoma cells to BALB/3T3 cells and their virus-tranformed derivatives by a monolayer-attachment assay. J Nat Cancer Inst 56:285–291, 1976.
40. Hart IR, Raz A, Fidler IJ: Effect of cytoskeletin-disrupting agents on the metastatic behavior of melanoma cells. J Nat Cancer Inst 64:891–900, 1980.
41. Hart IR: The selection and characterization of an invasive variant of the B16 melanoma. Am J Pathol 97:587–600, 1979.
42. Briles EB, Kornfeld S: Isolation and metastatic properties of detachment variants of B16 melanoma cells. J Nat Cancer Inst 60:1217–1222, 1978.
43. Varani J, Orr W, Ward PA: Comparison of subpopulations of tumor cells with altered migratory activity, attachment characteristics, enzyme levels and *in vivo* behavior. Eur J Cancer 15:585–592, 1979.
44. Varani J, Orr W, Ward PA: Hydrolytic enzyme activities, migratory activity and *in vivo* growth and metastatic potential of recent tumor isolates. Cancer Res 39:2376–2380, 1979.
45. Varani J, Orr W, Ward PA: Adhesive characteristics of tumor cell variants of high and low tumorigenic potential. J Nat Cancer Inst 64:1173–1178, 1980.
46. Varani J, Lovett EJ, Elgebaly S, Lundy J: Characteristics of tumor cell clones with varying malignant potential. In: Metastasis, clinical and experimental aspects, Hellmann K, Hilgard P, Eccles S (eds). The Hague: Martinus Nijhoff, pp 189–193.
47. Varani J, Lovett EJ, Elgebaly S, Lundy J, Ward PA: *In vitro* and *in vivo* adherence of tumor cell variants correlated with tumor formation. Am J Pathol 101:345–352, 1980.
48. Coman DR: Decreased mutual adhesiveness, a property of cells from squamous cell carcinoma. Cancer Res 4:625–629, 1944.
49. McCutcheon M, Coman DR, Moore FB: Studies on invasiveness of cancer: adhesiveness of malignant cells in various human adenocarcinoma. Cancer I:460–467, 1948.
50. Tjernberg B, Zajicek J: Cannulation of lymphatics leaving cancerous nodes in studies on tumor spread. Acta Cytol 9:197–202, 1965.
51. Postlethwaite AE, Kang AH: Characterization of the guinea pig lymphocyte-derived chemotactic factor for fibroblasts. J Immunol 124:1462–1466, 1980.

52. Chiang TM, Postlethwaite AE, Beachey EH, Seyer JM, Kang AH: Binding of chemotactic collagen-derived peptides to fibroblasts: the relationship to fibroblast chemotaxis. J Clin Invest 62:916–922, 1978.
53. Ozaki T, Yoshida K, Ushijima K, Hayashi H: Studies on the mechanisms of invasion in cancer. II. *In vivo* effects of a factor chemotactic for cancer cells. Int J Cancer 7:93–100, 1971.
54. Koono M, Ushijima K, Hayashi H: Studies on the mechanisms of invasion in cancer. III. Purification of a neutral protease of rat ascites hepatoma cells associated with production of a chemotactic factor for cancer cells. Int J Cancer 13:105–115, 1974.
55. Koono M, Katsuya H, Hayashi H: Studies on the mechanisms of invasion in cancer. IV. A factor associated with release of a neutral protease of tumor cells. Int J Cancer 13:334–342, 1974.
56. Agostino D, Cliffton EE: Trauma as a cause of localization of blood-borne metastases: preventive effect of heparin and fibrinolysin. Ann Surg 161:97–102, 1965.
57. Alexander JW, Altermeier WA: Susceptibility of injured tissue to hematogenous metastases: an experimental study. Ann Surg 159:933–944, 1964.
58. Black JW: The localization of metastatic Brown-Pearce Carcinoma in granulation tissue. Br J Cancer 18:143–145, 1964.
59. Crowley JD, Still WJS: Metastatic carcinoma at the site of injection of iron-dextran complex. Br Med J 1960 1:1411–1412.
60. Fisher B, Fisher ER: Experimental studies of factors influencing hepatic metastases. III. Effect of surgical trauma with special reference to liver injury. Ann Surg 150:731–744, 1959.
61. Fisher ER, Fisher B: Experimental studies on factors influencing the development of hepatic metastases: XIII. Effect of hepatic trauma in parabiotic pairs. Cancer Res 23:896–900, 1963.
62. Fisher B, Fisher ER, Feduska N: Trauma and the localization of tumor cells. Cancer 20:23–30, 1967.
63. Jewell WR, Romsdahl MM: Recurrent malignant disease in operative wounds not due to surgical inplantation from the resected tumor. Surgery 58:806–809, 1965.

8. Antimetastatic concomitant immunity

E. GORELIK

Metastatic spread and growth are the most crucial manifestations of malignancy in human cancer. If tumors were nonmetastatic their surgical removal would effect complete recovery. Unfortunately, surgical excision of the malignant tumor in many patients does not prevent the metastatic growth in different anatomic locations and therefore death. In experiments it was found that the excision of the transplanted tumor in mice may render mice immune to a subsequent graft of the same tumor cells [1, 2]. By using murine metastasizing tumors it was found that the surgical exision of the primary tumor was accompanied by accelerated growth of pulmonary metastases. Tyzzer [3] and Tadenuma and Okogoni [4] were the first to describe this puzzling phenomenon. Further, using inbred strains of mice and syngeneic tumors, Schatten [5] and Ketcham et al. [6] confirmed this observation.

Dramatic acceleration of metastatic growth was also found in hamsters following the removal of the locally growing lymphoma [8]. The mechanism of this phenomenon is obscure. Gershon [7] suggested that the removal of the locally growing tumor led to a diminution in concomitant immunity, as a result of an increased activity of suppressor cells, thus leading to acceleration in the growth of distant metastases.

An alternative explanation was based on the assumption that the locally growing tumor secreted inhibitory factor(s) which might suppress the growth of the metastatic cells. Once the primary tumor was excised, its inhibitory influence was abolished, permitting the uncontrolled growth of metastatic cells [5, 6, 9, 12].

The present chapter summarizes the results of investigations of the relationship between a locally growing tumor and its pulmonary metastases, growth characteristics of the postoperative metastases in mice, and the role of the immunological and nonimmunological mechanisms in the control of growth of the pulmonary metastases in mice [9, 10, 11]. Experiments were carried out relevant to the mechanisms involved in tumor 'concomitant immunity,' e.g., suppression of the second tumor graft growth in the presence of the first growing tumor. This mechanism may help in understanding the mechanism of inhibition of metastatic growth by the primary tumor and accelerated growth of postoperative metastases in mice following the excision of the primary tumor [11]-

L.A. Liotta and I.R. Hart (eds.), Tumor Invasion and Metastasis. ISBN-13: 978-94-009-7513-2.
© 1982 Martinus Nijhoff Publishers, The Hague/Boston/London.

1. Growth characteristics of postoperative metastases

The investigations were performed using mainly highly metastasizing Lewis lung carcinoma (3LL) transplanted into C57BL/6 mice. This tumor after transplantation intramuscularly (i.m.), subcutaneously (s.c.), or intrafootpad (i.f.p.) gives metastases preferentially in the lungs. Metastatic growth was assessed by determining the incidence of metastases, the volume of individual metastases, total metastatic volume per lungs, uptake of ^{125}IdUrd by highly proliferating metastatic cells, and total weight of lungs with metastases [9, 10].

In the first set of experiments constant doses (10^5) of 3LL tumor cells were inoculated into the footpad. Local tumors that reached 10 mm in diameter were removed and at various times the metastatic growth in the lungs was analyzed (Table 1). Shortly after tumor excision (5 days) the weights of lungs in operated and nonoperated mice were similar. However 10 days later a higher rate of growth of metastases in the lungs of tumor-excised mice resulted in the dramatic increase in the weight of lungs with metastases (697 mg versus 231 mg in tumor-bearing mice).

These data indicated that differences in the metastatic growth increase with time following tumor excision. However, the survival of tumor-bearing mice is a factor that restricts the period of observation of metastatic growth in operated and nonoperated tumor-bearing mice. Usually the mean survival time of tumor-bearing mice was shorter than that of operated tumor-excised mice. In all tumor-amputated mice severe dyspnea appeared and until their death the thoracic cavity was filled with tumor mass and the weight of lungs with metastases reached 1100 mg. At this time the differences in the volume of metastatic mass in operated and nonoperated mice reached their maximum. The tumor-bearing mice died of the local tumor rather than metastases which were too small to account for death.

In order to avoid the differences in the survival of operated and nonoperated mice we assessed the metastatic growth in these mice during the 9–11 days following tumor excision when most of the tumor-bearing mice were still alive.

Table 1. Excision of local tumor increases growth of lung metastases.*

Group no.	Treatment	Weight of lungs (mg) 5 days after amputation	10 days after amputation	At time of death	Mean survival (days)
1	Amputed	204 ± 8 (5)**	697 ± 94 (5)	1100 ± 54 (10)	34 ± 2
2	Non-amputated	186 ± 9 (5)	231 ± 13 (5)	286 ± 16 (10)	30 ± 2.1

* 1×10^5 3LL tumor cells were inoculated into right hind footpad. Twenty-one days later legs with tumors 10 mm in diameter were amputated.

** Number of mice examined in each group.

Table 2. Effect of size of local tumor at time of excision on the increase of progression of lung metastasis*.

Group no.	No. of mice	Treatment	Diameter of local tumor at time of amputation (mm)	No. of metastases per lung	Volume of metastases (mm^3)	Total metastatic volume per lung**	Weight of lungs (mg)	Weight of spleen (mg)
1	9	Amputated	8–10	29***	2.8 ± 0.4***	81.2***	215 ± 24***	159 ± 16***
2	10	Amputated	6–8	19	4.1 ± 0.8***	77.9***	248 ± 22***	163 ± 5***
3	10	Amputated	4–6	5***	3.4 ± 1.1***	17.0***	171 ± 11***	143 ± 5***
4	11	Non-amputated		11	.4 ± 0.09	4.4	141 ± 7.2	325 ± 42

* 1×10^5 3LL tumor cells were inoculated into the right footpad. Fifteen days later mice were divided into groups according to the diameter of their primary tumors. Nine days following excision of the primary tumor the development of pulmonary metastases was examined.

** Total metastatic volume per lung = mean no. of visible metastases times mean volume of metastases.

*** Significantly different from group 4, $p < 0.05$.

Increased growth of metastases in the lungs following removal of the primary tumor indicates that tumor cells migrate to the lungs. Yet their proliferation there is arrested when the primary tumor grows progressively. The number of metastatic cells settled in the lungs correlates positively with the mass of the primary tumor [13].

It is expected that the size of amputated local tumor is a crucial factor responsible for the metastases resulting in the lungs of tumor-excised mice. We tested this by measuring the incidence of lung metastases as a function of size of the primary tumor at the time of excision. Following i.f.p. inoculation of 10^5 3LL tumor cells, some differences in tumor growth were found in mice. Fifteen days following inoculation mice were separated into three groups according to their tumor size (Table 2). Following surgical removal of relatively small tumors (4–6 mm in diameter), the number of lung metastases was lower than in non-amputated tumor-bearing mice. The number of metastases increased above control when larger tumors (6–8 or 8–10 mm in diameter) were excised. In all tumor-excised mice, the volume of the individual pulmonary metastases was strikingly larger (2.8–4.1 mm^3) than in the tumor-bearing mice (0.4 mm^3). This increased growth of the metastases in operated mice was reflected also in the increase in total metastatic volume and the weight of lungs (Table 2). The total increase of the metastatic mass in the lungs was higher in mice from which larger local tumors (6–10 mm) were removed. Although the tumor removal was performed on the same day following tumor cell transplantation, the size of the local tumor developing at this time was responsible for the number of metastatic cells settled in the lungs. Their unrestricted growth in operated mice was reflected in a dramatic increase in the total metastatic mass. Therefore, in the next series of experiments local tumors were removed when they reached a certain size (8–10 mm in diameter), although the tumor excision was performed at various periods following tumor cell transplantation. We had found that mice in which tumor reached this size after a short period had less metastatic volume than did mice in which tumor grew slowly. This observation suggested that growth kinetics of 3LL tumor may influence the metastatic growth. In order to analyze this assumption we studied the development of the lung metastases in C57BL/6 mice inoculated i.f.p. with different doses of 3LL tumor cells ($3 \times 10^4 - 5 \times 10^6$).

In these mice the length of the latency period prior to the appearance of a detectable tumor was inversely related to the inoculum size. The growth rate of established tumor in all mice was equal and independent of the initial size. The shortest latent period was in mice inoculated with $5 \times 10^6 - 1 \times 10^6$ 3LL tumor cells and 8–10 mm tumors in these mice were removed 6–8 days following tumor cell inoculation. In mice transplanted with 3×10^4 3LL tumor cells the same tumor size was reached 21–23 days following inoculation. In spite of the removal of tumors of the same size, striking differences in the metastatic growth were observed in operated mice. After excision of tumors produced by inoculation of 5×10^6 or 1×10^6 cells, the incidence of metastases was lower, although the diameters of the individual metastases were larger those in nonoperated mice [10]. Total metastatic volumes in

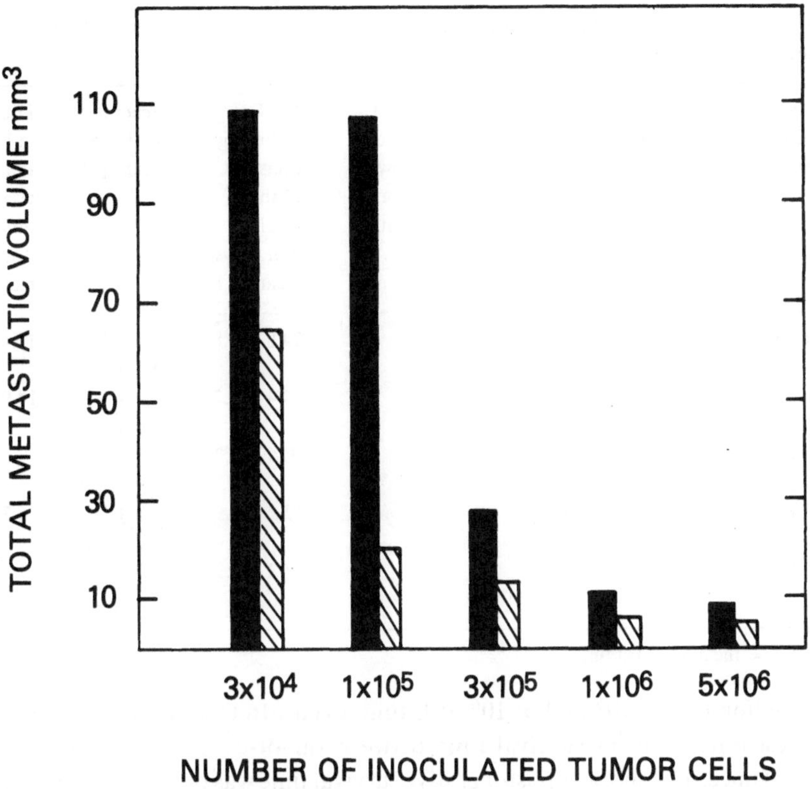

Figure 1. Effect of tumor excision on development of lung metastases in mice inoculated with different doses of tumor cells. Total metastatic volume = mean number of visible metastases times mean volume of metastases. ■ tumor-excised mice; ▧ nonoperated tumor-bearing mice.

these mice (operated and nonoperated) were similar (Figure 1). A dramatic increase in metastatic growth following tumor excision was observed in mice inoculated with 1×10^5 and 3×10^4 tumor cells (Figure 1).

In tumor-bearing mice inoculated with the lowest dose of tumor cells (3×10^4) the metastatic volume was higher than that in mice transplanted with increased numbers of tumor cells ($1 \times 10^5 - 5 \times 10^6$). The same results were obtained when metastatic growth was assessed by the ^{125}IdUrd uptake by highly proliferating metastatic cells in the lungs [10]. The growth of postoperative metastases determines the survival of operated animals. It is expected that in mice with high rates of growth of postoperative metastases the survival time would be shorter.

The results (Table 3) indicate that the survival of nonoperated tumor-bearing mice was a function of the number of inoculated cells. Apparently, tumor-bearing mice died of the local tumors rather than of metastases, which were too few and too small to account for death. The tumor-excised mice died after development of severe dyspnea, and their lungs were full of metastases. The longest postoperative survival time was recorded among mice in which the excised tumor developed as a result of

Table 3. MST of tumor-excised and tumor-bearing mice inoculated with different numbers of 3LL tumors cells*.

No. of inoculated tumor cells	Tumor excision	No. of mice/ group	Day of excision following tumor inoculation	MST following excision of the local tumor, days, mean $\pm$ SE	General MST, days, mean $\pm$ SE	Differences in MST of tumor-excised and tumor-bearing mice, days
5×10^6	+	12	6	24.8 ± 1.8	30.8 ± 1.8	15.4
	−	11			15.4 ± 1	
1×10^6	+	11	8	24.4 ± 1.7	32.4 ± 1.7	14.9
	−	12			17.5 ± 1.5	
3×10^5	+	13	13	20.5 ± 1.2	33.5 ± 1.2	8.6
	−	11			24.9 ± 1.9	
1×10^5	+	12	16	17.2 ± 0.9	33.2 ± 0.9	4.7
	−	10			28.7 ± 2.3	
3×10^4	+	10	21	17.2 ± 0.9	38.2 ± 0.9	4.0
	−	10			34.2 ± 2.4	

* MST = mean survival time.

inoculation of 5×10^6 or 1×10^6 3LL tumor cells. In these groups we found the greatest differences in survival time between tumor-excised and tumor-bearing control mice. The shortest postoperative survival time was observed among mice in which the tumors were produced by inoculation of 1×10^5 or 3×10^4 tumor cells (Table 3).

In all of these experiments the size of tumor was kept constant at the time of surgery. However, in mice inoculated with low doses of tumor cells, tumor reached 8–10 mm in diameter after longer periods than in mice transplanted with high doses of tumor cells ($5 \times 10^6 - 1 \times 10^6$).

In order to analyze the metastatic growth of postoperative metastases as a function of the time interval following tumor inoculation, we inoculated i.f.p. 1×10^5, 1×10^6, and 3×10^6 3LL tumor cells into C57BL/6 mice. In each group, mice were subjected to surgical removal of the local tumor every 2–3 days after tumor cell inoculation regardless of tumor size. Metastatic growth was assayed 11 days after tumor excision. The results (Table 4) show that for each of the inoculum sizes there were three periods of local tumor growth, each characterized by a different effect of tumor removal on metastatic growth. After removal of local tumors of relatively small sizes (up to 6.1 or 5.3 mm for tumors produced by the $1 \times 10^5 - 3 \times 10^6$ cells, respectively), ^{125}IdUrd incorporation in the lungs was smaller than in mice bearing local tumors. This stage was followed by a stage at which the removal of tumors resulted in ^{125}IdUrd uptake in the lungs similar to that of nonoperated mice. Finally, a third stage of local tumor growth occurred at which tumor removal was followed by a dramatic acceleration of metastatic growth.

Table 4. Development of postoperative metastases in the lungs as a function of initial tumor inoculum and size of the tumor at surgery*.

	Initial tumor inoculum, no. of 3LL cells								
	3×10^6			1×10^6			1×10^5		
Day postinoculation, when amputation was performed	Diameter of amputated tumor, mm ± SE	Weight of lungs, mg	^{125}IdUrd uptake, cpm	Diameter of amputated tumor, mm ± SE	Weight of lungs, mg	^{125}IdUrd uptake, cpm	Diameter of amputated tumor, mm ± Se	Weight of lungs, mg	^{125}IdUrd uptake, cpm
3	4.1 ± 0.15	200	448**						
5	6.1 ± 0.25	181	583**	4.7 ± 0.2	206	700**	2.0***	182**	541**
7				6.8 ± 0.2	205	908			
8	9.3 ± 0.37	298	1 702				3.1 ± 0.2	189**	563**
9				8.2 ± 0.23	274	1 194			
10	10.8 ± 0.5	583**	14 107***				5.3 ± 0.3	181**	513**
11				10.3 ± 0.27	540**	5 679**			
12	12.7 ± 0.5	1 003**	42 482**				7.1 ± 0.3	271	1 995
13				12.5 ± 0.4	749**	25 506**			
14							8.5 ± 0.35	416**	5 954**
17							10.9 ± 0.57	805**	29 519**
Tumor-bearing mice	>15	220	1 213	>15	227	1 078	>15	289	2 038
Normal mice		189 ± 12	507						

* Mice were inoculated i.f.p. with 3×10^6, 1×10^6, or 1×10^5 3LL tumor cells. At different periods after tumor transplantation, established tumors were removed. After 10 days, mice were inoculated with 25 μm FdUrd and 1 μCi ^{125}IdUrd, and on the 11th day the lungs were weighed and their ^{125}IdUrd incorporation was determined. Ten mice were used in every group of amputated mice.

** Significantly different from tumor-bearing mice ($P < 0.05$).

*** At that time, no tumors were visible in the footpad.

These three distinct periods were found for local tumors produced by each of the different inoculum sizes tested. Acceleration of metastasis in mice inoculated with 1×10^5 tumor cells was observed when the excised local tumor reached a diameter of 8.5 mm ($>310\,mm^3$), whereas animals inoculated with 1×10^6 or 3×10^6 cells manifested acceleration only when the excised local tumor reached a diameter of more than 10.3 mm ($>550\,mm^3$). After the same 10-day period, tumors produced by inoculation of 10^5 cells were 5.3 mm in diameter, and their removal did not result in acceleration of metastatic growth.

It seemed, therefore, unlikely that the differences in metastatic growth, observed in Figure 1 and Table 3, between mice inoculated with low compared to high cell inocula should be attributed merely to the differences in the latency period of tumor growth. Rather, differences in metastatic growth following excision seemed to reflect differences in the incidence of surviving viable tumor cells in the lungs. This in turn may be a function of the intensity of immune response elicited by the tumor cells, as a function of the inoculum size. The initial high cell dose may evoke a higher level of immune reaction and, subsequently, a lower level of tumor cell survival in the lungs. If this is true, then inoculation of low and high tumor cell doses to animals that are immunologically suppressed should result in the same of metastatic growth.

To study the effect of the host's immune reactivity on metastatic progression, we tested metastatic growth in normal compared to immunologically impaired mice given transplants of 3×10^6 or 1×10^5 3LL tumor cells.

In immunosuppressed B mice, the growth of the local tumors that developed after inoculation of 3×10^6 or 1×10^5 tumor cells was retarded compared to intact control tumor-bearing groups. However, in Cy-treated (200 mg/kg) mice, the local tumor showed accelerated growth [10]. Here again the development of the postoperative metastasis was strikingly higher in normal mice given transplants of 1×10^5 tumor cells than of 3×10^6 3LL tumor cells (Table 5). Compared to normal recipients, metastatic growth in immunosuppressed mice was significantly accelerated, and further acceleration of metastasis development was obtained after surgical excision of the local tumors. Unlike normal recipients, immunologically suppressed mice demonstrated a similar level of metastatic growth, irrespective of the size of the initial inoculum (Table 5). Thus the progression of lung metastasis in B mice inoculated with 3×10^6 cells was similar to that of mice inoculated with 1×10^5 cells, though the latency period before tumor appearance was significantly shorter in mice inoculated with the high inoculum dose. The results presented in Tables 4 and 5 indicated that differences in the latency periods of tumor development could not account for the differences in metastatic growth following excision of the local tumors produced by inoculation of different doses of tumor cells. The size of the local tumor at surgery was found to be of crucial importance. Dependent on the size at surgery, the level of postoperative metastatic growth could be either lower, identical, or higher than in non-operated tumor-bearing mice. When relatively small local tumors were excised, the lungs were left with too few metastatic cells in comparison to those in lungs in nonoperated tumor-bearing mice in which

Table 5. Development of metastases in immunologically intact and immunoimpaired tumor-bearing and tumor-excised mice*.

			Tumor-bearing mice						
Group no.	Host	No. of tumor cells inoculated	Amputated				Non-amputated		
			No. of mice	Days of amputation	Weight of lungs, mg	^{125}IdUrd uptake cpm	No. of mice	Weight of luNgs, mg	^{125}IdUrd uptake cpm
1	Normal	3×10^6	10	8	245	1 074	7	251	1 133
2	B mice	3×10^6	7	11	578^b	16 236**	8	400***	9 481***
3	Cy-treated	3×10^6	14	8	445^b	11 634**	12	326***	4 190***
4	Normal	1×10^5	10	18	439^b	7 612**	8	286	2 200
5	B mice	1×10^5	10	21	530^b	13 473**	12	407***	6 407***
6	Cy-treated	1×10^5	10	16	497^b	11 124**	8	380***	4 722***
7	Intact non-tumor-bearing		11		207	469			

* Local tumors (8–10 mm in diameter) were excised. After 10 days, tumor-bearing and tumor-excised mice were inoculated with 25 μg of FdUrd and 1 μCi of ^{125}IdUrd. Mice were killed on the next day; their lungs were weighed and radioactivity was measured.

** Significantly different from all tumor-bearing mice ($P < 0.05$) according to the Mann-Whitney *U* test.

*** Significantly different from normal tumor-bearing mice in groups #1 and #4 ($P < 0.05$) according to the Mann-Whitney *U* test. B mice had been thymectomized (at age of 2 mo), lethally irradiated and reconstituted with 2×10^6 bone marrow cells. Two months later mice were used in experiments.

the local tumor continued to shed numerous cells. Their growth at this stage exceeds the growth of the fewer cells existing in the lungs of the operated mice. At the next stage of medium-sized tumors, an equilibrium was reached between the effect of suppression exerted by the local tumor and the shedding of cells. Although the removal of the local tumor stopped the continuous shedding of metastatic cells, it removed also the suppressive effect of the local tumor on its metastases. The continuous supply of metastatic cells in the tumor-bearing mouse resulted in a metastatic mass similar to that reached by the fewer metastatic cells in the lungs of tumor-amputated mice because of the accelerated growth after removal of the suppressive effect of the local tumor. At this stage, tumor-amputated mice may show fewer metastatic foci in the lungs, but each focus is of a larger mass. At the third stage, when the local tumor reaches a larger mass, more metastatic cells settle in the lungs and they are subjected to a greater suppressive effect by the local tumor. Hence tumor excision resulted in larger metastatic masses than those found in tumor-bearing mice. However, this accelerated growth of postoperative metastases in mice inoculated with low doses of 3LL cells (1×10^5) was observed following removal of the local tumors of more than 310 mm^3. The same effect was observed in mice given transplants of high doses of 3LL cells ($1 \times 10^6 - 3 \times 10^6$) only when the removed local tumors had reached a volume of more than 550 mm^3. These differences in metastatic growth could be attributed to differences in survival of metastatic cells in the blood and lungs. This could result from the capacity of high cell inocula to produce a more efficient immune response and subsequently a lower level of survival of tumor cells in the lungs. This is deduced from the observation that in immunosuppressed B mice or in Cy-treated mice, the same level of metastatic growth was obtained irrespective of the inoculum size (Table 5). Immunosuppression clearly accelerated metastatic growth. Yet an additional stimulus for metastatic development was observed following tumor excision in such immunosuppressed mice.

2. Mechanisms controlling growth of postoperative metastases in the lungs

The experiments described indicate that, from one side, the local growing tumor is a source of the metastatic cells which may spread in different anatomic locations. From the other side, locally growing tumor may exert a suppressive effect on the proliferation of the metastatic cells. Once the local tumor was excised, its inhibitory influence was abolished and permitted the uncontrolled growth of metastatic cells [5, 6, 9, 12]. Indeed, this inhibitory effect can be restored by retransplantation of the second tumor graft into mice from which the first local tumor was removed. As a result of the growth of the retransplanted tumor, the acceleration of the metastatic growth in the lungs was abrogated [9]. This inhibitory effect of the local tumor on the growth of the pulmonary metastases is a function of the size of a tumor mass. Different doses of 3LL tumor cells ($1 \times 10^5 - 3 \times 10^6$) were retransplanted i.f.p.

Table 6. Suppression of pulmonary metastases in tumor-amputated mice is a function of dose of reinoculated 3LL tumor cells.

Group no.	Treatment		No. of mice	No. of metastases in lungs	Volume of metastases 1mm^3)	Total metastatic volume per lung	Weight of lungs (mg)	Diameter of reinoculated tumor		Weight of spleen (mg)
	Ampu-tation	Reinoc-ulation of tumor cells						5 days post amput.	10 days post. amput.	
1	–	—	11	7.5	0.2 ± 0.05	1.5	226 ± 25	—	—	314 ± 28
2	+	—	15	19.7**	2.2 ± 0.38**	43.3**	381 ± 36**	—	—	163 ± 13*
3	+	1×10^5	10	13	1.8 ± 0.3**	23.4**	300 ± 28**	2.6	6.4	170 ± 18*
4	+	3×10^5	10	16**	1.8 ± 0.32**	28.8**	340 ± 32**	4.4	8.7	195 ± 13*
5	+	1×10^6	10	5.8	1.0 ± 0.2**	5.8**	250 ± 17	6.1	10.4	259 ± 20*
6	+	3×10^6	11	7.4	0.5 ± 0.09	3.7	244 ± 20	7.2	11.8	266 ± 21

* 1×10^5 3LL tumor cells were inoculated into the third right footpad. Tumors 8–10 mm in diameter were amputated and 1×10^5–3×10^6 3LL tumor cells were reinoculated simultaneously into the left footpad. Lungs of these mice were examined 10 days later.

** Differs significantly from Group 1 ($p < 0.05$).

into C57BL/6 mice simultaneously with excision of the first growing 3LL tumor (Table 6). Small inocula of tumor cells (1×10^5 and 3×10^5) failed to inhibit the metastatic growth of tumor-amputated mice. Mice reinoculated with 1×10^6 and especially with 3×10^6 tumor cells showed rapid growth of the local tumor. So even after 5 days following tumor excision retransplanted tumors reached the size of 6.1–7.2 mm in diameter. Growth of these tumors inhibited the proliferation of metastatic cells in the lungs. In comparing with tumor-amputated mice the incidence of metastases, their volume and total weight of lungs with metastases were lower and similar to those in the nonoperated tumor-bearing control mice (Table 6).

The inhibitory effect exerted by a local tumor on the progression of the pulmonary metastases seems not to be based solely on immunological mechanisms. Using different immunosuppressive procedures, we found a dramatic acceleration of metastatic growth (Table 5). Nevertheless, even under these conditions excision of the local 3LL tumor was followed by a further acceleration of metastatic growth. The highest weight of lungs due to metastases was observed in immunosuppressed mice from which the local tumor had been removed. These data indicated that suppression of metastatic growth might be due to both immunological and non-immunological factors.

Involvement of the immune system in the control of metastatic spread and growth is supported by the fact that immunosuppression or immunostimulation led to acceleration or inhibition of metastatic growth, respectively [14–16]. Gatenby and Basten [17] had found that stimulation of the immune system by *C. parvum* can reduce the enhanced growth of lung metastases produced by amputation of the primary B16 melanoma or 3LL tumor.

The data presented in Tables 2 and 6 show that in mice with the surgically removed 3LL tumor the spleen weight was considerably lower than that in nonoperated tumor-bearing mice. Retransplantation of 3LL tumor cells to the tumor-excised mice abrogated the accelerated growth of pulmonary metastases and concomitantly increased the weight of spleen of these mice (Table 6). These data suggest that the spleen may participate in the control of the growth of postoperative metastases. Indeed, simultaneously performed splenectomy and tumor excision may abrogate the accelerated growth of pulmonary metastases [18]. However, this inhibitory effect of splenectomy was observed only in mice from which relatively small tumors (6–9 mm in diameter) were removed. When splenectomy was performed simultaneously with removal of larger 3LL tumors [9–11 mm], the accelerated growth of postoperative metastases was not abrogated.

As we showed above, the abrogation of the accelerated growth of postoperative metastases in the lungs can be achieved by retransplantation of the tumor cells. The same effect can be achieved by splenectomy performed simultaneously with tumor excision. Therefore, the next set of experiments was designed to test whether the two phenomena, i.e., splenectomy and reinoculation, are related; namely, if the reduction in metastatic growth following reinoculation of a second tumor is dependent on the presence of a functional spleen.

Table 7. The effect of splenectomy and/or reinoculation of fresh tumor cells on the progression of lung metastases following excision of the primary tumor.

No. of group	Treatment			Mice per group		Volume of reinoculated tumor (mm^3)		Weight of lungs (mg)		^{125}IUdR uptake** cpm	
	Amp.	Splx.	Reinoc.	Exp. 1	Exp. 2	Exp. 1 M ± SE	Exp. 2 M ± SE	Exp. 1	Exp. 2	Exp. 1	Exp. 2
1	—	—	—*	10	10	—	—	258	243	1995	1361
2	—	+	—	8	10	—	—	275	300	2661	2615
3	+	—	—	9	15	—	—	554[a]	417[a]	8842[a]	4575[a]
4	+	+	—	8	12	—	—	464[ab]	343	4686[ab]	2443[b]
5	+	—	+	9	11	684 ± 92	579 ± 57	463[ab]	303[b]	5351(4263)[ab]	2560(1008)[b]
6	+	+	+	9	12	429 ± 59	256 ± 30	362[abc]	241[bc]	3058(1970)[bc]	1811(347)[bc]
7	intact mice		+	12	10	1000 ± 119	1098 ± 135	189	182	1088	1464
8	normal mice		—	—	7	—	—	—	191	—	499

Mice were injected with 10^5 3LL tumor cells into the right hind footpad. Amputation and splenectomy were performed simultaneously when tumor reached 63–108 mm^3 in volume. Some of the mice (as indicated in the table) were reinoculated with 3×10^6 3LL cells into the other footpad. Eleven days later all mice were killed and their lungs assayed for the presence of metastases.

** The numbers in parentheses are the calculated net numbers. They are obtained by deducting the number of cpm of the intact, reinoculated mice from the relevant cpm.

* These control animals underwent amputation of their right healthy leg.

[a] Significantly different from Groups 1 and 2 ($P < 0.05$).

[b] Significantly different from Group 3 ($P < 0.05$).

[c] Significantly different from Groups 4 and 5 ($P < 0.05$).

Mice were inoculated with 10^5 tumor cells into the right hind footpad. When tumors reached 5–7 mm in diameter, amputation, splenectomy and reinoculation of 3×10^6 tumor cells to the other footpad were performed in different combinations as shown in Table 7. The results summarized in this table demonstrated again that amputation of the tumor-bearing leg caused a marked increase in the metastatic growth and that this increase was abolished by either splenectomy or reinoculation of fresh tumor cells. When splenectomy and reinoculation of tumor cells were performed simultaneously, a clear additive inhibitory effect was observed, leading to a dramatic reduction in the weight of lungs and the ^{125}IUdR uptake by the metastases in the lungs.

In the tumor excised and reinoculated mice, some of the metastatic foci in the lungs have probably derived from the reinoculated tumor. In intact mice inoculated with the same number of tumor cells (3×10^6) a large tumor developed (1000–1098 mm^3) and the ^{125}IUdR uptake in the lungs of these mice was 1088–1464 cpm (versus 499 cpm in normal mice). If one calculates the 'net' level of radioactivity in the lungs of the tumor excised, splenectomized and reinoculated mice, the inhibitory effect on the metastatic growth seems even more dramatic (Table 7). In mice, tumor excision performed simultaneously with splenectomy might increase the activity of antitumor cell-mediated immunity probably by the removal of suppressor cells. This assumption can be supported by the fact that tumor excision only slightly increased the resistance to the 3LL tumor cells retransplanted into the secound leg. The inhibition of growth of retransplanted tumor was more profound in mice that underwent tumor excision and splenectomy (Table 7).

These data suggest that immunological and nomimmunological mechanisms are involved in the control of growth of distant metastases in mice. Gershon [7] supposed that the removal of the locally growing tumor diminishes the concomitant immunity, as a result of an increased activity of suppressor cells, thus leading to acceleration in the growth of distant metastases. Concomitant suppression of the second tumor graft in the presence of the first progressively growing tumor has been known since the description by Ehrlich [19]. Indeed, spontaneous metastases can be considered as the second tumor graft, naturally developed in the presence of the primary tumor. We assumed that the relationships existing between the first growing tumor and the second tumor graft might, in principle, mimic the complex relationships that exist during the growth of a malignant tumor and its distant metastases. Therefore, the analysis of the mechanism of concomitant immunity might be relevant to the understanding of the complex interactions existing between the primary tumor and its metastases [11].

For these purposes we reinoculated different doses of 3LL tumor cells (2×10^5 – 5×10^6) i.f.p. mice bearing s.c. 3LL tumor. We found that suppression of the second tumor graft growth is a function of the tumor mass developed at the moment of retransplantation. This inhibitory effect was most expressed in mice in the latest period of tumor growth. Mice bearing large tumor masses were able to completely prevent growth of the second graft even following reinoculation of 5×10^6 3LL

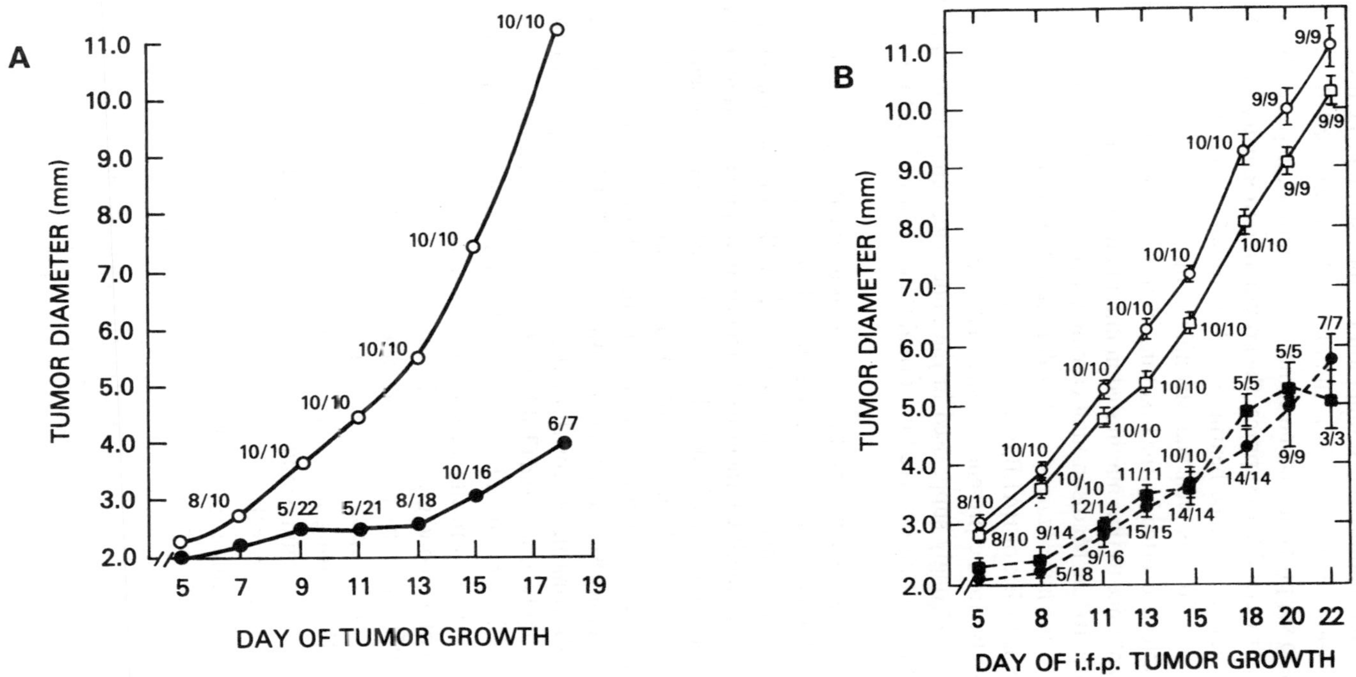

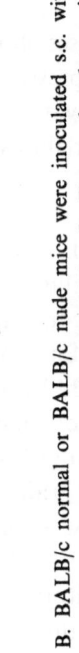

Figure 2. Suppression of the second tumor graft in tumor-bearing nude mice.

A. 3×10^6 3LL tumor cells were inoculated s.c. into ICR nude mice. When tumors reached more than 1.5 cm in diameter, mice were reinoculated i.f.p. with 1×10^6 3LL tumor cells. I.f.p. growth in nude (o) or in tumor-bearing nude mice. Numbers indicate the incidence of mice bearing i.f.p. tumor.

B. BALB/c normal or BALB/c nude mice were inoculated s.c. with 0.5×10^6 Madison lung carcinoma (M109) cells. Twenty days later mice bearing s.c. tumor more than 2.0 cm in diameter were retransplanted i.f.p. with 0.5×10^6 M109 tumor cells. Nontumor-bearing normal BALB/c (o) or BALB/c nude mice (□) inoculated i.f.p. with M109 tumor cells, (•) normal BALB/c or nude (■) mice bearing s.c. M109 tumor and retransplanted i.f.p. with M109 cells.

tumor cells. The resistance of mice bearing smaller tumor can be overcome by increased doses of the reinoculated 3LL tumor cells [10]. Since we had found that in immunosuppressed B mice additional stimulation for metastatic growth was observed following excision of the local 3LL tumor (Table 6), we used B mice to analyze their ability to suppress the second tumor graft. Immunoimpaired B mice bearing s.c. 3LL tumor were able to suppress the growth of reinoculated i.f.p. 3LL tumor cells [11]. In ICR nude mice bearing s.c. 3LL tumor the growth of reinoculated 3LL cells (1×10^6) as well was strongly suppressed (Figure 2A). To compare inhibitory effects exerted by the first tumor on the second tumor graft in the immunocompetent mice to that manifested in immunodeficient nude mice, we inoculated i.f.p. 0.5×10^6 or Madison lung carcinoma (M109) cells into normal BALB/c or BALB/c nude mice bearing s.c. M109 tumor 2 cm in diameter (Figure 2B). In control intact BALB/c or BALB/c nude mice inoculated with M109, tumor cells grew progressively. In the presence of s.c. M109 tumor, the growth of the second i.f.p. graft was strongly suppressed in the nude mice, and the extent of suppression was similar to that observed in normal tumor-bearing BALB/c mice (Figure 2B).

The inhibitory effect exerted by the first tumor graft on the subsequent retransplanted tumor is a nonspecific phenomenon. Mice bearing s.c. 3LL carcinoma, B16 melanoma, EL-4 lymphoma were inoculated i.f.p. with nonhomologous tumors, which differ in their kinetic characteristics. Hence, to obtain a s.c. tumor of a certain size at a certain period, different initial doses of tumor cells were inoculated.

C57BL/6 mice were inoculated with 1×10^6 of 3LL tumor cells or 5×10^6 B16 melanoma cells. When the s.c. tumor reached more than 2 cm in diameter, both tumor-bearing and intact mice were injected i.f.p. with 1×10^6 of 3LL or 5×10^6 B16 tumor cells. In tumor-bearing mice growth of the second tumor i.f.p. was completely prevented or strongly suppressed (Table 8). 3LL tumors developed s.c. were very effective in suppressing growth of tumor cells isolated from pulmonary metastases (M-3LL) and inoculated i.f.p. Similarly, metastatic tumor cells inoculated s.c. suppressed the growth of a second graft of 3LL from a local tumor (Table 8).

(C3H/DiSn $\times$ C57BL/6)F_1 mice bearing s.c. methylcholanthrene-induced T-10 tumor were able to strongly suppress the growth of 3LL tumor cells inoculated i.f.p. into these mice. Mice bearing 3LL tumors s.c. were resistant to the growth of 5×10^6 EL-4 lymphoma cells and, similarly, mice bearing i.m. EL-4 lymphomas strongly suppressed the i.f.p. growth of 1×10^6 3LL cells (Table 8). Furthermore, immunocompetent and immunosuppressed B mice bearing s.c. 3LL or B16 melanoma were equally effective in preventing the i.f.p. growth of 3LL cells [10].

Thus, the suppression of growth of a second tumor graft in tumor-bearing animals seems to be tumor nonspecific. In our previous study we suggested that inhibition of the metastatic growth by the local tumor is a tumor-specific phenomenon. This suggestion was based on the fact that retransplantation of the 3LL tumor, but not B16 melanoma or EL-4 lymphoma cells, was effective in the abrogation of the accelerated growth of the 3LL lung metastases, following 3LL tumor exision. The

Table 8. The inhibitory effect exerted by progressively growing tumors on a subsequent tumor graft is tumor-nonspecific.

First s.c. tumor	Second inoculated tumor	No. of i.f.p. inoculated cells	% inhibition* of i.f.p. growth
3LL	3LL	1×10^6	100
3LL	B16	5×10^6	35
B16	B16	5×10^6	60
B16	3LL	1×10^6	100
3LL	M-3LL**	1×10^6	100
M-3LL**	3LL	1×10^6	100
3LL	EL-4	5×10^6	100
EL-4	3LL	1×10^6	55
T-10***	3LL	1×10^6	62

Tumor cells were inoculated s.c. When the s.c. tumor reached more than 2 cm in diameter, both tumor-bearing and intact mice were retransplanted i.f.p. with tumor cells as indicated in the table. Each group contained 10 mice.

* Percent inhibition was determined: $\frac{a-b}{a} \times 100$, where a = tumor diameter i.f.p. of control mice, b = i.f.p. tumor diameter of mice bearing s.c. tumor.

** M-3LL: metastatic 3LL tumor cells derived from the metastatic nodules in the lungs and inoculated s.c. or i.f.p. (1×10^6).

*** 1×10^6 T-10 methylcholanthrene-induced tumor cells were inoculated s.c. into (C3H/DiSn x C57BL/6)F_1 mice.

apparent specificity of the inhibitory effect exerted by 3LL tumor on the 3LL pulmonary metastases may be partly attributed to the high growth rate of 3LL retransplanted tumor cells, compared to other tumors (B16 and EL-4), hence its stronger inhibitory capacity. In addition, the complexity of different specific and nonspecific mechanisms involved in the control of metastatic growth should be taken into consideration. Our results demonstrate that 'concomitant immunity', namely the resistance of tumor-bearing animals to a second tumor challenge, is not a T cell-mediated tumor-specific immunological phenomenon. Macrophages and NK cells could theoretically also be involved in the nonspecific resistance of tumor-bearing animals to implantation of a second tumor graft. Yet such suggestions seem unlikely. a) In many experiments it was found that at the latest stages of tumor growth both the function of macrophages and the cytotoxic activity of NK cells are suppressed [20, 21]. b) In silica-treated mice the macrophages and NK cell were activity inhibited [21]. However, normal C57BL/6 or silica-treated tumor-bearing mice were equally efficient in the suppression of growth of the second tumor grafts (Gorelik, to be published). c) By using ^{125}IdUrd labeled 3LL or M109 tumor cells, it was found that in tumor-bearing mice the radiolabeled tumor cells inoculated i.f.p. were not eliminated and persisted as dormant tumor cells. Proliferation of these cells in the presence of the first tumor is strongly inhibited (Gorelik, to be published).

It is thus necessary to differentiate specific antitumor immune responses which are T cell mediated from nonspecific resistance of tumor-bearing mice to the second tumor graft ('concomitant immunity'). During tumor growth, weakly immunogenic tumors like 3LL failed to induce strong specific immune responses, but they were able to express tumor nonspecific concomitant resistance to the proliferation of the retransplanted tumor cells. Strongly antigenic tumor may induce immune response which might be responsible for the specific resistance to the same retransplanted tumor cells. At the latest period of the primary tumor growth the specific resistance decreased and nonspecific resistance to nonhomologous tumor cells became apparent [22].

We suggest that tumor cells of the first graft produce or induce inhibitory factor(s) which suppress the replication of tumor cells of the second inoculum. This inhibitory factor(s) is nontumor specific and functions independently of the components of the immune system, hence its effect in immunosuppressed mice. This inhibitory effect appears only when the tumor mass reaches a certain critical size [9, 10]. The production of such factors may explain the suppressive effect which the local tumor exerts on its metastases and hence the accelerated growth of metastases manifested following removal of the primary tumor mass [5, 6, 9, 12]. Alternative and additional immunological factors also participate in the control of the spread and growth of the distant metastases in mice.

References

1. Prehn R, Main J: Immunity to methylcholanthrene-induced sarcomas. J Natl Cancer Inst 18:769–778, 1957.
2. Klein G, Sjorgen H, Klein E, Hellström K: Demonstration of resistance against methylcholanthrene-induced sarcomas in the primary autochthonous host. Cancer Res 20:1561–1572, 1960.
3. Tyzzer E: Factors in the production and growth of tumor metastases. J Med Res 28:309–332, 1913.
4. Tadenuma K, Okonogi S: Experimentelle Untersuchungen über Metastasen bei Mäusecarcinoma. Z Krebsforsch 21:168–172, 1924.
5. Schatten W: An experimental study of postoperative tumor metastases. I. Growth of pulmonary metastases following total removal of primary leg tumor. Cancer 11:455–459, 1958.
6. Ketcham A, Kinsey D, Wexler M, Mantel N: The development of spontaneous metastases after removal of a 'primary' tumor. II. Standardization protocol of five animal tumors. Cancer 14:875–882, 1961.
7. Gershon R: Regulation of concomitant immunity. Activation of suppressor cells by tumor excision. Isr J Med Sci 10:1012–1023, 1974.
8. Green H, Harvey E: The inhibitory influence of a transplanted hamster lymphoma on metastasis. Cancer Res 20:1094–1100, 1960.
9. Gorelik E, Segal S, Feldman M: Growth of a local tumor exerts a specific inhibitory effect on progression of lung metastases. Int J Cancer 21:617–625, 1978.
10. Gorelik E, Segal S, Feldman M: Control of lung metastasis progression in mice: role of growth kinetics of 3LL Lewis lung carcinoma and host immune reactivity. J Natl Cancer Inst 65:1257–1264, 1980.
11. Gorelik E, Segal S, Feldman M: On the mechanism of tumor 'concomitant immunity'. Int J Cancer 27:847–856, 1981.

12. Sugarbaker E, Thornthwaite J, Ketcham A: Inhibitory effect of a primary tumor on metastasis. In: Progress in cancer research and therapy, Vol. 5, Day S, et al. (eds). New York: Raven Press, 1977, pp 227–240.
13. De Wys W: Studies correlating the growth rate of a tumor and its metastases and providing evidence for tumor-related systemic growth retarding factors. Cancer Res 32:374–379, 1972.
14. Alexander P, Eccles S: The contribution of immunological factors to the control of metastatic spread of sarcomata in rats. In: Critical factors in cancer immunology, Vol 10, Schultz J, Leif R (eds). New York: Academic Press, 1975, pp 159–173.
15. Pimm M, Baldwin R: Immunology and immunotherapy of experimental and clinical metastases. In: Secondary spread of cancer, Baldwin R (ed). New York: Academic Press, 1978, pp 163–210.
16. Fidler I, Gersten D, Hart I: The biology of cancer invasion and metastasis. Adv Cancer Res 28:149–189, 1978.
17. Gatenby P, Basten A: A mouse model for immunotherapy of osteosarcoma. II. Corynebacterium parvum immunotherapy. Cancer Immunol Immunother 8:103–111, 1980.
18. Ron J, Gorelik E, Segal S, Feldman M: Involvement of the spleen in the control of tumor growth and development of metastases. Immunological aspects of experimental and clinical cancer. Tel Aviv (Abstract), 1979, p 137.
19. Ehrlich P: Experimentelle Karzinomstudien an Mäusen. Arb Inst Exp Ther Frankfurt 1:65, 1906.
20. Kano J, Friedman H: Immunosuppression and the role of suppressive factors in cancer. Adv Cancer Res 25:271–322, 1977.
21. Herberman R, Holden H: Natural cell-mediated immunity. Adv Cancer Res 7:305–377, 1978.
22. Kearney R, Nelson D: Concomitant immunity to syngeneic methylcholanthrene-induced tumors in mice. Occurrence and specificity of concomitant immunity. Aust J Biol Med Sci 51:723–735, 1973.

9. Immunobiological diversity of metastatic cells

E. GORELIK, M. FOGEL, P. DE BAETSELIER, S. KATZAV, M. FELDMAN and S. SEGAL

The analysis of antigenic and immunogenic properties of tumor cells and of mechanisms of antitumor response should furnish the basis for the investigation of methods aimed at immunotherapy of malignant diseases. One may expect that such methods will be especially effective in the prevention of metastatic progression following surgical removal of the primary tumor mass. Immunotherapeutic approaches are based either on nonspecific stimulation of the host's immune system or on the specific immunization of the organism against tumor cells originating in the surgically removed tumor. These immunization procedures are expected to stimulate the development of cytotoxic lymphocytes or antibodies which are capable of inhibiting tumor growth and destroying metastatic tumor cells. Another experimental approach to immunotherapy is based on the adoptive transfer to the diseased host of lymphocytes sensitized *in vitro* against tumor cells [1].

The specific immunotherapeutic methods formerly were based on the assumption that tumor cells originating in metastases are phenotypically identical copies of cells found in the primary tumor tissues and therefore they share with the primary tumor identical tumor-associated cell surface antigens. Despite that attractive assumption, given the fact that most of the malignant tumors are heteroploid, one is forced to reexamine the validity of this concept. Obviously the question is raised whether indeed metastatic cells are random representatives of the primary tumor cell population or whether they are selected out of a diverse population. The fact that tumor cells are characterized by impaired chromosome replication and segregation furnishes the basis for the generation of diversity among the primary tumor cell population. Such diversity may determine heterogeneity in genetic and phenotypic properties which in turn may furnish the basis for selective processes. Variant cells with a higher probability of metastasis formation could be selected out from parental tumors [2]. Such an increased capacity for metastatic growth could be based on an increased probability of cell migration, on increased affinity for certain tissues, on preferential growth in the new tissue environment [2–4], and on resistance of the metastatic cells to the host's immune response directed against the primary tumor [5].

Recent studies have indeed indicated that metastases may differ from the primary tumor cell population in a number of properties. Thus, differences in drug susceptibility [6], affinity to various organs [2, 7, 8], chromosome number [9, 10], and some biochemical properties [2, 11] have been observed.

L.A. Liotta and I.R. Hart (eds.), Tumor Invasion and Metastasis. ISBN-13: 978-94-009-7513-2.
© 1982 Martinus Nijhoff Publishers, The Hague/Boston/London.

The progression of metastasis may be a function of properties both of the host and of the neoplastic cells. Thus, it has been demonstrated that activation or suppression of the host's immune reactivity may result in decrease or increase of metastatic progression [12–14].

Metastatic spread may conceivably take place in organisms which respond immunologically against the primary tumor. Antigenic heterogeneity of tumor cell populations is the basis for immunoselection of tumor cell clones which may survive under this immunological pressure. The initial small populations of metastatic cells could escape immune destruction if their cell surface tumor antigens were different from those of the primary cell population. Immunoselection would then predict that cells of tumor metastases differed antigenically from cells of the primary tumor. In the present paper we summarize our investigations of the antigenic diversity of tumor cells relevant to their metastatic properties [5, 15–18].

1. Antigenic differences between tumor cells derived from the local 3LL tumor and its pulmonary metastases

In a previous study [19] we found that *in vitro* sensitization of lymphocytes against monolayers of syngeneic tumors carried out in culture media containing xenogeneic serum such as fetal calf serum (FCS) results in cytotoxic lymphocytes (CL) directed mainly against FCS determinants rather than against the actual cell surface tumor-associated antigens. We therefore studied the generation of CL when sensitization against syngeneic tumors was carried out in the presence of syngeneic mouse serum. We demonstrated [19] that sensitization in syngeneic serum results in CL manifesting strict specificities against the tumor antigens.

Having found such antitumor specificities, we turned to test whether cells of the

Table 1. Specificity of cytotoxic activity of syngeneic C57BL/6 spleen cells sensitized *in vitro* against local (L-3LL) or metastatic derived (M-3LL) tumor cells.

Sensitizing tumor cells	Target tumor cells	% Cytotoxicity at lymphocyte-to-target-cell ratio of:				
		Expt. 1		Expt. 2		Expt. 3
		25:1	12.5:1	25:1	12.5:1	25:1
L-3LL	L-3LL	54.6	57.6	49.3	31.1	45.7
L-3LL	M-3LL	13.1	4.4	5.2	0.4	3.7
M-3LL	M-3LL	21.5	31.4	47.1	46.5	37.1
M-3LL	L-3LL	9.2	4.2	7.0	9.5	8.2

Normal C57BL/6 spleen cells were sensitized *in vitro* for 5 days on monolayers of L-3LL and M-3LL tumor cells. Cytotoxic activity of sensitized lymphocytes was tested *in vitro* by ^{51}Cr end labeling technique.

Table 2. Anti-M-3LL lymphocyte suppression of the development of lung metastases.

Spleen cells sensitized against tumor cells	Transplanted tumor cells	No. of pulmonary metastasis in mice inoculated with sensitized lymphocytes and tumor cells at ratio:		
		25:1		12.5:1
Control,	L-3LL cells alone		19.6	
None	L-3LL	21.7		27.3
L-3LL	L-3LL	28.6		35.2
M-3LL	L-3LL	3*		17.8
Control,	M-3LL cells alone		21.1	
None	M-3LL	42.4		N.T.
L-3LL	M-3LL	52*		42
M-3LL	M-3LL	7.7*		3.5*

Normal C57BL/6 syngeneic spleen cells were sensitized *in vitro* for 5 days on monolayers of primary local 3LL (L-3LL) and pulmonary metastasis-derived (M-3LL) carcinoma cells, in the presence of 1% syngeneic mouse serum. Sensitized cells were collected and transplanted at various ratios, together with either M-3LL or L-3LL tumor cells, intrafootpad. The number of lung metastases was counted 21 days later. Each experimental group contained 10 mice.

* Differs significantly from control group according to Mann-Whitney U test ($P < 0.05$).

local growth of the 3LL tumor (L-3LL) possess antigenic specificities different from those of the metastatic population (M-3LL). We examined the specificity of the cytotoxic activity manifested by lymphocytes sensitized against monolayers of M-3LL compared to lymphocytes sensitized against L-3LL monolayers. The results described (Table 1), summarizing three separate experiments, indicated that lymphocytes sensitized in fresh syngeneic mouse serum against monolayers of L-3LL lysed L-3LL targets significantly more than they lysed M-3LL cells. The activity against the L-3LL targets was very high, since even at ratios of lymphocytes to targets of 12.5 : 1 we got high levels of cytotoxicity. Conversely, lymphocytes sensitized against M-3LL cells lysed M-3LL targets significantly more than they lysed L-3LL targets. It appears, therefore, that each of these tumor populations is characterized, in addition to shared determinants, by specific cell surface antigens.

The specificity we obtained against metastatic cells, using *in vitro* cytotoxicity assays, raised the question of whether anti-M-3LL cytotoxic lymphocytes generated *in vitro* or anti-M-3LL lymphocytes in M-3LL tumor-bearing mice (TBM) are capable of suppressing the development of metastases *in vivo*. To test this we injected into the footpad either anti-L-3LL or anti-M-3LL *in vitro*-sensitized lymphocytes admixed with 2×10^4 L-3LL or M-3LL cells, at lymphocytes-to-tumor-cell ratios of 25:1 or 12.5:1. We found no significant differences in growth of the local tumor at these cell ratios. However, when testing for the incidence of lung metastases at 21 days following cell inoculation, we found (Table 2) that anti-L-3LL cytotoxic lymphocytes did not reduce the incidence of metastases produced by L-

3LL cells (if anything, they increased the number of lung metastases). On the other hand, anti-M-3LL caused a significant reduction of metastases produced following the inoculation with L-3LL. A dramatic reduction was obtained at ratios of 25:1 lymphocytes to tumor cells. The effect of anti-L-3LL and anti-M-3LL cytotoxic lymphocytes on the production of metastases by M-3LL cells was also tested. Here again, anti-L-3LL cells did not reduce the incidence of lung metastases, whereas anti-M-3LL cytotoxic lymphocytes caused a reduction at lymphocyte-to-tumor-cell ratios of 25:1 and 12.5:1.

The existence of antigenic differences between a local growing methylcholanthrene-induced tumor and its pulmonary metastases was demonstrated by Sugarbaker and Cohen [20]. Using the method of cross grafting of syngeneic mice with cells from the primary tumor and its metastasis these authors had found that some metastases possessed specific antigenic determinants not shared by the primary tumor cells. In some cases, metastatic cells lost their immunogenicity. Shirrmacher et al. [21] reported that a methylcholanthrene-induced nonmetastasizing lymphoma Eb and its metastasizing variant ESb carry distinct antigens. Lymphocytes immunized against the metastasizing subline ESb, but not against the nonmetastasizing Eb tumor, were able to prevent the development of metastases in the mice bearing ESb lymphoma [21].

2. Cells from pulmonary metastasis are less susceptible than cells of the 3LL local tumor to the cytotoxic activity of natural killer (NK) cells

Recent studies have suggested that nonspecific mechanisms mediated by naturally occurring killer cells (NK cells) may have a decisive function in controlling tumor development [22, 23]. We therefore suggest that metastatic cells are not exempt from such defense mechanisms and therefore only NK resistant tumor cells which survive in the blood and in various organs may be the main cellular source for initiation of distant metastases. Hence, it seemed of interest to investigate whether, indeed, cells of tumor metastases and those of the local tumor manifest differences with regard to susceptibility to the cytotoxic activity of NK cells. For that purpose experiments using different *in vitro* and *in vivo* approaches were performed to test the relative resistance of M-3LL and L-3LL tumor cells to injury by normal lymphoid cells.

The data described in Table 3 show that normal spleen cells are capable of killing 3LL tumor cells. The cytotoxic effect was exhibited by both freshly isolated normal spleen cells and by spleen cells cultured *in vitro* for 2 or 5 days [16].

In parallel, experiments performed with M-3LL target cells clearly show that metastasis-derived tumor cells were more resistant to the cytotoxic activity of normal spleen cells than L-3LL tumor cells (Table 3).

Resistance of M-3LL cells to NK cells of freshly isolated spleen cells was similar to the resistance against spleen cells cultured for 2 or 5 days [16].

To test whether the differences in sensitivity of M-3LL and L-3LL tumor cells to

Table 3. Sensitivity of L-3LL and M-3LL tumor cells to the cytotoxic action of fresh unsensitized normal spleen cells of C57BL/6 mice.

Expt. No.	Ratio between tumor and spleen cells	% cytotoxicity against target cells	
		L-3LL	M-3LL
1	1:200	57.5	19.0
	1:100	35.6	21.9
	1:50	33.6	14.9
	1:25	28.8	18.3
2	1:50	40.0	11.4
	1:25	12.0	7.0
3	1:50	17.0	14.0
	1:25	6.0	0.5
4	1:50	35.8	16.0
	1:25	21.9	5.2
5	1:200	29.3	15.4
	1:100	23.3	13.7

Fresh normal spleen cells of C57BL/6 mice were put into the wells on the monolayer of L-3LL or M-3LL tumor cells. Following 18 h survival, part of monolayers were labeled with ^{51}Cr.

the cytotoxic effects of NK cells observed *in vitro* have any *in vivo* significance, we tested the capacity of spleen cells derived from normal animals to inhibit the development of either M-3LL or L-3LL cells in intact syngeneic mice. M-3LL and L-3LL tumor cells were prepared and 2×10^4 cells of each tumor cell suspension were admixed with syngeneic normal spleen cells at a ratio of 1:25–1:100 tumor to spleen cells.

The mixture was inoculated into the hind footpads of syngeneic recipients. The development of tumors was assayed by recording the day of tumor appearance and tumor diameter, at various time intervals. An inhibition of L-3LL tumor growth was observed when the ratio of inoculated tumor to spleen cells was 1:50 and 1:100. The growth of M-3LL tumor cells was inhibited only when the ratio of spleen to tumor cells was 1:100. Yet even at this ratio (1:100) normal spleen cells inhibited L-3LL cells significantly more than they inhibited M-3LL tumor cells. The percentage of inhibition of L-3LL tumors was 51–57%, whereas that of M-3LL tumors was only 25–26%.

These data suggest that the relative resistance of M-3LL cells to NK cells might be a result of selection of metastatic cells during their circulation in the blood. If resistance to natural effector cells increases the probability of production of metastases by tumor cells, then selection for resistance to NK cells could concomitantly select tumor cells for increase in metastatic potency. In the next series of experiments 0.5×10^6 3LL cells were transplanted s.c. with 5×10^6 of normal spleen cells of

C57BL/6 mice for eight transplant generations. The resulting tumors were designated 3LLN. Cells from these tumors of the third, fifth and eighth transfers were tested for their susceptibility to the cytotoxic activity of normal spleen cells. The results presented in Table 4 show that after three passages of 3LL cells with normal spleen cells the 3LLN cells acquired relative resistance to the *in vitro* cytotoxic activity of spleen cells. We then studied the metastatic capacity of the selected tumor cell populations.

One $\times$ 10^5 3LL cells or 3LLN cells were inoculated intra-footpad (i.f.p.). The local tumors were excised when they reached 8–10 mm in diameter and both the local growth and the development of lung metastases were examined. We found no significant differences in the growth of the local 3LL and 3LLN tumors in the C57BL/6 mice. On the other hand, the 3LLN tumor cells were significantly more efficient in developing lung metastases than the original 3LL tumor cells (Table 4). Thus, the weight of lungs with metastases and the level of ^{125}IUdR incorporation were higher in mice inoculated with 3LLN than in mice inoculated with 3LL tumor cells. This increased metastatic potency appeared after three s.c. passages of tumor

Table 4. Development of metastases in mice following excision of the local 3LL or 3LLN tumor.

Generation	Tumor	% Cytotoxic activity of normal spleen cells**	Weight of lungs (mg)	cpm per pair of lungs
I	3LL	NT***	452	9299
	3LLN	NT	447	9215
II	3LL	NT	518	11593
	3LLN	NT	484	11140
III	3LL	23	379	5265
	3LLN	9	510*	11436*
IV	3LL	NT	731	15973
	3LLN	NT	820	22594
V	3LL	25	554	12128
	3LLN	14	706*	20162*
VI	3LL	NT	547	10769
	3LLN	NT	699*	16719*
VII	3LL	NT	628	8664
	3LLN	NT	748*	14644*
VIII	3LL	31	598	15813
	3LLN	4	775*	30616*
Normal lungs			202	488

1 $\times$ 10^5 3LLN or 3LL tumor cells were inoculated intra-footpad into C57BL/6 mice. 8–10 mm tumors were removed. Eleven days later, 1 μCi of ^{125}IUdR was inoculated i.p. After 24 h the weight of lungs and their radioactivity were determined. 10–19 mice per group.

* The weight of lungs and their ^{125}IUdR incorporation significantly higher (P <0.05) according to Mann-Whitney U test.

** Cytotoxicity at effector: target ratio 100:1 in 18 h ^{51}Cr end labeling assay.

*** NT – not tested.

cells admixed with normal spleen cells and was maintained during the subsequent transplantation generations.

It has been known for years that i.v. inoculated tumor cells are eliminated from the circulation very quickly and only 0.1% of initial population of inoculated cells may develop metastatic nodules in the lungs [2, 3, 24]. Riccardi et al. [25] found that it is mostly NK cells which are involved in this elimination of tumor cells. Depression of NK activity resulted in decrease of tumor cell destruction in the lungs and subsequently increases in development of artificial metastases in the lungs. Relatively high levels of NK activity in nude mice and low levels of NK activity in beige mice positively correlate with their ability to prevent the development of spontaneous or artificial lung metastases. Following serial incubation *in vitro* of tumor cells with spleen cells of nude mice, an NK resistant variant was selected [27]. Only this resistant subline displayed a metastatic ability in the nude mice. These data support our suggestion that NK or NK-related cells may participate in the elimination of circulating tumor cells and in the selection of cells which would survive and further develop tumor metastases [16]. Yet by using different metastasizing tumors, or their clones, it appears that resistance to NK cell destruction is not the only property required for the metastatic process [26, 27].

3. H-2 antigenic differences between local and metastatic tumor cells

The 3LL Lewis lung carcinoma arose spontaneously in a C57BL mouse, but during its sucessive passages the tumor lost its strain specificity and can grow progressively in allogeneic mice. We found that tumor cells derived from lung metastases (M-3LL) have greater ability to grow in F_1 hybrids and even across the allogeneic barrier than L-3LL tumor cells [28]. These findings stimulated a study of the expression of H-2 antigens on the cell surfaces of the local tumor and on it metastasis. The cell surface antigen expression was analyzed by fluorescence serology, using a fluorescence activated cell sorter (FACS-II). H-2^b antigen expression was determined on the surface of M-3LL tumor cells obtained from the individual metastatic nodules. Some M-3LL nodules expressed very low levels, some M-3LL nodules had higher levels of H-2^b antigens on the cell surface (Figure 1). The i.f.p. growth of M-3LL tumor cells with relatively low level of H-2^b expression was retarded in comparison with either L-3LL or with M-3LL which manifested high concentrations of expressed H-2^b antigens. Furthermore, following excision of the local tumors of 8–10 mm in diameter high H-2^b M-3LL tumors generated more metastatic tumors in the lungs than H-2^b low M-3LL or than original l-3LL tumor—weight of lungs metastasis was 807 mg, 251 mg and 300 mg, respectively.

Since subcutaneous and pulmonary M-3LL cells were shown to consist of H-2^b low and H-2^b high tumor cells with distinct tumorigenic properties it was of interest to analyse the behavior of H-2^b low and H-2^b high 3LL cells isolated from a L-3LL population. This was performed using the FACS-II to sort out H-2^b low and H-2^b

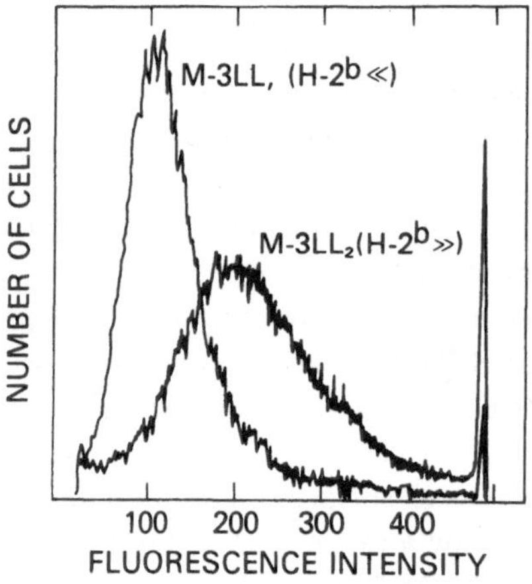

Figure 1. Fluorescence distribution of M-3LL cells isolated from two different metastatic nodules in the lungs stained with anti-H-2^b serum.

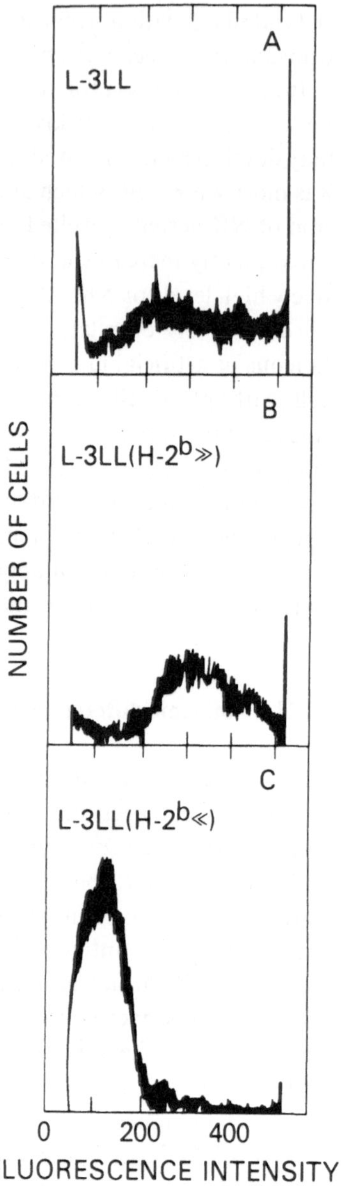

Figure 2. Fluorescence distribution of initial L-3LL cells and L-3LL cells sorted by FACS-II for high and low expression of H-2^b on their cell surfaces.

high 3LL cells from a heterogeneous L-3LL cell suspension (Figure 2). These different populations were injected i.f.p. to syngeneic C57BL/6 recipients, and both tumor appearance and tumor diameter were recorded. On the 16th day after inoculation of 5×10^4 L-3LL (H-2^b high) tumor cells 90% of C57BL/6 mice had established tumors, while only 55% of the mice inoculated with 5×10^4 L-3LL (H-2^b low) tumor cells showed palpable tumors. In addition, H-2^b low L-3LL cells generated fewer metastases in the lungs (mean of lung weight 12 days post amputation = 410 mg) than H-2^b high tumors (mean of lung weight 12 days post amputation = 605 mg).

Using antisera directed against both H-2K and H-2D encoded antigens of the H-2^b haplotype, we have found that the 3LL tumor cells do not express H-2K encoded antigens of the H-2^b haplotype at least detected serologically. It is possible that disproportional expression of H-$2K^b$ and H-$2D^b$ antigens on the cell surface of 3LL tumor cells could provide their local growth even in allogeneic mice. Immune responses evoked in these mice against H-$2D^b$ antigens were unable to prevent the local growth, but were efficient in the complete suppression of the metastatic growth in the lungs [28, 29]. Experiments performed in our laboratory [29] have indeed demonstrated that 3LL tumors which grow progressively across allogeneic barriers did not generate metastasis in allogeneic mice unless the animals had shared with the tumor gene products of the H-2D region of the MHC. In immunosuppressed mice metastatic growth was observed in spite of the incompatibility between allogeneic host and 3LL tumor cells in H-2D region.

All these studies were carried out using a 3LL tumor which has originated in a homozygous H-2^b mouse. To get closer to the human situation we were interested in studying the role of MHC in metastatic processes using metastatic tumor originated in F_1 hybrids bearing two distinct H-2 haplotypes. We have therefore chosen the T-10 sarcoma which was induced by methylcholanthrene in (C3Heb x C57BL/6)F_1

Table 5. Parental H-2 haplotype expression on L-T10 and M-T10 tumor cells.

Experiment no.	Tumor cells (origin)	Relative no. of cells stained with:			
		αH-2^b	αH-2^k	αH-$2D^k$	αH-$2K^k$
1	L-T10	85	0	0	0
	M-$T10_1$	44	71	74	42
	M-$T10_2$	45	78	80	38
	M-$T10_3$	40	71	60	45
2	L-T10	93	24	8	7
	M-T10	55	85	86	50
	M-$T10_1$	61	86	87	42
	M-$T10_3$	40	82	73	53
3	L-T10	84	16	—	—
	M-$T10_1$	47	90	—	—
	M-$T10_2$	37	75	—	—

The T10 sarcoma tumors from the original local tumor (L-T10) or from different metastatic pulmonary nodules (M-$T10_{1,2,3}$) were maintained by subcutaneous transfers of 1×10^6 viable cells in (C3Heb × C57BL/6)F_1 mice. The fluorescence stainings of the L-T10 and M-T10 tumor cells were analyzed on the FACS-II (Becton-Dickinson Electronics Laboratory).

mice [30]. The data presented in Table 5 indicate that cells from locally growing T-10 tumor (L-T10) cells express mainly or exclusively the H-2^b parental haplotype while cells from pulmonary metastases (M-T10) cells express both the H-2^b haplotype (although at a lower level than L-T10 cells) and the H-2^k haplotype. These differential characteristics in H-2 expression were found to be stable despite several serial transfers. In addition, different M-T10 clones (obtained from single metastatic nodules) showed identical staining patterns, implying the homogeneous nature of this variant. The H-2^k-encoded molecules expressed on the M-T10 cells consisted of serological determinants encoded by the different subregions of the H-2 locus, since the M-T10 cells were stainable with anti-H-2^k antisera directed against both the H-2D and H-2K end products of the H-2^k haplotype (Table 5). Again, L-T10 tumor cells were found to be serologically negative when analyzed with these specific antisera. In order to test whether the M-T10 cells were preexisting variants in the local tumor population, the L-T10 tumor cells were cloned in semi-solid agar, and individual clones which were passaged in F_1 recipients were analyzed for the presence of H-2^k or H-2^b membrane antigens. As shown in Table 6, the fluorescence analyses of 10 randomly chosen T10 clones revealed the presence of two clones (i.e., IE7 and IB9) expressing both the H-2^k and the H-2^b parental haplotypes. The remaining clones were found to be H-2^k negative but H-2^b positive.

These last findings suggested that the original local T10 tumor consisted of a mixture of H-2^k positive and H-2^k negative cells, with a predominance of H-2^k negative cells. To approach the question of whether the expression of the H-2^k determinants on the T10 tumor cells is related to the metastatogenic potency of the cells, the capacity of the different L-T10 clones to produce lung metastasis was tested by injecting 10^6 viable tumor cells intravenously and two weeks later examining the organs for the appearance of tumor nodules. From the data outlined in Table 6, it is obvious that the H-2^k positive clones are potentially able to survive in the peripheral blood stream and to develop subsequently in one organ, i.e., in the lungs. Such features were not observed at all with the H-2^k negative clones. These two concomitant characteristics, namely, membrane expression of the H-2^k parental haplotype and the production of lung metastases, were stable and remained unchanged even after ten serial passages in syngeneic F_1 mice.

Evidence for the ability of H-2^k positive T10 tumor cells to circumvent host's resistance mechanisms was obtained by analyzing the growth capacities of L-T10 and M-T10 cells in parental recipients. When 10^6 viable L-T10 cells or M-T10 cells were grafted i.f.p. to C57BL/6 (H-2^b) mice or C3H/eb (H-2^k) mice, differential growth patterns were observed, depending on the origin of the T10 tumor cells. M-T10 cells were found to grow both in an H-2^b and in an H-2^k environment, while L-T10 cells grew only in H-2^b mice and were completely rejected in H-2^k mice.

The high metastatic properties of H-2^b/H-2^k T-10 tumor clones could be attributed to their ability to survive in the blood stream and in the lungs in spite of the action of nonspecific natural cell-mediated immunity or/and specific antitumor response. This notion is strengthened by our observation that H-2^k negative T-10 tumor cells

Table 6. Parental H-2 haplotype expression and metastatic potential of T10 clones.

No. of transfer *in vitro*	Tumor cells (origin)	Relative no. of cells stained with		Experimental metastases after i.v. inoculation	
		Anti-H-2^b	Anti-H-2^k	Presence of nodules in lung	Weight of lungs (mg)
1	L-T10	84	23	±	300
	T10 clone IC9	66	14	—	212
	IG2	67	16	—	214
	IIF3	73	8	—	241
	IG3	81	11	—	232
	IB9	93	65	+++	655
	IE7	97	73	+++	759
	IF7	94	17	n.d.	n.d.
	IID6	77	14	n.d.	n.d.
	IID9	82	15	n.d.	n.d.
	IB7	85	14	n.d.	n.d.
5	L-T10	87	12	±	241
	T10 clone IE7	91	93	+++	765
	IID6	77	10	—	214
	IB9	73	74	+++	704
	IC9	71	7.8	—	205
10	L-T10	82	13	±	256
	T10 clone IE7	80	77.4	+++	960
	IB9	89	94	+++	803

T10 cells were cloned in soft agar, H-2 antigen expression and capacity to form the metastatic nodules in the lungs was analyzed. 10^6 cloned T10 tumor cells were inoculated i.v. of (C3Heb × C57BL/6)F_1 mice. The weight of lungs and number of metastatic nodules was determined two weeks following tumor cell inoculation. Weight of normal lungs 202 ± 8 mg.

—, no metastases; ±, <10 nodules; +++, extensive involvement by tumor, numerous metastasis.

n.d. – not done.

could generate pulmonary metastases when injected i.v. into sublethally irradiated recipients.

Metastatic growth is a function of numerous properties of both the tumor cells and the host. Selective processes might be operating, resulting in the selection of tumor cell variants which survive in the circulation in spite of the action of specific or nonspecific (natural cell-mediated) immune processes and which are able to settle and grow progressively in a particular organ. The absence of one of the involved properties may block the completion of the cascade of events involved in the metastatic process. The participation of natural or specific T-cell mediated immunity in these selection processes might be dependent on their susceptibility to NK cells or on the immunogenicity of the tumor cells. Thus, from a diverse tumor cell population strongly immunogenic migrating variants could be eliminated or suppressed during the early phases of tumor growth by the immune reaction which they themselves evoke; clones of different antigenic determinants could then be selected out. One may also expect that in addition to preexistence of diversity, new antigenic variants may be generated during the progression of the local tumor.

Our results indicated that metastatic tumor cells may differ from the locally growing tumor cell population in the expression of tumor-associated or/and of H-2 antigens. Antigenic modulation of the H-2 coded antigens can be an additional mechanism associated with tumor's escape from host's immune destruction. H-2 restricted mechanisms of the antigen recognition and tumor cell destruction by immune lymphocytes might obviously be relevant to these processes [31, 32].

The participation of the natural cell-mediated immunity in the immunoselection of the metastatic variants would result in the formation of an NK resistant tumor cell population. The extent of the immunoselective process might change during the progression of the malignant disease. At the latest phases of tumor growth specific and nonspecific immunity decrease and their participation in the antimetastatic defense diminish. In these conditions more tumor cells are able to survive and develop metastatic nodules. It may be one of the mechanisms responsible for the heterogeneity which exists among different metastatic nodules developed in the lungs.

Our own results and those of others [2] indicate that the development of malignant metastases is the result of a multifactorial process depending on many different phenotypic properties of the tumor cells themselves as well as on a variety of both immunologic and nonimmunologic mechanisms in the tumor-bearing host, whatever the relevance of the different antigenic properties of the metastatic cells to their biologic characteristics, such properties might be of extreme importance with respect to any future rational approach to the problem of immunotherapy of malignancies and may contribute to a better understanding of the unique physiologic characteristics of tumor metastases.

References

1. Rosenberg S, Terry W: Passive immunotherapy of cancer in animals and man. Adv Cancer Res 25:323–388, 1977.
2. Fidler I, Gersten D, Hart I: The biology of cancer invasion and metastasis. Adv Cancer Res 28:149–250, 1978.
3. Fidler I, Nicolson G: Organ selectivity for implantation survival and growth of B16 melanoma variant tumor lines. J Natl Cancer Inst 57:1199–1202, 1976.
4. Liotta L, Tryggvason K, Garbisa S, Gehron Robey P, Murray J: Interaction of metastatic tumor cells with basement membrane collagen. In: Cancer campaign, Vol. 4, Metastatic tumor growth. Grundmann, E (ed). New York: Gustav Fisher Verlag, 1980, pp 21–30.
5. Gorelik E, Fogel M, Segal S, Feldman M: Tumor-associated antigenic differences between the primary and the descendant metastatic tumor cell populations. J Supramol Struct 12:385–402, 1979.
6. Trope C: Different sensitivity to cytostatic drugs of primary tumor and metastasis of the Lewis carcinoma. Neoplasma 22:171–180, 1975.
7. Nicolson G: Cell surfaces and blood-borne tumor metastasis. In: Cancer invasion and metastasis: biological mechanisms and therapy. Day SB et al. (eds). New York: Raven Press, 1977, pp 168–174.
8. Hart L, Talmage J, Fidler I: Metastatic behavior of a murine reticulum cell sarcoma exhibiting organ-specific growth. Cancer Res 41:1281–1287, 1981.
9. Rabotti G: Ploidy of primary and metastatic human tumors. Nature 183:1276–1277, 1959.
10. Chu E, Malmgren R: Microspectrophotometric determination of deoxyribonucleic acid in primary and metastatic mouse mammary tumors. J Natl Cancer Inst 27:217–220, 1961.
11. Chatterjee S, Kim U: Fucosyl-transferase activity in metastasizing and nonmetastasizing rat mammary carcinomas. J Natl Cancer Inst 61:151–162, 1978.
12. Gershon R, Carter R: Facilitation of metastatic growth by antilymphocyte serum. Nature 226:368–370, 1970.
13. Jones P, Castro J: Immunological mechanisms in metastatic spread and the antimetastatic effects of C. parvum. Br J Cancer 35:519–527, 1977
14. Alexander P, Eccles S: The contribution of immunological factors to the control of metastatic spread of sarcomata in rats. In: Critical factors in cancer immunology, Vol. 10, Shultz J, Leif E (eds). New York: Academic Press 1975, pp 159–171.
15. Fogel M, Gorelik E, Segal S, Feldman M: Differences in cell surface antigens of tumor metastases and those of the local tumor. J Natl Cancer Inst 62:585–588, 1979.
16. Gorelik E, Fogel M, Feldman M, Segal S: Differences in resistance of metastatic tumor cells and cells from local tumor growth to cytotoxicity of natural killer cells. J Natl Cancer Inst 63:1397–1404, 1979.
17. Gorelik E, Feldman M, Segal S: Selection of 3LL tumor subline resistant to natural effector cells concomitantly selected for increased metastatic potency. Immunol Immunother Cancer (in press).
18. Baetselier P, Katzav S, Gorelik E, Feldman H, Segal S: Differential expression of the H-2 gene products in tumour cells is associated with their metastatogenic properties. Nature 288:179–181, 1980.
19. Fogel M, Segal S, Gorelik E, Feldman M: Specific cytotoxic lymphocytes against syngeneic, but not xenogeneic, serum. Int J Cancer 22:329–334, 1978
20. Sugarbaker E, Cohen A: Altered antigenicity in spontaneous pulmonary metastases from an antigenic murine sarcoma. Surgery 72:155–161, 1972.
21. Schirrmacher V, Bosslet K, Shantz G, Clauer K, Hubsch D: Tumor metastases and cell-mediated immunity in a model system in DBA/2 mice. IV. Antigenic differences between a metastasizing variant and the parental tumor line revealed by cytotoxic T lymphocytes. Int J Cancer 23:245–252, 1979.
22. Herberman R, Holden H: Natural cell-mediated immunity. Adv Cancer Res 7:305–377, 1978.
23. Kiessling R, Wigzell H: An analysis of the murine NK cell as to structure, function and biological

relevance. Immunol Rev 44:166–208, 1979.
24. Liotta L, Vembu D, Saini R, Boone C: *In vivo* monitoring of the death rate of artificial murine pulmonary micrometastases. Cancer Res 38:1231–1236, 1978.
25. Riccardi C, Puccetti P, Santoni A, Herberman R: Rapid *in vivo* assay of mouse natural killer (NK) cell activity. J Natl Cancer Inst 63:1041–1045, 1979.
26. Hanna N, Fidler I: The role of natural killer cells in the destruction of circulating tumor emboli. J Natl Cancer Inst 65:801–809, 1980.
27. Hanna N, Fidler I, Relationship between metastatic potential and resistance to NK cell mediated cytotoxicity in three murine tumor systems. J Natl Cancer Inst 66:1183–1190, 1981.
28. Gorelik E, Fogel M, Segal S, Feldman M: Antigenic differences between local 3LL tumor and its metastases. III. Difference in growth rate in syngeneic, semiallogeneic and allogeneic hosts. Ninth Annual Meeting of the Israel Immunological Society 35: 1978.
29. Isakow N, Feldman M, Segal S: Genetic regulation of metastatic progression: the development of pulmonary metastases of the 3LL lung carcinoma is controlled by both non H-2 gene(s) and gene(s) linked to the H-2D region of the mouse MHC. Transp Proc 13:778–782, 1981.
30. Brodt P, Gordon J: Anti-tumor immunity in B lymphocyte-deprived mice. I. Immunity to a chemically induced tumor. J Immunol 121:359–365, 1978.
31. Zinkernagel R, Doherty P: H-2 compatibility requirement for T cell mediated lysis of target cells infected with lymphocytic choriomeningitis virus. Different cytotoxic T cell specificities are associated with structures coded for in H-2K or H-2D. J Exp Med 141:1427–1436, 1975.
32. Meruelo D, Nimelstein S, Jones P, Lieberman M, McDevit H: Increased synthesis and expression of H-2 antigens on thymocytes as a result of radiation leukemia virus infection: a possible mechanism for H-2 linked control of virus-induced neoplasia. J Exp Med 147:470–487, 1978.

10. Methods and models for studying tumor invasion

G. POSTE

1. Introduction

1.1. Invasive cells

Invasion is the process whereby cells of one type penetrate into the interior of a tissue containing cells or a different type.

Invasiveness is exhibited by a variety of cells in both normal and pathological phenomena. Neural crest cells, primordial germ cells, nerve axon cones, presumptive hepatocytes, sternal mesenchymal cells and cardiac endothelium each show periods of invasive behavior during embryonic development [review, 1].

In post-natal life, certain neural crest derivatives (e.g. dermal melanocytes), capillary endothelial cells and several classes of motile white blood cells (neutrophils, eosinophils, lymphocytes and macrophages) retain their invasive properties. However, the majority of cells in the coherent tissues of the body are stationary and do not invade adjacent tissues or emigrate to distant sites elsewhere in the body. This behavior, though essential for the stability of organotypic structure, is not irreversible and most tissue cells are potentially mobile as shown by their migratory behavior during wound healing and when explanted *in vitro* and grown as two-dimensional monolayer cultures. Important information on the control of cellular invasion may thus come from a better understanding of the factors responsible for 'stabilizing' intercellular relationships in normal tissues. Mechanisms of possible importance in this regard are: cell specific adhesive and cognitive interactions via specific topographic arrangements of cell surface molecules; intercellular cohesive interactions involving various classes of cell junctions; contact inhibition of locomotion; and mechanical barriers and constraints provided by basement membranes and other impenetrable intercellular matrices [review, 2].

The other major category of invasive cells comprises malignant tumor cells. Malignant cells arising in diverse tissues are capable of invading host tissues and this process, though not always correlated with metastatic ability, is important in the dissemination of malignant cells to establish secondary tumors (metastases) at sites in the body distant from the primary tumor.

The purpose of this paper is to provide a critical survey of the adequacy of the experimental systems presently used to study tumor cell invasion *in vivo* and *in vitro*. Information concerning the mechanism(s) of tumor invasion will not be discussed

L.A. Liotta and I.R. Hart (eds.), Tumor Invasion and Metastasis. ISBN-13: 978-94-009-7513-2.
© 1982 Martinus Nijhoff Publishers, The Hague/Boston/London.

other than to indicate the potential value of particular experimental systems in identifying the role of specific cellular properties in the invasive process.

1.2. Terminology

Much of the terminology used to classify tumor cells and their behavior has its origin in the clinical literature. Thus, the terms 'tumor' and 'neoplasm' were coined (and used interchangeably) to describe lesions resulting from unchecked proliferation of host cells and the terms 'benign', 'invasive' or 'malignant' were adopted as prefixes to describe the ability or inability of tumors to invade and/or metastasize. Most important, the term malignant was applied only to lesions that were able to metastasize. Although invasiveness is an invariant feature of malignant (i.e. metastatic) tumors, invasiveness and metastatic ability are not always correlated and certain tumors, for example, human basal cell carcinoma, are highly invasive and produce extensive local tissue destruction but rarely metastasize.

The terms 'transformation' and 'transformed' are of more recent origin. They were first introduced to describe the spontaneous morphologic 'transformation' undergone by certain rodent cell populations following prolonged cultivation *in vitro*. Compared to their 'untransformed' counterparts, such cells had a different morphology, grew to higher densities, were able to grow when plated onto other cells and did not require attachment to a solid substrate in order to proliferate (loss of anchorage dependence). With the finding in the 1960s that the same alterations occurred after exposure of cultured cells to tumor viruses or chemical carcinogens, these properties came to be interpreted as representing *in vitro* correlates of the neoplastic state *in vivo*. An unfortunate legacy of the uncritical acceptance of this correlation is that in far too many instances these *in vitro* criteria have been used as the *sole* basis for assuming that a cell population has undergone neoplastic conversion without parallel studies being done to verify that they are tumorigenic *in vivo*.

The shortcomings inherent in reliance on *in vitro* parameters of transformation is adequately illustrated by the widespread use of heteroploid established cell lines such as BHK-21, NIL-B and NIL-8 hamster cells as so-called 'normal' control cells to compare with cells of the same type after 'transformation' by tumor viruses even through all of these lines are tumorigenic before 'transformation'!

In the last few years an increasing number of papers have begin to employ the term 'malignant transformation' to describe the various *in vitro* alterations in cell morphology and growth behavior seen following exposure of cells to oncogenic agents *in vitro*. This is not only unwarranted but also has led to considerable confusion. The most cursory examination of the literature reveals numerous examples in which the term 'malignant' or 'malignant transformation' is used, albeit incorrectly, as a synonym for 'neoplastic' or 'tumorigenic.' Equally common are references to the 'malignant transformation' of cells *in vitro* by a particular virus or chemical. In far too many instances this description is used to refer to changes in cell behavior *in vitro* and experiments to determine whether the cells are even tumorigenic *in vivo* (i.e. neoplastic transformation) yet alone capable of metastasizing *in vivo* (i.e. malignant transformation) are never done. Although some, but not all, of the *in vitro* properties typically referred to as 'transformed properties' show a reasonably consistent correlation with tumorigenicity, there is presently no evidence that they correlate with metastatic ability (i.e. malignancy). Indeed, the converse may be true. Ossowski and Reich [3] have reported that acquisition of increased metastatic potential in HEp-3 cells is accompanied by low or reduced expression of several *in vitro* markers of the so called 'transformed' phenotype.

I therefore consider that it would be useful if the term 'transformed' were used only to describe cells that have been shown to be tumorigenic *in vivo* or, if not used in this sense, that the term should at least be qualified with respect to the type of cellular changes being monitored *in vitro*, e.g. morphologic, antigenic, neoplastic and so on. By the same rationale, the use of the prefix 'malignant' should be applied only to cells shown to be capable of causing metastases.

1.3. Choice of tumor systems

In order to study tumor invasion it is necessary to work with a tumor that is invasive. This may seem to be stating the obvious to the point of absurdity. However, the most cursory examination of the literature reveals numerous examples where the stated purpose of the work claims to be to identify the cellular properties associated with 'invasion' or 'metastasis', yet the cells being studied do not exhibit either of these behavioral traits *in vivo*.

With the prerequisite of an invasive tumor, the next question concerns whether spontaneous or transplanted tumors are preferable. No single tumor system stands out as providing an all inclusive experimental model and the choice will depend on the question(s) being asked. It could be argued, for example, that to evaluate optimally the effect of therapeutic modalities on the natural course of invasion and/or metastasis studies on spontaneous tumors would be preferable. However, the relative rarity of spontaneous neoplasms in most laboratory animal species [review, 4] dictates that transplanted tumors have of necessity been used extensively in experimental studies of the invasive phenotype.

I do not propose to discuss the many questions relating to the respective value of spontaneous versus induced tumors and the equally important problem of the emergence of highly selected, atypical tumor cell populations during serial passage of tumors *in vivo* or *in vitro*. These have been debated at length and undoubtedly merit careful consideration [see references 5–9 for reviews].

Finally, the importance of rigorous characterization of the experimental methods used in passaging and preparing tumor cell populations cannot be overemphasized (see [6], for a detailed survey of technical issues pertaining to the preparation of uniform tumor cell populations from tumor tissue *in situ* and from cultured cell lines and the importance of standardizing conditions for assaying tumor cell behavior *in vivo*).

1.4. Phenotypic heterogeneity in tumor cell populations: implications for experimental analysis of the invasive phenotype

Experimental efforts to identify the cellular and subcellular properties responsible for the invasive behavior of tumor cells requires comparison of invasive tumor cells with tumor cells of similar origin that lack this property.

Studies done in many laboratories over the last few years have shown that by the time many human and animal tumors are of sufficient size to be detectable clinically they contain a variety of tumor cell subpopulations [review, 10].

This heterogeneity is demonstratable irrespective of whether the original carcinogenic insult involved neoplastic conversion of a single cell (monoclonal tumor) or multiple cells (polyclonal tumor). Generation of phenotypically diverse subpopulations of cells within tumors is believed to result from the phenomenon of tumor progression in which progressive growth of a tumor is accompanied by emergence of variant tumor cell clones whose phenotype(s) differs from the parent cells from which they were derived [11].

With time this process creates a diverse panel of clonal subpopulations within the tumor. At any given time during tumor progression the number of subpopulations present, and the extent of their phenotypic diversity, will depend on the selection pressures encountered during the lifetime of the tumor. Selection pressures can be natural (e.g. assault from host defense mechanisms; limiting nutritional conditions etc.) or artificial (e.g. clinical therapy).

Cells populating human and animal neoplasms have been shown to be heterogenous with respect to their immunogenicity, antigenic properties, growth rate, metabolic properties, hormone receptors, karyotype, radiosensitivity and susceptibility to cytotoxic drugs [reviews 10, 12]. Of more relevance to this chapter is the finding that tumors contain subpopulations of cells with differing invasive and metastatic capacities. Invasive and metastatic heterogeneity in subpopulations of cells isolated from the same tumor has been identified in several experimental animal tumors [review, 10].

Efforts to demonstrate similar heterogeneity in human tumors has been hindered by the lack of a suitable experimental system for analyzing the *in vivo* behavior of these cells. Transplantation into athymic nude mice has been used widely to assay the tumorigenic potential of human tumor cells [review, 12]. However, a consistent finding has been that the resulting tumors fail to invade or metastasize. The same situation applies to experimental animal tumors implanted into nude mice, including tumors that are invasive and metastatic in immunocompetent hosts. Recently, however, it has been shown that the absence of invasion and metastasis in tumors implanted in nude mice is an age dependent phenomenon [13] and tumors which are non-metastatic in nude mice 10 weeks of age or older will metastasize when inoculated into 3-week-old animals. This important finding opens the way for experimental analysis of the important question of whether of human tumors contain subpopulations of cells with differing invasive and metastatic capacities in analogous fashion to experimental animal tumors.

Identification of significant variation in the invasive/metastatic properties of cells isolated from the same tumor has important implications for experimental attempts to define which cellular properties correlate with invasiveness. Hitherto, the question has been investigated by analyzing tumor cells isolated at random from cultured tumor cell lines or from biopsies of tumor tissue *in vivo*. This is valid only if the tumor cell population being studied is uniform and the cells are phenotypically homogenous. If, however, extensive cellular heterogeneity exists, and cell subpopulations endowed with invasive properties are only a minor fraction of the total population, random analysis of the entire population will mean that non-invasive subpopulations may present a 'background noise' which obscures features unique to invasive subpopulations.

Continued experimental efforts to characterize the invasive phenotype using heterogenous tumor cell populations may therefore be less productive than studies in which invasive/metastatic subpopulations are isolated and compared with non-invasive/non-metastatic subpopulations from the same tumor.

Whereas the experimental strategy adopted for identifying tumor cell properties that correlate with tumorigenicity involves comparison of non-neoplastic and neoplastic cells, analysis of the invasive and/or metastatic phenotypes is more complicated and will require comparison of the following cell populations (preferably isolated from the same parent tumor cell population):

tumorigenic, non-invasive
versus
tumorigenic, invasive, non-metastatic
versus
tumorigenic, invasive, metastatic

Three different experimental approaches have been used to date to isolate tumor cell subpopulations with differing invasive and/or metastatic abilities.

The first involves *enrichment* of the fraction of invasive/metastatic subpopulations present in heterogeneous tumor cell populations and subsequent comparison with the original parent population. This approach has been used by Hart and Fidler [14], Hart [16] and Poste et al [16] to select B16 melanoma sublines with enhanced tissue invasive capacities (see section 2.2.4.).

A related approach is to select for (or against) cells which exhibit properties considered important for successful invasion (e.g. production of tissue lytic enzymes; locomotion etc.). As in the first approach, the selection procedures are applied to heterogeneous (uncloned) tumor cell populations and variants displaying (or lacking) the property of interest are recovered and assayed to determine whether

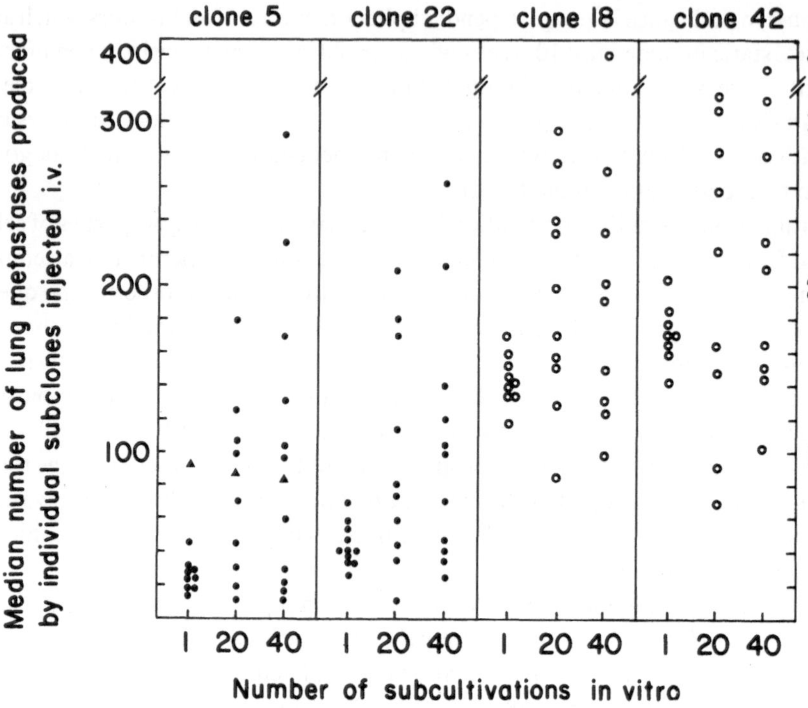

Figure 1. Incidence of lung metastases produced by subclones isolated after serial subcultivation of four clones derived from the murine B16-F10 cell line. The metastatic activity of the uncloned parental B16-F10 cell line is also shown (▲). Metastasis formation was assayed by injection of 2.5×10^4 viable cells as a single cell suspension in 0.2 ml HBBS. Mice were killed 18 days later, the lungs removed, rinsed in water, fixed in formalin and the number of melanotic lung tumor colonies (experimental metastases) counted under a dissecting microscope. Reproduced with permission from Poste et al. [21].

their invasiveness differs significantly from that of the original parent cell population. Selection *in vitro* for tumor cell variants with reduced adhesive properties, resistance to lysis by cytotoxic lymphocytes, resistance to lectin-mediated toxicity and altered attachment to collagen have been used successfully to isolate variant tumor cell lines with altered metastatic capabilities [review, 10].

The third approach involves cloning of heterogeneous tumor cell populations to identify clones with desired invasive/metastatic properties which can be compared with clones from the same population that fail to express these properties. This approach was used by Fidler and Kripke [17] to isolate B16 melanoma clones with highly different metastatic properties from the same parent cell population. Similar demonstrations of the presence of clones with widely differing invasive and/or metastatic properties within the same tumor have been made in several other animal tumors [10, 16, 18–20].

Phenotypic analysis of tumor cell clones is the most direct and satisfactory of the three approaches. In the other two, selection to enrich the subpopulations showing the desired phenotype, though useful, still carries the difficulty that several subpopulations with differing phenotypes persist within the population and may complicate interpretation of experimental data.

The value of tumor cell clones in analyzing any aspect of tumor cell behavior requires that the phenotypic character(s) of interest are stable during serial passage of the clones whether *in vivo* or *in vitro*. Although many cellular properties are highly stable in cloned cells in the absence of specific selection pressures, recent work in my laboratory [21] and by Fidler and Nicolson [22] has revealed that the invasive and metastatic properties of B16 melanoma clones are highly unstable during serial passage and subclones with different invasive and metastatic properties are generated rapidly on serial passage *in vitro* or *in vivo*. The instability of these properties in clones propagated in isolation contrasts with the apparent stability of these traits in the heterogeneous polyclonal parent cell populations from which they were isolated (Figure 1). Observations on individual B16 clones carrying a variety of stable biochemical markers have revealed that whereas the invasive/metastatic phenotype is unstable when clones are grown singly, mixing and cocultivation of clones to create artificially a polyclonal population eliminates this phenotypic instability and formation of variant subclones with altered properties is reduced dramatically (Figure 2). This suggests that some form of 'interaction' is occurring between the various cellular subpopulations in polyclonal populations which somehow 'stabilizes' not only their invasive/metastatic properties but also their relative proportions within the total population. This type of interaction would conserve clonal diversity within a tumor cell population and prevent domination of the population by a few subpopulations, or even a single subpopulation.

Introduction of a new selection pressure can alter the 'equilibrium' between different clonal subpopulations and restrict subpopulation diversity by eliminating unfit clones. We have shown that if the majority of the subpopulations are eliminated, the 'stabilizing' interaction between subpopulations is lost and the surviving subpopulations become phenotypically unstable and quickly generate a new panel of variant subpopulations with different invasive/metastatic properties. This was demonstrated by showing that in polyclonal populations produced by mixing three wild type (*wt*) and three drug-resistant B16 melanoma clones subsequent treatment with drug to eliminate *wt* clones stimulated phenotypic instability within the surviving drug-resistant clones and new panel of subclones with different invasive/metastatic properties emerged rapidly (Figure 2). This amplification of subpopulation diversity did not proceed indefinitely but eventually 'stabilized,' presumably a result of the establishment of a new equilibrium between the recently generated subpopulations. This would presumably persist until another selection pressure is encountered and the cycle repeated.

Although these experiments were concerned specifically with the effect of interactions between tumor cell subpopulations on their invasive and metastatic properties, work by Heppner and het colleagues [23, 24] using murine mammary tumors has shown that cell subpopulations within the same tumor can exert growth

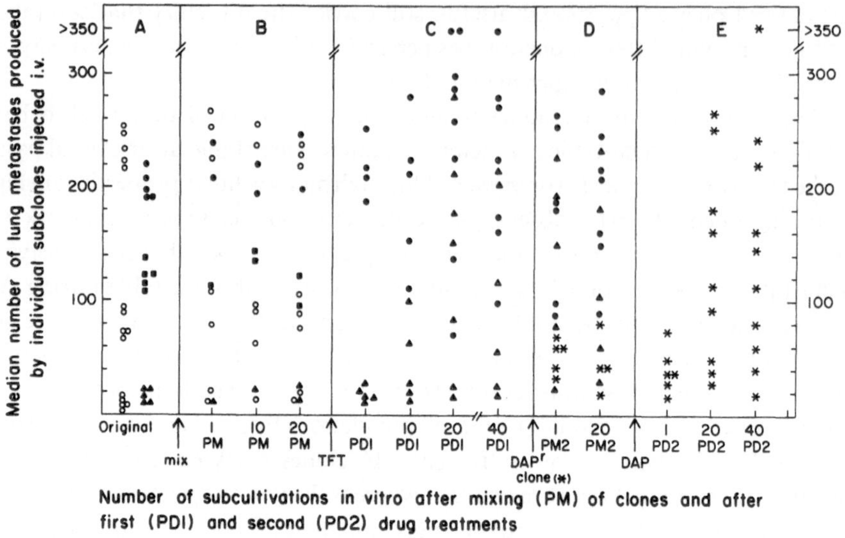

Figure 2. Stability of the metastatic phenotype in polyclonal cultures prepared by cocultivation of a series of clones isolated from the murine B16-F10 melanoma cell line. Wild-type, drug-sensitive B16-F10 clones (wt; ○) were mixed with clones resistant to trifluorothymidine (TFT^r; ▲), oubain (Oua^r; ■) or to both drugs (TFT^r/Oua^r; ●) (panel A). Subclones were isolated after 10 or 20 subcultivations (panel B) and assayed for their metastatic properties and drug-sensitivities. After 20 subcultivations the cultures were treated with TFT. The surviving cells were then passaged (panel C) and subclones isolated and tested for metastatic properties and for resistance to 2 μg/ml TFT (▲) or TFT and 1 × 10^{-3}M oubain (●). After 40 subcultivations a new clone of DAP^r cells (*) were added. Subclones were isolated from this mixed cell population after 20 subcultivations (panel D) and their metastatic properties and susceptibility to TFT (2 μg/ml), oubain (1 × 10^{-3}M) and DAP (4.7 × 10^{-5}M) evaluated. Replicate cultures were treated with DAP (4.7 × 10^{-5}M). The surviving cells were passaged (panel E) and subclones isolated at the indicated intervals and tested for their metastatic properties and their ability to grow in HAT medium (DAP^r variants (*) grow; TFT^r variants fail to grow).

regulatory restraints on each other and also on their immunogenicity and sensitivity to cytotoxic drugs [24]. The numerous reports showing that the presence of the primary tumor can restrict the growth of metastases in certain tumors may represent an analogous phenomenon [25–28 and Gorelik, chapter 9; this volume].

Irrespective of the mechanism(s) responsible for these fascinating phenomena, identification of interactions occurring between clonal subpopulations within the same tumor introduces an additional level of complexity to the experimental analysis of tumor cell properties since it suggests that a full understanding of the behavior of tumors may not be possible by analysis of individual component cells but may require more sophisticated analyses of subpopulation interactions.

Cloning provides the most direct and efficient method for the identification of tumor cells with differing invasive and/or metastatic properties. However, if the data described above concerning phenotypic instability in B16 melanoma clones is applicable to tumor cells in general, then cloning alone will not guarantee uniform experimental material. By eliminating the interaction between subpopulations, cloning provides a potent stimulus for emergence of variant subclones with differing phenotypes. If this proves to be a general feature of malignant tumor cells it will be essential to practice the additional step of recloning tumor cell clones at regular intervals to ensure that cell preparations with uniform properties are being studied. The alternative would be to 'stabilize' the invasive/metastatic phenotype in clones by artificially creating polyclonal populations via cocultivation of a series of clones. In this case the most logical approach would seem to be first to identify a series of clones with similar invasive properties and mix them. This population could then be compared with a polyclonal population prepared by mixing a similar number of non-invasive clones isolated from the same parent cell population.

2. Current research approaches

2.1. Strategies for experimental analysis of tumor cell invasion

Before reviewing the various methods used as models for tumor invasion I will discuss briefly three issues that are pertinent to any experimental attempt to correlate specific cellular properties with invasiveness. These focus on the obvious, yet frequently ignored, requirement that the tumor cells being used be shown to be invasive *in vivo* and that any heterogeneity in the expression of this trait by cells within the same population be identified. These requirements can be fulfilled only by using a combination of *in vitro* and *in vivo* techniques and by the availability of methods which permit quantatation of invasion and/or recovery of invasive cells for further study.

2.1.1. The correlation of in vitro and in vivo data. Cultured cell populations provide the major source of experimental material used in cancer research laboratories. The relative simplicity of *in vitro* cell culture systems, the opportunities for detailed analyses of large numbers of cells under controlled conditions and the ability to study directly the cellular and subcellular changes produced by exposing cells to oncogenic agents *in vitro* are powerful approaches that would be very difficult or impossible to duplicate *in vivo*. Nonetheless, awareness of the phenotypic changes that may be imposed on cells by cultivation *in vitro* is crucial if *in vitro* culture techniques are to be used effectively in correlating specific cellular properties with invasiveness. The myriad changes that cells undergo when initiated in culture; the effect of prolonged cultivation in promoting further phenotypic shifts; and the role of environmental conditions in producing subtle yet important changes in cellular properties have been discussed fully elsewhere [review, 29].

In analyzing the neoplastic phenotype it is also necessary to consider the technical implications of the level of cellular heterogeneity encountered in many tumor cell populations (section 1.4.) and take appropriate steps to ensure that the cells being studied are as uniform as possible or, if not, that the extent of cellular heterogeneity be known.

Finally, the importance of parallel studies to correlate the *in vitro* and *in vivo* properties of all cell populations selected for study cannot be overemphasized. Also, in seeking to correlate a property detected in cells *in vitro* with invasive behavior *in vivo* it is necessary to show that the same property is still expressed by cells *in vivo* and is not subject to phenotypic modulation *in vitro*.

2.1.2. Quantitation of tumor cell invasion. The single greatest difficulty that has beset experimental efforts to study tumor invasion has been the lack of methods for rigorous quantitation of invasion.

In the majority of published papers, tumor invasion has been assayed by descriptive, semi-quantitative observations of fixed histologic tissue sections, with invasion being scored on a + to + + + + scale based on the distance that identifiable tumor cells penetrate into host tissue. The accuracy of histologic methods requires, of course, that tumor cells can be reliably identified. Differences in tumor and host cell morphology, karyotype, histochemistry and radioautographic methods have been used for this purpose with varying degrees of success. Accurate quantitation of invasion from histologic sections requires tedious and demanding reconstruction of the invading lesion from serial sections. Even then it is exceptionally difficult, if not impossible, to determine what proportion of a tumor cell population has invaded successfully.

These shortcomings have prompted efforts to quantify invasion using radiolabeled tumor cells. Measurements of cell-associated radioactivity recovered from host tissues exposed to radiolabeled tumor cells permits accurate quantitation of the fraction of a tumor cell population that is invasive. Radiolabeled materials used for this purpose include: ^{51}Cr, ^{99m}Tc, ^{3}H-thymidine and ^{125}I-IUDR. The latter offers several significant advantages.

^{125}I-IUDR is incorporated into the DNA of proliferating cells and is released only after cellular DNA breaks down following cell death. Most important, unlike ^{3}H-thymidine or ^{51}Cr, radiolabel released from dead cells (largely as free ^{125}I) is not reincorporated into nearby cells and measurements of cell-associated radioactivity thus provide an accurate estimate of the number of viable tumor cells present. The short half-lives of ^{99m}Tc and ^{51}Cr preclude their use in long-term experiments but ^{125}I-UDR has a moderately long half-life (60 days) and can be used for experiments of 2–3 weeks duration. Another major disadvantage of ^{51}Cr is that it does not bind firmly to cells and high levels of spontaneous 'background' release of isotope from viable cells is a constant problem. Elution of ^{51}Cr from tumor cells is particularly rapid, with rates of 30–60% in 24 h having been reported [see, 30]. Thus when used to label tumor cells the high level of spontaneous release hinders detection of small numbers of tumor cells in tissues. Similarly, when used to label host cells, release of radiolabel cannot be reliably correlated with tumor-mediated tissue destruction. For example, in the study of Mareel et al. [31], changes in the release of ^{51}Cr from labeled fragments of embryonic chick heart accompanying tumor invasion did not correlate with the extent of invasion and host cell destruction determined by histology. As mentioned, a further complication of using ^{51}Cr is that released radiolabel is readily reincorporated by nearby cells leading to falsely high measured levels of cell-associated radioactivity.

A full description of the factors affecting the efficiency of labeling of tumor cells by ^{125}I-IUDR and the methods for achieving optimal labeling without altering the biological behavior of tumor cell populations are given in the review by Fidler [6].

Hart and Fidler [14] and Poste et al. [16] have used ^{125}I-IUDR as a cellular label to quantify the ability of B16 melanoma lines with differing metastatic properties to invade *in vitro* preparations of chick CAM, mouse bladder and canine and bovine veins. Liotta et al. [32] in an elegant study correlating clearance of ^{125}I-IUDR labeled tumor cells from the pulmonary microcirculation of mice with the morphologic development of micrometastases in the lung showed that the kinetics of clearance of labeled cells could be used to distinguish between initial tumor cell arrest and the subsequent invasion of cells into the lung parenchyma. This procedure was used later by Poste and Nicolson [33] to demonstrate that experimental manipulation of the surface properties of B16 melanoma cells produced by fusion of plasma membrane vesicles from B16 cells with differing metastatic properties caused significant alterations in the efficiency of tumor cell arrest and invasion in the lung microcirculation.

2.1.3. Recovery of invasive tumor cells from host tissues. Until recently there was no compelling reason to attempt to recover invasive tumor cells from within solid host tissue. However, with the finding that many tumor cell populations display extensive cellular heterogeneity, it cannot be assumed that because invasive cells are demonstratable within a population that all cells express this property. Accurate definition of the extent of heterogeneity of invasive phenotypes present within a cell population is thus an essential prerequisite for attempts to correlate specific cellular characteristics with invasiveness. If extensive heterogeneity exists, procurement of uniform cellular material for study dictates that the invasive subpopulations must be isolated. This can be achieved in two different ways. The first is to clone the population to identify clones within the desired invasive profile. The second is to isolate invasive cells directly from host tissues.

Several groups have described methods whereby invasive tumor cells can be recovered from a variety of tissues maintained *in vitro* and subsequently compared with noninvasive cells from the same population [14–16, 34]. In these methods, which are discussed in more detail in section 2.2.4, tumor cells are confronted with a barrier of host tissue and only those cells capable of traversing the entire barrier are harvested. This method thus yields tumor cells of proven invasive ability with the additional advantage that there is little or no contamination with host cells. This approach also avoids the technically more demanding feat of isolating tumor cells from within solid host tissues. The latter has been somewhat neglected and the problem deserves more attention than it has received to date. Several methods have been developed for enzymic and/or mechanical dispersal of tumor tissue to tumor and host cell fractions [reviews 35, 36]. However, the sensitivity of these methods and their usefulness in detecting very small numbers of tumor cells within host tissues and in quantitating changes in the proportion of invasive cells at different stages of tumor growth have still to.be evaluated.

2.2. *Experimental models of tumor invasion*

In surveying the methods used in studying tumor invasion it can be stated at the outset that no single system offers an all embracing model of the invasive process. All of the methods in current use are very far removed from the natural situation. Invasion of a spontaneous tumor is undoubtedly different from the events examined in the majority of experimental systems where host tissues are typically challenged with massive numbers of tumor cells. For technical convenience most of the experimental work on invasion to date has used tumor cell lines that have been highly selected by serial passage for long periods *in vitro* or *in vivo* and it is unclear as to how far their properties are atypical. Similar questions concerning relevance must be directed to experimental systems in which tumor-host cell interactions are studied using cells from different species, different genetic strains within a species and tissues which tumor cells would not ordinairly encounter during the pathogenesis of the natural disease. All *in vitro* models suffer from the absence of host defense reactions and how far this influences the observed tumor-host cell interactions has still to be clarified. Models of tumor invasion *in vivo* avoid this problem but even here the recipient is almost invariably a completely healthy animal without the many, and so far largely uncharacterized, changes which take place in a tumor-bearing host.

The utility of any particular experimental model thus depends on the question(s) being asked. Assay systems that evaluate the entire invasive process either *in vivo* or in organotypic cultures *in vitro* may be so complex as to hinder study of more specific aspects of tumor cell behavior and the contribution of particular cellular activities to the invasive process. On the other hand, highly simplified *in vitro* models such as monolayer cultures lend themselves to detailed analysis of specific cell functions such as locomotion yet do not offer a suitable system for predicting whether a tumor cell population will be invasive *in vivo*.

In presenting a critique of current methods and models used in studying tumor invasion I have accorded particular priority to the following two requirements: 1) the ability to quantify the kinetics and extent of tumor invasion in an accurate and reproducible manner; and 2) the ability to recover invasive tumor cells for further study and comparison with non-invasive tumor cells derived from the same cell population.

2.1.1. Monolayer cell cultures. The behavior of tumor cells when mixed with non-neoplastic cells in two-dimensional monolayer cultures *in vitro* has been studied extensively with the purported aim of providing information on host-tumor cell interactions in invasion [review, 37]. The belief that this highly simplified system is a valid model for invasion stems from the finding that neoplastic and non-neoplastic cells differ in their ability to infiltrate confluent monolayers of normal cells, with tumor cells showing a greater tendency to exhibit this behavior. This has been interpreted as indicating that tumor cells are less responsive than normal cells to contact inhibition of locomotion and that infiltration of tumor cells between adjacent cells in the monolayer is analogous to tumor penetration of host tissues *in situ*. The validity of these assumptions has still to be confirmed.

Critical appraisal of the merit of the monolayer infiltration assay as a model for invasion is hindered by the general failure of investigators using this system to undertake parallel studies to determine the invasive properties of the same cells *in vivo*. The study by Mareel et al. [38] stands as an exception and demonstrates the value of using a variety of assays to screen for invasive activity. Mareel et al. found that mouse fibrosarcoma cells were unable to infiltrate or destroy two-dimensional monolayer cultures of chick heart cells even though they were highly invasive and rapidly destroyed three-dimensional organotypic cultures of chick heart *in vitro* and produced invasive lesions in syngeneic mice *in vivo*. Conversely, a number of non-neoplastic cells have been shown to infiltrate monolayers of normal cells [39, 40].

Review of the available evidence indicates that the ability to infiltrate between cells in monolayer cultures is undoubtedly found more frequently in tumor cells than normal cells. Significant exceptions exist, however, and the validity of infiltrative behavior as an *in vitro* correlate of invasiveness *in vivo* remains questionable.

The relevance of monolayer culture systems as models for invasion must also be questioned from the standpoint of how far cellular interactions in two-dimensional monolayers are representative of events in complex three-dimensional tissue matrices. Among the issues that merit consideration in this context are: 1) possible differences in the type of intercellular adhesive and cohesive forces operating in the two situations; 2) the possibility that the profound alterations in cell geometry imposed by cultivation in two-dimensional monolayers cause changes in cell surface properties that alter cellular responses to the 'signals' involved in control of cell locomotion and/or proliferation; 3) the effect of disruption of three-dimensional tissue architecture and removal of extracellular structures such as basement membranes and supporting tissue stroma in predisposing monolayers to invasion by cells that would be incapable of doing so in intact tissues; and 4) the role of the substratum to which cells adhere in determining the outcome of host-tumor cell interactions in monolayer cultures.

A further criticism, though not unique to the monolayer model and equally applicable to other *in vitro* models of invasion, is that the emphasis to date has been on the infiltration and invasion of single tumor cells. Although serial section histologic studies of tumor invasion *in vivo* indicate that single tumor cells can undoubtedly participate in this process, invasion by multicellular 'tongues' or 'cords' of tumor cells is equally, and perhaps more, common [review, 41]. Progress of tumor tongues or whole tumor fronts is probably mediated by movement of cells at the edges of the cell sheet in analogous fashion to the morphogenetic cell movements seen during epiboly in the early embryo [see, 41]. Invasion and locomotion of aggregates of tumor cells must also be considered. *In vitro* models of these phenomena have yet to be devised.

Although the simplified nature of the monolayer cell culture may preclude its use as a model for studying the complete spectrum of events in invasion, the monolayer system has made a major contribution to the experimental analysis of tumor cell locomotion. The validity of studying this aspect of tumor cell behavior *in vitro* has been evaluated by studies showing that the locomotion of tumor cells in monolayer cultures does not differ in any significant way from tumor cells observed moving within transparent host tissues *in vivo* [41, 42 for refs.].

2.2.2. Tumor cell deformability and invasion: studies with single cell suspensions. The capacity of tumor cells to undergo mechanical deformation may be of considerable importance in determining their capacity to infiltrate into narrow tissue spaces and between adjacent host cells. Circumstantial support for this view is provided by evidence showing that cytoskeletal disruptive drugs produce significant alterations in the organ distribution and extravasation of circulation tumor cells [43]. Although the interpretation that these effects result from drug-induced enhancement of cell deformability seems reasonable, strict correlation of cellular deformability with invasive capacity is hindered by the lack of suitable methods for direct measurement of this property.

Efforts to determine 'deformability' by measuring the negative pressure required to draw a hemispheric cellular bulge into the tip of a micropipette [44] are not only technically tedious but are difficult to interpret. The negative pressure required for hemisphere formation may relate only to the elastic limit of the cell cortex and its relationship to the deformability of the entire cell is unclear.

Sato and Suzuki [45] have attempted to characterize tumor cell deformability by measuring the flow characteristics of cell suspensions through membrane filters of defined pore size under positive pressure. This approach offers several advantages over the micropipette technique: 1) rapid measurements can be made on entire cell populations; 2) the use of positive pressure better approximates events during extravasation; and 3) 'filterability' is influenced by both intrinsic (i.e. inherent deformability of the kind measured by the micropipette) and extrinsic cell properties (i.e. surface to volume ratios) and also by the flow conditions. The only drawback to Sato and Suzuki's apparatus in its present form is that the pressure required to induce trans-filter passage of cells is monitored only on one side of the filter. Their assumption that the pressure above and below the filter are equal is valid only if every pore in the filter is occupied by cells every time a measurement is made. Also, since cellular 'filterability' varies with flow rates, the question of how far the pressure/flow conditions chosen approximate those in the microcirculation is unclear. A further complication is that if tumor cells are like erythrocytes in showing non-linear filterability under different pressure/flow conditions [46], the question of the precise conditions used in comparing different cells becomes crucial, since differences detected under one set of pressure/flow conditions *in vitro* may be non-existent under other conditions (e.g. *in vivo*).

2.2.3. Cultured cell aggregates. Formation of three-dimensional cell aggregates by rotation-mediated aggregation of single cell suspensions of cultured cells has been used in developmental biology for many years as a tool for studying adhesive and cognitive interactions between embryonic cells [47]. More recently aggregates prepared in this way, and the closely related three-dimensional cell spheroid system, have been used as in vitro models of tumor invasion. This topic is covered fully elsewhere in this volume by Mareel (chapter 13) and Gershman (chapter 14) and no mention of these techniques will be made other than to acknowledge their existence.

2.2.4. Organ cultures. Organ cultures of a variety of host tissues have been used as substrates for tumor invasion *in vitro*. These include: rodent omentum, scrotal sac, neonatal calvaria, mesonephros, lung, bladder; human prostate and amnion; and avian skin, mesonephros, heart, amnion, blastoderm and chorioallantois [reviews 28, 48]. Typically, organ culture blocks are placed in direct contact with either single tumor cells or tumor cell aggregates and penetration of tumor cells at the zone(s) of confrontation measured. The obvious advantage of organ cultures over cell monolayers and aggregates is that they reproduce to a large degree the complex three-dimensional cellular relationships found in tissues *in situ*.

In many studies the zone of initial confrontation between tumor cells and host cells is at the exposed cut edge of the organ culture. This raises the obvious question of how far tumor cell penetration is facilitated by the disruption of normal tissue architecture in this region. Although certain investigators [31, 49] preincubate organ cultures for up to 72 h in an effort to allow healing of dissection trauma before challenge with tumor cells, the zone of confrontation is still different from that in intact tissue. This problem is eliminated, however, if the region of confrontation is at areas of the organ culture block which have not been traumatized. For example, in organ cultures of CAM [14, 16], amnion [34] and bladder [16] tumor cells are placed onto the upper, intact (non-traumatized) epithelium and penetration of tumor cells into sub-epithelial regions requires that they breach the integrity of the epithelium and its associated basement membrane.

The majority of observations on tumor invasion in organ cultures have been descriptive and merely document that invasion has taken place. The extensive reliance on histologic techniques to define invasion, frequently without serial sec-

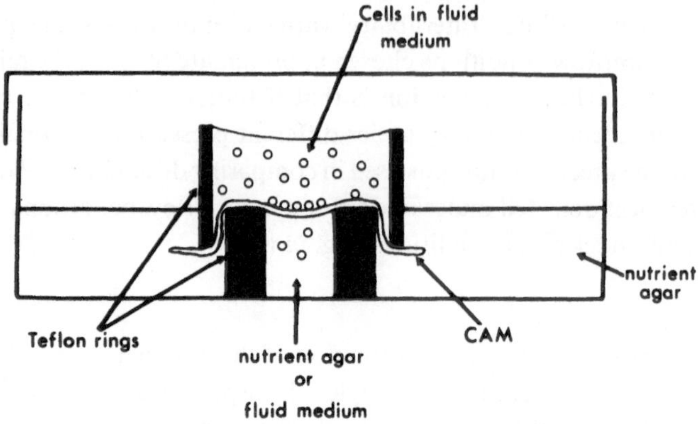

Figure 3. Cross-section of an invasion chamber system for quantitation of tumor cell invasion in the chick CAM and for recovery of cells that traverse the full thickness of the CAM. (Reproduced from Poste et al. [16]; this is a modification of a chamber devised by Hart and Fidler [14] in which cells traversing the CAM were harvested in a block of photographic sponge rather than agar.)

tion reconstructions, dictates that little quantitative information has been obtained regarding either the kinetics of invasion or the fraction of tumor cells that are invasive. These deficiencies have stimulated attempts to devise new methods for accurate quantitation of invasion and the recovery of invasive cells.

The first of this new generation of methods was developed by Hart and Fidler [14] (Figure 3). By immobilizing sections of chick CAM on a mechanical support they were able to apply radiolabeled tumor cells to the non-traumatized endodermal epithelium and monitor invasion by measuring the cell-associated radioactivity present in the CAM at intervals. Another innovative feature of this method is that invasive tumor cells which traverse the entire thickness of the CAM are recovered within a sponge matrix placed beneath the eccodermal epithelium. This technique was modified by Poste et al. [16] who devised a two chamber system in which tumor cells traversing the CAM were recovered in a layer of agar underlying the CAM. The use of agar rather than photographic sponge not only avoids the toxicity problems encountered with certain batches of sponges but also enables penetrating tumor cells to be distinguished from desquamated host cells since the latter do not show loss of anchorage dependence and thus cannot grow in agar.

The aim of being able to quantify tumor invasion and achieve simultaneous recovery of invasive cells has also been fulfilled in another *in vitro* system described by Poste et al. [16] in which tumor cells interact with segments of vein maintained in a perfusion apparatus (Figure 4). This method has several useful features. First, by allowing tumor cells to interact with either the outer adventitial elements of the vessel or the lumenal endothelial surface (by using everted vessels) it is possible to study both intravasation and extravasation. Second, cells that successfully invade and cross the wall of the vein are immediately recovered in the internal perfusion circuit and can be compared with non-invasive cells harvested from the outer injection chamber.

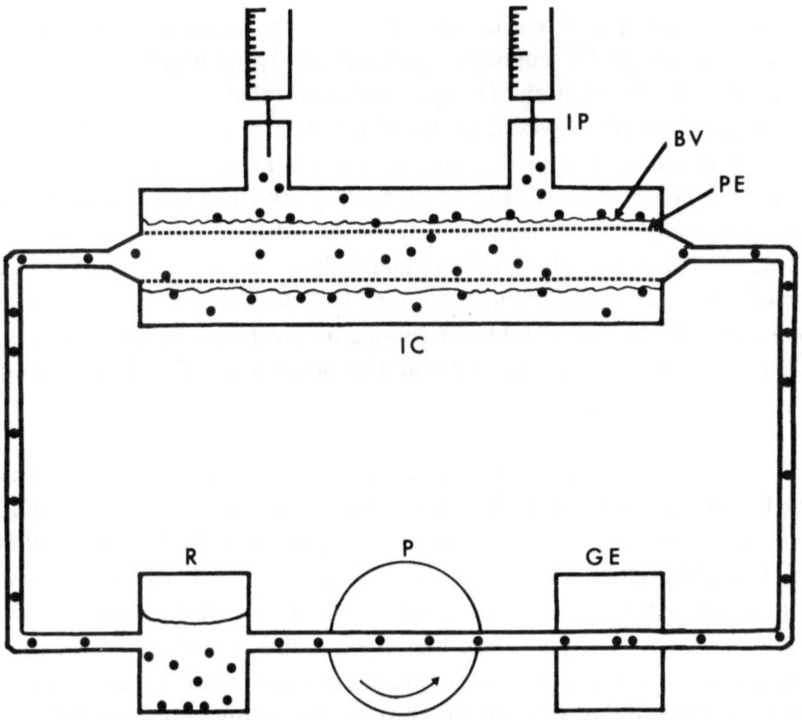

Figure 4. Cross-section of a perfusion invasion chamber system for quantitating invasion of tumor cells in blood vessels and for recovery of tumor cells that successfully invade and penetrate the vessel wall (Reproduced from Poste et al. [16]). Portions of blood vessel (BV), typically vein, are fitted onto a central tube of porous ultra high molecular weight polyethylene (PE) with a defined pore size (typically 20 or 50 μm). Culture medium is perfused through the cente of the tube from a reservoir (R) by a peristaltic pump (P) at flow rates of 2–4 ml/min and passage through a gas exchanger (GE). Tumor cells (•) are injected into the outer chamber surrounding the vessel via injection ports (IP) fitted with self sealing rubber caps. The injected cells attach to the surface of the vessel. Segments of vein can be placed with either the endothelium facing inwards or as everted segments in which the endothelium is facing the injection ports. Invasion of cells into the vessel wall can be determined using radiolabeled cells and measuring the radioactivity associated with the vessel after washing to detach non-invasive cells. Cells that successfully traverse the entire wall of the vessel will then pass across the pores in the central PE tube and can be recovered in the internal perfusion circuit.

Despite the importance of tumor invasion of blood vessels and lymphatics in the pathogenesis of metastasis, information on the mechanisms involved is scant. This reflects both the formidable technical difficulties associated with studying these events *in vivo* and the lack hitherto of suitable *in vitro* models. The blood vessel perfusion system in Figure 4 thus offers new opportunities for studying the following questions: are the events involved in initial penetration of tumor cells into vessels (intravasation) identical to those in passage of arrested cells into extravascular tissues (extravasation)?; do intra- and extravasation occur via destruction of the endothelium and other elements of the vessel wall or by active tumor cell locomotion?; do the mechanisms of intra- and extravasation vary between different types of tumor cells and in different regions of the circulation?; and what role do host cells such as PMN leukocytes, platelets and lymphocytes play in facilitating the arrest and extravasation of circulating tumor cells?

In its present form, however, the blood vessel perfusion system suffers from one major shortcoming. The process of tumor cell intravasation *in vivo* and the subsequent arrest and extravasation of circulating cells take place in the microcirculation and rarely involve large diameter vessels of the kind used in the perfusion system. Unfortunately, the small size and delicate structure of capillary networks precludes their use in this perfusion system. Even large vessels from mice and other small mammals are not suitable for routine use. Miniaturization of the perfusion system shown in Figure 4 to eliminate this deficiency is therefore an important priority.

2.2.5. Tumor invasion in vivo. Experimental efforts to study tumor invasion *in vivo* have been hindered by the technical problems of how to detect small numbers of tumor cells within host tissues and to recover them for study. A further difficulty in using transplanted tumors is that the practice of injecting relatively large numbers of tumor cells direct into tissues is very different from the events in initial invasion of spontaneous tumors. Apart from the large number of cells typically injected in many published experiments, the tissue damage produced by injection may predispose the tissue to invasion. However, transplanted tumors can probably be used as valid models of the invasion processes that occur subsequent to successful establishment of the initial transplant. For example, there is no evidence to indicate that the processes of intravasation and extravasation during hematogenous spread of transplanted tumor cells are significantly different from that in spontaneous tumors. Thus, in testing potential therapeutic agents for anti-invasive activity it may be more appropriate to screen for their ability to modify intra- and extravasation or local tissue invasion in the vicinity of metastases than for activity against invasion at the initial site of tumor inoculation.

Direct observation of tumor cells within tissues is virtually impossible in most tissues since they are opaque. The few studies in which tumor cell behavior has been followed *in situ* have used transparent tissues such as mesentery, CAM, rabbit ear chamber, hamster cheek pouch, tadpole tail fin or teleost embryos [41, 42]. These technically demanding studies have yielded esthetically impressive cinematographic evidence of the movement of tumor cells within tissues, and the vasculature in particular, but have provided little insight into the mechanism of invasion.

Information on tumor cell invasion in opaque tissues has come exclusively from histologic and ultrastructural studies of fixed tissue sections. The problem of analyzing a dynamic process such as invasion from static tissue sections need not be belabored. However, when done carefully, including the use of serial sections to reconstruct the topography of the tumor-host tissue margin, these methods can give some notion of the presence and extent of tumor cell invasion, particularly if invasion is extreme and tissues are examined at carefully staged intervals. The limitation, of course, is that each new time interval involves a different set of cells.

Invasion *in vivo* can also be assessed from indirect evidence. The obvious example is metastasis formation following injection of tumor cells. Metastases can be formed only by successful completion of one or more sequences of invasion (the exact number depending on the route of tumor inoculation). Although mere documentation of metastasis formation does not provide insight into the mechanism(s) of invasion, recovery of cells from metastases provides a useful method for obtaining cells of proven invasive capacity for further study. By comparing the properties of cells harvested from metastases in different organs it may also be possible to determine if different cellular properties are needed for successful colonization of different organs [33].

A number of body sites have been used to assay tumor cell invasion *in vivo*. As with *in vitro* assays, the choice of site, the route of tumor inoculation and the methods used to identify tumor cells in tissues will depend on the question(s) being asked.

Histologic and ultrastructural observations of tumor invasion following s.c. or i.m. injection of tumor cells have been valuable in documenting the routes of initial tumor penetration. Similarly, studies with tumor cells injected i.v. have identified important morphologic aspects of host-tumor cell interactions in extravasation and metastatic colonization of various organs [reviews, 8, 50].

The chorioallantoic membrane (CAM) of the developing chick embryo deserves special mention in this section since it has been used by many investigators as a model for tumor invasion *in vivo* and its validity thus merits examination. This system has the advantage that eggs are cheap and readily available and tumor formation on the CAM can be observed directly via a window created in the shell. Also, invasion of the CAM by certain tumors is accompanied by penetration of the CAM vasculature and metastasis formation in various organs of the developing embryo.

On the negative side, the thickness and histology of different regions of the CAM can vary significantly, making histologic comparison of different CAM preparations difficult. Inadequate attention to the incubation conditions, notably humidity, can produce extensive keratinization of the ectodermal epithelium and fibroblastic hyperplasia of the mesoderm, both of which can modify the course of tumor invasion and also complicate histologic interpretation. Lack of care in removing the overlying egg shell can deposit microscopic particles of shell on the CAM and evoke marked inflammatory reactions that hinder evaluation of the extent of tumor growth and invasion.

The large number of published studies comparing the growth of neoplastic cells and their 'normal' counterparts when plated onto the CAM have established that, with the exception of normal cells such as macrophages that possess tissue infiltrative abilities, normal cells are unable to invade the CAM. In contrast, tumor cells of diverse tissue origins from a wide range of species rapidly form tumors within the mesodermal layer of the CAM. Although the presence of tumor cells in the mesoderm means that they have invaded across the ectodermal epithelium, this is not a reliable correlate of invasive potential in other tissues. Thus, many tumor cell lines that are non-invasive in their natural host will form large invasive tumors in the CAM and the degree of invasion produced by these tumors is often indistinguishable from that caused by tumors that are highly invasive in their natural host.

Additional evidence indicating that tumor invasion in the CAM does not correlate with invasive behavior in other tissue comes from recent studies using B16 melanoma cell lines selected for enhanced ability to invade either the CAM or organ cultures of murine bladder and canine femoral vein [16]. Variants selected for invasiveness in the CAM are non-invasive in both bladder and vein but variants selected for invasiveness in the latter two tissues are highly invasive in all three tissues. Evaluation of the *in vivo* properties of these cell lines revealed that selection for increased invasiveness in bladder or vein was accompanied by significant enhancement of invasive and metastatic activities in syngeneic mice but these in vivo properties were unchanged in the CAM-selected variants.

These data suggest that sucessful penetration of the CAM may be a less demanding task than invasion of bladder or vein where the presence of thick basement membranes, dense collagenous stroma and muscle layers constitute a more formidable mechanical barrier to invasion.

2.2.6. Host defense reactions and invasion. One aspect of tumor invasion that can only be studied in tumors *in vivo* concerns the role of host inflammation and other defense reactions in promoting or retarding invasion. Current information on this question is both limited and ambiguous.

Development of an inflammatory response at sites of tumor infiltration could favor invasion by promoting the breakdown of normal tissue architecture as a result of edema and local release of tissue lytic enzymes. Similarly, release of mitogenic and angiogenic factors from infiltrating lymphocytes and macrophages could promote tumor cell proliferation. On the other hand, recruitment of cells endowed with non-specific tumoricidal activity (macrophages and NK cells) to sites of invasion might be expected to limit tumor growth. For example, the therapeutic usefulness of agents such as BCG and *C. Parvum* in cancer immunotherapy is believed to result from their ability to elicit inflammatory reactions and recruitment of tumoricidal activated macrophages.

Meaningful analysis of the role of non-specific and specific host defenses in the pathogenesis of invasion will require rigorous characterization of the type of host cells infiltrating primary and metastatic lesions. Correlation of the course of invasion with the type of the host response will also require examination of a range of tumors to assess the effect of differences in the site of tumor growth and variation in tumor growth rate and immunogenicity on the host response.

Solutions to these questions will not be forthcoming until methods for the recovery and identification of intratumoral host cell populations are improved significantly [see 36, for a critical survey of the current technical problems encountered in separation of host and tumor cells from neoplastic tissue].

Conclusions

Although the aim of *in vitro* models of invasion is to duplicate as far as possible events in spontaneous tumors *in vivo*, certain important differences must inevitably remain.

First, the majority of malignant neoplasms *in vivo* progress from a non-invasive state (e.g. carcinoma *in situ*) to an invasive and/or metastatic state. In contrast, *in vitro* systems employ tumor cells that have already acquired invasive capacity and are placed in direct contact, often in large numbers, with host tissues. In this respect, *in vitro* models may resemble more closely the process of tumor invasion in established metastatic lesions than invasion occurring in the vicinity of the primary tumor.

Second, although the use of tissue fragments and organ cultures enables tumor invasion to be studied *in vitro* in tissue matrices that for the most part retain organotypic structure, the various elements of host response to invasion are absent.

Third, in most model systems host tissues are obtained from normal donors and it is unclear whether this creates different patterns of tumor host cell interactions from those occurring in tissues from tumor-bearing individuals.

Critical survey of current in vitro models for invasion leads to the conclusion that inadequate attention has been given to five important issues:

1) Phenotypic heterogeneity in tumor cell populations and the problem created by the presence of subpopulations of cells with differing invasive properties within the same population.
2) The relationship of invasion assayed *in vitro* to the invasive behavior of the same cells *in vivo*.
3) Development of methods for quantitation of invasion *in vitro* and *in vivo*.
4) Development of techniques for recovery of invasive cells from host tissucs for comparison with non-invasive cells from the same population.
5) Evaluation of tumor cell invasion in tissues relevant to the natural pathogenesis of invasive tumors.

I consider that undue emphasis has been given to the use of cell monolayers and cell aggregates as models and that insufficient attention has been devoted to the technically more demanding task of studying invasion in complex three-dimensional tissue substrates. Only within the last few years has a concerted effort begun to change this situation and new methods devised that enable tumor invasion to be quantitated using radio-labeled cells instead of relying on semi-quantitative data from histologic analyses. Similarly, the development of methods whereby invasive tumor cells can be recovered from tissues offers future promise. So far this approach has been applied only to a limited number of tissues *in vitro* but there is no obvious reason why the same methods could not be modified for use with other tissues.

The tumor cells used in many published experiments on invasion have been of questionable relevance. The choice appears often to have been made on the grounds of technical convenience and/or availability rather than relevance to the pathogenesis of invasion. This problem is epitomized by the frequent use of cell lines whose invasive properties have never been tested *in vivo* or, worse still, lines that are known not to be invasive *in vivo*.

The problem of the cell system used has been complicated further in the last few years by the growing body of evidence indicating that many tumor cell populations are heterogenous and contain subpopulations of cells with differing phenotypes. This phenotypic heterogeneity extends to invasiveness and the demonstration of cells with differing invasive abilities within the same population has important implications for experimental efforts to identify the cellular properties responsible for invasiveness. If, as the weight of evidence now suggests, only certain subpopulations are invasive, accurate identification of properties peculiar to such cells will require rigorous comparison of non-invasive and invasive subpopulations isolated from the same parent population.

Recognition of the presence of tumor cell subpopulations with differing invasive properties within the same population also raises important questions concerning the factors that regulate the proportion of invasive cells in the population. For example, are invasive subpopulations present from very early in the life of a malignant tumor or do they emerge at some recognizable point in tumor progression? Similarly, once invasive subpopulations are present do they have adaptive advantage over non-invasive subpopulations so that their contribution to the overall population will increase with progressive growth of the tumor?

The question of relevance must also be raised in regard to the type of host tissues used as substrates for assaying invasiveness. Here again, the choice often appears to have been motivated by convenience rather than a desire to duplicate the type of tumor-host interactions that occur during invasion of spontaneous tumors. For example, the chick CAM has been used widely as a substrate for monitoring invasion but, as reviewed here, the capacity of cells to invade the CAM does not accurately predict their invasive potential *in vivo*. More attention must be given to the study of invasion in those tissues affected by tumor invasion *in vivo*. Given the importance of intravasation and extravasation in the metastatic process the lack of experimental work (other than descriptive morphology) on invasion of blood vessels and lymphatics is a serious deficiency. The technical challenge involved is not minimized but development of methods to address this problem deserves urgent priority.

It is also unclear whether the mechanism of invasion used by the same cell type varies in different tissues. For example, are events in intravasation and extravasation identical? Such questions are not without relevance to therapeutic attempts to frustrate tumor invasion. If, for example, the mechanisms of intravasation and extravasation are different, then therapeutic agents designed to prevent entry of cells into the vasculature may have little or no value in limiting metastasis formation by cells that reach the circulation. A further question concerns whether the mechanism and/or efficiency of tumor invasion in the same tissue alters with tumor progression and the emergence of increasingly invasive cells within the parent tumor.

In summary, only by using relevant host and tumor cell combinations, together with rigorous correlation of results from *in vitro* and *in vivo* assays, can we begin to define the essential features of the invasive phenotype and assess the functional importance of the various mechanisms discussed elsewhere in this volume.

References

1. Sträuli P, Barrett AJ, Baici A (eds): Proteinases and tumor invasion. New York: Raven Press, 1980.
2. Armstrong PB: Cellular positional stability and intercellular invasion. Bioscience 27:803–808, 1977.
3. Ossowski L, Reich E: Loss of malignancy during serial passage of human carcinoma in culture and discordance between malignancy and transformation parameters. Cancer Res 40:2310–2315, 1980.
4. Stewart HL, Dunn TB, Snell KC, Deringer MK: Tumours of the respiratory tract. In: Pathology of tumours in laboratory animals, Turusov VS (ed). Lyon: International Agency for Research, 1979, pp 251–268.
5. Alexander P: Back to the drawing board – the need for more realistic model systems for immunotherapy. Cancer 40:467–470, 1977.
6. Fidler IJ: General considerations for studies of experimental cancer metastasis. Methods Cancer Res XIV:399–439, 1978.
7. Fidler IJ, Kripke ML: Tumor cell antigenicity, host immunity and cancer metastasis. Cancer Immunol Immunotherapy 7:201–205, 1980.
8. Fidler IJ, Gersten DM, Hart IR: The biology of cancer invasion and metastasis. Adv Cancer Res 28:149–250, 1978.
9. Hewitt HB: The choice of animal tumors for experimental studies of cancer therapy. Adv Cancer Res 27:149–200, 1978.
10. Poste G, Fidler IJ: The pathogenesis of cancer metastasis. Nature 283:139–146, 1980.
11. Nowell PC: The clonal evolution of tumor cell populations. Science 194:23–28, 1976.
12. Fogh J, Giovanella BC (eds): The nude mouse in experimental and clinical research. New York: Academic Press, 1978.
13. Hanna N, Fidler IJ: Expression of metastatic potential of allogeneic and xenogeneic neoplasms in young nude mice. Cancer Res 41:438–444, 1981.
14. Hart IR, Fidler IJ: An *in vitro* quantitative assay for tumor cell invasion. Cancer Res 38:3218–3224, 1978.
15. Hart IR: The selection and characterization of an invasive variant of B16 melanoma. Am J Pathol 97:587–600, 1979.
16. Poste G, Doll J, Hart IR, Fidler IJ: *In vitro* selection of murine B16 melanoma variants with enhanced tissue invasive properties. Cancer Res 40:1636–1644, 1980.
17. Fidler IJ, Kripke ML: Metastasis results from pre-existing variant cells within a malignant tumor. Science 197:893–895, 1977.
18. Enders JF, Diamandopoulos GT: A study of variation and progression in oncogenicity in an SV 40-transformed hamster heart cell line and its clones. Proc Roy Soc (Biol) 171:431–443, 1969.
19. Kripke ML, Gruys E, Fidler IJ: Metastatic heterogeneity of cells from an ultraviolet light- induced murine fibrosarcoma of recent origin. Cancer Res 2962–2967, 1978.

20. Suzuki N, Withers RN, Koehler MW: Heterogeneity and variability of artificial lung colony-forming ability among clones from mouse fibrosarcoma. Cancer Res 38:3349–3351, 1978.
21. Poste G, Doll J, Fidler IJ: Interactions between clonal subpopulations affect the stability of the metastatic phenotype in polyclonal populations of B16 melanoma cells. Proc Nat Acad Sci USA.
22. Fidler IJ, Nicolson GL: The immunobiology of experimental metastatic melanoma. Cancer Biol Rev 2:1–53, 1981.
23. Miller FR, Heppner GH: Immunologic heterogeneity of tumor cell subpopulations from a single mouse mammary tumor. J Nat Cancer Inst 63:1457–1463, 1979.
24. Miller BE, Miller FR, Leith J, Heppner GH: Growth interaction *in vivo* between tumor subpopulations derived from a single mouse mammary tumor. Cancer Res 40:3977–3981, 1980.
25. DeWys WD: Studies correlating the growth rate of a tumor and its metastases and providing evidence for tumor-related systemic growth-retarding factors. Cancer Res 32:374–379, 1972.
26. Gorelik E, Fogel M, Segal S, Feldman M: Tumor-associated antigenic differences between the primary and the descendant metastatic tumor cell population. J Supramol Struct 12:385–402, 1979.
27. Greene HSN, Harvey GK: The inhibitory influence of a transplanted hamster lymphoma on metastasis. Cancer Res 20:1094–1100, 1960.
28. Yuhas JM, Pazmino NH: Inhibition of subcutaneously growing line 1 carcinomas due to metastatic spread. Cancer Res 34:2005–2010, 1974.
29. Poste G: The cell surface and metastasis. In: Cancer invasion and metastasis: biological mechanisms and therapy, Day SB (ed). New York: Raven Press, 1977, pp 19–46.
30. Van Rooijen N: Labeling of lymphocytes with various radioisotopes for *in vivo* tracer studies; a review. J Immunol Methods 15:267–277, 1977.
31. Mareel M, DeBruyne G, DeRidder L: Invasion of malignant cells into ^{51}Cr-labeled host tissues in organotypical culture. Oncology 34:6–9, 1977.
32. Liotta LA, Vembu D, Saini RK, Boone C: *In vivo* monitoring of the death rate of artificial murine pulmonary micrometastases. Cancer Res 38:1231–1236, 1978.
33. Poste G, Nicolson GL: Arrest and metastasis of blood-borne tumor cells are modified by fusion of plasma membrane vesicles from highly metastatic cells. Proc Natl Acad Sci USA 77:399–403, 1980.
34. Liotta LA, Lee CW, Morakis DJ: New method for preparing large surfaces of intact human basement membrane for tumor invasion studies. J Nat Cancer Inst (in press).
35. Pretlow TG, II, Pretlow TP: Separation of individual kinds of cells from tumors. In: Contemporary topics in immunobiology, Volume 10, Witz IP, Hanna MG, Jr (eds). New York: Plenum, 1980, pp 21–60.
36. Russell SW, Gillespie GY, Pace JL: Evidence for mononuclear phagocytes in solid neoplasms and appraisal of their nonspecific cytotoxic capabilities. In: Contemporary topics in immunobiology, Volume 10, Witz IP, Hanna MG, Jr (eds). New York: Plenum, 1980, pp 143–166.
37. Mareel MMK: Is invasiveness *in vitro* characteristic of malignant cells? Cell Biol Int Reports 3:627–640, 1979.
38. Mareel M, Bruyneel E, DeBruyne G, Dragonetti G: Methods for morphological and biochemical analysis of invasion *in vitro*. In: Cell movement and neoplasia, De Brabander M, Mareel M, DeRidder L (eds). Oxford: Pergamon Press, 1979, pp 87–95.
39. Armstrong PB, Lackie JM: Studies of intercellular invasion *in vitro* using rabbit peritoneal neutrophil granulocytes (PMNs) I. Role of contact inhibition of locomotion. J Cell Biol 65:439–462, 1975.
40. DeCossE JJ, Gossens C, Kuzuma JF, Unsworth BR: Embryonic inductive tissue interactions that cause histologic differentiation of murine mammary carcinoma *in vitro*. J Nat Cancer Inst 54:913–922, 1975.
41. Trinkaus JP: On the mechanism of metazoan cell movements. In: The cell surface in animal embryogenesis and development. Cell Surface Reviews, Volume 1, Poste G, Nicolson GL (eds). Amsterdam: North-Holland, 1976, pp 225–329.
42. Armstrong PB: Invasiveness of neutrophil leukocytes. In: Cell movement and neoplasis, De Bra-

bander M, Mareel M, De Ridder L (eds). Amsterdam: Elsevier, 1980, pp 131–151.
43 Hart IR, Raz A, Fidler IJ: Effect of cytoskeleton-disrupting agents on the metastatic behavior of malanoma cells. J Nat cancer Inst 64:891–900, 1980.
44. Weiss L: Cell deformability: some general considerations. In: Fundamental aspects of metastasis, Weiss, L (ed). Amsterdam: North-Holland, 1976, pp 305–310.
45. Sato H, Suzuki M: Deformability and viability of tumor cells by transcapillary passage, with reference to organ affinity of metastasis in cancer. In: Fundamental aspects of metastasis, Weiss L (ed). Amsterdam, North-Holland, 1976, pp 311–318.
46. Lessin LS, Kurantsin-Mills J, Weems HB: Deformability of normal and sickle erythrocytes in a pressure-flow filtration system. Blood Cells 3:241–262, 1977.
47. Maslow DE: *In vitro* analysis of surface specificity in embryonic cells. In: The cell surface in animal embryogenesis and development, Poste G, Nicolson GL (eds). Amsterdam: Elsevier, 1976, pp 697–745.
48. Easty DM, Easty GC: An *in vitro* model for studying cell invasiveness. In: Organ culture in biomedical research, Balls M, Monnickendam M (eds). Cambridge: Cambridge University Press, 1976, pp 379–393.
49. Schirrmacher V, Shantz G, Clauer K, Komitowski D, Zimmermann HP, Lohmann-Matthes M-L: Tumor metastases and cell-mediated immunity in a model system in DBA/2 mice I. Tumor invasiveness *in vitro* and metastasis formation *in vivo*. Int J Cancer 23:233–244, 1979.
50. Warren BA: The vascular morphology of tumors. In: Tumor blood circulation, Peterson H-I (ed). Boca Raton: CRC Press, 1980, pp 1–24.

11. *In vitro* quantitative assay of invasion using human amnion

R.G. RUSSO, U. THORGEIRSSON and L.A. LIOTTA

1. Introduction

The basic mechanisms by which tumor cells invade host tissue are poorly understood largely because this process has been difficult to study *in vitro*. Two major deficiencies have existed in past organ culture models of tumor cell invasion. The first is a lack of quantitation. The second is the use of non-human organs which contain multiple types of host tissue. A majority of the previous invasion assays have been qualitative studies in which fragments of organs are admixed with tumor cells (Table 1) [1–13]. The extent of invasion was judged by making histologic sections of the tissues after various incubation times. These previous methods provide an ideal system for visualizing the microscopic interactions between malignant and benign tissue. Unfortunately, they cannot be used to routinely quantitate the rate of tumor cell invasion during different experimental treatments. Investigators such as Hart [8] and Poste [12] have therefore developed quantitative assays for invasion using labeled tumor cells cultured on chicken chorioallantoic membrane or within the lumen of a perfused canine vein. The proportion of labeled tumor cells which traverse these tissue barriers is quantified by counting the radioactivity on each side of the barrier. In the systems described by Poste et al. [12], tumor cells which traverse the tissues can be collected for further study. However, a

Table 1. Examples of *in vitro* invasion assay systems.

1. Chick blastoderm (Mareel et al., 1975)
2. Human decidual tissue (Schleich et al., 1976)
3. Chick chorioallantoic membrane (Easty et al., 1976)
4. Chick chorioallantoic membrane (Scher et al., 1976)
5. Chick embryonic mesonephros (Pourreau-Schneider et al., 1977)
6. Chick embryonic skin (Noguchi et al., 1978)
7. Chick wing bud (Tickle et al., 1978)
8. Chick chorioallantoic membrane (Hart et al., 1978)
9. Mouse lung (Schirrmacher et al., 1979)
10. Chick embryonic heart (Mareel et al., 1979)
11. Rat embryo yolk sac (Maignan, 1979)
12. Canine vein (Poste et al., 1980)
13. Extracted bovine articular cartilage (Pauli et al., 1981)

L.A. Liotta and I.R. Hart (eds.), Tumor Invasion and Metastasis. ISBN-13: 978-94-009-7513-2.
© 1982 Martinus Nijhoff Publishers, The Hague/Boston/London.

disadvantage of these systems is the use of complex nonhuman organs. The chicken chorioallantoic membrane contains a series of multicellular and connective tissue layers (including endoderm and ectoderm) and is vascularized [3–8]. Host immune cells are present in the chorioallantoic membrane and its composition changes depending on the gestational age. The canine blood vessel perfusion system [12] is ingenious but suffers from the disadvantage of not being adaptable to routinely performing a large number of quantitative assays.

We have utilized human amnion in a new quantitative *in vitro* assay for invasion. The amnion is a transparent uniform membrane containing only two connective tissue layers. The human amnion obtained from one placenta measures approximately $1000\,cm^2$. An area of $10\,cm^2$ of amnion is used for each assay. Therefore, one amnion can be used for a large number of assays.

Invading tumor cells interact with a wide variety of cellular and noncellular components of the host. One experimental approach to explore this complex phenomenon is to prepare an *in vitro* organ culture system in which tumor cells interact with a limited number of defined host elements. Two important mechanical barriers to tumor cell invasion are basement membranes and collagenous connective tissue stroma. These extracellular matrix structures separate the blood vascular compartment from the organ parenchymal cells [14]. Basement membranes (BM) are continuous extracellular matrices composed of collagen type IV, glycoproteins and glycosaminoglycans [15]. Organ parenchymal cells are attached to one side of the BM and the connective tissue stroma is anchored to the opposite side [16]. The amnion membrane consists of a single layer of epithelium resting on a continuous BM which in turn is attached to a collagenous stroma [17]. The epithelium can be removed by brief alkali or detergent treatment resulting in a continuous surface of BM upon which to cultivate cells [18–19].

When used in the assay the amnion is clamped in a lucite holder with a separate

Table 2. Cultured cell lines tested in the amnion *in vitro* invasion assay.

I) Cells which do not invade the amnion within 6 days
  a) Human fibroblasts
  b) Human endothelial cells
  c) Bovine endothelium
  d) Rat hepatocytes

II) Cells which invade the amnion within 2 days
  a) Human MCF-7 breast carcinoma
  b) Human ZR-75-1 breast carcinoma
  c) Human Ewing's sarcoma
  d) Human A431 squamous carcinoma
  e) Human polymorphonuclear leukocytes
  f) Mouse M50-76 reticulum cell sarcoma
  g) Mouse BL6 (B16 variant) melanoma
  h) Mouse PMT sarcoma

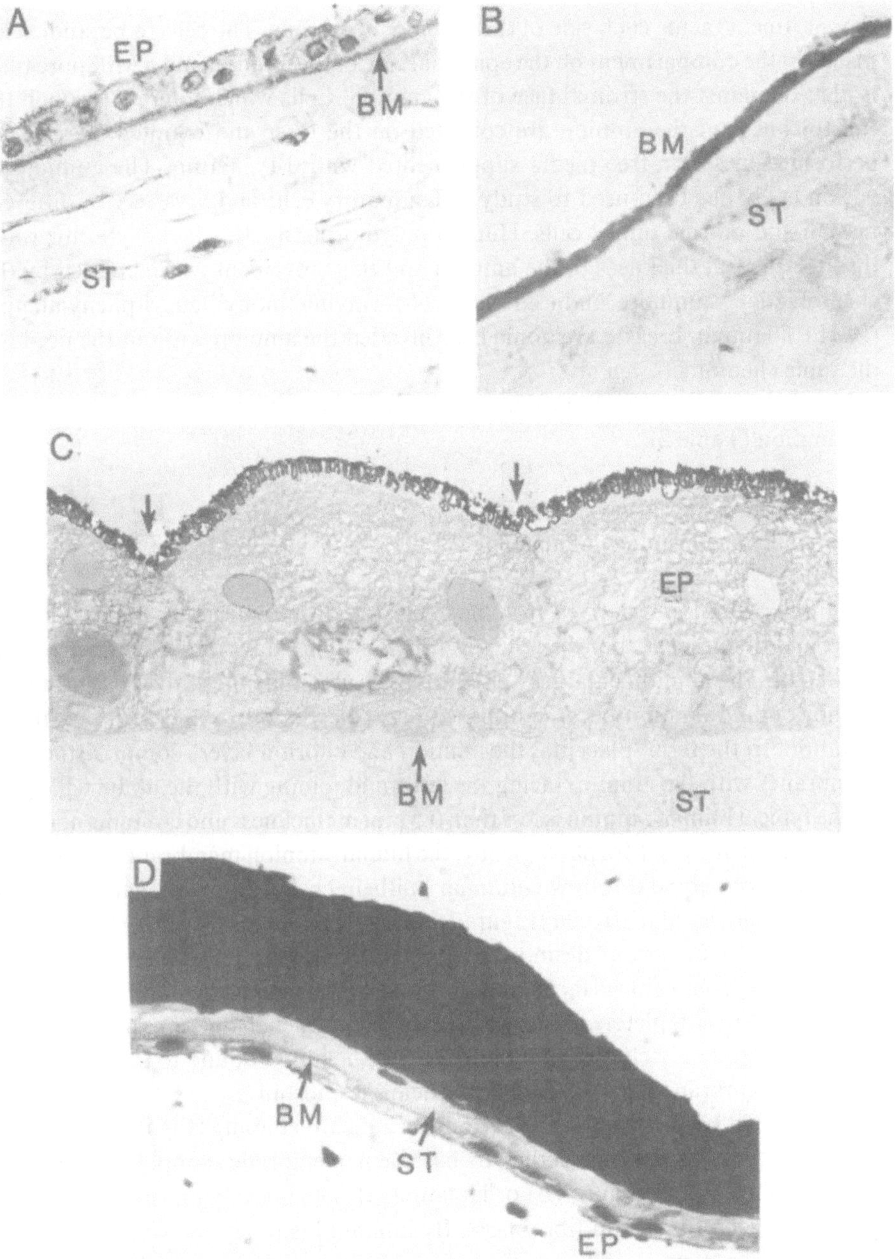

Figure 1. Morphology of normal amnion. (A) Periodic acid Schiff stain of normal amnion (400 ×). EP: epithelial cells; BM: basement membrane; ST: collagenous stroma. Occasional fibroblasts are present. (B) Anti-collagen type IV antibodies immuno-peroxidase stain of denuded basement membrane (BM); ST: collagenous stroma (630 ×). (C) Transmission electron micrograph of amnion epithelial intercellular junctions (arrows). EP: epithelium, BM: basement membrane, ST: collagenous stroma (3600 ×). (D) The collagenous stroma is nonpermeable to colloidal carbon (black layer). EP: epithelium, BM: basement membrane (Hematoxylin-eosin stain, 400 ×).

compartment facing each side of the amnion membrane. The cells to be studied are placed in the compartment on the epithelial side of the amnion and a Millipore filter is placed against the stromal face of the amnion. Cells which migrate through the full thickness of the amnion are collected on the filter and counted. Assays are performed in serum-free media supplemented with 0.1% fetuin. The amnion invasion assay has been used to study inflammatory cells and a variety of different human and murine tumor cells. Human polymorphonuclear leukocytes migrated through the full thickness of the amnion and this movement was increased by the chemotactic stimulus induced by N-formylmethionyl-leucyl-phenylalanine (FMLP). Human breast carcinoma cells invaded the amnion without the need for the same chemotactic agent.

Human endothelial and fibroblast cells or murine epithelial cells failed to invade the amnion (Table 2).

2. Anatomy and histology of amnion

The human amnion is derived from an extension of the extraembryonic somatopleure, and first appears between the seventh and eighth days of development of the ovum [20]. The amnion enlarges and gradually surrounds the embryo. Mesoblasts of chorion and amnion become opposed between the fourth and fifth months of gestation. In the term 'placenta' the amnion and chorion layers comprise the fetal membranes with the amnion facing the fetus and joining with the umbilical cord.

The typical human amnion is less than 0.5 mm in thickness and contains no blood vessels and no nerves. Morphologically, the human amnion membrane consists of a single layer of cuboidal to low columnar epithelial cells and basement membrane resting on nonvascular stroma (Figure 1A). Each epithelial cell is interlocked with its neighbor by numerous desmosomes (Figure 1C). Ruthenium red staining demonstrates a prominent surface glycocalyx and epithelial microvilli. The ruthenium red dye failed to completely penetrate between the epithelial junctions indicating the presence of tight or occluding junctions. The epithelium is bound to the continuous basement membrane (BM) by numerous hemi-desmosomes.

The BM can be identified using periodic acid Schiff staining (Figure 1A) or with immunohistology using antibodies to basement membrane components such as type IV collagen [21] (Figure 1B) or laminin [22]. The underlying stroma contains banded collagen fibers and fibroblasts. By immunohistology the stroma contains type I collagen, type V collagen, type III collagen and fibronectin [22, 23]. Even though the stroma connective tissue layer appears fibrillar it forms a dense barrier impermeable to colloidal carbon particles (Figure 1D) and therefore does not contain preformed channels through which cells can passively migrate.

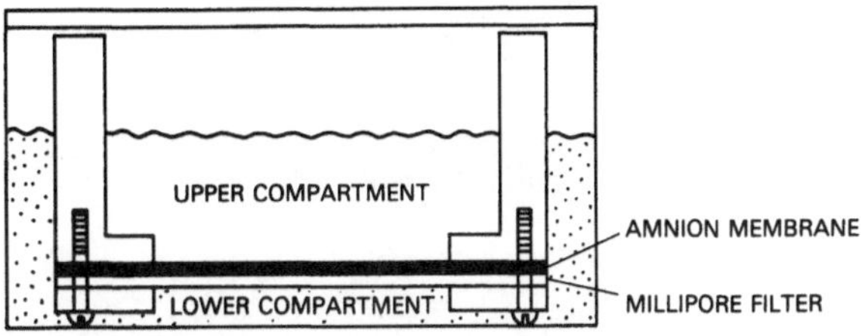

Figure 2. Amnion chemotaxis chamber: cross-sectional representation. The amnion membrane and filter are clamped between two Lucite rings creating two separate compartments. The amnion epithelium faces the upper compartment and the chemoattractant is placed in the lower compartment. Cells are placed in the upper compartment.

2.1 *Amnion invasion assay procedure*

Normal term placentas were obtained fresh after delivery. The transparent amnion was aseptically peeled away from the chorion by blunt dissection and rinsed twice with PBS solution containing 0.01% sodium hypochlorite. Then the membrane was immersed in PBS containing penicillin-streptomycin (PS) (50 IU/ml and 50 μg/ml, respectively). Amnions were finally immersed in Minimal Essential Medium (with Earle's salts) with glutamine (4 mM) and PS. For experiments requiring a living epithelium, the amnion was used immediately. For experiments using a denuded BM surface the epithelium was removed by treatment with 0.1% ammonium hydroxide (15 min, 25% C) and the amnions were stored refrigerated prior to use.

Two-compartment chemotaxis chambers (Figure 2) were constructed in the form of two Lucite rings. The rings measure 3.2 cm outside diameter and 1.2 cm inner diameter. The upper ring is 1.0 cm in height and the lower ring is 0.2 cm in height. Once clamped between the two halves of the chamber, the amnion divided the chamber into two compartments: upper and lower (Figure 2). A Millipore filter (5 or 8 μm pore size, 2.3 cm diameter) was sandwiched in the chamber so as to be in direct contact with the amnion stromal surface. The chambers are placed in 6-well cluster dishes (Costar, Cambridge, Mass.). The amnions were verified to be free of leaks as described previously. In some experiments a chemoattractant, N-formylmethionyl-leucyl-phenylalanine (FMLP), was introduced into the lower compartment. Cells were added to the upper compartment onto the amnion epithelial layer or onto the denuded BM surface at the concentration of 1×10^6 cells in a total volume of 1.5 ml. The chambers containing the cells were incubated at 37° C (5% CO_2, 95% air). Migration was observed periodically through an inverted microscope. Quantification of the cells which had traversed the full thickness of the amnion was done by staining the Millipore filter with standard hematoxyline -eosin solution. Cells trapped within or adherent to the filter were easily identified against the white filter background (Figure 3E). The whole filter (1.13 cm^2) was scanned (at 400× magnifi-

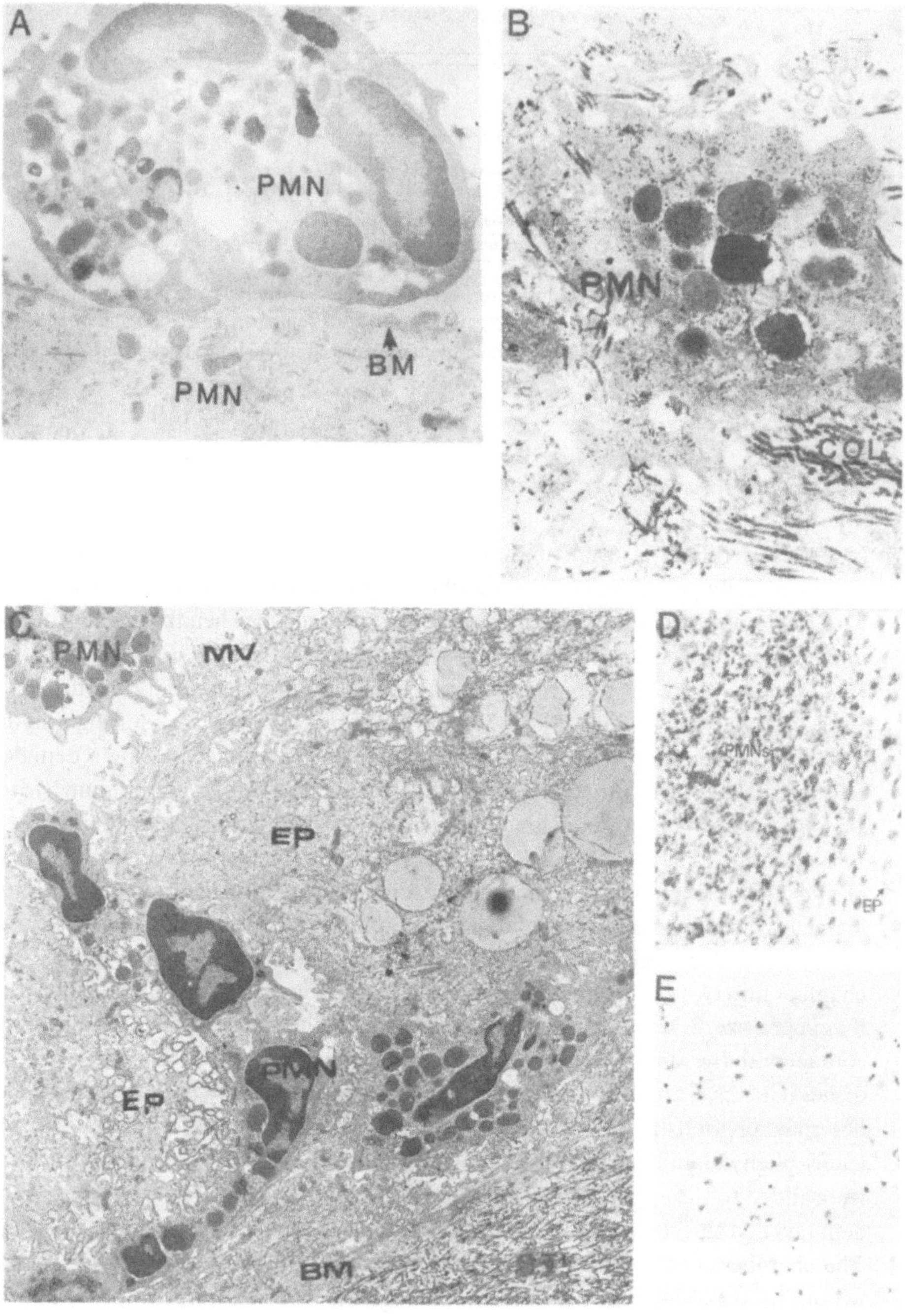

Figure 3. Polymorphonuclear leukocytes (PMN) chemotaxis through amnion in response to FMLP chemoattractant. (A) Transmission electron micrograph of PMN attachment to the continuous basement membrane (BM). Some PMN pseudopodia are visible beneath the BM (10 800 ×). (B) Transmis-

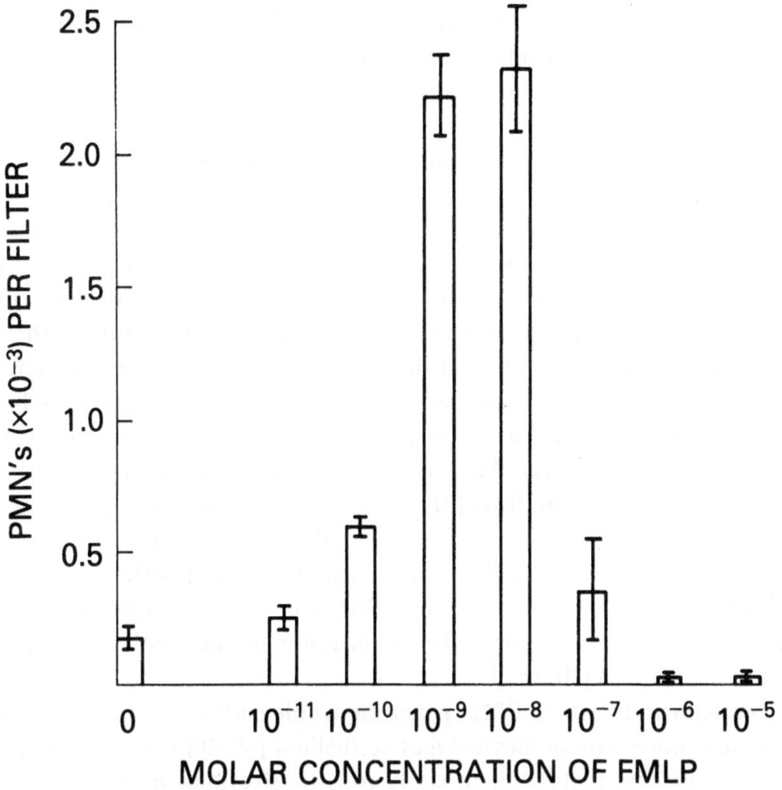

Figure 4. Concentration-dependent chemotaxis of PMN through human amnion. A series of different concentrations of FMLP was placed in the lower compartment. After 3 h the total number (mean ± range) of PMN traversing the amnion was counted on the filters. The optimal concentration is 10^{-8}M. Super-optimal concentrations (10^{-6} M, 10^{-5} M) induce less PMNmigration than controls without FMLP.

---

sion electron micrograph of PMN in the stromal collagen (COL) (3600 ×). (C) Transmission electron micrograph of the PMN breaking the intercellular junctions and migrating between the amnion epithelial cells (EP). Microvilli (MV) are visible on the upper surface of epithelial cells. BM: basement membrane. Collagen fibers are visible in the stroma (ST) (3600 ×). (D) Uniform distribution of PMN on amnion epithelium (EP) 3 h after the optimal concentration (10^{-8}M) of FMLP was placed in the lower compartment (Hematoxylin stain, 200 ×). (E) Filter containing PMN which have traversed the full thickness of the amnion to enter the Millipore filter (5 μm pore size) 3 h after the optimal concentration (10^{-8}M) of FMLP was placed in the lower compartment (Hematoxylin stain, 200 ×).

cation) and the total number of cells were counted on each filter. The means and ranges were recorded for triplicate experiments.

2.2. Polymorphonuclear leukocyte migration through amnion

Polymorphonuclear leukocytes (PMN) are normal host cells which migrate through host tissue barriers in response to inflammation [24, 25]. PMN adhere to the endothelial cell surface of post capillary venules, traverse the endothelium through interendothelial cell junctions and penetrate the basement membrane as they leave the vascular system to accumulate at the site of injury [25]. A variety of substances induce PMN chemokinesis and chemotaxis [26–28]. N-formylmethionyl-leucyl-phenylalanine (FMLP) has been demonstrated to be one of the most potent chemoattractants for phagocytic cells [29, 30]. This substance exerts its activity by binding to specific cell receptors on PMN [31, 32]. FMLP increases PMN adhesiveness to endothelial cells [33–35] and induces release of the granule bound enzymes [30, 34]. An optimal dose range exists for PMN chemotaxis by specific factors such as FMLP. At doses above the optimal range PMN homotypic aggregation is increased and migration is reduced. At doses below the optimal range both aggregation and migration are reduced [30, 36, 37].

The mechanism by which PMN penetrate whole endothelium basement membrane, collagenous stroma barriers and epithelium [38–40] is poorly understood because this process is difficult to study *in vitro*. Previous *in vitro* methods for investigating leukocyte migration and chemotaxis have utilized micropore filters alone [35, 41–44] or filters containing monolayers of cultured epithelial or endothelial cells [45, 46]. These previous systems are not optimal for simulating the actual physiological state because they do not include intact cell layers attached to normal continuous basement membrane, interfacing with connective tissue matrix.

The human amnion membrane contains all these three basic tissue components (epithelium, basement membrane and stroma [17, 47]) which can be traversed by leukocytes responding to an inflammatory stimulus. We have quantitated the rate of migration of PMN from the amnion epithelial side, through the basement membrane and the stroma, in the presence of different FMLP gradients. In addition, the histologic route of migration of PMN through the amnion was studied using light microscopy and transmission electron microscopy [19].

The numbers of PMN which have traversed the amnion to enter the filters after 3 hours are shown in Figure 4 for different concentrations of FMLP. Quantitation of the FMLP dose-response indicated that an optimal rate of migration occurred at 10^{-8}M and 10^{-9}M concentration of FMLP applied to the bottom compartment. At FMLP 10^{-8}M, the PMN were uniformly distributed as single cells and small aggregates (2–3 cells) at various stages of penetration within the epithelium (Figure 3D). PMN migration at this concentration was twelve-fold greater than spon-

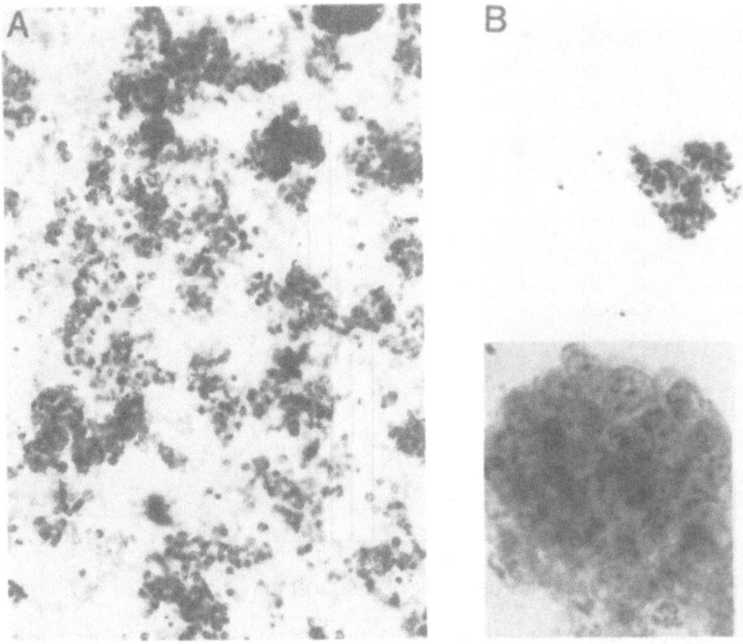

Figure 5. (A) Distribution of MCF-7 (human mammary carcinoma) cells on the surface of the denuded amnion basement membrane (Hematoxylin-eosin stain, 100 ×). (B) Hematoxylin-eosin stain (100 ×) of the filter containing MCF-7 cells which have traversed the full thickness of the amnion to enter the Millipore filter (8 μm pore size) after 48 h. The cells appear to be in single cell from or in clusters of various sizes (see insert: day 6: 630 ×).

taneous migration as detected without the addition of FMLP. At higher concentrations of FMLP (10^{-5}M, 10^{-6}M) the PMN were noted to aggregate into large clumps on the epithelial surface (greater than 50 cells) and migrate at a lower rate than the controls. Directed migration at low concentrations (10^{-10}–10^{-11}M) of FMLP showed only a three-fold increase over the controls. Thus at a concentration of FMLP optimal for chemotaxis, aggregation on the epithelial surface was minimal (Figure 4). Electron microscopy demonstrated that the route of migration of PMN through the amnion *in vitro* was similar to that reported for acute inflammation *in vivo*. Marchesi studied the time course of acute inflammation in rat mesentery venules [24]. Phillips and Mahler reported leukocyte migration through the rabbit vaginal epithelium [39]. Shaw studied lung inflammation in rabbits by intratracheal injection of chemotactic fragments from zymosan activated serum [48]. These investigators all found that the inflammatory cells first adhered to the epithelial or endothelial surface, then penetrated the intercellular junctions. After being held up at the basement membrane for a time period, the leukocytes were then noted to rapidly pass through local zones of basement membrane dissolution to enter the underlying collagenous stroma. In the amnion system the PMN placed on the epithelial layer adhered over the intercellular junctions. After extending pseu-

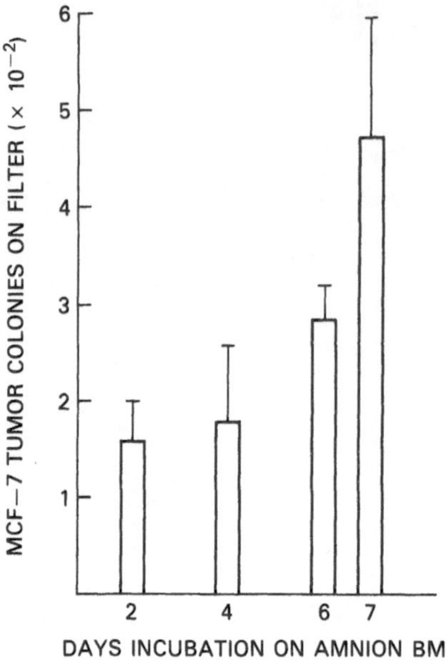

Figure 6. The migration of MCF-7 tumor cells through the whole thickness of the amnion is time dependent. The number of tumor colonies counted on the filter increases threefold between days 2 and 7. The whole filters in triplicate were stained with hematoxylin and eosin, and counted at 400 × magnification 2, 4, 6, and 7 days after the cells were put on the denuded basement membrane. The mean and the range are indicated.

dopods between adjacent epithelial cells, the PMN migrated in single file groups, around or through desmosomes connections and established, in some cases, an intimate contact with epithelial cells (Figure 3C). A focal dissolution of the basement membrane was observed at the front of PMN contact associated with cell pseudopodia (Figure 3A). After traversing the basement membrane, the PMN invaded the dense and loose collagenous stroma (Figure 3B). The amnion BM and stroma are impermeable to colloidal carbon. Therefore we suggest that the PMN actively disrupt the connective tissue to produce a migration tunnel. Since FMLP treatment induces the PMN to elaborate increased levels of type IV collagenolytic enzyme [49, 50] it is likely that proteolysis is involved in this process.

2.3. *Tumor cell migration through the amnion*

The amnion invasion assay was used to study a variety of murine and human tumor cell lines. Tumor cells grown in appropriate media were harvested from the log phase of growth and washed in serum free media. The cells were then placed into the upper compartment of the amnion holder (2×10^5 cells in 1.6 ml DMEM with 0.1% fetuin). In contrast to the PMN which showed rapid adherence to the living epi-

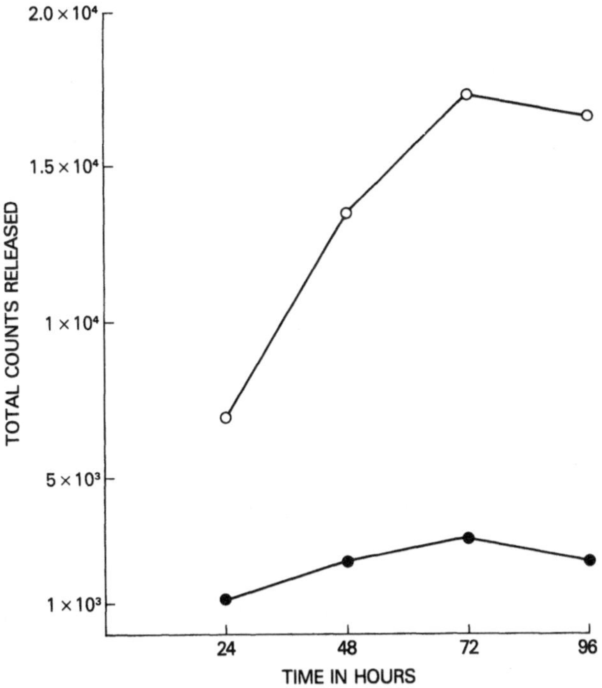

Figure 7. BM degradation by tumor cells cultured on the basement membrane surface. Four samples per time point. -o- mean of the counts released by 1 × 10^5 M50-76 cells. -•- mean of the counts released by 1 × 10^5 human fibroblasts.

thelial surface, all tumor cells tested exhibited a poor adherence to the epithelium. When the epithelium was denuded the tumor cells bound avidly to the intact basement membrane surface (Figure 5A). Within 24 h highly invasive tumor cells penetrated the full thickness of the denuded amnion basement membrane, the collagen stroma and entered the Millipore filter. Tumor cells trapped in the Millipore filter grew slowly in the filter as small colonies (Figure 5B). Tumor cells were quantitated on the filter as the total number of single cells and the total number of cell clumps or colonies. Time course studies suggested that most tumor cells traversed the amnion in single cell form and later grew as colonies on the filter. The number of tumor colonies on the filter increased with time as more tumor cells penetrated the amnion and reached the filter (Figure 6). Tumor cell colonies after penetrating the amnion could be subcultured. MCF-7 cells cycled through the amnion once showed a five-fold increase in the rate of invasion when they were again tested in the amnion assay.

A variety of normal human cells were tested in the amnion assay (Table 2). Human and bovine endothelium attached and grew on the BM surface, even in the absence of serum or growth factors other than fetuin. The endothelial cells did not invade the amnion up to 12 days in culture. Human fibroblasts or rat hepatocytes also did not invade the amnion membrane.

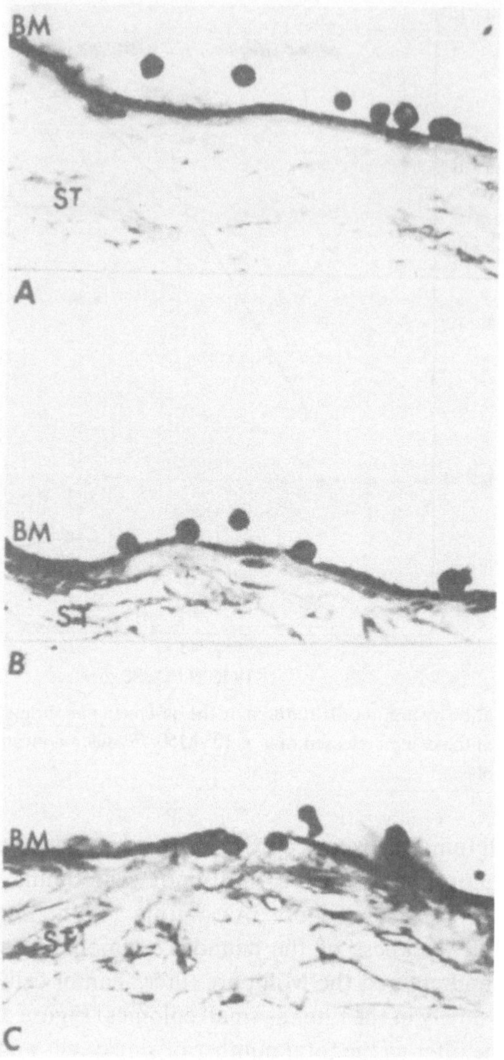

Figure 8. Tumor cells (M50-76) penetrate the amnion basement membrane (BM) to enter the collagenous stroma. Periodic acid Schiff (PAS) stain (630 ×). (A) Two hours after applying the tumor cells to the BM surface most tumor cells are attached. (Tumor cells and BM are both PAS positive.) (B) At 15 h incubation local thinning of the BM is noted beneath the attached tumor cells. (C) After 36 h the BM is ruptured and tumor cells have entered the collagenous stroma.

The amnion BM can be radiolabeled in organ culture. The labeled whole BM can then be used as a substrate for studying degradative enzyme activity in tumor cells. Whole, fresh amnion was preincubated for 1 h in media containing 20% dialyzed calf serum, ascorbate (50 μg/ml and beta amino-proprionitrile (25 μg/ml). [^{14}C] proline (50 mCi/ml) was then added to the organ culture media and incubation was continued for 24 h at 37° C. The ^{14}C proline was incorporated into collagenous and noncollagenous components of the basement membrane as verified by extraction of the labeled type IV collagen and laminin, immunoprecipitation and collagenase digestion [51]. M50-76 murine reticulum cell sarcoma cells were inoculated onto the [^{14}C] labeled amnion BM surface. Degradative activity was measured by the release of soluble radioactivity into the media. As shown in Figure 7, the radioactivity in the media increased significantly with time. In contrast, fibroblasts did not cause significant release of radioactivity. By comparing the maximum radioactivity released by purified collagenase or plasmin with the maximum radioactivity released by the tumor cells it was concluded that the tumor cells degraded both collagenous and glycoprotein [51] components of the BM. Histologic studies of the M50-76 cell invasion of the amnion showed local thinning of the BM at the point of cell attachment (Figures 8A, 8B). This was followed by penetration of the tumor cells through the BM into the stroma (Figure 8C). The histologic observations and the release of radioactive substrate are in keeping with the hypothesis of local active degradation of the connective tissue matrix by the invading tumor cells. Tumor cells are known to elaborate many types of latent and active proteases (see other chapters in this volume) [50, 52]. Tumor cells invaded the devitalized amnion connective tissue *in vitro*. Therefore, at least for the tumor cells studied here, active participation by living host cells is not required for tumor cell invasion.

In conclusion, the human amnion invasion assay is quantitative, simple to perform and utilizes readily available tissue. A large number of assays can be performed with a single amnion, therefore reducing experimental variability due to the tissue source. Assays are performed in serum-free media. This is an advantage because serum may interact with biochemical and pharmacologic agents used to experimentally modulate the invasion process. Finally, the chamber configuration of the amnion assay allows for many studies using chemotactic agents or selection of tumor cells which have penetrated the amnion.

References

1. Mareel M, De Ridder L, De Brabander M, Vakaet L: Characterization of spontaneous chemical and viral transformants of a C31+3T3 type mouse cell line by transplantation into young chick blastoderms. J Natl Cancer Inst 54:923–929, 1975.
2. Schleich AB, Frick M, Mayer A: Patterns of invasive growth in vitro. Human decidua graviditatis confronted with established human cell lines and primary human explants. J Natl Cancer Inst 56:221–225, 1976.
3. Easty DM, Easty GC: An in-vitro model for studying invasiveness. In: Organ culture in biomedical research, Balls M, Monnickendam M (eds). Cambridge: Cambridge University Press, 1976, pp 379–392.
4. Scher CD, Handenschild C, Klagsbrun M: The chick chorioallantoic membrane as a model system for the study of tissue invasion by viral transformed cells. Cell 8:373–382, 1976.
5. Pourreau-Schneider N, Felix H, Haemmerli G: The role of cellular locomotion in leukemic infiltration. An organ culture study on penetration of L 5222 rat leukemia cells into the chick embryo mesonephros. Virch Arch B Cell Pathol 23:257–264, 1977.

6. Noguchi PD, Johnson JB, O'Donnel R, Petricciani JC: Chick embryonic skin as a rapid organ culture assay for cellular neoplasia. Science 199:1980–1983, 1978.
7. Ticke A, Crawley A, Goodman M: Cell movement and the mechanism of invasiveness: a survey of the behavior of some normal and malignant cells implanted into the developing chick wing bud. J Cell Sci 31:293–322, 1978.
8. Hart IR, Fidler IJ: An in vitro quantitative assay for tumor cell invasion. Cancer Res 38:3218–3224, 1978.
9. Schirrmacher V, Shantz G, Clauer K, Komitowski D, Zimmermann HP, Lohmann-Matthes ML: Tumor metastases and cell mediated immunity in a model system in DBA/2 mice. I. Tumor invasiveness in vitro and metastasis formation in vivo. Int J Cancer 23:233–244, 1979.
10. Mareel M, Kint J, Meyvisch C: Methods of study of the invasion of malignant C3H-mouse fibroblasts into embryonic chick heart in vitro. Virch Arch B Cell Pathol 30:95–111, 1979.
11. Maignan MF: Étude ultrastructurale des interactions entre des cellules normales ou malignes et le sac vitellin de rat, explanté *in vitro*. Biologie Cellulaire 35:229–232, 1979.
12. Poste G, Doll J, Hart IR, Fidler IJ: In vitro selection of murine B16 melanoma variants with enhanced tissue-invasive properties. Cancer Res 40:1636–1644, 1980.
13. Pauli BU, Memoli VA, Kuettner KE: In vitro determination of tumor invasiveness using extracted hyaline cartilage. Cancer Res 41:2084–2091, 1981.
14. Liotta LA, Kleinerman J, Catanzaro P, Rynbrandt D: Degradation of basement membrane by murine tumor cells. J Natl Cancer Inst 58:1427–1431, 1977.
15. Kefalides NA, Denduchis B: Structural components of epithelial and endothelial basement membranes. Biochemistry 8:4613–4621, 1969.
16. Vrako R: Basal lamina scaffold-anatomy and significance for maintenance of orderly tissue structure. Am J Pathol 77:314–346, 1974.
17. Van Herendael BJ, Oberti C, Brosens I: Microanatomy of the human amniotic membranes. Am J Obstet Gynecol 131:872–880, 1978.
18. Liotta LA, Lee CW, Morakis DJ: New method for preparing large surfaces of intact human basement membrane for tumor invasion studies. Cancer Lett 11:141, 1980.
19. Russo RG, Liotta LA, Thorgeirsson U, Brundage R, Schiffman E: Polymorphonuclear leukocyte migration through human annion membrane. J Cell Biol 91:459–461, 1981.
20. Wynn RM: Development and morphology of the amnion. In: Amniotic Fluid, Vol I, Natelson S, Scommegna A, Epstein MB (eds). New York: J. Wiley & Sons, 1973, pp 5–21.
21. Garbisa S, Liotta LA, Tryggvason K, Siegal GP: Antibodies to collagenase-resistant terminal regions of pro-type IV collagen recognize whole basement membrane and 7S collagen. FEBS Lett 127:257–262, 1981.
22. Alitalo K, Kurkinen M, Vaheri A: Extracellular matrix components synthesized by human amniotic epithelial cells in culture. Cell 19:1053–1062, 1980.
23. Bentz H, Bachinger P, Glanville R, Kuhn K: Physical evidence for the assembly of A and B chains of human placenta collagen in a single triple helix. Eur J Biochem 92:563–567, 1978.
24. Marchesi VT: Ultrastructural aspects of acute inflammation. Pathol Ann 5:343–353, 1970.
25. Grant L: The sticking and emigration of white blood cells in inflammation. In: The inflammatory process, Vol II, Zweifach BW, Grant L, Mc Cluskey RT (eds). New York: Academic Press, 1973, pp 245–249.
26. Ryan GB, Majno G: Acute inflammation: a review. Am J Pathol 86:185–276, 1977.
27. Zigmond SH: Chemotaxis by polymorphonuclear leukocytes. J Cell Biol 77:269–287, 1978.
28. Niedel JE, Cuatrecasas P: Formyl peptide chemotactic receptors of leukocytes and macrophages. Curr Top in Cell Regul 17:137–170, 1980.
29. Becker EL: Some interrelations on neutrophil chemotaxis, lysosomal enzyme secretion, and phagocytosis as revealed by synthetic peptides. Am J Pathol 85:383–394, 1976.
30. Showell HJ, Freer RJ, Zigmond SH, Schiffmann E, Aswanikumar S, Corcoran B, Becker EL: The structure-activity relations of synthetic peptides as chemotactic factors and inducers of lysosomal

enzyme secretion for neutrophils. J Exp Med 143:1154–1169, 1976.

31. Williams LT, Snyderman R, Pike MC, Lefkowitz RJ: Specific receptor sites for chemotactic peptides on human polymorphonuclear leukocytes. Proc Natl Acad Sci USA 74:1204–1208, 1977.
32. Spilberg I, Mehta J: Demonstration of a specific neutrophil receptor for a cell-derived chemotactic factor. J Clin Invest 63:85–88, 1979.
33. Hoover RL, Briggs RT, Karnowsky MJ: The adhesive interaction between polymorphonuclear leukocytes and endothelial cells *in vitro*. Cell 14:423–428, 1978.
34. O'Flaherty JT, Showell HJ, Becker EL, Ward PA: Substances which aggregate neutrophils. Am J Pathol 92:155–166, 1978.
35. Smith CW, Hollers JC, Patrick RA, Hassett C: Motility and adhesiveness in human neutrophils. J Clin Invest 63:221–229, 1979.
36. O'Flaherty JT, Ward PA: Leukocyte aggregation induced by chemotactic factors. Inflammation 3:177–194, 1978.
37. Fehr J, Dahinden C: Modulating influence of chemotactic factor-induced cell adhesiveness on granulocyte function. J Clin Invest 64:8–16, 1979.
38. Anderson AO, Anderson ND: Lymphocyte emigration from high endothelial venules in rat lymph nodes. Immunology 31:731–748, 1976.
39. Phillips DM, Mahler S: Leukocyte emigration and migration in the vagina following mating in the rabbit. Anat Rec 189:45–60, 1977.
40. Seelig LL, Beer AE: Transepithelial migration of leukocytes in the mammary gland of lactating rats. Biol Reprod 17:736–744, 1978.
41. Boyden S: The chemotactic effect of mixtures of antibody and antigen on polymorphonuclear leukocytes. J Exp Med 115:453–466, 1962.
42. Keller HU, Borel JF, Wilkinson PC, Hess MW, Cottier H: Re-assessment of Boyden's technique for measuring chemotaxis. J Immunol Meth 1:165–168, 1972.
43. Gallin JI, Clark RA, Kimball HR: Granulocyte chemotaxis: an improved *in vitro* assay employing ^{51}Cr-labeled granulocytes. J Immunol 110:233–240, 1973.
44. Kawaoka EJ, Miller ME, Cheung ATW: Chemotactic factor-induced effects upon deformability of human polymorphonuclear leukocytes. J Clin Immunol 1:41–44, 1981.
45. Cramer EB, Milks LC, Ojakian GK: Transepithelial migration of human neutrophils: an *in vitro* model system. Proc Natl Acad Sci USA 77:4069–4073, 1980.
46. Taylor RF, Price TH, Schwartz SM, Dale DC: Neutrophil-endothelial cell interactions on endothelial monolayers grown on micropore filter. J Clin Invest 67:584–587, 1981.
47. King BF: A cytological study of plasma membrane modifications, intercellular junctions and endocytic activity of amniotic epithelium. Anat Rec 190:113–126, 1978.
48. Shaw JO: Leukocytes in chemotactic-fragment-induced lung inflammation. Am J Pathol 101:283–291, 1980.
49. Mainardi CL, Dixit SN, Kang AH: Degradation of (type IV) basement membrane collagen by a proteinase isolated from human polymorphonuclear leukocyte granules. J Biol Chem 255:5435–5441, 1980.
50. Liotta LA, Tryggvason K, Garbisa S, Hart I, Foltz CM, Shafie S: Metastatic potential correlates with enzymatic degradation of basement membrane collagen. Nature 284:67–68, 1980.
51. Timpl R, Rohde H, Gehron-Robey P, Rennard S, Foldart JM, Martin GR: Laminin – a glycoprotein of basement membranes. J Biol Chem 254:9933–9937, 1979.
52. Liotta LA, Goldfarb RH, Brundage RG, Siegal GP, Terranova VP, Garbisa S: Effect of plasminogen activator (urokinase), plasmin, and thrombin on glycoprotein and collagenous components of basement membrane. Cancer Res 41:4629-4636, 1981.

12. Experimental models of lymphatic metastasis

I. CARR and J. CARR

The common human cancers spread by lymphatic metastasis [1], but most experimental work on metastasis has been done with models of hematogenous metastasis since this occurs much more readily in animal systems. The classic work on lymphatic metastasis was that of Zeidman and Buss [2], but until 1970 the field was relatively unexplored. The present chapter describes work over a number of years on experimental lymphatic metastasis. Fuller reviews of the work of others have been published elsewhere [3, 4].

There were three initial aims: 1) to set up an adequate experimental model of lymphatic metastasis, 2) to identify the means of penetration of the lymphatic vessel, and 3) to identify the cells actually metastasizing.

The basic model is to inject tumor cells into the footpad and then to examine the draining popliteal lymph node histologically at varying times thereafter. Direct intralymphatic injection is excluded by serial histological section immediately and 6 h after injection of tumor cells. The footpad is examined by transmission electron microscopy after glutaraldehyde/osmium fixation; the blood vessels are marked and distinguished from lymphatic vessels by injecting an intravenous particulate tracer just before sacrifice.

A number of tumors have been examined in this way. The first to be studied was the Rd/3 tumor, originally induced by dimethylbenzanthracene and carried in an inbred strain of rats [5–8]. More recent work has been carried out on the Walker rat carcinoma [9], and on the syngeneic 13762 rat mammary adenocarcinoma [10]. The general pattern of the experiments is illustrated in Figures 1 and 2 which show the gross and histological appearance of metastasis of the Walker rat carcinoma in the popliteal lymph node after injection of tumor cells into the footpad. The rate and pattern vary somewhat from tumor to tumor.

1. RD/3 tumor

After injection of 5×10^6 Rd/3 cells, consistent lymphatic metastasis was present in the popliteal node (in over 95% of animals). Twenty-four hours after injection, a few tumor cells were present in the subcapsular sinus. Tumor cells were seen initially in the subcapsular sinus and spread down in the radial and medullary sinusoids. Tumor cells then distended and destroyed the sinusoids replacing the nodes at first

L.A. Liotta and I.R. Hart (eds.), Tumor Invasion and Metastasis. ISBN-13: 978-94-009-7513-2.
© 1982 Martinus Nijhoff Publishers, The Hague/Boston/London.

1

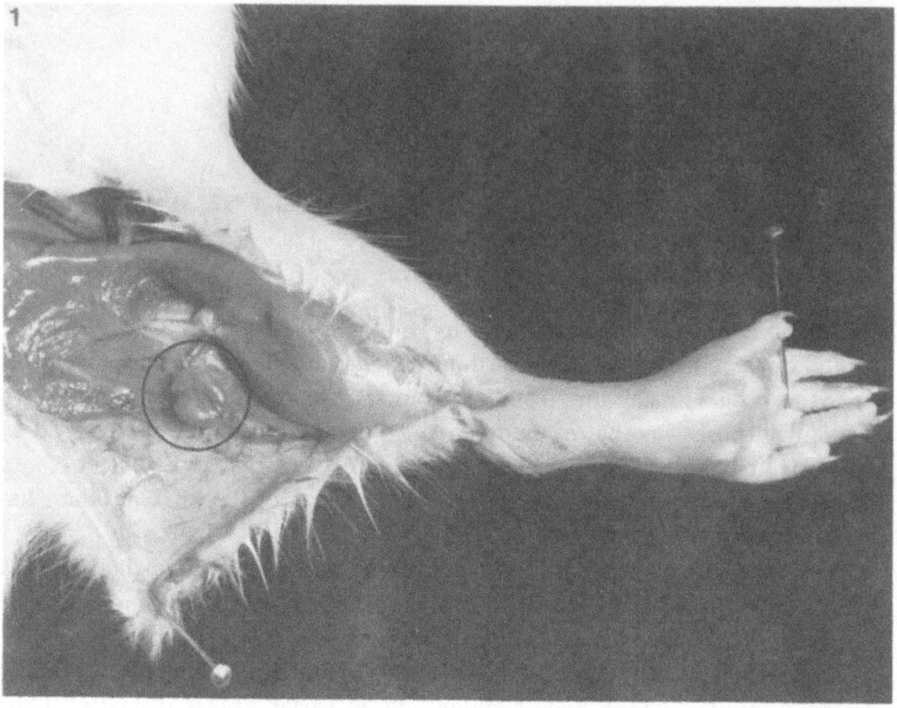

2

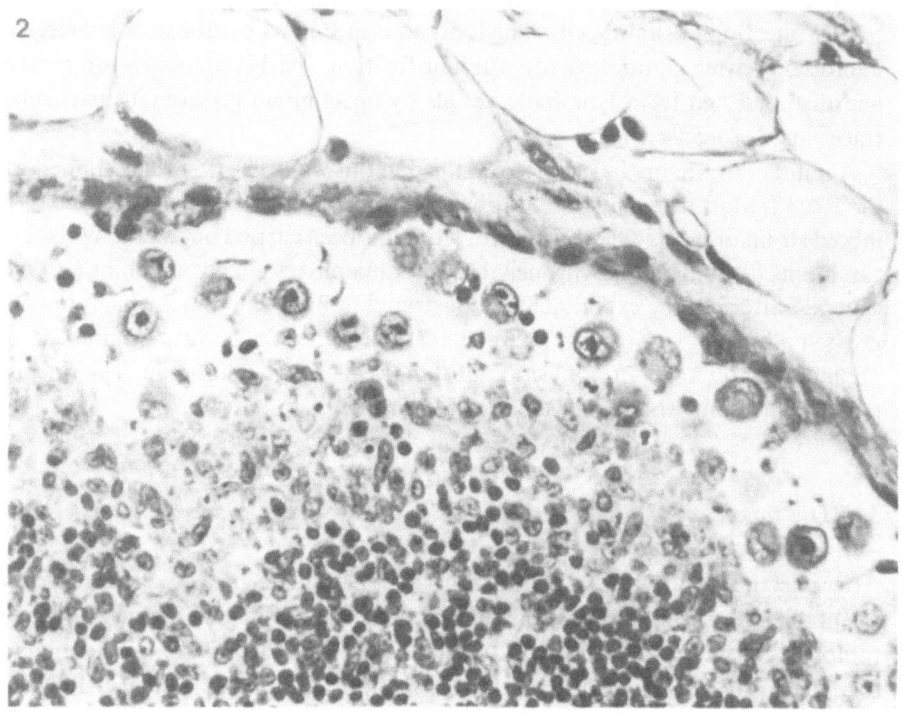

partially and then completely. Tumor cells were seen in the efferent trunks at 5 days and progressive metastasis to the para-aortic nodes followed thereafter. There was a high rate of tumor cells mitosis in the lymph node and also continuous recruitment from the footpad. Two components were observed in the lymph node reaction, an early proliferation of sinus macrophages (seen only with viable tumor and tumor extract), followed by marked germinal center enlargement and paracortical lymphocyte proliferation. When animals were allowed to survive beyond 14 days, they died with massive deposits of tumor in the para-aortic and lungs. The prior injection of 10 μl BCG into either footpad or lymph node was effective in inhibiting metastasis either partly or completely.

Macrophages did not proliferate in the lymph node after several nonspecific stimuli but did proliferate after injection of a freeze-dried tumor extract and in animals which had received whole body irradiation with lead-shielding of the left lower leg, including the node. It is likely that the resident lymph node macrophages were proliferating.

When metastasis was quantitated by counting cells in semiserial sections it was found that the rate was somewhat inconstant. After injection of 5×10^6 cells into the footpad, the lymph node contained about 1.5×10^2 tumor cells in 1 day, 2.3×10^4 in 2 days, 4.5×10^4 in 3 days and 5.0×10^5 in 4 days. If the footpad was removed any later than 24 h after implantation of 5×10^6 tumor cells, progressive metastasis occurred; while if the footpad was removed at 24 h or before progressive metastasis rarely occurred. It seems that the critical burden of tumor cells which could be destroyed in the popliteal node in this experiment was 2.5×10^2 cells – remembering that the accuracy of cell counts at the low level involved is not better than $\pm$ 10%. When 5×10^5 tumor cells were injected into the footpad and animals killed at 1, 2 and 3 weeks metastasis was present in the popliteal node in animals killed at 14 days and had disappeared by 21 days. It is likely, therefore, that small numbers of tumor cells can be destroyed in the lymph node.

A search was subsequently made for the actual process of invasion of lymphatics as seen in the footpad. Neoplastic cells were found indenting lymphatic endothelium and passing through gaps in the endothelium, probably between endothelial cells, because significant degeneration of lymphatic endothelium was not identified; lymphocytes and macrophages apparently passed through the same gaps. The cytoplasmic processes of tumor cells were identified lying in gaps in the endothelium (Figures 3, 4 and 5). There was no generalized patency of gaps between endothelial cells except where tumor cells, macrophages or lymphocytes were migrating through. These appearances were interpreted to mean that tumor cells

Figure 1. Hind limb of rat 5 days after injection of 20 million Walker rat carcinoma cells into the footpad. The swollen foot and grossly enlarged popliteal lymph node (circled) are evident.

Figure 2. Popliteal lymph node of rat 7 days after injection of 20 million Walker rat carcinoma cells into the footpad. Numerous tumor cells lie in the subcapsular sinus. × 180.

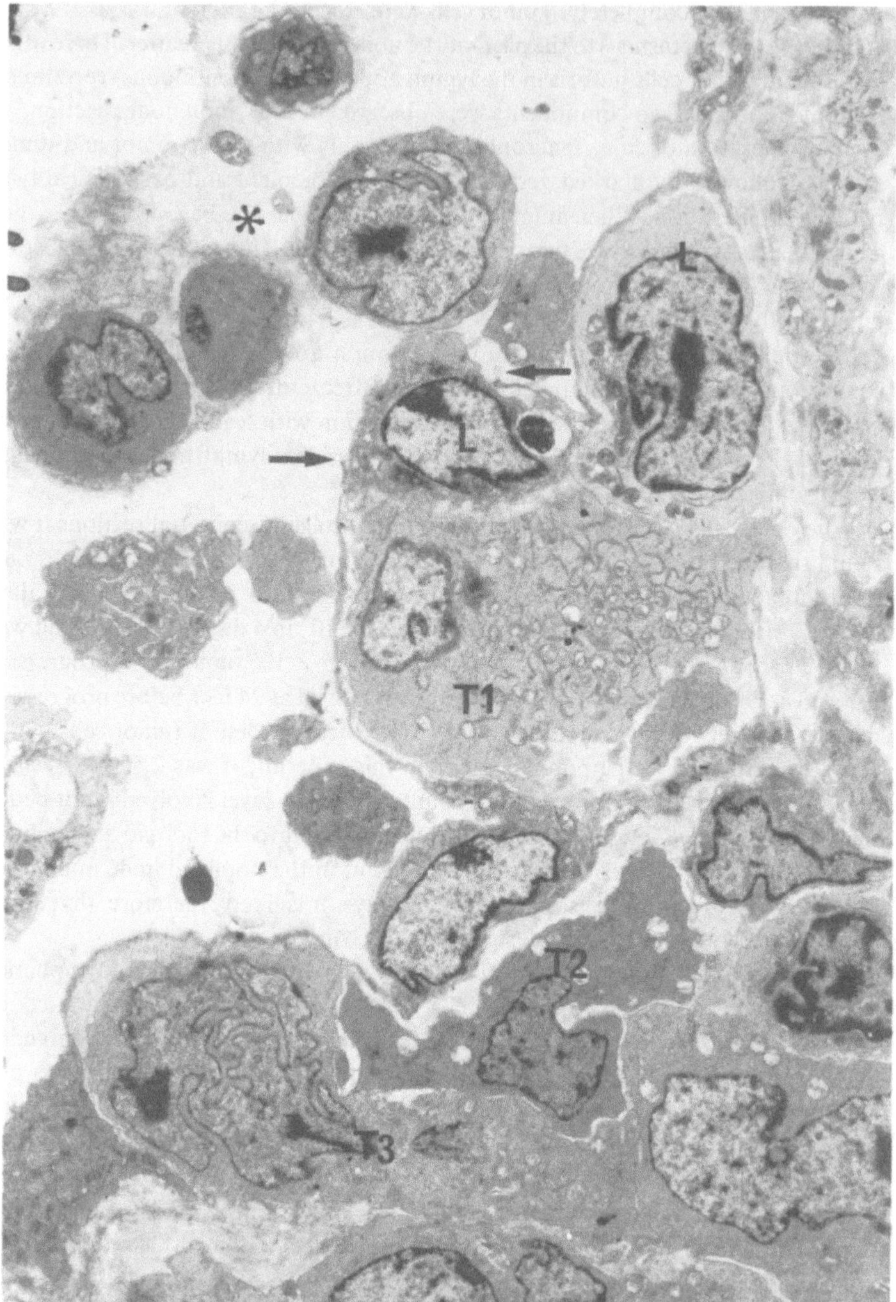

Figure 3. Tumor cell (T1) and lymphoreticular cells (L) passing through a gap (↑) in lymphatic wall in the footpad of a rat that had received 20 million Rd/3 cells into the footpad 5 days previously. The gap is arrowed. Numerous cells lie in the lumen (*). Elsewhere (T2, T3) elongated tumor cells are bulging the endothelium. × 3600.

migrated through gaps between endothelial cells and that macrophages and lymphocytes entered similarly. This process of 'reverse diapedesis' resembles the migration of leucocytes but is much harder to find. Either the tumor cells migrate through very quickly or relatively few do so. The direction of protrusion of cytoplasmic processes may determine the direction of movement of cells and may be related to the opening of previously closed endothelial cell junctions. No morphological evidence of secretion of toxins was seen.

2. Walker rat carcinoma

The next tumor system studied was the Walker rat carcinoma [9]. In 95% of newborn rats the injection of 5 million tumor cells resulted in metastasis to the draining popliteal node. In adult rats the injection of 20 million cells produced greater than 90% metastasis. Detailed histological evaluation showed a progression of metastasis similar to that seen in the Rd/3 tumor. A significant number of regressions did occur in adult rats, and the extent of metastasis at any given time varied considerably. This may be related to the fact that the tumor is not syngeneic.

The tumor cells in the lymph effluent from the tumor and afferent to the popliteal node were obtained by cannulating the popliteal lymph trunk with a 30G needle catched to a fine plastic cannula. With time there is a progressive rise in the number of tumor cells leaving the footpad (Figure 6). In general the later the stage of metastasis, the more tumor cells are found in the afferent lymph and the larger the metastatic deposit in the popliteal node. The normal (reactive) cells increase in number in parallel with the increase in number of tumor cells; there is no evident change in the proportion of different cell types. Tumor cells do not usually exceed 20 percent of the total cells present. Tumor cells were readily identified in lymph because they were large and had grossly pleomorphic and hyperchromatic nuclei (Figure 7). In all five animals where concurrent blood samples were taken from veins draining the primary, tumor cells were identified. Single tumor cells were seen in pulmonary capillarics but the animals were all killed before massive pulmonary metastasis had time to develop.

The flow of tumor cells may have been increased by the prior increase in tissue pressure induced by the introduction of 20 μl of Evans blue. It is not possible in this model to obtain significant amounts of lymph without delineation of the lymphatic with Evans blue, and gentle manipulation of the foot to stimulate lymph flow.

Migration of tumor cells through open gaps between adjacent endothelial cells was not identified. However, tumor cells indenting lymphatic endothelium seemed to produce degenerative changes in the endothelial cell cytoplasm. Such an indenting cell is seen in Figure 8. The tumor cell is elongated with nucleus at one end and a cytoplasmic tail at the other, appearances suggestive of cell movement. Numerous fine cytoplasmic processes of the tumor cell protrude towards the endothelium of the lymphatic vessel which has disintegrated. This is not a mechanical artifact

4

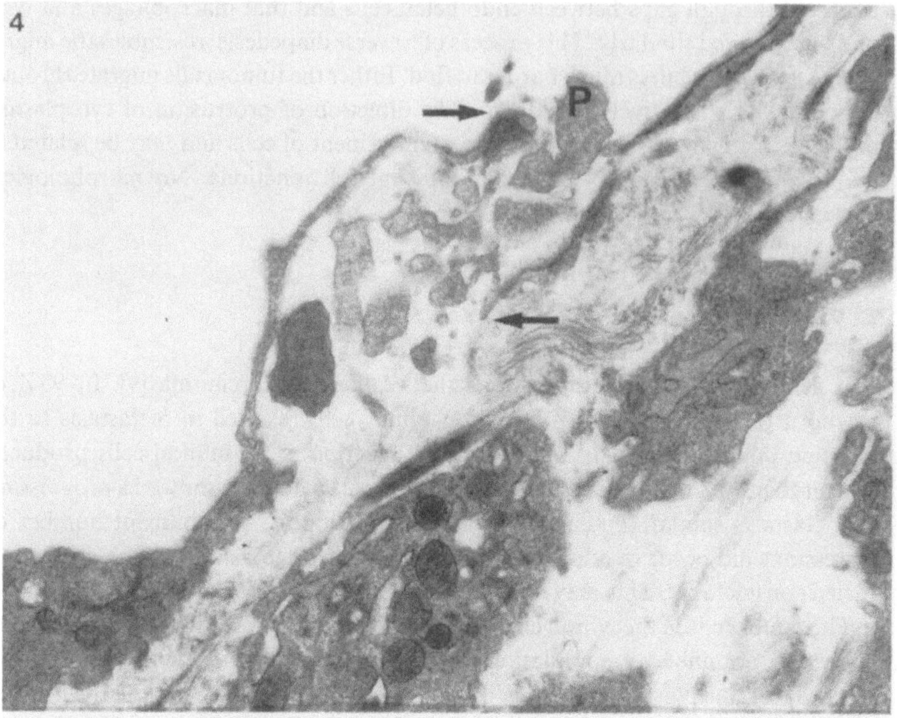

5

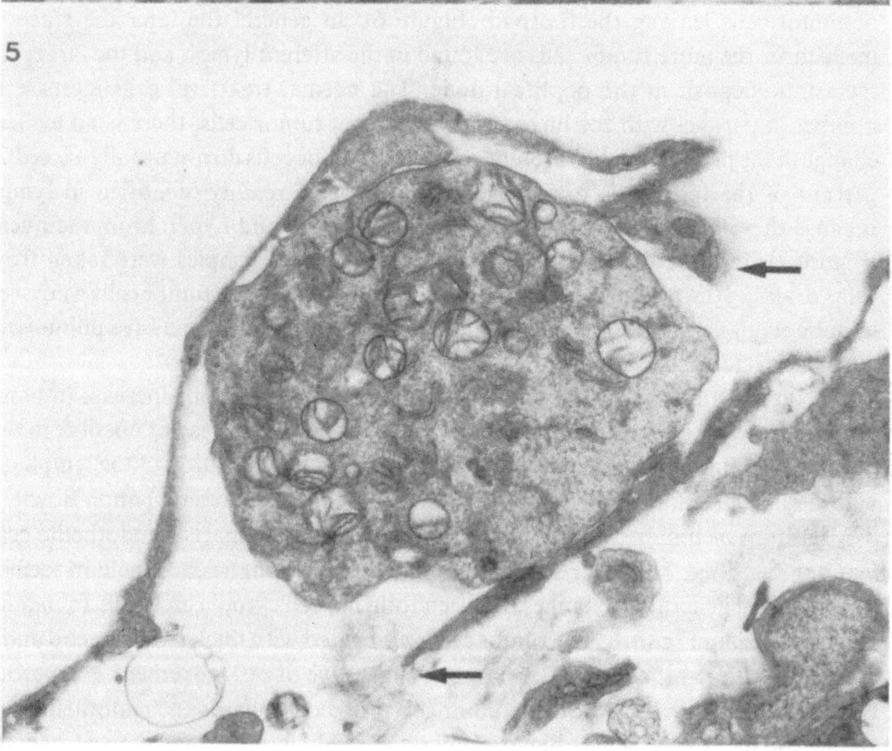

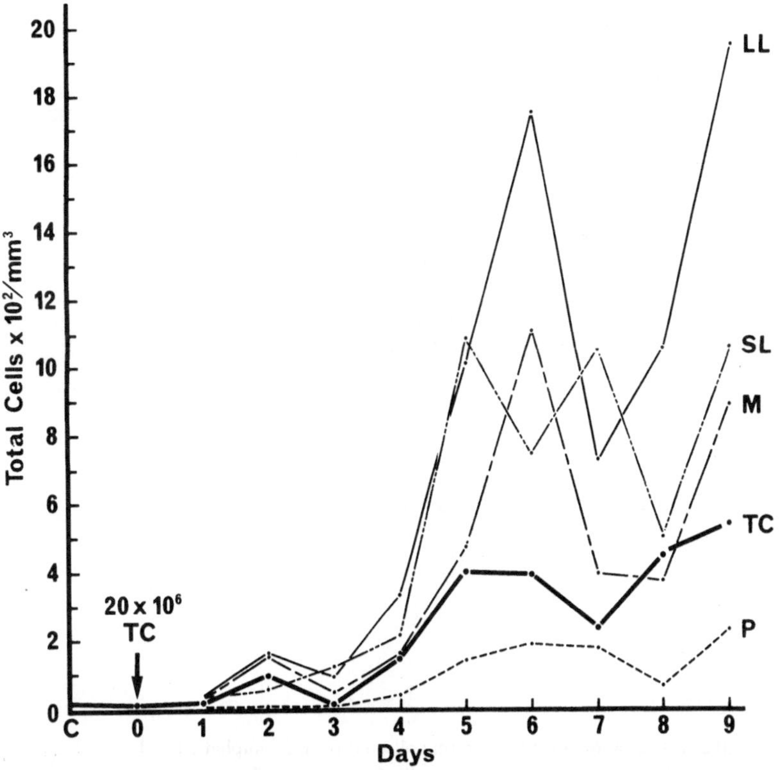

Figure 6. Cell output from lymphatic trunk during the progression of metastasis after injection of 20 million Walker rat carcinoma cells into footpad. Each point represents the mean of two animals. Additional animals killed at 7 and 9 days showed similar results. All the animals indicated had histologically confirmed metastasis in the popliteal node. LL = large lymphocytes, SL = small lymphocytes, M = macrophages, TC = tumor cells, P = polymorphs.

because the closely related endothelium on the other side of the lymphatic vessel is not disrupted. Elsewhere tumor cell processes can be seen protruding through gaps between endothelial cells. The endothelial cells show marked cytoplasmic and perinuclear vacuolation indicative of cell degeneration. In the last stage of this degenerative process a segment of the wall of the lymphatic disappears leading to an apparently open-ended lymphatic. This allows direct access from tumor to lymphatic lumen. Again the phenomenon of actual cellular penetration of the lymphatic is rare and difficult to identify.

Figure 4. Fine cytoplasmic processes of a tumor cell (P) protruding between endothelial cells of lymphatic into lumen without extensive lysis of collagen. An open gap exists (↑). The experimental circumstances are similar to those of Figure 3. × 9800.

Figure 5. Mass of tumor cell cytoplasm passing into lymphatic vessel between open endothelial cell junctions (↑). The endothelium shows no evidence of degeneration. The experimental circumstances are similar to Figure 3. × 10 600.

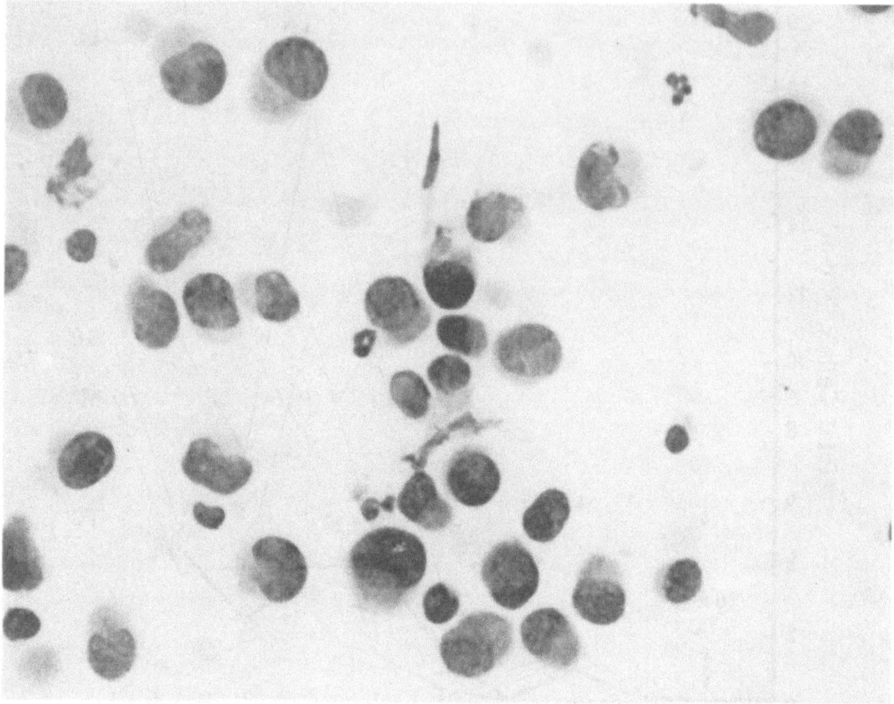

Figure 7. Walker rat carcinoma cells in lymph collected from a lymphatic trunk. The large cells with hyperchromatic nuclei are tumor cells (Hematoxylin-Eosin stain). The experimental circumstances were similar to those of Figure 8. × 410.

3. RMT 13762 mammary carcinoma

Recent experiments have been carried out with the solid variant of the RMT 13762 mammary carcinoma. Here metastasis is a little slower than with the previous tumors but even more highly reproducible. Failure to metastasize is very rare. A field at the edge of one of these tumors in the footpad is illustrated in Figure 9. A cluster of cells is seen migrating through the endothelium; these cells are adherent at binding sites (Figure 10). The lymphatic endothelium shows some areas of elevation or blebbing (Figure 9) possibly related to oedema, but there is no extensive evidence of endothelial cell degeneration. Tumor cells are found in clusters within the lumen of the lymphatic.

Cannulation of the lymphatic trunk yielded tumor cells, mainly in clumps (Figure 12) and in very much smaller numbers than in the case of the Walker rat carcinoma. There was no progressive increase in tumor cell output during the course of the experiment, and no increase in total cell output. These differences in the cells in the lymph may be due to the absence of massive destruction of lymphatic endothelium,

8

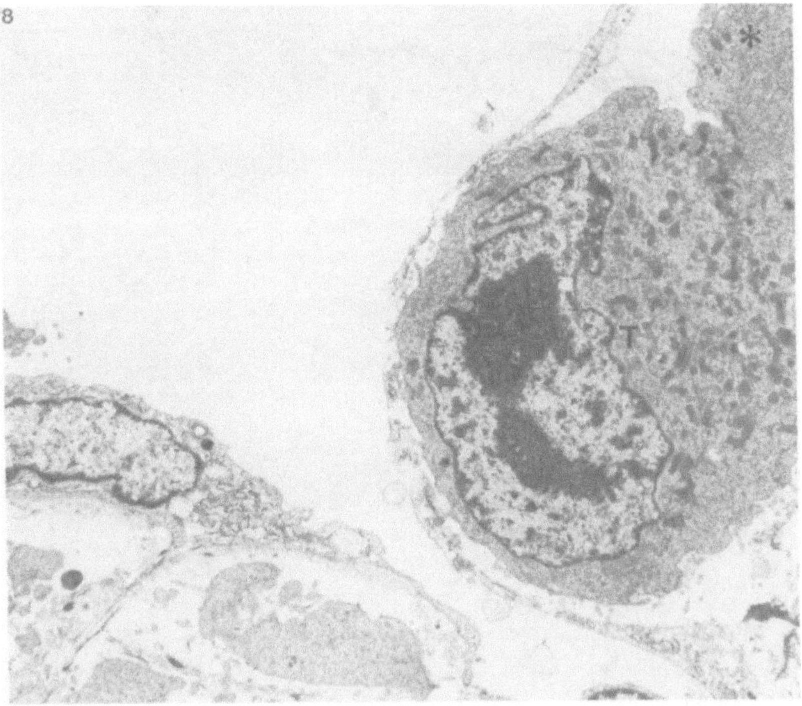

Figure 8. A tumor cell (T) deeply indents the endothelium of a lymphatic capillary 9 days after injection of 20 million Walker rat carcinoma cells into the footpad. Endothelium on the vessel wall away from the tumor cell is intact but over the tumor cell shows degeneration. A little of the 'tail' of the tumor cell is visible (*). × 5900.

and to the relatively minor lymphoreticular response which would be expected in the case of a syngeneic tumor.

These findings show that there are several ways in which tumor cells may penetrate lymphatic vessels. They may move by reverse diapedesis between the endothelial cells of lymphatic vessels, they may induce degeneration and necrosis of endothelial cells leaving an open-ended lymphatic, or clumps of tumor cells may push their way between endothelial cells, and metastasize as a group. The tumor cells then pass singly or in groups up to the draining node where they proliferate and migrate down the sinusoids, burst out of the sinusoid to destroy the node and migrate out of the proximal (efferent) lymphatic to metastasize to more proximal nodes and thence to the blood. Direct connections also exist between lymph and blood at the lymph node level.

There is a reaction in the node – variable early proliferation of sinus macrophages followed by paracortical immigration of lymphocytes and enlargement of and cell proliferation in germinal centers. These reactions have been described in detail by Van de Velde et al. [11–13] in a study of the lymphatic metastasis of a mouse

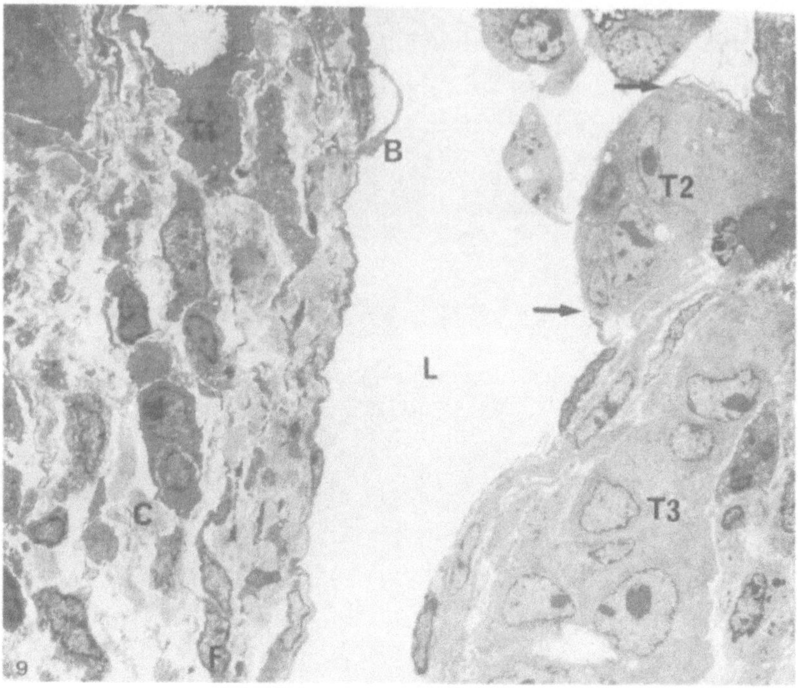

Figure 9. A lymphatic capillary at the edge of footpad tumor 15 days after injection of 5 million rat mammary tumor cells into the footpad. The capsule (C) is composed of fibroblasts (F) with occasional tumor cells (T1) with formation of acinar structures. The lymphatic (L) is lined by very thin endothelium occasionally blebbed into lumen (B) but showing no evidence of degeneration. There is a gap in the endothelium (↑) probably between two endothelial cells. Tumor cells (T2) lie in the gap, and are continuous in a deeper section, with a column of tumor cells with an acinus (T3). × 1900.

mammary adenocarcinoma. Morphometric analysis of the draining node showed an increase in paracortical area, cortical area and number of germinal centers. The reactions in distant nodes were similar. It seems clear [14, 15] that the first draining node is essential for the first step of the immune response but that later the whole lymphoreticular system reacts.

The tumor cells in the lymph are present in large numbers in the Walker rat carcinoma model – where presumably they enter into the disintegrating lymphatics in large numbers. Many fewer tumor cells are present in the lymph draining the syngeneic adenocarcinoma; and there is no progressive increase in the number of tumor cells exported over the course of the experiment. The large majority of the cells in lymph draining tumors are not neoplastic. In the case of the Walker rat carcinoma there is an enormous increase over the normal, probably representing an allograft reaction. The level of lymphoreticular cells in the lymph draining the syngeneic tumor does not rise above normal levels, nor is there evident change in the proportions of different cell types. This suggests that a less marked immune response occurs.

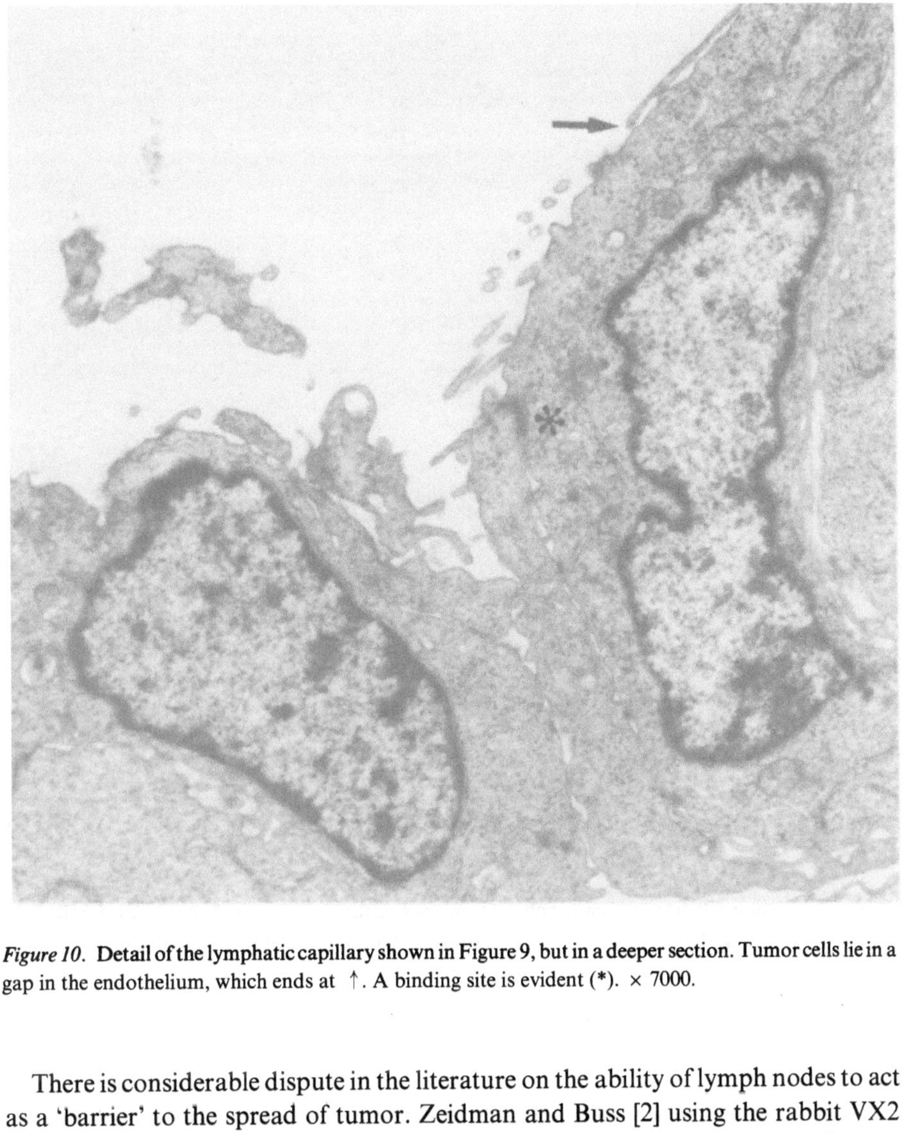

Figure 10. Detail of the lymphatic capillary shown in Figure 9, but in a deeper section. Tumor cells lie in a gap in the endothelium, which ends at ↑. A binding site is evident (*). × 7000.

There is considerable dispute in the literature on the ability of lymph nodes to act as a 'barrier' to the spread of tumor. Zeidman and Buss [2] using the rabbit VX2 carcinoma and infusing tumor cells into the lymphatic showed that tumor cells were held up for about 3 weeks. Most workers, however [5, 16–19], agree that tumor cells pass through quite quickly, in some circumstances within a few hours. Cortisone therapy and limb exercise reduce retention of tumor cells by the draining node and accelerate tumor dissemination [20, 21]. There is some dispute as to whether tumor cells can be destroyed in a node. In one model in which there was concomitant viral infection this certainly occurred [22] and there is good inferential evidence that it can occur during chemotherapy. In the absence of therapy both Zeidman [23] and Ludwig and Titus [24] suggested that it was possible. In our own experiments [5] there was good inferential evidence that about 250 tumor cells might be destroyed.

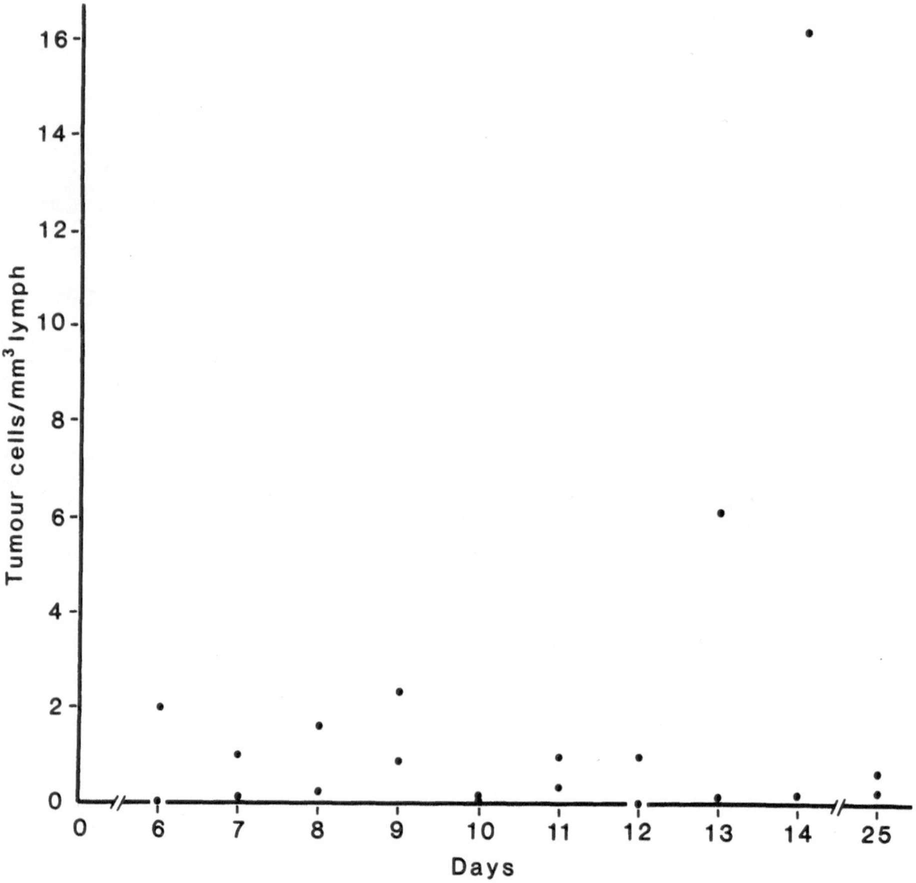

Figure 11. Tumor cell output from lymphatic trunk during the progression of metastasis after injection of 5 million rat mammary carcinoma cells into footpad. Each point represents lymph from one rat; two rats were examined at each time.

The node carrying a large burden acts as a new primary, shedding tumor cells into the blood [25].

There is now a variety of acceptable models of lymphatic metastasis of different types of neoplasm, hamster lymphomas [26, 27], a guinea pig hepatoma [28–32], rat hepatoma [33, 34], mouse mammary carcinomas [11–13, 17, 18], rat mammary adenocarcinoma [35–39], oesophageal carcinoma [40], prostatic carcinoma [41], mouse fibrosarcoma [42], and squamous carcinoma [43]. An interesting rat hepatic carcinoma [22] virally infected, shows spontaneous regression. The absence of a glycocalyx appears to be related to ability to metastasize [44, 45]. An ideal model would involve reproducible metastasis of a primary tumor to a defined lymph node that drained only that tumor, reproducible at a constant rate, metastasizing further to kill the animal by hematogenous spread. Such an ideal tumor would further be transplantable in a truly syngeneic strain, and its venous and lymphatic effluents

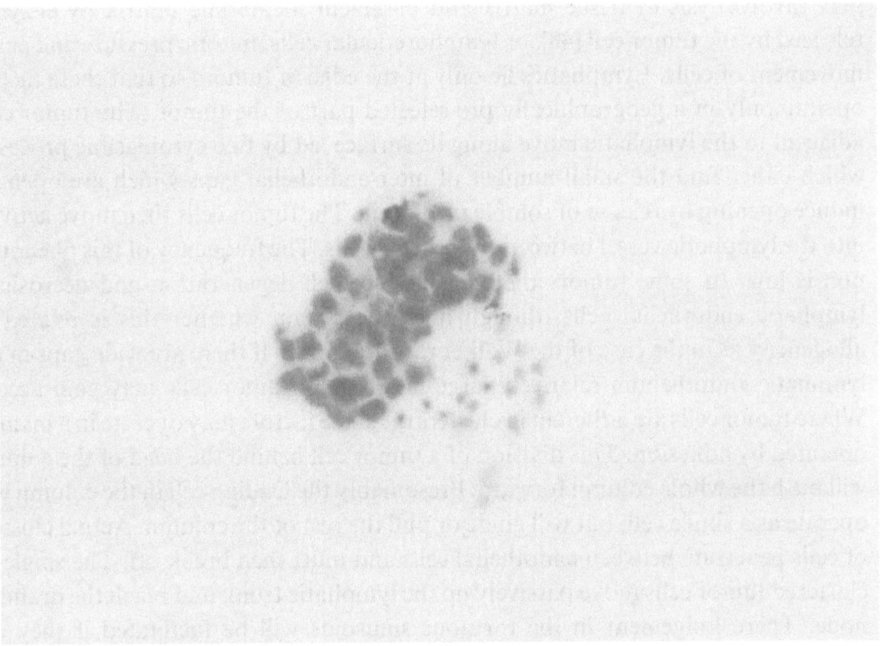

Figure 12. **Tumor cells obtained by cannulation of lymphatic trunk 5 days after implantation of 5 million rat mammary carcinoma cells into the footpad. The cells lie in a solid cluster more than one cell deep. H&E × 350.**

could be cannulated readily. Such a model does not presently exist.

Cancer cells metastatic in a lymph node in humans may produce extensive changes in the stroma and vasculature of the node but there has been little work on the corresponding changes in experimental metastasis. In a study of the allogeneic VX2 carcinoma in rabbits, Herman and others [46] have shown that for the first two weeks after tumor implantation there is an increase in vascularity. At about four weeks, the established metastasis is surrounded by plasma cells, and the vascular reaction subsides.

A number of questions can be asked using this type of model. Like other forms of metastasis, lymphatic metastasis can be regarded as a step-wise phenomenon. Is there one step more than another which can be regarded as rate-limiting? It is likely that a critical step is the transgression of the lymphatic endothelium. The local lymphoreticular reaction, or even inflammatory reaction may be important in limiting penetration of the lymphatic endothelium. Is it really true that tumor cells can be destroyed in lymph nodes? And if so, how, and how many?

An imaginative picture may be drawn of the situation around a lymphatic in a metastasizing neoplasm. Tumor cells may be singly or in clusters. Those which lie singly may be borne towards the lymphatic along prelymphatic pathways of orientation in connective tissue. Their transport may involve a tide of tissue fluid [47]. It may involve lysis of tissue matrix and basement membrane matrix by enzymes released by the tumor cell [48], or lymphoreticular cells, mitotic pressure and active movement of cells. Lymphatics lie only at the edge of tumors so that these factors operate only in a geographically pre-selected part of the tumor. The tumor cells adjacent to the lymphatic move along its surface led by fine cytoplasmic processes which either find the small number of inter-endothelial gaps which are open, or induce opening by release of soluble mediators. The tumor cells then move actively into the lymphatic vessel between endothelial cells. The frequency of this phenomenon is low. In some tumors they may induce cell degeneration and necrosis of lymphatic endothelial cells, though it is not certain whether this is related to allogeneity as in the case of the Walker rat carcinoma. If there are wide gaps in the lymphatic endothelium relatively large numbers of tumor cells may gain access. Where tumor cells are adherent in clusters the same factors may operate in a manner operated by adhesion. This division of a tumor cell behind the head of the column will push the whole column forward. Presumably the leading cell in the column will operate as a single cell, but will guide or pull the rest of the column. Actual clusters of cells penetrate between endothelial cells and must then break off. The single or clustered tumor cells move passively up the lymphatic trunk and reach the draining node. There lodgement in the tortuous sinusoids will be facilitated if they are clumped. The tumor cells proliferate (and it is not clear whether this is facilitated by the environment of the node), pass down the radial sinusoids and burst out of the sinusoids by mechanisms which must be similar to those involved in their penetration of the lymphatic. Within a few days tumor cells are found in the efferent sinusoids. Whatever tumor killing mechanisms operate in the node are effective only when a few cells are present.

There is now good evidence that pre-existing variants of tumor cells have a preferential ability to metastasize by the blood stream [49]. Is this also true of lymphatics? Fidler and Hoover [50] have submitted some evidence that this is so, but the case is far from proven. If there is such preferential ability it might be preferential ability to penetrate the lymphatic, due to increased mobility or preferential ability to survive in the lymph node. The latter seems more likely. Lymphatic metastasis is metastasis conditioned by the anatomy of the lymphatic capillary and the lymph node. Is there a way of modulating therapy to take advantage of this anatomy? There are scattered clinical studies suggesting that this may be so [51]. In animal models it is clear that after removal of the primary or simulated primary immunotherapy may produce cure but that the effect is optimal if the agent is introduced locally into or near the tumor, presumably so that it can act along the usual drainage paths of the tumor [29, 31]. The usual agent has been BCG or a derivative but other substances have been successfully used, e.g. corynebacterium parvum [37–39]. Systemic chemotherapy used as an adjuvant to surgery markedly improved survival in a rat mammary adenocarcinoma model [11, 12]. The effect on nodal metastasis was more marked than that on pulmonary metastasis, raising the possibility that metastases in different sites may be differentially sensitive. In some situations chemotherapy has actually accelerated tumor spread [53] presumably due to an effect on host resistance. Takahashi et al. [54–56] have studied the effects of chemotherapeutic agents suspended in lipid emulsions and either injected into tumors, or given orally in treatment of stomach cancer in man. Their results suggest that the drug has a local effect on the primary tumor, and is retained in the draining nodes producing degenerative changes in the tumor there. This interesting work requires further investigation. An optimal effect may be obtained by a combination of immunotherapy, radiotherapy and chemotherapy [57].

The application of such combined forms of therapy locally in animal models may yield results of significance in the treatment of lymphatic metastasis in human cancer.

Acknowledgments

Our own work quoted is supported by the National Cancer Institute of Canada. Figures 3, 4, 5, 6 and 8 are derived by permission from work published in the Journal of Pathology.

References

1. Weiss L, Gilbert HA, Ballon SC (eds): Lymphatic system metastasis. Boston: G.K. Hall, 1980.
2. Zeidman I, Buss JM: Experimental studies on the spread of cancer in the lymphatic system. I. Effectiveness of the lymph node as a barrier to the passage of embolic tumor cells. Cancer Res 14:403–405, 1954.
3. Van de Velde CJH, Carr I: Lymphatic invasion and metastasis. Experientia 33:837–84, 1977.
4. Carr I, Carr J: Experimental lymphatic invasion and metastasis. In: Lymphatic system metastasis, Weiss L, Gilbert HA, Ballon SC (eds). Boston: G.K. Hall, 1980, pp 41–73.
5. Carr I, McGinty F: Lymphatic metastasis and its inhibition: an experimental model. J Pathol 113:85–95, 1974.
6. Carr I, McGinty F: Neoplastic invasion and metastasis within the lymphoreticular system. Adv Exp Med Biol 73 (B): 319–329.
7. Carr I, Underwood JCE, McGinty F, Wood P: The ultrastructure of the local lymphoreticular response to an experimental neoplasm. J Pathol 113:175–182, 1974.
8. Carr I, McGinty F, Norris P: The fine structure of neoplastic invasion: invasion of liver, skeletal muscle and lymphatic vessels by the Rd/3 tumor. J Pathol 118:91–99, 1976.
9. Carr J, Carr I, Dreher B, Betts K: Lymphatic metastasis: invasion of lymphatic vessels and efflux of tumour cells in the afferent popliteal lymph as seen in the Walker rat carcinoma. J Pathol 132: 287–305, 1980.
10. Carr I, Carr J, Dreher B: Lymphatic metastasis of mammary adenocarcinoma: an experimental study in the rat with a brief review of the literature. Invasion and metastasis (in press).
11. Van de Velde CJH, Van Putten LM, Zwaveling A: A new metastasizing mammary carcinoma model in mice: model characteristics and applications. Eur J Cancer 13:555–565, 1977.
12. Van de Velde CJH, Van Putten LM, Zwaveling A: Effects of regional lymphadenectomy and adjuvant chemotherapy on metastasis and survival in rodent tumour models. Eur J Cancer 13: 883–895, 1977.
13. Van de Velde CJH, Meyer CJLM, Cornelisse CJ, Van der Velde EA, Van Putten LM, Zwaveling A:

A morphometric analysis of lymph node responses to tumors of different immunogenicity. Cancer Res 38:661–667, 1978.
14. Crile G, Jr: The effect of metastasis of removing or irradiating regional nodes of mice. Surg Gynecol Obstet 126:1270–1272, 1968.
15. Perez CA: Stewart CC, Palmer-Hanes LA, Powers WE: Role of the regional lymph nodes in the cure of a murine lymphosarcoma. Cancer 32:562–572, 1973.
16. Fisher B, Fisher ER: Transmigration of lymph nodes by tumor cells. Science 152:1397–1398, 1966.
17. Hewitt HB, Blake ER: Quantitative studies of translymphnodal passage of tumour cells naturally disseminated from a non-immunogenic murine squamous carcinoma. Br J Cancer 31:25–35, 1975.
18. Hewitt HB, Blake ER: Further studies of the relationship between lymphatic dissemination and lymph nodal metastasis in non-immunogenic murine tumours. Br J Cancer 35:415–419, 1977.
19. Kohno K, Tamaguchi T, Takahashi T: An experimental study of the spread of tumor cells through the lymph node. Tohoku J Exp Med 127:183–188, 1979.
20. Stoker TAM: The effect of cortisone therapy and limb exercise on the dissemination of cancer via the lymphatic system. Br J Cancer 23:132–135, 1969.
21. Stoker TAM: The effect of cortisone therapy and limb exercise on the retention of tumour cells by the regional lymph node. Br J Cancer 23:136–140, 1969.
22. Kodama T, Gotohda E, Takeichi N, Kuzumaki N, Kobayashi H: Histopathology of immunologic regression of tumor metastasis in the lymph nodes. J Natl Cancer Inst 52:931–939, 1974.
23. Zeidman I: Fate of circulating tumor cells. III. Comparison of metastatic growth produced by tumor cell emboli in veins and lymphatics. Cancer Res 25:324–327, 1965.
24. Ludwig J, Titus JL: Experimental tumor cell emboli in lymph nodes. Arch Path 84:304–311, 1967.
25. Crile Jr G, Isbister W, Deodhar SD: Demonstration that large metastases in lymph nodes disseminate cancer cells to blood and lungs. Cancer 28:657, 1971.
26. Carter RL: General pathology of the metastatic process. In: Secondary spread of cancer, Baldwin RW (ed). London: Academic Press, 1978, pp 1–52.
27. Carter RL: Lymphoreticular reactions and the metastatic process. In: Secondary spread of cancer, Baldwin RW (ed). London: Academic Press, 1978, pp 53–72.
28. Hanna Jr MG, Zbar B, Rapp HJ: Histopathology of tumor regression after intralesional injection of Mycobacterium bovis. I. Tumor growth and metastasis. J Natl Cancer Inst 48:1441–1455, 1972.
29. Zbar B, Bernstein ID, Bartlett GL, Hanna MG, Jr, Rapp HJ: Immunotherapy of cancer: regression of intradermal tumors and prevention of growth of lymph node metastases after intralesional injection of living Mycobacterium bovis. J Natl Cancer Inst 49:119–130, 1972.
30. Zbar B, Smith HG, Bast RC, Jr: Immunologic eradication of lymph node metastases. In: BCG in cancer immunotherapy, Lamoureux G, Turcotte R, Portelance (eds). New York: Grune and Stratton, 1976, pp 361–366.
31. Zbar G, Hunter JT, Rapp HJ, Canti GF: Immunotherapy of bilateral lymph node metastases in guinea pigs by intralesional or paralesional injection of Mycobacterium bovis (BCG). J Natl Cancer Inst 60:1163–1168, 1978.
32. Hanna MG, Jr, Peters LC: Specific immunotherapy of established visceral micrometastases by BCG-tumor cell vaccine alone or as an adjunct to surgery. Cancer 42:2613–2625, 1978.
33. Takazawa H, Shimizu S: An experimental model for lymphatic metastasis in rats. Gann 67:403–406.
34. Becker FF: Patterns of spontaneous metastasis of transplantable hepatocellular carcinomas. Cancer Res 38:163–167, 1978.
35. Bogden AE, Esber HJ, Taylor DJ, Gray JH: Comparative study on the effects of surgery, chemotherapy and immunotherapy alone and in combination, on metastases of the 13762 mammary adenocarcinoma. Cancer Res 34:1627–1631, 1974.
36. Sparks FC, O'Connell TX, Lee Y-T, N Breeding JH: Brief communications: BCG therapy given as an adjuvant to surgery: prevention of death from metastases from mammary adenocarcinoma in rats. J Natl Cancer Inst 53:1825–1826, 1974.
37. Kreider JW, Bartlett GL, Purnell DM: Suitability of rat mammary adenocarcinoma 13762 as a

model for BCG immunotherapy. J Natl Cancer Inst 56:797–802, 1976.

38. Kreider JW, Bartlett GL, Purnell DM, Webb S: Immunotherapy of an established rat mammary adenocarcinoma (13762A) with intratumor injection of Corynebacterium parvum. Cancer Res 38:689–692, 1978.
39. Kreider JW, Bartlett GL, Purnell DM, Webb S: Destruction of regional lymph node metastases of rat mammary adenocarcinoma 13762A by treatment with *Corynebacterium parvum*. Cancer Res 38:4522–4526, 1978.
40. Nakamura T, Mine G, Okudaira Y, Yaita A, Sugimachi M, Ueo H, Natsuda Y, Inokuchi K: Mode of lymphatic metastasis in the esophageal cancer using VX2 carcinoma in rabbits. Nippon Kyobu Geka Gakkai Zasshi 26:656–662, 1978.
41. Pollard M, Luckert PH: Transplantable metastasizing prostate adenocarcinoma in rats. J Natl Cancer Inst 54:643–649, 1975.
42. Finlay-Jones JJ, Bartholomaeus WN, Fimmel PJ, Keast D, Stanley NF: Biologic and immunologic studies on a murine model of regional lymph node metastasis. J Natl Cancer Inst 64:1363–1372, 1980.
43. Hagmar B, Ryd W: Metastasis spread from syngeneic murine tumours. Establishment of a test protocol for comparisons between ascites tumours and their progenitors. Acta Pathol Microbiol Scand (A) 86:231–239.
44. Kim U: Metastasizing mammary carcinomas in rats: Their induction and study of their immunogenicity. Science 167:72–74, 1970.
45. Kim U, Baumler A, Carruthers C, Bielat K: Immunological escape mechanisms in spontaneously metastasizing mammary tumors. Proc Nat Acad Sci USA 72:1012–1016, 1975.
46. Herman PG, Kim C-S, de Sousa MAB, Mellins HZ: Microcirculation of the lymph node with metastases. Am J Pathol 85:333–348, 1976.
47. Butler TP, Grantham FH, Cullino PM: Bulk transfer of fluid in the interstitial compartment of mammary tumors. Cancer Res 35:3084–3088, 1975.
48. Liotta LA, Tryggvason K, Garbisa S, Hart I, Foltz CM, Shafie S: Metastatic potential correlates with enzymatic degradation of basement membrane collagen. Nature 284 (5751):67–68, 1980.
49. Fidler IJ, Kripke KL: Metastasis results from pre-existing variant cells within a malignant tumor. Science 197:893–895, 1977.
50. Fidler IJ, Hoover HC: Lymph node and visceral metastasis of cloned murine fibrosarcoma cell lines. In: Lymphatic system metastasis, Weiss L, Gilbert HA, Ballon SD (eds). Boston: G.K. Hall, 1980, pp 80–90.
51. Plotkin D: Chemotherapy of lymph node metastases: differential response. In: Lymphatic system metastasis, Weiss L, Gilbert HA, Ballon SC (eds). Boston: G.K. Hall, 1980, pp 200–209.
52. Kreidler JW, Bartlett GL, Purnell DM: Immunotherapy of post operative metastases of 13762A rat mammary adenocarcinoma. Comparative effectiveness of BCG substrains and methods of preparation. Cancer 46:500–507, 1980.
53. Moore JV, Dixon B: Metastasis of a transplantable mammary tumour in rats treated with cyclophosphamide and/or irradiation. Br J Cancer 36:221–226, 1977.
54. Takahashi T, Mizuno M, Fujita Y, Ueda S, Nishioka B, Majima S: Increased concentration of anticancer agents in regional lymph nodes by fat emulsions, with special reference to chemotherapy of metastasis. Gann 64:345–350, 1973.
55. Takahashi T, Ueda S, Kono K, Majima S: Attempt at local administration of anticancer agents in the form of fat emulsion. Cancer 38:1507–1514, 1976.
56. Takahashi T, Kono K, Yamaguchi T, Watanabe S, Majima S: Enhancement of chemotherapeutic effect on lymph node metastasis by anticancer agents in fat emulsion. Gann Monograph on Cancer Research 20:195–206, 1977.
57. Bogden AE, Esber HJ: Influence of surgery, irradiation, chemotherapy and immunotherapy on growth of a metastasizing rat mammary adenocarcinoma. Natl Cancer Inst Monogr 49:97–100, 1978.

13. The use of embryo organ cultures to study invasion *in vitro*

M.M.K. MAREEL

1. Introduction

Amongst the reasons why cancers are so named, Gabriello Fallopio (1523–1562) cited that cancers seize on the surrounding parts with the tenacity of a crab seizing on its prey [1]. Seizing on the surrounding parts, called invasion, is indeed a characteristic of malignant tumors, distinguishing them qualitatively from their tissue of origin and from benign tumors and contributing to a considerable extent to their fatal outcome.

We discuss here some recent developments in the use of embryo organ culture to study the mechanisms of tumor invasion. Generally, in such experiments malignant cells (the tumor) are confronted with fragments of embryonic organs (the host tissue) and the confronting pairs are brought into organ culture. It is essential to make a distinction between organ culture and tissue culture [2]. In organ culture, small whole organs or fragments of organs are dissected from the intact animal and maintained *in vitro* in such a way that the three-dimensional histotypic structure which they possess *in vivo* is conserved. In tissue culture the organ fragments, either disaggregated or not, are explanted on an artificial substrate to which their cells can adhere. This leads to a rapid loss of the original histotypic structure, and, most importantly, to modifications of the relationship between the cells and their intercellular matrix.

As tissue culture was first developed, it was used in the earliest experiments about tumor invasion *in vitro*. These experiments were reviewed by Santesson [3]. This author studied the interaction between tumor explants and explants of normal tissue in plasma clot culture. To facilitate observations on living cultures, Santesson [3] avoided interactions within the three-dimensional central parts of the explants by placing them at such a distance from each other that the respective outwandering cells could not meet until after a few days. This way of investigation, which led to important new concepts [4], is beyond the scope of the present chapter. Three-dimensional tissue culture substrates have also been used by Leighton and coworkers [5, 6], who associated small clumps of human carcinoma cells with pieces of sponge matrix containing human fibroblasts.

Organ cultures were applied to the study of tumor invasion by Wolff and coworkers [7–9]. These investigators associated cells from tissue cultures of rodent and human tumors, or fragments from animal and human tumor biopsies, with

L.A. Liotta and I.R. Hart (eds.), Tumor Invasion and Metastasis. ISBN-13: 978-94-009-7513-2.
© 1982 Martinus Nijhoff Publishers, The Hague/Boston/London.

embryonic chick organs on top of a semisolid agar-agar medium. These experiments demonstrated the parasitism of malignant cells on normal tissues as compared to the parabiosis observed between normal cells of different types. In organ culture tumor cells organized in a way which was closer to their organization in the original tumor than when grown in tissue culture. Whereas Wolff and coworkers put much emphasis on the growth of the tumor cells, Easty and Easty [10], using adult or new-born mammalian organs as a host tissue, considered it as an advantage that the tumor cells did not grow extensively so that progressive stages of invasion depending on the motilities and contact behavior could be analyzed. The latter authors [10] maintained the confronting tissues on a rayon strip supported by a metal grid on top of fluid medium. A modification of this mixed culture technique was used by Lattner and coworkers [11]. They first allowed the tumor cells to establish as a monolayer on glass and then put small cubes of normal tissue on top of the monolayer.

Incubation of the culture vessels on a gyratory shaker at about 100 rpm has allowed submersion of organ fragments in fluid medium, avoiding their settling and subsequent outwandering on the artificial substrate. This technique has been used by Schleich and coworkers [12] to study the invasion of human tumor cells into human decidua graviditatis. We prefer the latter type of organ culture because it allows maintenance of a variety of organ fragments for periods of days to weeks. The fluid medium can be readily changed and drugs can be easily added and removed.

2. Invasion of tumor cells outside the body

2.1. Rationale

Taking malignant cells outside their natural environment and triggering them to invade tissues, other than those they were bound to invade, holds the risk of producing cellular activities which are not relevant to invasion inside the organism. Taking this risk is worthwhile only if the *in vitro* method offers serious advantages.

Analysis of invasion in organ culture is easier than *in vivo* where histology is the method of choice to describe invasion. Because of the heterogeneity of most tumors, serial sections of the whole area of contact between tumor cells and host tissue are advantageous. This is relatively easy in confrontations of a limited number of malignant cells with a small organ fragment, which can be folllowed sequentially from the onset until the moment of fixation. Eventual selection of subpopulations of malignant cells or areas of the host tissue which are not representative of the whole population, has to be controlled by making a number of cultures. Associations in embryo organ culture avoid the problems of transplantation immunity and this makes the method appropriate to study human tumor cells, for which suitable animals for transplantation are difficult to obtain. The method may offer a similar advantage for animal cell lines which are subject to antigenic modulation.

In vitro experiments allow separation of the various factors that act on invasion in the complex environment of the intact animal. For example, the fact that invasion occurs when malignant cells are confronted with foreign normal tissues *in vitro* has suggested that invasiveness is an inherent property of malignant cells, acquired somewhere during carcinogenesis, and does not depend primarily on alterations of the surrounding tissues. Furthermore, organ culture in combination with tissue culture techniques, where living cells can be directly observed, opens the possibility to analyse which activities of the malignant cells are vital for invasion.

The influence on invasion of metabolic alterations, hormones and temperature, which are subject to strict homeostasis *in vivo*, can be explored *in vitro*. Examination of the effect of experimental and clinical anticancer agents on invasion of malignant cells in organ culture may help us to understand their antitumoral activity *in vivo*, and lead to new therapeutic rationales and to new methods of drug screening.

Invasion *in vitro* may also prove to be useful in the study of the acquisition of invasiveness, a largely neglected area in the field of carcinogenesis. The technique offers the possibility to confront cells committed to malignant alteration at any moment from the application of the carcinogen until the appearance of overt malignancy.

2.2. Invasion in vitro as compared to in vivo

Against all the advantages listed above must be offset the fact that it is beyond doubt that invasion in organ culture differs from invasion *in vivo* [13].

Innervation, blood supply, cellular and humoral immunity, stromal reactions and neoangiogenesis are all absent *in vitro* and it is difficult to accept that none of these factors influences invasion. *In vitro* the malignant cells and the host tissue are new neighbours and the first contact between the malignant cells and the host tissue in many assays may be considered as a culture artefact. *In vivo* malignant cells usually do not encounter the edges of cut tissues or layers of cells comparable to those issued from the process of wound healing *in vitro*. However, these qualitative differences between invasion *in vivo* and *in vitro* do not necessarily constitute a drawback. On the contrary, they may indicate the contribution of the aforementioned factors to invasion.

More problematic might be quantitative differences due to increase or decrease of cellular activities, which result from the explantation *in vitro*. In this respect attention should be paid to any modification of the host tissue, which might

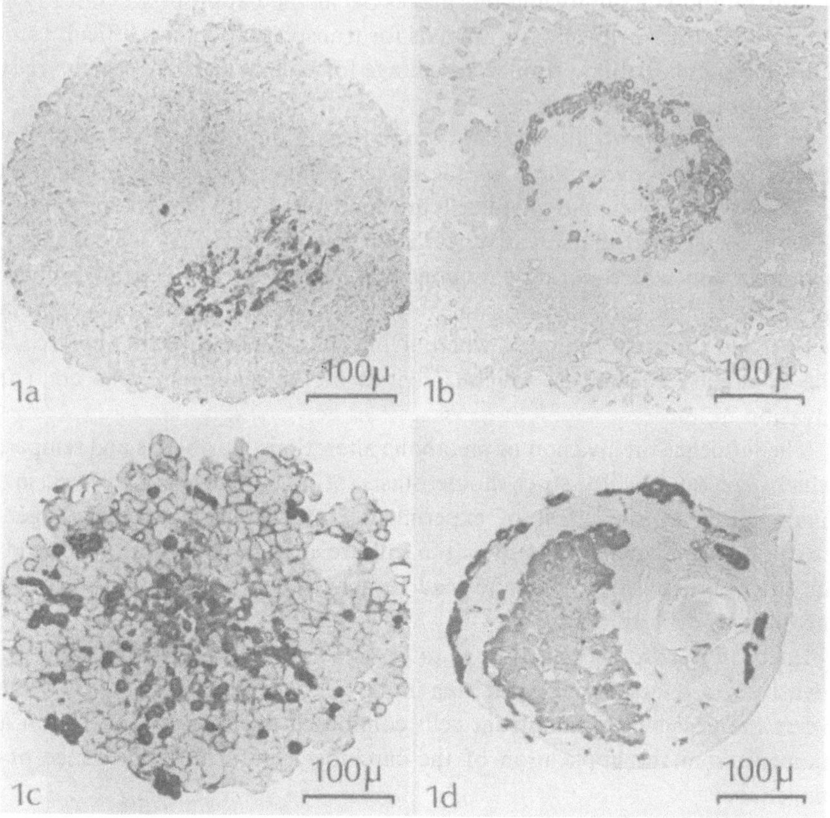

Figure 1. Light micrographs of sections from MO_4 cells (1a), HeLa cells (1b), B16-BL6 melanoma cells (1c) and cells from a human squamous cell carcinoma (1d) confronted with a fragment of chick cardiac muscle in organ culture and fixed after 4 days (1a), 7 days (1b), 14 days (1c) and 21 days (1d). Immunohistochemical staining with antiserum against embryonic chick heart. B16-BL6 melanoma cells were obtained from Dr. I.J. Fidler, Frederick Cancer Research Center, Frederick, Md., and human carcinoma cells from Drs. G. Easty and D. Easty, Ludwig Institute for Cancer Research, London, U.K. (from G. De Bruyne and M. Mareel, Unpublished results).

facilitate or prevent invasion or produce phenomena that resemble invasion, that renders the process not at all relevant to invasion as it occurs *in vivo*. It is therefore a good policy to rely on conclusions from *in vitro* experiments only when they have been confirmed by *in vivo* observations.

3. Methods to study invasion in organ culture

3.1. The host tissue

3.1.1. Histocompatibility. Since the experiments of Wolff and his school [9], it is well established that embryonic tissues exhibiting different histocompatibility profiles do not reject each other *in vitro*. Healthy chimaeras of tissues derived from different species have been maintained in organ culture. An exception to this rule was presented by the experiments of David [14], where incompatibility between embryonic chick liver and embryonic rabbit stomach epithelium resulted in lysis of the rabbit tissue after 6 days of coculture.

Although most of the tissues used as host in the invasion experiments are barely expected to contain immunocompetent cells, it cannot be excluded that the major histocompatibility complex influences to some extent the interaction *in vitro* of cells from different individuals. Curtis and Rooney [15], using Abercrombie's assay [4] found that contact inhibition of locomotion, measured as the degree of nuclear underlap between confronting areas of outwandering cells, was more marked in allogeneic than in syngeneic combinations. If we accept that contact inhibition of locomotion restricts invasion, it should be expected that the use of allogeneic or xenogeneic host tissues will hamper invasion. Unfortunately, very few experiments have been done to test this possibility and the assay developed by Abercrombie [4] for two-dimensional cultures can hardly be applied to three-dimensional cultures used for the study of invasion. On the basis of histologic examination no differences were observed between ESb2L tumor cells invading into fragments of lungs either from syngeneic DBA/2 mice or from allogeneic C57BL/10 mice [16]. An advantage of allogeneic or xenogeneic combinations that must be weighed against the theoretical objections listed above is the safe identification of the tumor cells inside the normal tissue by immunostaining with an antiserum either against the normal tissue (Figure 1) or against the tumor cells [16, 17].

3.1.2. Type of host tissue. Both *in vitro* and *in vivo* most tissues are susceptible to invasion by malignant cells. However, for the same type of malignant cells the pattern of invasion may vary when different types of host tissue are used. *In vitro* this pattern has to be inferred from the distribution of the malignant cells inside the host tissue and from the concomitant alterations of the host tissue in cultures fixed after various periods of incubation.

Comparison of various types of host tissue with the same kind of malignant cells in organ culture was made by Wolff and Schneider [8] and by de Ridder et al. [18]. In both series of experiments fragments from a large variety of chick embryonic organs were used. The authors concluded that invading cells first occupied the connective tissue and replaced the epithelial structures afterwards. In organs such as the mesonephros or the lung, containing much connective tissue, malignant cells invaded by strands, by fine files or by solitary cells; whereas a pattern of more bulk invasion by tumor cells was observed in liver, which contained little connective tissue. Whatever the structure of the host tissue invasion ultimately resulted in its replacement by malignant cells. In this respect cartilage is a remarkable exception.

Despite the apparent similarity of the ultimate result, variations in the behavior of malignant cells during their invasion into different tissues might help us to understand the mechanisms of invasion. Variations in the pattern of invasion have been explained on the basis of differences in the relative sensitivity or resistance of various structures towards the lytic action of invading cells. Thus, the resistance of cartilage has been ascribed to the presence of a collagenase inhibitor, neutralizing the collagenases which are considered to be vital for the process of invasion [20]. On the other hand the presence of 0.1% trypsin in the culture medium was found to stimulate the invasion of BHK21Py cells into foetal mouse heart in organ culture [21].

The propensity of different structures to serve as a substrate for the locomotion of invading cells offers an alternative explanation for the various patterns of invasion. Histologic examination of static pictures has indeed given the impression that the invading cells followed distinct pathways, which differed according to the structure of the host tissue. Haemmerli [quoted in 22] has analysed, by phase contrast cinemicrophotography, the locomotory behavior of L5222 cells invading into the rat mesentery isolated *in vitro* 3 days after intraperitoneal implantation of the tumor cells. The L5222 cells frequently changed their direction of movement and distinct pathways of individual invading cells could hardly be recognized. This observation does not necessarily contradict the idea that the pattern of invasion may be conditioned by the locomotory behavior of the malignant cells. It does however indicate that the direction of invasion is not determined uniquely by the interaction of individual cells with the substrate, but results from more complex phenomena including, for example, collisions between cells within the tumor cell population.

The above-mentioned explanations of the various patterns of invasion have assumed a passive role for the host tissue. A number of questions have to our knowledge not yet been investigated. To what extent does the host tissue trigger the activities of invading cells? Do malignant cells operate in different ways when they invade different tissues? Does the host tissue lay down extracellular material that creates a pathway for invading cells as it was shown for migrating cells during embryonic development [23]? How far is the pattern of invasion influenced by the locomotory capacity of the cells of the host tissue? Is degeneration of the invaded tissue only due to the activities of the malignant cells or does the behavior of the normal cells also lead to disorganization of the host tissue?

3.1.3. Invasion in embryonic as compared to adult host tissue. It has been known since the early days of tissue culture that embryonic cells adapt themselves to the conditions of *in vitro* life much more easily than adult cells. This is also the case for organ cultures, providing us with the main reason why most investigators have preferred fragments of embryonic organs for the study of invasion in organ culture. Provided the size of the fragment was limited and proper culture conditions were used, a large variety of embryonic organs maintained *in vitro* showed organized growth and differentiation patterns identical to those seen in the intact organism. One of the reasons, although most probably not the only one, why adult organ fragments are less well maintained *in vitro* is their higher sensitivity to conditions of hypoxia. For the design of experiments with adult tissues it is interesting to notice that among mammalia the inherent rate of oxygen consumption is inversely proportional to body size, so that material from humans might be more suitable than material from rodents or from fowls [24]. Central necrosis, presumably due to hypoxia, may also constitute a problem in organ cultures of both embryonic and adult tissues. It may be that malignant cells do not invade into the central necrotic area because the conditions of hypoxia paralyse the invading cells. Necrosis of the host tissue, whatever its cause, complicates the conclusions to be drawn from invasion experiments, because it is not clear whether or not malignant cells are able to invade into necrotic tissue. In the experiments of Lattner and coworkers [11] BHK21Py cells failed to invade into pieces of adult mouse kidney which were totally necrotic and when only part of the kidney fragment was necrotic the invading cells bypassed the necrotic area. Freeze-thawing of fragments of human amnion hampered their invasion by tumor cells in organ culture (Tchao and Schleich, personal communication). In contrast, when mouse fibrosarcoma cells were confronted with fragments of adult rat brain, which rapidly degenerated *in vitro*, they extensively invaded and completely replaced the brain tissue (Solheid and Titeca, personal communication). Whether or not the cause of necrosis was different in these three series of observations, so that different substrates were left for invasion, deserves further investigation.

Invasion of malignant cells in organ culture has been demonstrated using both embryonic and adult tissues [22]. To our knowledge, comparative experiments confronting the same organs in embryonic and in adult form with one type of malignant cells have not been described.

At the present time we prefer embryonic to adult tissues for the study of invasion in organ culture for the following reason. Invasion occurred in embryonic chick organs *in vivo* when tumor cells were injected into the vitelline vein or inoculated onto the chorioallantoic membrane [25, 26] and from the histopathologic point of view the process bore a close resemblance to the invasion in adult organs *in vivo*. Since embryonic organ fragments are maintained *in vitro* in a way that resembles their behavior *in vivo* more closely than it occurs with adult tissues, we use embryonic material as host tissue in our *in vitro* assays of invasion.

3.1.4. Preparation of the host tissue. When organs were cut into an appropriate size for maintenance in culture, they were traumatized and histologic examination showed necrotic cells at the cut surfaces (Figure 2). Such necrotic sites may not be ideal for the study of the invasive behavior of tumor cells [19]. This potential drawback has been avoided either by allowing the trauma to heal before the tumor cells were added to the tissue, or by confronting the tumor cells with the intact surface of so-called natural membranes.

When fragments of embryonic [27] or adult [16] organs were cultured for a short

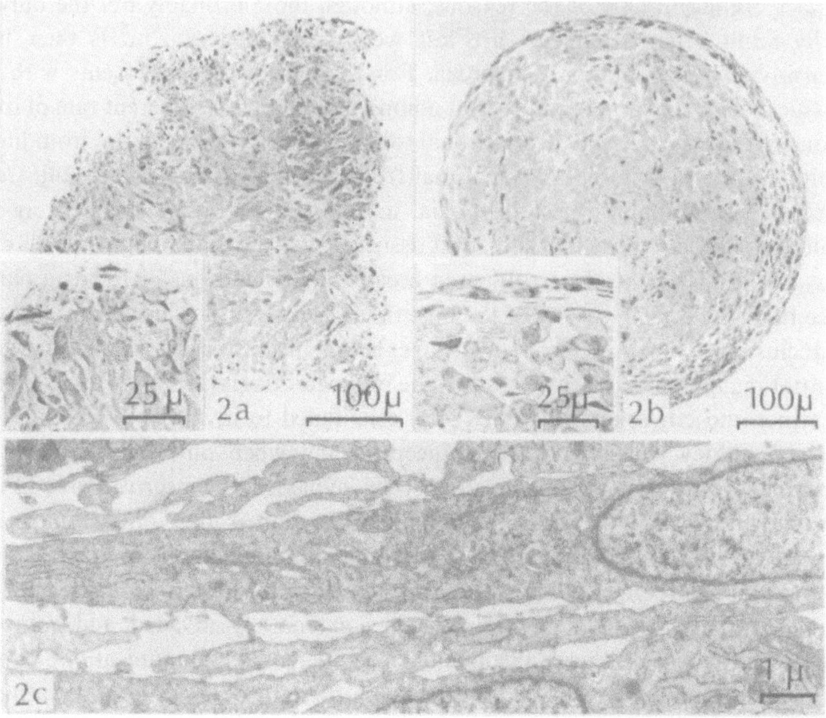

Figure 2. Light micrographs of 2 μm thick sections from a freshly cut (2a) and from a precultured (2b) fragment of 9-day-old embryonic chick heart, stained with hematoxylin and eosin. Insets: details of the periphery of the fragments. Fig. 2c is a transmission electron micrograph of a fibroblastic cell at the periphery of a precultured fragment of heart.

while they became surrounded by cells that migrated from certain parts of the cut surfaces. These cells formed one or a few layers of flattened cells, which in histological sections looked like fibroblasts (Figure 2). It is likely that cells other than fibroblasts participated in this type of wound healing and indeed with the chick mesonephros it has been shown that some of the cells involved were epithelial cells from the cut edges of the tubules [27]. The phenomenon did not seem to be excluselively a reaction to wounding, but could also be interpreted as the reorganization of a tissue, which now faces a new environment. In this respect the layers of fribroblastic cells would constitute the natural lining of the miniature organ. This explains why the formation of this natural lining could be prevented by wrapping the freshly cut organ fragment in a piece of vitelline membrane [27], and why the fibroblastic cells disappeared whenever the cultured fragment came into contact with another organ fragment or with other cells, invasive or not. We have confronted malignant cells with freshly cut and with precultured fragments of embryonic chick heart, but have observed no differences in the patterns of invasion [28]. Nevertheless we have continued to use precultured fragments because they presented a more homogeneous substrate for the study of the early steps of invasion *in vitro* [29].

The intact surface of so-called natural membranes consists of endothelia or epithelia. From the experiments published so far, one might wonder whether malignant cells are able to attach to the apical side of endothelia or epithelia and consequently invade into them.

HeLa cells, hepatoma cells and BHKPy cells failed to attach to the apical side of the epithelium of skin or stomach taken from 9-day-old chick embryos. If the epithelia were accidentally or intentionally wounded the malignant cells attached and invaded [30]. Similarly, tumor cells failed to attach to the epithelium of the embryonic chick trachea [19] or to the epithelium of the adult human fallopian tube [31]. On the contrary, B16 melanoma cells were found to attach to and/or penetrate into the transitional epithelium of the mouse urinary bladder within 12 h [32]. For epithelia, which are not more than one cell layer thick, or endothelia, this controversy does not seem to exist. The chick chorioallantoic membrane has allowed attachment and invasion of tumor cells in a number of experiments [19, 32, 33]. Tumour cells were also shown to invade into the human chorionic epithelium (Figure 3) and into the rat omentum [19].

The use of the rat omentum as a substrate for the study of invasion *in vitro* was not pursued, because of the frequently occurring holes in this tissue. It is, however, unlikely that accidental wounds could solely explain why tumor cells attached to one type of epithelium and not to the other. Although differences due to the use of different types of tumor cells cannot be excluded, it is most likely that the apparent contradictions were due to discrete differences in the structure and function of the living substrates. The latter opinion was supported by experiments using the ventral side of young chick blastoderms as a substrate. After about 12 h of incubation of the fertilized egg, the lining of the ventral side of the young blastoderm contained at the level of the area pellucida two generations of epithelium, the hypoblast and the endoblast [34]. Tumor cells readily attached to and penetrated the hypoblast but failed to do so when laying on top of the endoblast (Figure 4). Penetration through the hypoblast was not a specific characteristic of malignant cells since a series of non-malignant cells or small fragments of normal tissue also did so.

Recent cinematographic analysis of explanted hypoblast in tissue culture showed that cells put on top of the hypoblast produced extensions, which penetrated between the hypoblast cells. As a consequence the hypoblast cells retracted towards the borders of the foreign cell mass. The reaction of the hypoblast after this initial retraction differed whether they were confronted with malignant cells or with non-malignant cells [35, 36]. Non-malignant cells allowed the hypoblast to migrate over their free surface, to close the wound and in this way to restore its condition as a natural lining. Malignant cells appeared to continuously push aside the hypoblast, preventing closure of the wound (Figure 5). The same phenomena were observed when aggregates of malignant or of non-

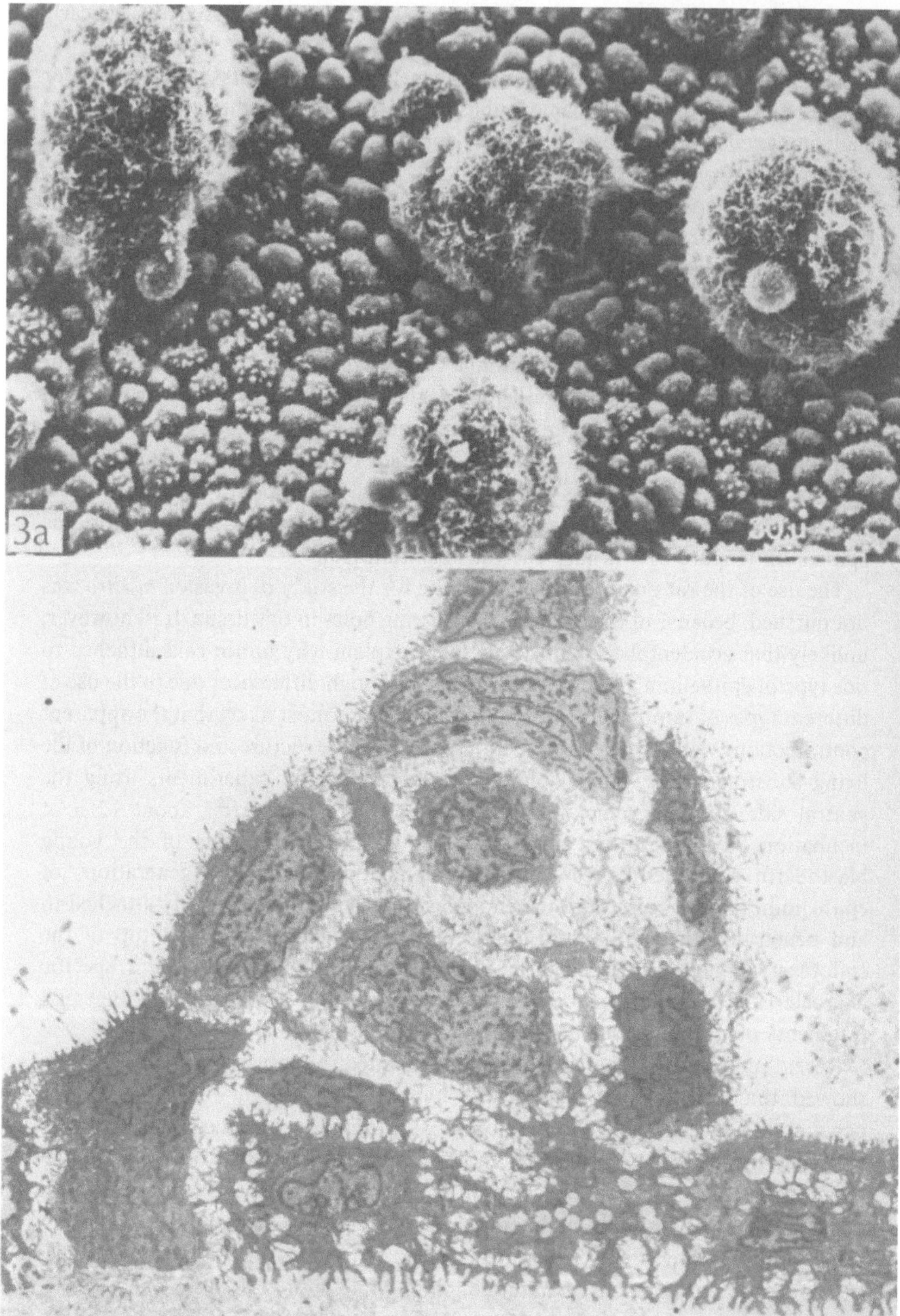
3a
3b
10 µ

malignant cells were put on the chorionic epithelium *in vitro* (A. Schleich and R. Tchao, personal communication).

3.2. Preparation of the tumor

How and in what form will the tumor sample be confronted with the organ fragment?

Biopsy specimens from animal and human tumors have been used by a number of investigators [37]. The biopsy specimens were cut into appropriate sizes and put on the host tissue without delay. For human tumors it has been our policy to prepare the cultures in the operating theater so that the tumor fragment came into contact with the host tissue less than 15 min after removal from the body.

When tissue culture cells served as the tumor, they had to be removed from the bottom of the culture flask either mechanically or by enzymatic treatment. Then, a monolayer fragment or a cell suspension could be dropped on the host tissue [19, 28]. There were no indications that in these experiments the organization of the tumor influenced invasion per se. In other experiments the fragments of normal tissue were incubated with a suspensions of tumor cells on a gyratory shaker [12, 28]. Here the tumor cells, either as single cells or as small aggregates, were more or less randomly trapped by the host tissue. In our experiments [28] with ^{3}H-thymidine labeled mouse MO_4 fibrosarcoma cells the fraction of MO_4 cells trapped by fragments of embryonic chick heart within 4 days was less than 1% of the total amount of cells added to the culture medium. A potential drawback of this method of confrontation is that lack of attachment may be interpreted as lack of invasiveness. In the experiments of Lohmann-Matthes and coworkers [16], cell suspensions from locally growing mouse tumors did not affect fragments of adult mouse lung in cocultures on gyratory shaker. In our opinion this observation demonstrated that the tumor cells were unable to attach to the normal tissue, but did not tell us whether they were invasive or not.

We prefer to use aggregates of cells, rather than cell suspensions for the following reasons.

Formation of the aggregate allows the cells to recover from the treatment applied to remove them from the tissue culture substrate. The diameter of the aggregate provides us with an index of the number of cells. The organization of the tumor cells as an aggregate, called a miniature tumor [12], usually mimics the

---

Figure 3. Interaction between aggregates of squamous cell carcinoma and human amnion *in vitro*. 3a: Scanning electron micrograph of aggregates attached to the epithelium of the amnion, fixed 24 h after association. 3b: Transmission electron micrograph, showing an aggregate on the amnion fixed after 48 h culture. One cell on the left hand side has invaded the epithelium and established contact with the underlaying basement membrane (from H. Felix and A. Schleich, unpublished results).

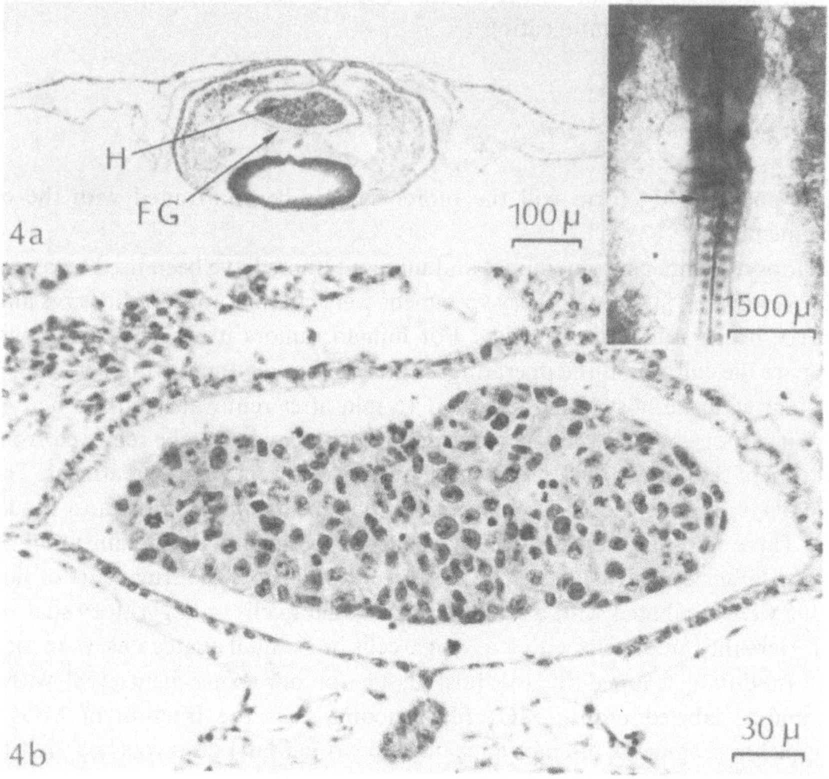
H
FG
100 μ
4a
1500 μ
4b
30 μ

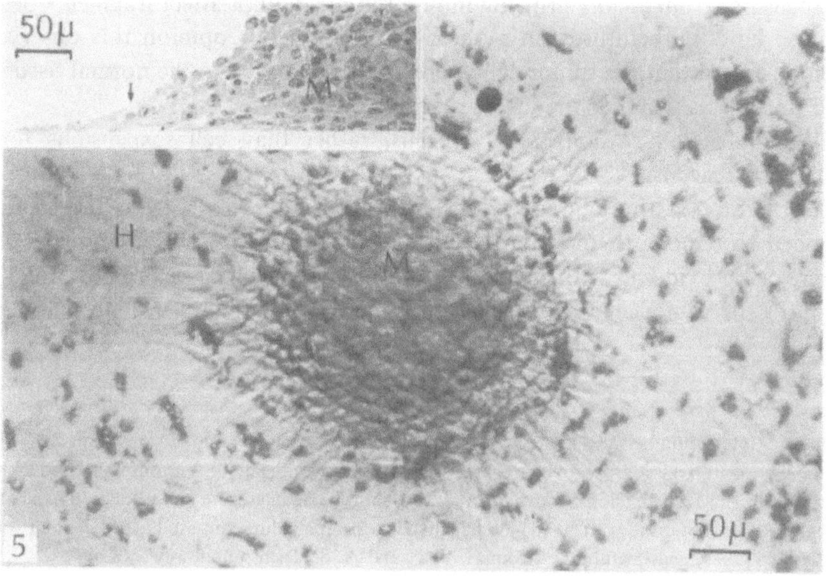
50μ
M
H
M
50μ
5

situation *in vivo* more closely than a single cell suspension or a monolayer fragment. One aspect of this organization may influence invasion. Aggregates with a large diameter consist of a peripheral layer of proliferating cells and a central part of interphase cells which afterwards become necrotic (Figure 6). Necrosis of the tumor rather than the host tissue may promote invasion [38].

Confrontation of an aggregate with a host tissue not only demonstrates the new relationship the tumor cells established with the host tissue, but also alterations of the intercellular relationship between the neoplastic cells of the miniature tumors themselves (Figure 7). Finally, confronting pairs of aggregates and tissue fragments can be followed under the stereomicroscope at regular intervals during incubation, providing useful data about their interaction, about the moment of fixation and about the method of histologic analysis. The fact that not all tissue culture cells produce aggregates of an appropriate size is a restriction to this method.

3.3. The organ culture technique

Organ culture techniques used for the study of invasion have been briefly reviewed in section 1. The method actually used in our laboratory is presented in Figure 8. We would again like to stress here that at least some aspects of invasion might be different in organ culture as compared to tissue culture.

When an aggregate (diameter = 0.2 mm) of MO_4 cells was confronted with a precultured fragment of embryonic chick cardiac muscle (diameter = 0.4 mm) in organ culture, the cardiac muscle degenerated and the whole fragment was replaced by the malignant cells within 5 days. When a similar fragment of cardiac muscle was allowed to establish as a monolayer on an artificial substrate in tissue culture and an aggregate of MO_4 cells with a diameter of 0.2 mm was put on top of the monolayer, the cardiac muscle cells survived and little or no degeneration was observed [28]. So far, we can only speculate about the reasons why in tissue culture the cardiac muscle cells escaped from the deleterious effect of the malignant cells.

Figure 4. Light micrographs of a transverse section through a chick blastoderm cultured during 24 h. An aggregate of HeLa cells (H) was initially layed on the endoblast and is now enclosed in the foregut (FG). Figure 4b is a detail from Figure 4a. Staining with hematoxylin and eosin. Inset: stereomicrograph of the blastoderm from which the histologic sections were made. The arrow indicates the position of the HeLa cell aggregate in the foregut (from M. Mareel, unpublished).

Figure 5. Aggregate of MO_4 mouse fibrosarcoma cells (M) put on top of a fragment of chick hypoblast (H) in tissue culture, photographed under the stereomicroscope after 48 h. The hypoblastic cells contain yolk (dark vacuolated spots). Inset: light micrograph of a 2 μm thick section from a similar culture, showing the relationship between the hypoblast (arrow) and the MO_4 cells (M) at the rim of the outwandering aggregate. Hematoxylin and eosin. (From M.C. Van Peteghem, unpublished results).

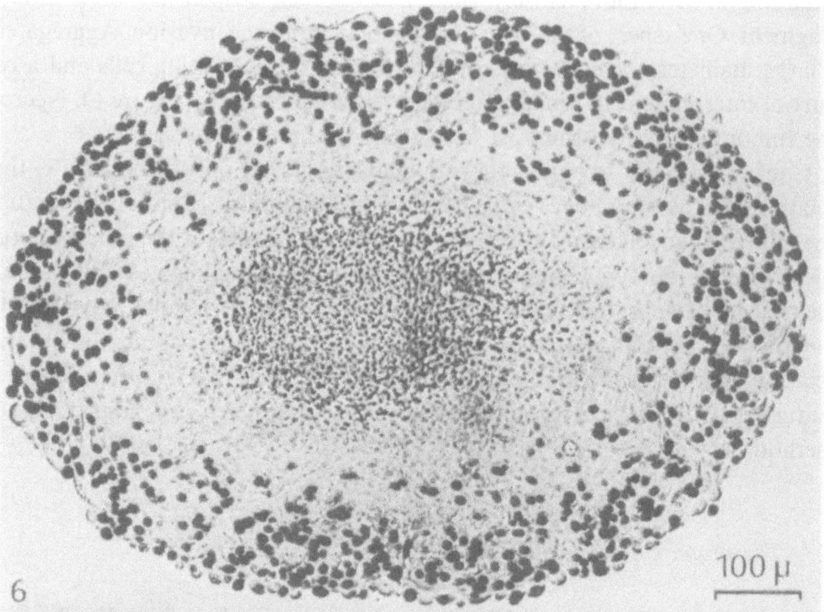

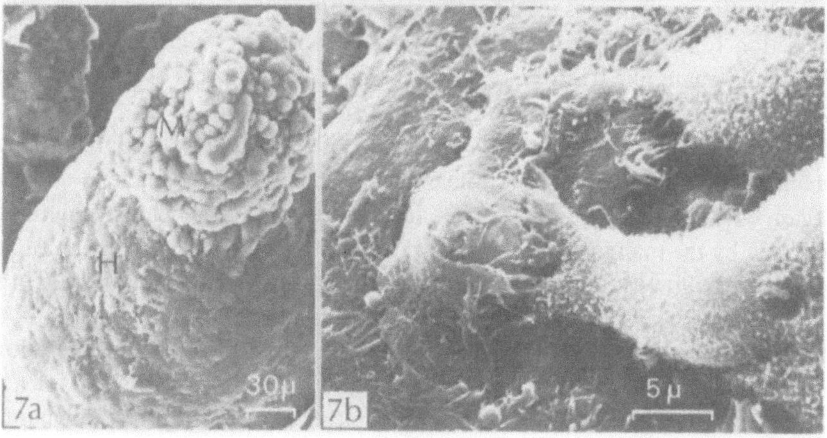

Figure 6. Histoautoradiograph of a section through the equator of a large aggregate of MO_4 cells, to which ^3H-thymidine was added 24 h before fixation (from C. Dragonetti, unpublished results).
Figure 7. Scanning electronmicrographs of an aggregate of MO_4 cells (M) confronted with a precultured fragment of embryonic chick cardiac muscle (H) and fixed after 2 h. Fig. 7b is a detail of a MO_4 cell attaching to the heart tissue (from L. Vakaet, Jr. and E. Bruyneel, unpublished results).

It appeared as if the normal cells retracted when confronted with invading malignant cells, provided a suitable substrate for locomotion was available. If they could not actively migrate as was the case when maintained in organ culture, they degenerated. A similar impression was gained from the behavior of the chick hypoblast confronted with malignant cells in tissue culture as compared to organ culture (see 3.2.). It is our opinion that a comparative study of the interaction of

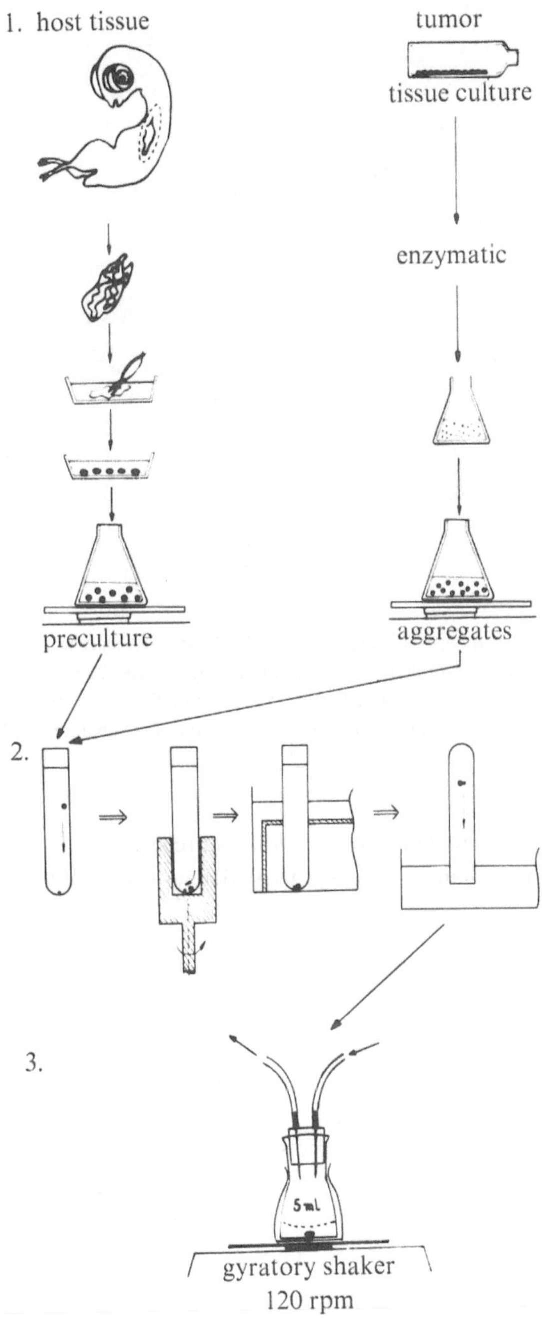

Figure 8. Outline of our method to study invasion in embryo organ culture. 1: Preparation of the host tissue and of the tumor. 2: Attachment of the tumor to the host tissue. 3: Three-dimensional culture of confronting pair. Not drawn to scale.

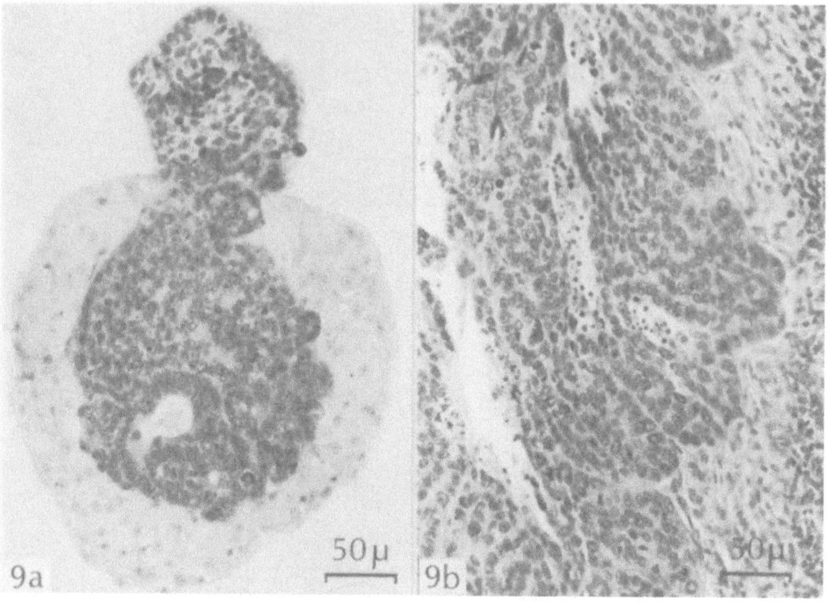

Figure 9. Lightmicrographs of an aggregate of K12 rat adenocarcinoma cells confronted with a fragment of chick cardiac muscle in organ culture and fixed after 21 days (9a), and implanted in the pinna of a syngeneic BDIX rat and fixed after 14 weeks (9b). Staining with hematoxylin-eosin (9a) and with hematoxylin-phloxin-safranin (9b) (from G. Storme, D. Schallier, C. Meyvisch, unpublished results).

malignant cells with normal cells in both culture systems may provide information how invading malignant cells exert their deleterious effect on the host tissue.

4. Testing the assay

The question of whether invasion of malignant cells into embryonic tissues in organ culture is relevant for invasion of tumor cells in the body is critical for the further use of this *in vitro* method.

Three arguments favoured this method. First, the criteria of invasion of tumor cells *in vivo* also applied to invasion in organ culture. Invasive malignant cells occupied the host tissue. The host tissue degenerated. Both processes were progressive in time and in space. The last criterion distinguished invasion by malignant cells from invasion by non-malignant cells, e.g. during nidation of the trophoblast or in rheumatoid arthritis, both of which processes are limited in time and/or in space [39].

Second, for a number of cell lines examined so far, the histopathology of invasion *in vitro* resembled that of invasive tumors in syngeneic animals. The resemblances pertained to both the manner and the rate of invasion. An example is presented in Figure 9. We have recently tested in organ culture the invasiveness into cardiac muscle of a number of human cell lines derived from squamous cell carcinomas of the head and neck. Because in the *in vitro* assay these populations of epithelial cells showed both invasiveness and terminal differentiation with formation of keratin (visible in Figure 1d), the histology of the cultures remarkably resembled that of the tumor from which the cell lines were derived.

Third, invasiveness in embryo organ culture appeared to correlate with the capacity of cells to produce invasive and eventually metastasizing tumors after implantation into syngeneic animals [37]. The correlation was particularly convincing in cell lines, that were tested before and after malignant alteration. 3T3-type C3H mouse fibroblastic cells (MO), at early passages, did not invade into embryonic chick skin and were not tumorigenic. 'Spontaneous' transformants at later passages and viral and chemical transformants did invade and also produced invasive fibrosarcomas in syngeneic mice [35]. Similar results were obtained with ST-L cells, established from single cultures derived from normal lung tissue of 3 to 5 months old ST/aFib H-2b mice [40]. 'Spontaneous' acquisition of tumorigenicity by ST-L cells corresponded with the acquisition of invasiveness in organ culture. These observations were confirmed using fetal brain cells (BT) removed from BDIX rats, 20 to 90 h after exposure to a transplacental pulse of N-ethyl-N-nitrosourea and established in tissue culture. At regular intervals after explantation in tissue culture aggregates of these cells, committed to malignant alteration, were confronted with chick cardiac muscle in organ culture or implanted into syngeneic rats. These comparative assays demonstrated a strict correlation between invasion *in vitro* and formation of invasive tumors *in vivo* [41]. The results from these experiments with the MO, the ST-L- and the BT-cell lines appeared to confirm the opinion of Barski and Wolff [42] that malignancy was essentially due to the fact that cells acquired new mechanisms that enabled them to invade normal histologic structures.

When normal cells, from primary tissue cultures or from early passages, were confronted with fragments of normal tissue in organ culture they usually have not survived for more than a few days. Therefore some authors [42, 43] have considered the capacity of tissue culture cells to survive in organ culture as an additional criterion of malignancy, next to invasiveness. One exception was present in the experiments of de Ridder and Laerum [41]: RE-E cells, an epitheloid variant of a fibroblastic cell line from Sprague-Dawley rats, which were not tumorigenic, organized around the normal tissue, proliferated but failed to invade (Figure 10).

Contrary to many so-called normal cells derived from cultured lines, tissue fragments from an organ associated with tissue fragments from another organ, either autogeneic, syngeneic, homogeneic or xenogeneic, easily formed healthy chimaeras, which could survive for considerable periods. Many examples of this can be found in the work of Wolff and his school [9]. Why, in this respect, tissue fragments differed from cells was not clear.

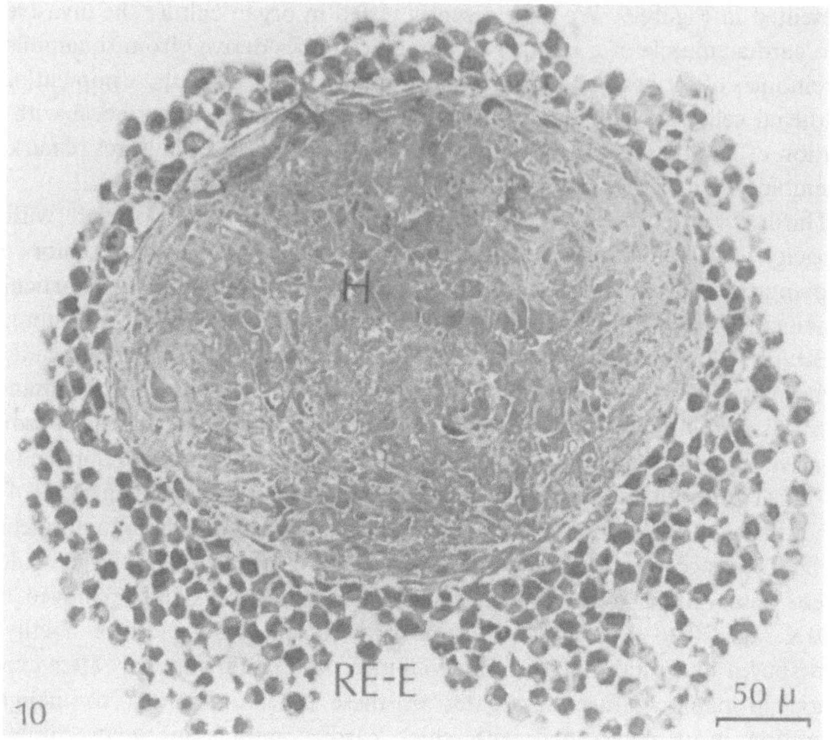

Figure 10. Lightmicrograph of a 2 μm thick section from RE-E cells confronting a fragment of chick cardiac muscle (H), fixed after 4 days in organ culture. Hematoxylin and eosin. (from L. de Ridder and O.D. Laerum, unpublished results).

5. Invasion of MO_4 cells into chick cardiac muscle in organ culture

An example of the kind of investigations which can be done in organ culture, is demonstrated by the invasion of MO_4 mouse fibrosarcoma cells into embryonic chick cardiac muscle. The preparation of the organ fragments and of the miniature MO_4 tumors and the method of confronting both tissues with each other are shown in Figure 8.

5.1. The early steps of invasion in vitro [29, 44]

MO_4 cell aggregates consisted of about 1×10^4 cells, most of which were polygonal to round with short villous extensions. After contact with the heart tissue, MO_4 cells became polarized. They produced long cytoplasmic extensions, anchoring between the peripheral fibroblastic cells of the heart fragment, and became spindle shaped (Figure 7). Shortly after contact, polarization was limited to the site of immediate contact with the heart tissue, but later the tendency to flatten extended towards cells at the opposite pole of the aggregate. We suggest that the cytoplasmic extensions produced by the MO_4 cells were responsible for the attachment of the MO_4 cell aggregate to the fragment of heart. The rate of attachment was quantitated in the following way: The test tube in which the confronting pairs were incubated was turned upside down so that they sedimented (Figure 8), and the rate of attachment was expressed as the number of pairs remaining together after sedimentation, divided by the total number tested. This rate of attachment was about 40% after 15 min of incubation and reached 100% after 45 min [29]. Attachment did not occur at 4° C and was reduced by treatment with KCN or with cytochalasin B. Attachment was not sensitive to treatment of the tissues with Nocodazole, with 5-fluorouracil, with ionizing radiation or with cycloheximide. These experiments indicated that attachment was an active cellular process depending on ATP-energy and for which an intact microfilament system was necessary.

Measurement of the rate of attachment in various experimental conditions together with ultrastructural analysis of the area of contact allowed us to distinguish between various steps during the early interaction of MO_4 cells and peripheral fibroblastic heart cells [44]. It is suggested that the following sequence of events determined the observed interaction. First, the glycoproteins at the external side of the plasmamembrane of MO_4 cells interacted with these of the peripheral fibroblastic heart cells or with their extracellular matrix. This process, called adhesion, might be the key event triggering all the subsequent activities of the MO_4 cells. Second, MO_4 cells produced cytoplasmic extensions with a diameter of 0.1 to 0.2 μm containing microfilaments but no other organelles. These extensions anchored between the peripheral heart cells. Both adhesion and anchorage occurred when the heart fragment was prefixed with glutaraldehyde. Third, larger extensions or parts of the cytoplasm of MO_4 cells, penetrated between the fibroblastic heart cells. Fourth, penetration was accompanied by widening of the intercellular spaces between the peripheral fibroblastic heart cells, which started to retract and had a tendency to become rounded. This sequence of adhesion, anchorage and penetration also occurred when aggregates of non-invasive cells were confronted with precultured heart fragments. However, with non-invasive cells the peripheral heart cells reorganized and started to circumvent the confronting aggregate. With invasive cells, the peripheral heart cells showed degenerative alterations: swelling of the endoplasmic reticulum, lowering of the electrondensity of the cytoplasm and disruption of the plasma membrane.

5.2. Occupation of the cardiac muscle by invading MO_4 cells

After 1 day of incubation MO_4 cells had started to occupy the cardiac muscle. This process was progressive, leading to complete replacement of the heart tissue within

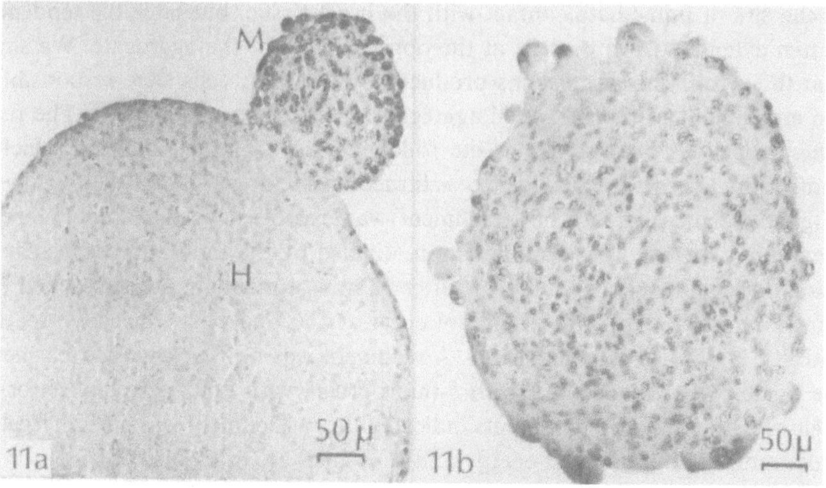

Figure 11. Lightmicrographs of 8 μm thick sections from MO_4 cell aggregates (M), irradiated with 16 Gy, and confronted with heart fragments (H) in organ culture. Fixation after 3 h (11a) and after 14 days (11b) (from G. Storme, unpublished results).

the next 4 days, and appeared to be a unique characteristic of malignant cells (see 4.).

Progressive disappearance of the heart tissue was not only obvious from the routine histology of fixed cultures after various periods of incubation, but also from immunohistochemical staining with an antiserum prepared against embryonic chick heart (Figure 1). These morphological observations were confirmed by the LDH-isozyme pattern in cellulose-acetate electrophorograms of homogenates prepared from confronting tissues after various periods of culture.

Degenerative changes of cardiac muscle cells, observed in transmission electron micrographs, were aspecific and provided no indications about the causes of degeneration. Central necrosis of the cardiac muscle due to hypoxia occurring before complete replacement was observed in some cultures, where the rapidly proliferating MO_4 cells had a tendency to occupy the periphery of the heart fragment. This could be avoided by irradiation of the MO_4 cell aggregate with a sublethal dose of X-rays, inducing a delay in proliferation. In these experiments complete replacement of the cardiac muscle invariably occurred without central necrosis (Figure 11), showing that bulk hypoxia was not responsible for degeneration of the heart tissue.

Phagocytosis of heart material by invading MO_4 cells seemed, at least partly, responsible for the disappearance of the invaded tissue. Using ^{51}Cr-labeled host tissues [45] we were surprised to find that disappearance of the invaded tissue was not accompanied by an increased release of the isotope into the culture medium. We inferred from these experiments that chromium was taken up by the invading cells via endocytosis of labeled macromolecules or labeled fragments of cells. This opinion was later confirmed by immunohistochemical staining with an antiserum against chick heart, showing phagosomes with immunoreactive material inside MO_4 cells at the fore-front of invasion.

The activity of many malignant tumors has been described as invasive growth, suggesting that growth and invasion were causally related. However, no firm evidence has been presented that invasion of malignant tumors, which is quite different from the expansive growth of benign tumors, is the consequence of growth alone. In organ culture invasion of MO_4 cells into the cardiac muscle was not directly related to the growth of the MO_4 cell population. Invasion has been demonstrated in presence of agents that completely inhibited the growth of the MO_4 cells [46, 47, 48]. The rate of invasion in these cultures was slower, possibly because the number of invasive cells was lower than in control cultures. When aggregates, containing approximately the same number of MO_4 cells as was expected to be present in control cultures after 4 days, were confronted with heart fragments in the presence of 5-fluorouracil invasion hardly differed from that in controls. These experiments indicated that invasion and growth were not causally related, but rather that growth influenced the rate of invasion through increases of the number of invasive cells. These conclusions have been criticized because they were believed to have no bearing on the *in vivo* situation [49]. Even if we accept that invasive tumors usually do also grow, it is not hard to imagine that drug treatment controls proliferation of a tumor whilst invasion, and eventually metastasis, continues. The results of both processes might become clinically apparent when therapeutic control is lost and growth resumes.

Some inhibitors of growth, known to interfere with the formation of the mitotic spindle, also inhibited the invasion of MO_4 cells in organ culture [46, 50]. The main argument that interference with the mitotic spindle was not responsible for inhibition of invasion was provided by combined treatment of confronting tissues. Treatment with 5-fluorouracil inhibited growth but allowed invasion. Consequent addition of microtubule inhibitors interfered with the invasion of these non-proliferating MO_4 cells. Since 5-fluorouracil blocked the mitotic cycle in early S-phase, it was difficult to accept that the anti-invasive activity of the microtubule inhibitors was due to their effect on the mitotic spindle. Inhibition of invasion by microtubule inhibitors appeared to be due to abolishment of the cytoplasmic microtubule complex, a structure necessary for directional migration, a vital, though not the only, activity of invading cells. The arguments were: First, a series of microtubule inhibitors, with different structures, different tubulin-binding sites and sometimes different mechanisms of action, all interfered with the function of the cytoplasmic microtubule complex at anti-invasive doses [50]. Second, for the vinca alkaloids, vinblastine, vincristine and vindesine (Eli Lilly & Co, Indianapolis, Indiana) inhibition of invasion and inhibition of directional migration, measured by explantation of MO_4 cell aggregates on glass [47], showed the same dose-responsiveness. Third, inhibitors of growth, which left the cytoplasmic microtubule complex unaltered, did not interfere with directional migration and allowed invasion. Recent experiments by Schallier and Storme (unpublished), confronting aggregates of K12 rat colonic adenocarcinoma cells with precultured heart fragments in the presence of microtubule inhibitors, have shown that the cytoplasmic microtubule complex is involved in the invasion of epithelial malignant cells as well as in the fibroblastic MO_4 cells.

6. Conclusions and prospects

I have discussed the advantages and the limitations of embryo organ culture for the study of invasion. The histopathology of invasion in this model and the good correlation between invasion *in vitro* and formation of invasive tumors *in vivo*, justify the use of embryo organ culture for the further exploration of the vital activities of invading tumor cells. Current research in our laboratory concentrates on the following aspects of invasion: 1) Study of the cellular alterations accompanying the acquisition of invasiveness during the course of carcinogenesis, 2) Dissection of the cellular activities of invading tumor cells, 3) Definition of the factors, both extracellular and intracellular, that regulate the cellular activities of invading tumor cells, and 4) Systematic analysis of the anti-invasive effect of currently used and new anticancer agents.

Despite the obvious similarities between invasion *in vivo* and invasion in embryo organ culture, it remains our policy to rely on conclusions from *in vitro* experiments only when they have been confirmed by *in vivo* observations.

Acknowledgments

Research in the author's laboratory is supported by the Kankerfonds van de Algemene Spaar- en Lijfrentekas, Brussels, Belgium, and by Grants (20093 and 3.009.80) from the Fonds voor Wetenschappelijk Geneeskundig Onderzoek, Brussels, Belgium. The author thanks G. De Smet-Matthys for typing, the Staff of the Laboratory of Experimental Cancerology for reviewing the manuscript and J. Roels van Kerckvoorde for preparing the illustrations.

References

1. Rather LJ: The genesis of cancer. A study in the history of ideas. Baltimore: The Johns Hopkins University Press, 1978.
2. Schaeffer WI: Proposed usage of animal tissue culture terms (revised 1978). TCA Manual 4:779–782, 1978.
3. Santesson L: Characteristics of epithelial mouse tumour cells *in vitro* and tumour structures *in vivo*. A comparative study. Acta Pathol Microbiol Scand (Suppl XXIV):1–227, 1935.
4. Abercrombie M: Contact inhibition and malignancy. Nature (London) 281:259–262, 1979.
5. Leighton J, Klein I: Studies on human cancer using sponge matrix tissue culture. II. Invasion of connective tissue by carcinoma (strain HeLa). Texas Rep Biol Med 12:868–873, 1954.

6. Leighton J, Klein I, Belkin M, Tetenbaum Z: Studies on human cancer using sponge-matrix culture. III. The invasive properties of a carcinoma (strain HeLa) as influenced by temperature variations, by conditioned media, and by contact with rapidly growing chick embryonic tissue. J Natl Cancer Inst 16:1353–1365, 1956.
7. Wolff ET, Haffen K: Sur une méthode de culture d'organes embryonnaires '*in vitro*'. Texas Rep Biol Med 10:463–472, 1952.
8. Wolff ET, Schneider N: La culture d'un sarcome de souris sur des organes de poulet explantés *in vitro*. Arch Anat Microsc Morphol Exp 46:173–198, 1957.
9. Wolff EM: Organ chimaeras and organ culture of malignant tumors. In: Organ culture. Thomas JA (ed). New York: Academic Press, 1970, pp 459–505.
10. Easty GC, Easty DM: An organ culture system for the examination of tumor invasion. Nature 199:1104–1105, 1963.
11. Lattner AL, Longstaff E, Lunn JM: Invasive properties of histone transformed cells. Br J Cancer 25:568–573, 1971.
12. Schleich AB, Frick M, Mayer A: Patterns of invasive growth *in vitro*. Human decidua graviditatis confronted with established human cell lines and primary human explants. J Natl Cancer Inst 56:221–237, 1976.
13. Mareel MMK, Meyvisch C: Invasion of malignant cells *in vivo* and *in vitro*: similarities and differences. Arch Geschwülstforsch 51:20–27, 1981.
14. David D: Evolution de l'épithélium gastrique isolé de son mésenchyme et cultivé *in vitro* au contact du foie. Experientia 26:1001–1003, 1970.
15. Curtis ASG, Rooney P: H-2 restriction of contact inhibition of epithelial cells. Nature (London) 281:222–223, 1979.
16. Lohmann-Matthes M-L, Schleich A, Shantz G, Schirrmacher V: Tumor metastases and cell-mediated immunity in a model system in DBA/2 mice. VII. Interaction of metastasizing and nonmetastasizing tumors with normal tissue *in vitro*. J Natl Cancer Inst 64:1413–1425, 1980.
17. De Bruyne G, Mareel M: Immunohistochemistry of invasion in threedimensional culture. Arch Geschwulstforsch 51:15–19, 1981.
18. de Ridder L, Mareel M, Vakaet L: Invasion of malignant cells into cultured embryonic substrates. Arch Geschwulstforsch 47:7–27, 1977.
19. Easty DM, Easty GC: Measurement of the ability of cells to infiltrate normal tissues *in vitro*. Br J Cancer 29:36–49, 1974.
20. Kuettner KE, Pauli BV, Soble L: Morphological studies on the resistance of cartilage to invasion by osteosarcoma cells *in vitro* and *in vivo*. Cancer Res 38:277–287, 1978.
21. Yarnell MM, Ambrose EJ: Studies of tumour invasion in organ culture. Eur J Cancer 5:265–269, 1969.
22. Mareel M: Recent aspects of tumor invasiveness. Int Rev Exp Pathol 22:65–129, 1980.
23. Solursh M: Glycosaminoglycan synthesis in the chick gastrula. Dev Biol 50:525–530, 1976.
24. Moscona A, Trowell OA, Willmer EN: Methods. In: Cells and tissues in culture. Methods, biology and physiology, Vol. 1, Willmer EN (ed). London: Academic Press, 1965, pp 19–98.
25. Locker J, Goldblatt PJ, Leighton J: Ultrastructural features of invasion in chick embryo liver metastasis of Yoshida ascites hepatoma. Cancer Res 30:1632–1644, 1970.
26. Ossowski L, Reich E: Experimental model for quantitative studies of metastasis. Cancer Res 40:2300–2309, 1980.
27. Wolff Et: Utilisation de la membrane vitelline de l'oeuf de poule en culture organotypique. I. Technique et possibilités. Dev Biol 3:767–786, 1961.
28. Mareel M, Kint J, Meyvisch C: Methods of study of the invasion of malignant C3H-mouse fibroblasts into embryonic chick heart *in vitro*. Virchows Arch [Cell Pathol] 30:95–111, 1979.
29. Mareel MM, Bruyneel E, Storme G: Attachment of mouse fibrosarcoma cells to precultured fragments of embryonic chick heart. An early step to invasion *in vitro*. Virchows Arch [Cell Pathol] 34:85–97, 1980.

30. de Ridder L, Mareel M, Vakaet L: Adhesion of malignant and nonmalignant cells to cultured embryonic substrates. Cancer Res 35:3164–3171, 1975.
31. Vakaet L, Vandekerckhove D, Mareel M: Association de cellules HeLa avec de l'épithélium tubaire humain adulte. C R Soc Biol 165:2225–2226, 1971.
32. Poste G, Doll J, Hart I, Fidler IJ: *In vitro* selection of murine B16 melanoma variants with enhanced tissue-invasive properties. Cancer Res 40:1636–1644, 1980.
33. Hart I, Fidler IJ: An *in vitro* quantitative assay for tumor cell invasion. Cancer Res 38:3218–3224, 1978.
34. Sanders EJ, Bellairs R, Portch PA: *In vivo* and *in vitro* studies on the hypoblast and definitive endoblast of avian embryos. J Embryol Exp Morph 46:187–205, 1978.
35. Mareel M, de Ridder L, De Brabander M, Vakaet L: Characterization of spontaneous, chemical, and viral transformants of a C3H/3T3-type mouse cell line by transplantation into young chick blastoderm. J Natl Cancer Inst 54:923–929, 1975.
36. Van Peteghem MC, Mareel MM, De Bruyne G: Phagocytic capacity of invasive malignant cells in three-dimensional culture. Virchows Arch [Cell Pathol] 34:193–204, 1980.
37. Mareel MMK: Mini-review: Is invasiveness *in vitro* characteristic of malignant cells? Cell Biol Int Rep 3:627–640, 1979.
38. Turner GA, Weiss L: Some effects of products from necrotic regions of tumours on the *in vitro* migration of cancer and peritoneal exsudate cells. Int J Cancer 26:247–254, 1980.
39. Armstrong PB: Cellular positional stability and intercellular invasion. Bioscience 27:803–809, 1977.
40. Kieler J, Briand P, Van Peteghem MC, Mareel M: Comparative studies of two types of 'spontaneous' malignant alteration of ST/A mouse lung fibroblasts propagated *in vitro*. *In Vitro* 15:758–771, 1979.
41. de Ridder LI, Laerum OD: Invasion of rat neurogenic cell lines into embryonic chick heart fragments *in vitro*. J Natl Cancer Inst 66:723–728, 1981.
42. Barski G, Wolff EM: Malignancy evaluation of *in vitro* transformation of mouse cell lines in chick mesonephros organ cultures. J Natl Cancer Inst 34:495–510, 1965.
43. Noguchi PD, Johnson JB, O'Donnell R, Petricciani JC: Chick embryonic skin as a rapid organ culture assay for cellular neoplasia. Science 199:980–983, 1978.
44. Bruyneel E, Mareel M: Early activities of invasive malignant cells *in vitro*. Arch Geschwulstforsch 51:34–39, 1981.
45. Mareel M, De Bruyne G, de Ridder L: Invasion of malignant cells into ^{51}Cr-labeled host tissues in organotypical culture. Oncology 34:6–9, 1977.
46. Mareel M, De Brabander M: Effect of microtubule inhibitors on malignant invasion *in vitro*. J Natl Cancer Inst 61:787–792, 1978.
47. Storme G, Mareel M: Effect of anticancer agents on directional migration of malignant C3H mouse fibroblastic cells *in vitro*. Cancer Res 40:943–948, 1980.
48. Storme G, Mareel M: Effect of anticancer agents on invasion of mouse fibrosarcoma cells *in vitro*. Oncology 38:182–186, 1981.
49. Sträuli P: A concept of tumor invasion. In: Proteinases and tumor invasion, Sträuli P, Barrett EJ, Baici A (eds). New York: Raven Press, 1980, pp 1–15.
50. Mareel M, Storme G, De Bruyne G, Van Cauwenberge R: Antiinvasive effect of microtubule inhibitors *in vitro*. In: Microtubules and microtubule inhibitors, De Brabander M, De Mey J (eds). Amsterdam: Elsevier/North-Holland Biomedical Press, 1980, pp 535–544.

14. Three-dimensional models for the study of invasion and metastasis

H. GERSHMAN

1. Introduction

1.1. Scope of this discussion

Over the last several decades, research into the possible causes and preventions of malignant invasion and metastasis has vastly increased in scope and magnitude. Concurrent with this increased interest, a number of model systems for the examination of invasion and metastasis have been presented. The purpose of this paper is to review a related group of these model systems and to evaluate their relevance to the *in vivo* condition they are intended to model. The group of model systems to be examined in detail are the three-dimensional culture models, in which cellular aggregates and fragments, maintained as spherical masses in liquid or semi-solid culture medium, serve as the substrate for invasion by single cells or masses of malignant cells. Some related models and assays for malignancy, particularly the rate of attachment of single cells to aggregates, the rate of aggregation of single cells, and the inhibition of cellular aggregation will be discussed briefly. The range of model systems to be examined in this review is therefore a fairly limited one; however, discussions of other model systems, some more complex (for example, entire organs studied *in vitro*) and others more simple (for example, monolayer cultures) will be dealt with in other papers is this volume.

1.2. Rationale for the use of model systems

The rationale for the use of a model system for the study of invasion or metastasis is to provide a simplified, more manipulable experimental material than the intact organism. From this simplification directly spring both the strengths and the weaknesses of this approach. On the one hand, the problem may be dissected into a series of discrete steps which can be examined individually or in groups. At the same time, the investigator must decide which of these subprocesses are important for further and detailed study. For example, the process of metastasis can be subdivided into a series of discrete stages. [See reference 1 for a comprehensive review on this subject.] Different culture models can be devised that yield specific information concerning cell detachment, cell attachment, random cell movements in masses, intermixing of

L.A. Liotta and I.R. Hart (eds.), Tumor Invasion and Metastasis. ISBN-13: 978-94-009-7513-2.
© 1982 Martinus Nijhoff Publishers, The Hague/Boston/London.

apposed cell masses, etc. The ability to examine each of these events in the absence of the others is the invaluable feature of model systems. In fact, a great deal of valuable basic information about cellular properties related to cell movement and cell interaction has been gained from these experiments. Interpretive difficulties arise, however, when the investigator attempts to relate these subprocesses to the original, *in vivo* process of invasion and metastasis.

The ability to deal with homogenous cell populations which can be cloned and examined in detail, and from which specific variants can be selected was also originally seen as a major advantage of *in vitro* model systems. Recent data, unfortunately, suggest that the cells that have been most commonly used in these studies are rather poor representatives of malignant cells. Even more disturbingly, recent data suggest that tumor cells growing *in vivo* consist not of a series of discrete populations undergoing selective pressures that tend to decrease their heterogeneity, but may in fact be capable of continuously generating subpopulations that express new phenotypic properties in response to population pressures.

Still, the ability to control the cellular environment must be viewed as a very positive attribute of *in vitro* culture models. Distinct advantages for such studies include the ability to vary the composition of extracellular matrix proteins; the ability to control the size and shape of the cell masses; and the elimination of the immune system, thus allowing the examination of cells of various genetic compositions in co-culture. As a final note, however, I would like to re-emphasize that the onus is upon the investigator to note where these culture systems simplify, or fail to possess, attributes of the *in vivo* condition, and to temper his interpretations and conclusions accordingly.

1.3. Culture models to be discussed

The three-dimensional culture models which are aimed at elucidating mechanisms of cell movement fall into two categories based on the method of obtaining three-dimensional masses for study. In the first technique, single cells are obtained from tissues, usually embryonic but occasionally adult, or from conventional monolayer cultures of established cell lines and are formed into cellular aggregates, also called reaggregates or multicellular spheroids. In the second technique, fragments are cut directly from normal embryonic or adult or tumor tissue. The limited data available suggest that results obtained using these two alternative techniques are similar. In either case, aggregates or fragments, the masses are maintained in agitated liquid medium or semisolid medium to prevent attachment and spreading of the cells on solid surfaces.

The movements of cells in aggregates or fragments are assayed in one of two ways. In the first procedure, two masses, typically a mass of cells of tumor origin and a second mass of cells of non-tumor origin, are brought into contact and cellular intermixing is measured histologically. Alternatively, a few individual cells are allowed to attach to a mass of cells and the extent of their penetration into the mass is determined histologically. Comparison of the cellular events that occur in these two assays would seem to suggest that they model different stages in the metastatic or invasive process, and for that reason they will be dealt with separately here. A third group of assays that utilize masses or aggregates involves the attachment of cells to each other or to masses, or the attachment of masses to monolayers. These group of assays would appear to model still another subprocess in invasion or metastasis and again will be dealt with separately. In addition, a few other assays not so easily classified will also be discussed here.

2. Assays for cell movement and invasion

2.1. Homotypic intermixing of cells in aggregates and tissue fragments

The first experiments attempting to estimate the rates of cellular intermixing in three-dimensional masses were carried out by Weston and Abercrombie [2] in 1967. In these studies, the authors fused two fragments of embryonic chick heart ventricle, one of which had been pre-labeled by exposure to [^{3}H]thymidine *in ovo*. After a period of culture, during which time the two fused fragments rounded up into a single spherical mass, the mass was subjected to histology and autoradiography and the border between radiolabeled and unlabeled cells was examined. It was found that minimal mixing across the fusion border had occurred. It should be noted, however, that all subsequent studies that have probed this problem have obtained different results and drawn different conclusions. For example, Armstrong and Armstrong [3] carried out a similar series of experiments using fragments of chick embryonic mesonephric mesenchyme. In contrast to the results of Weston and Abercrombie, Armstrong and Armstrong found substantial intermixing across the fusion border with this tissue. In addition, a later study by the same authors provided similar results and conclusions for aggregates of chick fibroblasts from several tissue sources, including heart ventricle [4].

Wiseman and Steinberg also reexamined this problem, again using chick embryonic cells, but with a different assay procedure [5]. They prepared suspensions of cells from chick embryonic tissues by trypsin-mediated dissociation, allowed the dissociated cells to reaggregate, and then incubated the unlabeled aggregates with a suspension of cells of the same tissue prelabeled with [^{3}H]thymidine. After a three hour period to allow the radiolabeled cells to attach to the aggregates, the non-attached cells were washed away and the aggregates cultured for varying periods of time. Histological examination and autoradiography subsequently located the radiolabeled cells. The theory was that the rate at which the radiolabeled cells penetrated to the interior of the mass of unlabeled cells would be indicative of the rate of cellular intermixing or movement. Since the radiolabeled cells and unlabeled aggregates were of the same type, the penetration should be due to random cell movements, analogous to diffusion, rather than a directed migration. Their data indicated that intermixing was suprisingly rapid. In the case of embryonic heart or liver, radiolabeled cells were often found more than three cell diameters from their original position at the periphery of the aggregate. The study by Wiseman and Steinberg [5] provided only marginal improvement in the quantitation of the rates of intermixing as compared to the study of Weston and Abercrombie [2]; other studies, carried out in my laboratory [6, 7], provided improved quantitation and arrived at similar conclusions: that embryonic cells in these masses were in rapid random motion. In the study by Wiseman and Steinberg [5], interestingly, radiolabeled cells diffused into fragments of embryonic tissue about as well as they intermixed with cells of aggregates. Again we confirmed these data in a subsequent study using embryonic heart cells [7]. In addition, Wiseman has reported that non-living cell-sized particles of metal, glass and plastic are also translocated to the interior of aggregates of liver and heart [8], and also provided some evidence that this rapid intermixing is not due to trypsin-treatment of the cells [9]. A more recent report has also suggested that lipid vesicles can penetrate to the interior of aggregates of V79 Chinese hamster lung cells [10]. The apparent discrepancy between the original Weston and Abercrombie study and the large number of studies that followed it thus remains unresolved. The weight of the evidence, however, clearly suggests that both in fragments and reaggregates of chick embryonic cells, the rate of cellular intermixing is rapid.

Taken together these data are particularly interesting in that they suggested from the outset that aggregates or fragments of chick embryonic tissues from the ages commonly used (5–9 days of gestation) might be poor models of normal adult tissues, since the cells appeared to be in continuous random motion. This rapid intermixing is perhaps not surprising in that morphogenesis might require such mobility of embryonic cells. The movement of the corresponding adult cells might very well be considerably less. A study from my own laboratory [7] has provided support for this notion. The movement of chick embryonic heart cells was examined over the range 5 to 19 days of gestation, and was found to decrease about three-fold over this period. These data suggest that fragments from adult tissues or from older embryos might be a much better model substrate for the study of invasion *in vitro* than the young embryonic tissues used to date. Another alternative is the use of aggregates of cells of established lines which are non-tumorigenic or minimally tumorigenic *in vivo* and which have a low degree of cellular movement in aggregates.

We have carried out such studies using non-embryonic cells [6, 11] and we have found that the rapid movement characteristic of young embryonic cells is not a universal property of cells in aggregates. Cells of some established lines, BALB/c 3T3 cells, for example, do not intermix rapidly in aggregates [6]. On the other hand, SVT-2, NIL B, SV-NIL, and NH32, NH37, NH38, and NH40 cells intermix at a rapid rate [6, 11]. We have also recently carried out a survey of a number of other established cell lines and found that several lines in addition to BALB/c 3T3 display modest to low rates of intermixing in this system. Among the lines that displayed limited intermixing were WI-38 (1.42 cell diameters/day), and MRC-5 (0.73 cell diameters/day; (unpublished). As compared to 5–6 cell diameters/day for 5-day embryonic chick heart cells this represents a substantial decrease. The possibility for using aggregates of cells of established lines or perhaps fragments of adult tissues in this assay therefore seems reasonable. On the other hand, studies using young chick embryonic cells as the substrate for investigating invasion *in vitro* must be considered questionable, due to the intrinsic rapid movement of these cells.

Despite the problems noted above, this technique for assaying cell movement appears to have some potential for comparisons of metastatic or invasive cells with their non-invasive counterparts. Using BALB/c 3T3 cells as our control, we have carried out several studies comparing the intermixing of cells in aggregates as a function of viral transformation. In these studies, the 3T3 cells intermixed at a very low rate (less than 0.33 cell diameters/day) while the SVT-2 cells (SV40 virus transformant of 3T3) intermixed much more rapidly (as much as 8 cell diameters/day). On the other hand, a comparison of NIL B cells (moderately tumorigenic in syngenic hamsters [11]) and SV40 transformed NIL B cells (highly tumorigenic) showed no dramatic increase [6], or only a modest increase [11]. A comparison of the NIL 8 and SV-NIL lines with strains selected for tumor growth from the primary site in hamsters injected with NIL 8 cells also showed only a modest increase in intermixing [11]. We have also found that the enhanced mobility of the SVT-2 cells is completely suppressed by agents that increase intracellular cyclic AMP levels and that this effect is associated with a characteristic morphological alteration of the transformant to a more '3T3-like' appearance [12, 13].

The results of these experiments hint at an increase in intermixing as the result of oncogenic transformation or tumorigenecity. It should be noted, however, that the critical property of cells that needs to be examined in this type of assay is not transformation, or even tumorigenecity, but rather invasive or metastatic ability. There is little reason to suppose that tumor formation *per se* need be associated with rapid cellular movements. There is good reason, on the other hand to ask if invasive or metastatic ability is associated with this property. It seems doubtful, however, that this can be adequately tested using the sorts of established cell lines used in the studies cited above. These lines have been highly selected for their ability to grow in monolayer culture. They probably represent poor models of either 'normal' cells, tumorigenic cells or metastatic cells. While this technique may be useful, any definitive conclusions concerning its validity must await the critical test of the correlation of intermixing to *in vivo* invasiveness or metastasis. The point of correspondance of these studies of homotypic intermixing to metastasis and invasion *in vivo* is difficult to determine. The assay would appear to best examine cellular events that occur in the interior of the primary tumor. It might be postulated that the degree of intermixing is related to the probability of tumor cells leaving the mass and either penetrating into surrounding tissues (invasion) or to entering the circulation (intravasation). While this postulate is not without its logic, it would seem, as noted above, that the simplest and most satisfying way to validate this assay would be to directly test the correlation between intermixing and invasion or metastasis. To date, this has not been attempted.

2.2. *Heterotypic interactions of cells in aggregates and fragments*

The experiments described in the previous section were based on the measurement of random intermixing of cells in homogeneous aggregates or tissue fragments. A second class of assays has examined a more complex series of interactions in which a tissue mass of one cell or tissue type is confronted with either single cells, or another mass of cells but of a different type. Most typically, for purposes of examining invasion or metastasis, one cell type is of normal (primary) embryonic origin, while the cell type confronting it is considered to be neoplastic. As compared to homotypic intermixing, these heterotypic models provide the potential for the interplay of other factors, such as differential adhesion, haptotaxis, chemotaxis, etc. They are thus simultaneously more like conditions that obtain *in vivo*, and also more difficult to interpret. Heterotypic interactions may be postulated to model different subprocesses in the metastatic sequence depending on whether: (1) a mass is exposed to single cells of a different type, or (2) two different masses are apposed. Specifically, the penetration of single cells into a mass has been suggested as a model of the penetration of metastatic cells into normal tissues prior to intravasation and following extravasation. On the other hand, the interactions that occur at the fusion border of two apposed adherent masses has been suggested as a model of invasion or a primary of secondary tumor into surrounding normal solid tissues.

The behavior of populations of cells of different origins has been most extensively studied in aggregates and fragments of chick embryonic cells. Two basic techniques have been employed to this end. In the first, apposed masses of different tissue origins were examined. In the second, aggregates were constructed in which the cells of the two tissue types are randomly intermixed as a starting point. The segregation of the cells of the randomly intermixed mass into tissue-specific concentric spheres has been described extensively by Moscona [14, 15], Steinberg [16, 17], Trinkaus and Lentz [18], and Curtis [19] and referred to as histotypic segregation, sorting-out, or tissue reconstruction. This random intermixed starting point does not have any obvious counterpart *in vivo*, however the behavior of the same cells caused to confront each other as apposed masses produces identical results: concentric spheres of cells of different types. Workers in the field have therefore concluded that both processes are reflections of the same basic cellular properties. Steinberg has proposed that these rearrangements are energetically driven by differences in energies of the various adhesive bonds between cells [16, 17].

The importance of the adhesion-driven cellular movements observed in three-dimensional cultures of embryonic cells in the process of tumor invasion has not been extensively studied. Only a single study from my own laboratory [20] has examined the sorting-out behavior of normal and transformed cells in aggregates in a systematic manner. One of the results of this study was the observation that SV40 virus-transformed 3T3 cells segregated externally to BALB/c 3T3 cells in aggregates. Interpreted in terms of the differential adhesiveness hypothesis of Steinberg [17], these data suggest that the transformed cells are less adhesive than their non-transformed counterparts. This is consistent with the notion, first set forth by Coman [21], that malignant cells are less adhesive than their non-malignant counterparts. In addition, Carter [22] has proposed that decreased adhesiveness results in increased motility. The potential significance of a decrease in adhesiveness and concomitant increase in mobility with neoplastic transformation is that such alterations might increase the rate at which cells leave the primary tumor and either invade surrounding tissues or enter the circulation. On the other hand, such an external segregation, if extrapolated to *in vivo* invasiveness would appear to act to prevent penetration and intermixing of malignant cells with surrounding tissues. However, as with the studies previously described, no studies of sorting-out have been carried out using defined invasive or metastatic variants and their parent lines. A possible correlation between decreased adhesiveness and either invasiveness or metastatic potential, therefore, has not been shown.

A number of recent studies have combined fragments of chick tissues and fragments of tumor (either obtained directly, or by reaggregation of monolayer-grown cells) in artificial medium. The pioneering study in this regard was that of Wolff and Schneider [23] who studied the penetration of mouse sarcoma 180 cells into various chick tissues. Later studies, such as those of Easty and Easty [24] have followed this basic plan, in which two fragments were combined and supported on an agar base or a floating raft, with access to the culture medium, such as an agar base, or a floating raft. This last study is noteworthy because the authors attempted to use adult tissue fragments or fragments of neonatal mammalian organs as the substrate for *in vitro* invasion. In neither of these two studies, which are otherwise commendable, were attempts made to quantitate invasion or to test pairs of tumors which differed in their invasive potential. Yarnell and Ambrose [25, 26] have reported the results of studies of co-culture of fragments of fetal mouse heart with suspensions of polyoma virus-transformed BHK cells and BHK cells. Although a comparison was made here between cells of a virally transformed line and cells of the parent (BHK) line, both of these, like the NIL B/SV-NIL combination tested in my own laboratory [11] are tumorigenic. BHK cells have also been tested by Latner, Longstaff and Pradham for their ability to cause release of host tissue proteins from mouse kidney explants [27]. Again the major interpretive difficulty arises from the use of embryonic masses as a model of adult tissues, a model so far unvalidated.

Mareel and co-workers have also recently examined several similar culture systems in which heterotypic interactions have been suggested to model invasion *in vivo*. Mareel, de Bruyne and de Ridder [28] allowed fragments of HeLa cell monolayers to adhere to fragments of embryonic chick heart and mesonephros which had been prelabeled with $[^{51}Cr]Na_2CrO_4$. Although the HeLa cell fragments appeared to invade both the heart and mesonephros, no significant release of radiolabel was seen as compared to fragments of heart and mesonephros not in contact with HeLa cells. No quantitation of the degree of intermixing of the HeLa and embryonic cells was attempted in this study. The authors concluded that they were unable to account for the failure of chromium release to reflect the 'cytocidal process brought about by malignant invasion.' The simplest explanation for this failure is that the intermixing of embryonic and HeLa cells was not, in fact, cytocidal, and perhaps not representative of invasion as it occurs *in vivo*. This explanation is supported by studies described in the previous section which indicate that chick embryonic fragments consist of cells that are already in relatively rapid random motion [3, 4, 5, 6, 7, 9], and therefore no cell destruction need be postulated in order to explain penetration by the tumor cells. Although the age of the chick tissue is a potential factor in this analysis, in this study 9-day-old embryos were the donors and previous studies have shown that this is sufficiently young to provide rapid intermixing [7]. In a later study, Mareel, Kint and Meyvisch [29] confronted fragments of embryonic chick heart (9-day) with suspensions of virally transformed mouse cells. The transformed cells adhered to and penetrated into the chick fragments to form a central core reminiscent of the results of sorting-out of two embryonic tissues. However, the rapid growth of the transformed cells quickly created a central necrotic zone, as described by Folkman, Hochberg and Knighton [30], which is probably due to the failure of oxygen to penetrate more than 150–200 microns into solid tissues [31]. The authors also carried out studies in which fragments of monolayers or reaggregates of virally transformed mouse cells were allowed to adhere to fragments of chick heart. The results of these studies were basically similar to those of the first series, except that since the total number of transformed cells was more carefully controlled, necrosis was less of a confounding variable. Again, penetration of the tumor cells into the embryonic mass was seen and described in some detail. As an interesting minor point, the authors concluded that static cultures (on semisolid agar) were less suitable due to increased central necrosis as the result of anoxia than were fragments and aggregates suspended in agitated liquid medium. In another study using a somewhat different system, Mareel and de Brabander showed that treatment with an inhibitor of microtubule polymerization suppressed the expected penetration of the transformed mouse cells into fragments of 9-day embryonic chick heart and mesonephros [32]. In this study, however, the two fragments were cultured on chick vitelline membrane lying on semisolid medium. More recently, Mareel, Storme, de Bruyne and van Cauwenberge [33] have examined a larger number of microtubule inhibitors, including colchicine, and the vinca alkaloids. Eight of these agents were tested and found to inhibit the penetration of virally transformed mouse cells into fragments of embryonic chick heart (9-day) when cocultured on semisolid medium or in agitated liquid medium [33, 34]. These studies confirm previous observations on the inhibition of cell movements in homotypic chick cell aggregates by antimicrotubule agents [35], as well as other studies examining the effects of cytoskeletal disruptors such as cytochlasin B on histotypic segregation (sorting-out) of chick tissue cells in heterotypic aggregates [36, 37, 38]. The interpretation of these experiments appears to be the obvious one: that an intact cytoskeleton is as necessary for active cell movements in three-dimensional cultures as it is for movements on solid artificial surface [39].

Mareel has also reviewed a number of culture model system studies [40] and has concluded that some *in vitro* systems have some validity as judged by the fact that cells of known malignancy display active penetration of the host tissue. However, none of these studies have fully validated the utility of any of these various models by a comparison of known invasive or metastatic variants with their parent lines. In addition, all of the studies described in detail above have utilized chick embryonic tissues as the substrate, and as discussed above, the apparent rapid random movements of these young embryonic cells suggest the possibility that much of the 'invasion' observed may be due to the host tissues. There is no compelling reason to assume that the penetration observed in these masses is a valid model of *in vivo* malignant invasion.

Another group of assays has employed membranes or fragments of membranes as the substrate for invasion. These membranes are highly evolved multilayered structures and their use introduces another level of complexity into these assays. Because many of these studies will be covered elsewhere in this volume they will not be considered in detail here. Most of them have employed chicken egg membranes [e.g. 41–44], especially the chorioallantoic membrane, or chicken skin [e.g. 45] as the substrate. One of these studies, reported by Hart and Fidler [46], is of particular importance to the evaluation of culture models because it introduced, for the first time, a method of quantitating CAM invasion. When the CAM invasion assay was later re-examined by Poste, Doll, Hart, and Fidler, using B16 melanoma variants, it was found that penetration of the CAM did not correlate with metastatic potential [47], although penetration of mouse bladder did show such a correlation. This result clearly underlines the major problem with the three-dimensional *in vitro* assays discussed above; none have been validated by *in vivo* studies.

A yet more complex group of assays involves the implantation of tumor tissues into normal developing embryonic tissues, especially the limb of the chick [48, 49, 50], but also into the auricles and outer ear of the mouse [e.g. 51]. The fate of these cells is then followed histologically. Again, a detailed analysis of the results of these studies is beyond the scope of this review. However, it should be noted that despite the fact that the implants are being made into whole living animals, they are not made at normal sites. In addition, the use of young chick embryonic tissues as receptors for the implants introduces the possiblity that rapid random or morphogenetic movements might bias the results.

2.3. Aggregation of tumor cells

A large number of studies have been carried out in which the rate, extent, or pattern of reaggregation of tumor cells have been tested. The point of relevance of these studies to specific subprocesses in invasion or metastasis appears to be that larger emboli of potentially metastatic cells which are already blood-borne have an increased probability of arrest as compared to smaller emboli or single cells. Although most of these emboli appear to consist of a few tumor cells plus fibrin or platelets, the possibility that homotypic aggregation might occur cannot be discounted. Fidler, Gersten and Hart [1] have clearly reviewed these data and arguments. Most of the more recent aggregation rate studies have utilized electronic particle counting as a method of quantitation. Many of these studies have been summarized in a report by Whur et al. [52]. Alternatively, the final size of aggregates produced has been taken as a measure of the strength of adhesion. Generally, these studies have assumed that the rate or extent of aggregation is a reflection of the strength of adhesion of tumor cells to each other or to other cells. Theoretical arguments in favor and against this view have been presented by Curtis [53] and Steinberg [17], respectively. Despite the difficulty in interpreting these studies relative to tumor invasiveness or metastasis, some interesting observations have been reported particularly at the ultrastructural and biochemical level. In addition, some attempts to correlate aggregation with *in vivo* properties of tumor cells have been carried out and are described below.

The initial reports of the aggregation of tumor cells by Moskowitz noted that the serum content of the medium in which the cells had been grown as monolayers had observable effects on the size of aggregates formed [54]. More recent reports by Maslow, Mayhew, and Feldman [55] have suggested that the presence of cells of high metastatic sublines of B16 melanoma may inhibit the aggregation of chick embryonic cells to a greater degree than the presence of a similar number of cells of the low metastatic variant, as judged by final aggregate diameters. Similarly, they report that SV40 virus-transformed BALB 3T3 cells are more effective in this process than a similar number of 3T3 cells [56]. Whether this process is mediated by direct cell-cell contact or via diffusible factors is not known, although a number of workers have reported the purification or identification of factors that inhibit or stimulate aggregation [e.g. 57, 58, and summarized by Curtis in reference 53 and more recently by Culp and by Jones in references 59 and 60]. As early as 1965, Curtis reported the purification to homogeneity of a serum factor that that inhibited aggregation [61]. To date, however, no *in vivo* significance has been shown for any of these inhibitory or stimulatory factors. This may be due in large part to the fact that aggregation is essentially a laboratory phenomenon; embyronic morphogenesis and tissue maintenance do not normally proceed by disaggregation and reaggregation in mammalian or avian organisms. That is, although aggregation rate may reflect basic and vital cellular properties, no specific *in vivo* event has been shown to depend on the same combination of behaviors and properties.

Some studies have been carried out which suggest that transformation, invasiveness or tumorigenicity may be reflected in alterations in the rate of aggregation. Edwards, Dysart, Edgar and Robson [62] report that transformation of BHK21 cells by polyoma or Rous sarcoma viruses results in reduction of rate of aggregation as compared to the virally transformed parent line. It is worth repeating here that BHK21 cells are already tumorigenic. In an experiment of similar design, Wright, Ukena, Campbell and Karnovsky [63] report that a selection of clones of Swiss 3T3 cells and primary mouse fibroblasts display low rates of aggregation. In contrast SVT2 (SV40 virus transformed BALB 3T3), SVPy 3T3 (Swiss 3T3 doubly transformed with SV40 and polyoma viruses), Kirsten leukemia virus transformed 3T3, B16 melanoma and several lines of murine fibroblasts transformed by oncogenic viruses, all displayed increased rates of aggregation. These data support the notion that transformed cells are less adhesive than non-transformed cells, assuming that aggregation rate is a reflection of strength of adhesion. On the other hand, this study also found that A31 BALB 3T3 cells aggregated at a high rate, while a spontaneously transformed line of hamster fibroblasts aggregated less rapidly than any other cell line tested. In general (excepting the A31 3T3 cells), a low rate of aggregation correlated with ability to grow in semisolid medium and with tumorigenecity. These correlations, although not absolute, are still impressive. In an interesting study, Lackie and Armstrong co-aggregated embryonic chick heart fibroblasts with rabbit neutrophil granulocytes and found that the two populations tended to aggregate homotypically and independently of each other; that is, little heart-granulocyte aggregation was observed [64]. In a previous study [65], the neutrophil granulocytes had been shown to readily penetrate aggregates of chick embryonic fibroblasts and the authors therefore identified them as 'invasive' although they are also clearly non-malignant. Although penetration of chick heart aggregates does not appear to be a rigorous test of invasiveness, the properties of the neutrophils in other systems (specifically their failure to display contact paralysis in monolayer culture) support this notion. These data may explain, at least in part, the observations of Maslow and Mayhew [55, 56]: if heterotypic adhesions are disfavored during aggregation of suspended cells, addition of melanoma cells or transformed mouse cells to aggregating chick embryonic cells might inhibit aggregation by lowering the effective rate of aggregation-competent collisions.

In summary, the studies using aggregation rate or extent as a probe have yielded little information applicable to the study of invasion or metastasis. The primary reason for this failure is by now familiar to the reader: no systematic attempts to correlate aggregation properties with *in vivo* invasion or metastasis have been made. In addition, the cells which were examined were often compared to similar ones (tumorigenic parent lines compared to the same lines transformed by oncogenic viruses). As a further complication, aggregation assays are artificial and sensitive to a variety of experimental manipulations such as concentration of cells, viscosity and macromolecular composition of the medium, method by which the single cell suspensions were obtained, temperature, speed and method of agitation, and the method of determining the rate of aggregation. In all fairness, however, few if any of these studies drew specific conclusions regarding invasion or metastasis. Instead, most of these studies were directed at elucidating basic mechanisms of intercellular adhesion.

2.4. *Other studies using three-dimensional cultures*

Besides the three classes of assays already described, a number of others have been used and applied as models of invasive or metastatic subprocesses. In addition, cellular aggregates of tumor cells have been used in a variety of other studies not closely related to the study of invasion and metastasis, but still important to other areas of oncology.

2.4.1 Other assays for metastasis and invasion in vitro. De Ridder et al. have reported studies [66] in which the initial attachment of fragments of monolayers of HeLa, hepatoma, and PY cells as examples of malignant cells and BHK, used here as an example of a non-malignant line, were allowed to attach to fragments of chick blastoderm. In this study, the fraction of monolayer fragments that attached to the chick tissues was used as the assay for adhesion. A difference in adhesion to the upper and lower surfaces of the blastoderm was noted, with the dorsal surface being less adhesive. In addition, the apical surface of chick embryonic tissue fragments from skin and stomach were much less adhesive than the basal surfaces. Fragments cut from non-epithelial organs such as lung, heart, liver, etc, all supported adhesion of tissue fragments. Wounding was reported to allow adhesion to surfaces not previously adhesive. Although these data do provide some interesting insights into adhesions of tumor cells to embryonic cells, they do not appear to shed any light on the mechanisms of invasion or metastasis. A more recent study from the same laboratory has examined the attachment of aggregates of mouse fibrosarcoma cells to fragments of embryonic 9-day chick heart ventricle [67]. Attachment failed to occur at reduced temperature, in the presence of KCN, and was reduced after treatment with Cytochalasin B. Radiation and 5-fluuorouracil did not affect attachment. Although this study again provides some information on cell attachment, despite the author's claims that it models an early step in invasion, there is little that can be done to extrapolate these results to the *in vivo* situation, primarily because of the choice of tumor cells tested and of an embryonic tissue fragment as substrate.

Cassiman and Bernfield have carried out a series of experiments using somewhat similar techniques in order to test differences between non-transformed and transformed cells [68]. In this experiment, aggregates of BALB/c 3T3 cells and an SV40 virus-transformed derivative (3T3SV) were allowed to attach to tissue culture plastic or to monolayers of either of the two cell types. It was shown that binding of the aggregates to the monolayers was first order and essentially irreversible under the conditions comployed. Aggregates of both 3T3 and 3T3SV bound to plastic at similar rates, and both bound to 3T3 monolayers at similar rates. However, when 3T3SV monolayers were tested, they bound 3T3 aggregates about two-fold more rapidly than they bound 3T3SV aggregates. Although this carefully done study does avoid one of the most troublesome of the problems of dealing with embryonic or tissue culture cells – treatment with proteases or chelators to obtain single cells or reaggregates, it generates several other ambiguities. For example, it is well known that cells adherent to polystyrene expose a relatively non-adhesive surface to the medium [69], and in addition, the peripheral cells of aggregates of BALB/c 3T3 cells and SV40 virus-transformed 3T3 cells are also morphologically distinguishable from cells in the interior of the mass [12, 13]. In addition, although some differences between non-virally transformed and transformed cells are evident, this does not necessarily imply that similar differences exist between invasive and non-invasive cells, or that any such differences have a functional significance in invasion or metastasis.

One additional study, by Umbreit and Erbe [70], introduced a novel system for studying cell interactions in cellular aggregates, and which the authors suggest is relevant to the study of metastasis. In this system aggregates of two different cell types are incubated in the same medium but separated by a nylon screen with a mesh size small enough to pass single cells, but not aggregates. Radiolabeled aggregates of hamster melanoma cells were placed on one side of the screen and unlabled aggregates of BHK cells placed on the other. The appearance of radiolabeled cells adherent to the unlabeled BHK aggregates was then measured with time. The rate of transfer in this system was impressively high: up to 16% of the starting melanoma cells were associated with the BHK aggregtes after 4 h. In a control experiment, BHK aggregates transfered about one half as many cells in the same time period. These data are extremely interesting in that the system intuitively seems to model some of the more important aspects of metastasis in a manner that admits of experimental manipulation. Specifically, the series of subprocesses involved in detachment from a primary tumor and readherence elsewhere would seem to be tested without interference from the intra- and extravasation steps. The authors are modest in their conclusions and caution against extrapolation to *in vivo* conditions; they also suggest that this model requires testing with different cell lines. In this regard, they have pointed out the primary weakness in this otherwise very interesting study: the choice of cell lines. While the hamster melanoma may very well be a highly metastatic line, BHK, despite claims from a number of workers, is clearly a tumorigenic line, and probably malignant as well. They have not noted that the normal substrate for attachment of blood-borne metastatic cells is probably endothelial cells, or perhaps the subendothelial layer. It would seem that a combination of the assays of Umbreit and Erbe [70], which may model detachment fairly well, and a modification of that of Cassiman and Bernfield [68], using collecting monolayers of endothelial cells which might model the interior of blood vessels, may be worth testing.

2.4.2 Other studies involving tumor cell aggregates. Several other groups of studies have employed cellular aggregates of tumor cells to examine various aspects of malignancy not directly related to invasiveness. One such group are studies of the proliferative potential of tumor cells in three-dimensional masses [e.g. 30, 71–77]. These studies have established the ability of many transformed or tumorigenic cells to proliferate in aggregates under conditions in which non-transformed cells do not

[72, 78]. In addition, a number of other features of cells in aggregates which appear to have applicability to tumor growth have been examined in detail, particularly the development of necrotic zones [e.g., 74], as originally described by Folkman [30].

A second use of tumor cell aggregates has been in the study of their interaction with the mobile cells of the immune system. In these studies, tumor cell aggregates are formed, and then implanted into the peritoneal cavity of host animals, usually mice. After several days the masses are recovered and assayed for the presence of macrophages and lymphocytes, for evidence of cytotoxicity (by release of radioactive chromium), and for response to various therapies (such as radiation therapy) [79–92].

3. Conclusions

A large number of studies have been carried out in recent years using three-dimensional tissue cultures of tumor cells as models of invasion and metastasis. These have been somewhat arbitrarily grouped in the discussion above according to the type and complexity of interactions between the cells involved. A number of these studies have provided valuable information about the interactions of tumor cells with each other and with some other cell types, usually of embryonic orign. In general, unfortunately, little information about the processes of invasion and metastasis *in vivo* has thus far been obtained. I perceive a number of reasons for this failure:

First, the choice of tumor cells to be tested has often been made for reasons of convenience rather than systematically. In many cases the cells chosen have not been proven to be metastatic or invasive. In nearly every case cited above, no fully equivalent control cells have been used and often none were available. One exception to this are studies in which cells have been examined before and after viral transformation. In these studies, therefore, it has been possible to draw some conclusions regarding the effects of transformation. Unfortunately, transformation is not necessarily related to metastasis or invasion. Very often the non-transformed cells are tumorigenic in syngenic animals and the viral transformation serves to increase the tumorigenecity. For data that clearly bears on the mechanisms of invasion or metastasis, it will be necessary to compare cells that have a known metastatic or invasive potential with a parallel or parent line with an increased or decreased potential. This approach requires not only testing in an *in vitro* system, but also parallel *in vivo* studies. In the last few years, however, parallel lines with differing metastatic potential have been developed and are available. Therefore, this particular problem appears to be soluble.

This argument is not without its logical flaws, however. For example, if metastasis is really to be considered as a series of subprocesses as Fidler and Cifone strongly argue [83], a non-metastatic variant may be deficient in any one of several properties. The simultaneous advantage and disadvantage of culture models is that they simplify the *in vivo* condition. The particular deficiency thus may not be tested by the model culture assay in question. Because of this, a positive result in the culture model for both the metastatic and non-metastatic variant does not invalidate the model. A negative test result for a cell known to be metastatic should, however, cast serious doubts on the utility of the model. The solution to this dilemma may be to approach the testing in the opposite fashion: to test a number of lines of known metastatic potential in the culture model; upon finding one or more that fail the *in vitro* test, they should also fail to invade or metastasize *in vivo*. Validation of the model system would then come if a sufficient series of such tests were accumulated. In summary, for any culture model to provide information relevant to *in vivo* conditions, it must be validated by correlating its measurements with the actual *in vivo* event.

Second, the choice of the substrate for invasion or metastasis *in vitro* has also been generally made without sufficient analysis of its properties. The use of embryonic chick tissue fragments is a good example. These fragments have been shown in a number of studies to consist of cells in rapid random motion. Their inability to resist 'invasion' by a mass of tumor cells or a few isolated tumor cells therefore says little about the properties of the tumor cells. If metal spheres, lipid vesicles, and other embryonic cells penetrate these masses, what can be concluded from noting that tumor cells also invade? Future studies must employ masses whose intrinsic mobility has been tested and found to be satisfactorily low.

A third point of controversy with many model system studies is one of semantics. The use of the terms 'invasion' and 'malignant invasion' to describe cell behaviors in tissue cultures has substantially confused the literature. I suggest that these terms be reserved exclusively for the *in vivo* events. The behaviors of cells in monolayers or three-dimensional cultures should be described in operational terms as devoid as possible of any *in vivo* or mechanistic connotations. For example, intermixing to describe movements of cells in aggregates or tissue fragments is a neutral term. Directed migration is probably acceptable, providing the directional nature of the movement has, in fact, been established. This last term has been commonly misused to describe radial outgrowth from explants, which is not directed in the sense that chemotaxis or haptotaxis direct movement. Penetration can be used to describe a process by which one cell type displaces cells in the interior of a mass of the second type, and is far preferable to describing it as invasion.

In addition, terms used to describe the properties of tumor cells are often used incorrectly. The terms 'invasive', 'metastatic', and even 'tumorigenic' should not be used unless these specific properties have been demonstrated for the cells in question. The term 'malignant' implies all of these properties: malignant cells can form tumors, invade and also metastasize. The term 'transformed' should be qualified when used, as in virally transformed, chemically transformed, or spontaneously transformed. In addition, the criteria for applying the term should be noted at some point. Even more importantly, the terms 'normal', 'non-tumorigenic', and 'non-transformed' are not synoymous. The bulk of the established tissue culture lines which have been adequately tested are tumorigenic to some degree and are probably spontaneously transformed. Many of these are routinely referred to in the literature as 'normal' and are commonly used as the baseline for studies of 'transformed' counterparts. This is probably an example of the unfortunate situation in which confused terminology actually creates bad experiments; investigators unfamiliar with the field assume that a cell line referred to as 'normal' is actually non-tumorigenic and use it as such in their own experiments. Similar and more detailed recommendations on correct terminology have already been made by Poste and Fidler [84].

Lest this review end on a pessimistic note, I should like to note with some satisfaction, that the studies cited above have yielded a considerable body of useful information on the behavior of cells in three-dimensional masses. The criticisms I have leveled at them are not uniquely applicable to three-dimensional culture models; most can be easily translated for use with monolayers or organ cultures. A number of these studies of three-dimensional models show exceptional promise; the large body of work by Mareel and his collaborators, the assays of Umbreit and Erbe and of Cassiman and Bernfield, and the careful observations of Armstrong and his co-workers, as well as other studies, all show promise of attacking the basic mechanisms of invasion and metastasis. The availability of simplified, experimentally manipulable model culture systems will continue to be an important tool in the study of malignant invasion and metastasis, particularly if they are properly used and the data obtained carefully interpreted.

Acknowledgments

This manuscript was prepared with funding provided by grants CA20323 from the National Cancer Institute, and PCM 80-17858 from the National Science Foundation.

References

1. Fidler IJ, Gersten DM, Hart IR: The biology of cancer invasion and metastasis. Adv Cancer Res 28:149–250, 1978.
2. Weston JA, Abercrombie M: Cell mobility in fused homo- and heterotypic tissue fragments. J Exp Zool 164:317–324, 1967.
3. Armstrong PB, Armstrong MT: Are cells in solid tissues immobile? Mesonephric mesenchyme studied *in vitro*. Dev Biol 35:187–209, 1973.
4. Armstrong MT, Armstrong PB: Cell motility in fibroblast aggregates. J Cell Sci 33:37–52, 1978.
5. Wiseman LL, Steinberg MS: The movement of single cells within solid tissue masses. Exp Cell Res 79:468–471, 1973.
6. Gershman H, Drum J: Mobility of normal and virus-transformed cells in cellular aggregates. J Cell Biol 67:419–435, 1975.
7. Gershman H, Weis G, Barstow N: Dibutyryl cyclic AMP supresses mobility in embryonic chick heart cells in aggregates. J Cell Sci 37:243–256, 1979.

8. Wiseman LL: Contact inhibition and the movement of metal, glass, and plastic beads within solid tissues. Experentia 33:734–735, 1977.
9. Wiseman LL, Gorbsky GJ, Melester TS: Is the movement of single cells within solid tissue masses induced by trypsinization? Exp Cell Res 103:426–431, 1976.
10. Sridhar R, Barratt DG, Grant CWM: Infiltration of multicellular spheroids by lipid vesicles. Fed Proc 38:370, 1979.
11. Gershman H, Katzin W, Cook RT: Mobility of cells from solid tumors. Int J Cancer 21:309–316, 1978.
12. Gershman H, Drumm J, Rosen JJ: Dibutyryl cyclic AMP treatment of 3T3 and SV-40 virus transformed 3T3 cells in aggregates. Effects on mobility and cell contact ultrastructure. J Cell Biol 72:424–440, 1977.
13. Gershman H, Rosen JJ: Cell adhesion and cell surface topography in aggregates of 3T3 and SV-40 virus transformed 3T3 cells. Visualization of interior cells by scanning electron microscopy. J Cell Biol 76:639–651, 1978.
14. Moscona A: Cell suspensions from organ rudiments of chick embryos. Exp Cell Res 3:535–539, 1952.
15. Moscona A, Moscona H: The dissociation and aggregation of cells from organ rudiments of the early chick embryo. J Anat 86:287–301, 1952.
16. Steinberg MS: Reconstruction of tissues by dissociated cells. Science 141:401–408, 1963.
17. Steinberg MS: Does differential adhesion govern self-assembly processes in histogenesis? Equilibrium configurations and the emergence of a heirarchy among populations of embryonic cells. J Exp Zool 173:395–434, 1970.
18. Trinkaus JP, Lentz JP: Direct observation of type-specific segregation in mixed cell aggregates. Dev Biol 9:115–136, 1964.
19. Curtis ASG: The specific control of cell positioning. Arch Biol (Bruxelles) 85:105–121, 1974.
20. Gershman H, Drumm J, Culp L: Sorting out of normal and virus-transformed cells in cellular aggregates. J Cell Biol 68:276–286, 1976.
21. Coman DR: Decreased mutual-adhesiveness, a property of cells from squamous cell carcinomas. Cancer Res 4:625–629, 1944.
22. Carter SB: Principles of cell motility: the direction of cell movement and cancer invasion. Nature 208:1183–1187, 1965.
23. Wolff E, Schneider N: La culture d'un sarcome de souris sur des organs de poulet explantés *in vitro*. Arch Anat Micros 46:173–197, 1957.
24. Easty GC, Easty DM: An organ culture system for the examination of tumor invasion. Nature 199:1104–1105, 1963.
25. Yarnell MM, Ambrose EJ: Studies of tumour invasion in organ culture I. Effects of basic polymers and dyes on invasion and dissemination. Eur J Cancer 5:255–263, 1969.
26. Yarnell MM, Ambrose EJ: Studies of tumour invasion in organ culture II. Effects of enzyme treatment. Eur J Cancer 5:265–269, 1969.
27. Latner AL, Longstaff E, Pradham K: Inhibition of malignant cell invasion *in vitro* by a proteinase inhibitor. Br J Cancer 27:460–464, 1973.
28. Mareel M, de Bruyne G, de Ridder L: Invasion of malignant cells into ^{51}Cr-labeled host tissues in organotypical culture. Oncology 34:6–9, 1977.
29. Mareel M, Kint J, Meyvisch C: Methods of study of the invasion of malignant C3H mouse fibroblasts into embryonic chick heart *in vitro*. Virchow Arch B Cell Pathol 30:95–111, 1979.
30. Folkman J, Hochberg M, Knighton D: Self-regulation of growth in three dimensions: the role of surface area limitation. Cold Spring Harbor Conf Cell Prolif 1:833–842, 1974.
31. Tomlinson RH, Gray LH: The histological structure of some human lung cancers and the possible implications for radiotherapy. Br J Cancer 9:539–549, 1955.
32. Mareel M, de Brabander M: Methyl(5-(2-thienylcarbonyl)-1H-benzimidazome2-yl) carbamate, (R17934), a synthetic microtubule inhibitor, prevents malignant invasion *in vivo*. Oncology 35:5–7, 1978.

33. Mareel M, Storme G, de Bruyne G, van Cauwenberge R: Anti-invasive effect of microtubule inhibitors *in vitro*. In: Microtubules and microtubule inhibitors, de Brabander M, de Mey J (eds). Amsterdam: Elsevier/North Holland Biomedical Press, 1980, pp 535–543.
34. Mareel M, de Brabander MJ: Effect of microtubule inhibitors on malignant invasion *in vitro*. J Nat Cancer Inst 61:787–792, 1978.
35. Armstrong MT, Armstrong PB: The effects of antimicrotubule agents on cell motility in fibroblast aggregates. Exp Cell Res 120:359–364, 1979.
36. Armstrong PB, Parenti D: Cell sorting in the presence of cytochalasin B. J Cell Biol 55:542–553, 1972.
37. Steinberg MS, Wiseman LL: Do morphogenetic tissue rearrangements require active cell movements? The reversible inhibition of cell sorting and tissue spreading by cytochalasin B. J Cell Biol 55:606–615, 1972.
38. Maslow De, Mayhew E: Cytochalasin B prevents specific sorting of reaggregating embryonic cells. Science 177:281–282, 1972.
39. Carter SB: Effects of cytochalasins on mammalian cells. Nature 213:261–264, 1967.
40. Mareel M: Is invasiveness *in vitro* characteristic of malignant cells? Cell Biol Int Reports 3:627–640, 1979.
41. Mareel M, de Ridder L, de Brabander M, Vakaet L: Characterization of spontaneous, chemical, and viral transformants of a C3H/3T3-type mouse line by transplantation into young chick blastoderms. J Nat Cancer Inst 54:923–927, 1975.
42. Van Peteghew MC, Mareel MM, de Bruyne GK: Phagocytic capacity of invasive malignant cells in 3-dimensional culture. Virchows Arch B Cell Pathol 34:193–204, 1980.
43. Scher CD, Haudenschild C, Klagsbrun M: The chick chorioallantoic membrane as a model system for the study of tissue invasion by viral transformed cells. Cell 8:373–382, 1976.
44. Easty DM, Easty GC: Measurement of the ability of cells to infiltrate normal tissues *in vitro*. Br J Cancer 29:36–49, 1974.
45. Noguchi PD, Johnson JB, O'Donnell R, Petricciani JC: Chick embryonic skin as a rapid organ culture assay for cellular neoplasia. Science 199:980–983, 1978.
46. Hart IR, Fidler IJ: An *in vitro* quantitative assay for tumor cell invasion. Cancer Res 38:3218–3224, 1978.
47. Poste G, Doll J, Hart IR, Fidler IJ: *In vitro* selection of murine B-16 melanoma variants with enhanced tissue invasive properties. Cancer Res 40:1636–1644, 1980.
48. Tickle C, Crawley A, Goodman M: Mechanisms of invasiveness of epithelial tumours: ultrastructure of the interactions of carcinoma cells with embryonic mesenchyme and epithelium. J Cell Sci 33:133–155, 1978.
49. Tickle C, Goodman M, Wolpert L: Cell contacts sorting out *in vivo*: the behavior of some embryonic tissues implanted into the developing chick wing. J Embryol Exp Morphol 48:225–237, 1978.
50. Tickle C, Crawley A, Goodman M: Cell movement and the mechanism of invasiveness: a survey of the behaviour of some normal and malignant cells implanted into the developing chick wing bud. J Cell Sci 31:293–322, 1978.
51. Meyvisch C, Mareel M: Invasion of malignant C3H mouse fibroblasts from aggregates transplanted into the auricles of syngenic mice. Virchows Arch B Cell Pathol 30:113–122, 1979.
52. Whur P, Koppel H, Urquhart C, Williams DC: Quantitative electronic analysis of normal and transformed BHK-21 fibroblast aggregation. J Cell Sci 23:193–210, 1977.
53. Curtis ASG: Cell adhesion. Prog Biophys Mol Biol 27:317–386, 1973.
54. Moskowitz M: Aggregation of cultured mammalian cells. Nature 200:854–856, 1963.
55. Maslow DE, Mayhew E, Feldman J: Differential inhibition of *in vitro* malignant cell assays by B6 mouse melanoma variants. J Nat Cancer Inst 64:635–638, 1980.
56. Maslow DE, Mayhew E: Inhibition of embryonic cell aggregation by neoplastic cells. J Nat Cancer Inst 54:1097–1102, 1975.
57. Hanaoka Y, Kudo K, Ishimaru Y, Hayashi M: Biochemical and morphological comparison of 2

tumor cell aggregation factors from rat ascites hepatoma cells. Br J Cancer 37:536–544, 1978.

58. Pessac-Pejsachowicz B, Alliot-Mayet F: Mise en évidence d'un 'facteur' diffusible facilitant l'aggregation de cells cancerèuses *in vitro*. CR Acad Sci Paris (D) 266:1809–1812, 1968.
59. Culp LA: Biochemical determinants of cell adhesion. In: Current topics in membranes and transport, Volume 11, Juliano R, Rothstein A (eds). New York: Academic press, 1978, pp 327–396.
60. Jones BM: Regulation of the contact behavior of cells. Biol Rev Camb Philos Soc 55:207–235, 1980.
61. Curtis ASG, Greaves MF: the inhibition of cell aggregation by a pure serum protein. J Embryol Exp Morphol 13:309–326, 1965.
62. Edwards JG, Dysart JM, Edgar DH, Robson RT: On the reduced adhesiveness of virally transformed BHK-21 cells. J Cell Sci 35:307–320, 1979.
63. Wright TC, Ukena TE, Campbell R, Karnovsky MJ: Rates of aggregation, loss of anchorage dependence, and tumorigenicity of cultured cells. Proc Nat Acad Sci USA 74:258–262, 1977.
64. Armstrong PB, Lackie JM: Studies of intercellular invasion *in vitro* using rabbit peritoneal neutrophil granulocytes (PMNs) I. Role of contact inhibition of locomotion. J Cell Biol 65:439–462, 1975.
65. Lackie JM, Armstrong PB: Studies of intercellular invasion *in vitro* using rabbit peritoneal neutrophil granulocytes II. Adhesive interactions between cells. J Cell Sci 19:645–652, 1975.
66. de Ridder L, Mareel M, Vakaet L: Adhesion of malignant and non-malignant cells to cultured embryonic substrates. Cancer Res 35:3164–3171, 1975.
67. Mareel M, Bruyneel E, Storme G: Attachment of mouse fibrosarcoma cells to precultured fragments of embryonic chick heart. An early step of invasion *in vitro*. Virchows Arch B Pathol 34:85–98, 1980.
68. Cassiman JJ, Bernfield MR: Transformation induced alterations in adhesion binding of preformed cell aggregates to cell layers. Exp Cell Res 103:311–320, 1976.
69. DiPasquale A, Bell PB: The upper cell surface: its inability to support active cell movement in culture. J Cell Biol 62:198–214, 1974.
70. Umbreit JN, Erbe RW: Transfer of tumor cells between cell aggregates as a model for adhesive changes in metastasis. Cancer Res 39:2001–2005, 1979.
71. Yuhas JM, Tarleton AE, Molzen KB: Multicellular tumor spheroid formation by breast cancer cells isolated from different sites. Cancer Res 38:2486–2491, 1978.
72. Carrino D, Gershman H: Division of BALB/c mouse 3T3 and SV-40 transformed 3T3 cells in cellular aggregates. Proc Nat Acad Sci USA 74:3874–3878, 1977.
73. Moskowitz M, Amborski GF, Wieker CH: Structure development in aggregens. Nature 211:1047–1049, 1966.
74. Carlsson J: A proliferation gradient in three-dimensional colonies of cultured human glioma cells. Int J Cancer 20:129–136, 1977.
75. Freyer JP, Sutherland RM: Selective dissociation and characterization of cells from different regions of multicell tumor spheroids. Cancer Res 40:3956–3965, 1980.
76. Sigdestad CP, Grdina DJ, Ando K: Density gradient centrifugation of cells separated from multicellular tumor spheroids. Experentia 35:815–817, 1979.
77. Putnam DL, Park DK, Rhim JS, Stuer Af, Ting RC: Correlation of cellular aggregation of transformed cells with their growth in soft agar and tumorigenic potential. Proc Soc Exp Biol Med 155:487–494, 1977.
78. Gershman H, Crissman HA, Carrino DA: Cell cycle parameters of 3T3 cells cultured as aggregates. In Vitro 17:143–149, 1977.
79. Lord EM, Penney DP, Sutherland RM, Cooper RA: Morphological and functional characteristics of cells infiltrating and destroying tumor multicellular spheroids *in vivo*. Virchows Arch B Cell Pathol 31:103–116, 1979.
80. Yuhas JM, Culo F, Harmon J, Tarleton AE: A hybrid *in vivo/in vitro* system for the study of multicellular tumor spheroid responses. Radiat Res 74:533, 1978.
81. Lord EM, Landry J, Sutherland RM: Use of the multicellular spheroid system for assaying the immune responses to tumors and the effects of therapy modalities on these responses. Radiat Res

74:471, 1978.
82. Macdonald HR, Howell RL, McFarlane DL: The multicellular spheroid as a model tumor allograft. Part 2. Characterization of spheroid infiltrating cytotoxic cells. Transplantation 25:141–145, 1978.
83. Fidler IJ, Cifone MA: Properties of metastatic and non-metastatic cloned subpopulations of an ultraviolet-light-induced murine fibrosarcoma of recent origin. Am J Pathol 97:633–648, 1979.
84. Poste G, Fidler IJ: The pathogenesis of cancer metastasis. Nature 283:139–146, 1980.

15. *In vitro* assay of invasion using endothelial and smooth muscle cells

P. A. JONES

1. Introduction

The process of extravasation is one of the key steps in the hematogenous spread of malignant cells from one site to another. The successful establishment of a secondary tumor requires that circulating tumor cells escape the inhospitable environment of the blood stream, cross the endothelium and underlying basement membranes and establish themselves in the extravascular tissues. Most extravasation from the blood stream occurs through thin-walled venules and capillaries, since arteries and arterioles are rarely invaded [1, 2]. Metastasis can also occur through the lymphatic system [1] but this route will not be considered in the present review, since most *in vitro* assays have utilized model systems derived from vascular cells.

One of the important events in the escape of malignant cells from the circulation is therefore the penetration of the endothelium and underlying basement membrane, and this process would seem to lend itself to study by tissue culture techniques. Indeed, several reports on interactions between tumor cells and cultured endothelial cells have recently been published [3–7]. These systems are promising, since they suggest that this aspect of the metastatic process can now be studied in a more controlled environment than was previously possible.

In this review, morphological aspects of extravasation *in vivo* will first be discussed since these morphological studies provide an essential frame of reference for the *in vitro* systems. The fidelity of the differentiated phenotype displayed by cultured endothelial cells will then be reviewed. Subsequently, the results obtained for the interactions of tumor cells with cultured endothelial cells will be discussed and compared to the *in vivo* findings for extravasation. Finally, the limitations of current experimental design will be presented in the hope that this important field of research may continue to advance to systems which more accurately reflect extravasation as it occurs in humans and animals.

2. Extravasation *in vivo*

The exit of circulating malignant cells from the blood stream into host tissues is a rare event in the tumor-bearing patient [1]. Most of our knowledge of this process

L.A. Liotta and I.R. Hart (eds.), Tumor Invasion and Metastasis. ISBN-13: 978-94-009-7513-2.
© 1982 Martinus Nijhoff Publishers, The Hague/Boston/London.

comes from morphological studies utilizing animal tumor models, but little is known of the biochemical events responsible for extravasation. The ability of tumor cells to cross the endothelial layer and underlying subendothelial matrix *in vivo* has received special attention because of its potential importance to metastasis. These data will first be reviewed so that results obtained with cultured cell types may be seen in perspective.

Analysis of the blood of tumor-bearing experimental animals [8, 9] and humans [10, 11] indicates that malignant cells are almost constantly entering the vascular system in a number which far exceeds the total number of metastases. The enormous majority of these cells perish within the blood stream which led Willis [12] to conclude that 'tumor embolism is not metastases,' a concept first proposed by Goldmann in 1897 [13]. Thus, the mere presence of large numbers of tumor cells in the circulation does not necessarily indicate a bad prognosis [14]. However, once tumor cells have been released into the circulation, there are direct correlations between the size of the embolus, the rate of its arrest in blood vessels, and the formation of secondary tumors [15–17].

When circulating tumor cells or emboli have adhered to the vascular endothelium the process of extravasation and transcapillary migration can begin. The mechanisms by which tumor cells penetrate the endothelial layer appear to vary and have been investigated in several experimental systems. Wood [18] made direct cinematographic observations on the intravascular behavior of V2 carcinoma cells injected slowly into the auricular artery of rabbits with vascularized ear chambers. Intracapillary thrombus formation, which tended to enmesh the cancer cells and obstruct blood flow, occurred after attachment of the V2 carcinoma cells. Part of this peritumoral thrombus was often fragmented and dislodged, although tumor cells destined to penetrate the endothelium remained adherent. The endothelium adjacent to these cells appeared damaged and leukocytes accumulated in the areas within 30 min to several hours. Leukocytes migrated through the endothelial wall and appeared to leave behind defects through which other leukocytes and later cancer cells migrated. Tumor cells were observed in the perivascular connective tissue after 3 h and tumor growth was observed after 6 h. Those tumor cells which had penetrated the endothelium incompletely were covered by endothelial proliferation within 24 h and flow through the parent vessel was therefore re-established. The possibility that tumor cells might follow the migration of lymphocytes or macrophages was also suggested by Sherwin and Richters [19].

The mode of penetration of mouse lung endothelium by a chemically-induced murine fibrosarcoma was the subject of a transmission electron microscope study by Sindelar et al. [20]. Tumor cells which had become arrested in the pulmonary vessels initiated penetration of the endothelium by 24 h after arrest. The actual breaching of the vessel wall took place between the junctions of adjacent endothelial cells with the penetrating tumor cells appearing to cause some separation of the endothelial cytoplasmic processes. These findings substantiated earlier proposals that vascular penetration by embolized tumor cells occurred directly between adjacent endothelial cells [21, 22] in a similar manner to that observed for leukocytes [23]. The fibrosarcoma cells were observed to invade the perivascular pulmonary parenchyma after vascular penetration, and viable cells underwent mitosis to form cell nests that presumably gave rise to metastatic foci. Carr et al. [24] also observed that cells of a rat neoplasm (Rd/3) appeared to pass through gaps between endothelial cells in the liver following injection into the portal vein.

These studies do not show whether tumor cells actively induce the breakage of junctions between adjacent endothelial cells or whether they take advantage of naturally occurring gaps in the endothelium to gain entrance to the extravascular tissues. Such gaps do occur under normal circumstances and the endothelial cells of the postcapillary venules of rat diaphragm, for example, often display open intercellular spaces of approximately 60 Å [25]. Normal gaps in endothelium resulting from wear and tear might also provide a route through which tumor cells could migrate [26, 27]. Intracellular junctions between endothelial cells may open during cell division [28], and this may also prove to be a possible invasion pathway. The exposure of the subendothelium through naturally occurring gaps may also increase the adherence of circulating tumor cells to the vessel wall [29, 30], increasing the relative importance of this mode of extravasation.

Other investigators have suggested that arrested tumor cells might cause the cytotoxic or enzymatic lysis of endothelial cells [31, 32]. Such damage to the endothelium could lead to the accumulation of neutrophils so that tumor cells might infiltrate the extravascular tissues by folllowing the pathway set by migrating leukocytes [33]. Destruction of the vessel wall by arrested tumor cells was also observed by Baserga and Saffioti [34], Locker et al. [35] and Warren and Gates [36]. However, the possible roles of proteolytic enzymes or pressure atrophy in this process are completely unknown.

There is also evidence that platelets and other coagulation factors could play a role in extravasation [37]. Adherence of platelets to subendothelial connective tissues is the first observable response to vascular injury [38] and such damage could be induced by the temporary blockage of capillaries by tumor emboli [39]. The release of ADP, and generation of other biologically active substances such as the platelet derived growth factor may well also influence extravasation. The intracapillary growth of tumor emboli can also lead to the 'explosive' extravasation of the malignant cells [39].

There have also been proposals that mouse mammary carcinoma and lymphosarcoma cells might migrate directly through the endothelial cell cytoplasm without breaching endothelial junctions in liver tissue [40, 41]. The mode of endothelial penetration by lymphosarcoma cells was compared to the migration of leukocytes through liver sinusoid endothelium, and it was concluded that both types of extravasation were essentially transcellular. DeBruyn and Cho [42] studied the entry of metastatic acute myelogenous leukemia cells into the circulation, and concluded that these cells penetrated the endothelial cell body by making a temporary migration pore, which closed after the malignant cells entered the vascular lumen, so that the endothelium remained continuous.

There therefore seem to be several routes by which metastasizing cells can gain access to the subendothelial zone. Whatever route is taken, the invading tumor cells often appear to be covered by regrowth or healing of the endothelium [18, 22, 35] and may be held up at the site between the endothelium and subendothelial basement membrane. Warren [43] has suggested that this may be a site where they are protected from the inhospitable environment of the blood and also a potential site for tumor dormancy.

The breaching of the endothelium *in vivo* is a complex process involving tumor cells, endothelial cells, basement membrane components, blood cells and clotting factors. Thus, while *in vitro* experiments are normally designed to minimize the number of components, the complexity of the process in the animal or patient should not be forgotten. The suitability of such *in vitro* systems will be discussed in the next section.

3. Suitability of *in vitro* assays for tumor cell – blood vessel interactions

The succesful establishment of a secondary tumor occurs with a low frequency since most embolised tumor cells perish in the circulation, and it is virtually impossible to study the process of extravasation at the biochemical level in whole animal experiments. The use of organ cultures of blood vessels would represent a lower order of complexity. However, blood vessels are not easy to maintain *in vitro* [44] and until recently there was only one report in the literature on the culture of veins [45].

Poste et al. [46] have successfully utilized explants of dog femoral veins to select for B16 melanoma variants with enhanced tissue invasive properties. This technique also allowed for the quantitation of the number of cells penetrating the vessel wall as well as for the recovery of more invasive variants. Despite the usefulness of the organ culture technique, it is difficult to establish on a routine basis and does not allow for biochemical experiments requiring large numbers of reproducible substrates. Also, since most hematogenous metastasis occurs through capillaries and venules rather than through large vessels, the vein may provide a more formidable barrier than that successfully transversed by a tumor cell in an animal.

Several investigations have therefore attempted to study the process of extravasation by the utilization of endothelial cell cultures. However, before discussing these experiments, the literature will be reviewed which suggests that endothelial cells display a phenotype in culture which is similar to that exhibited by endothelia *in vivo*.

Endothelial cells have been cultured from human umbilical cord [47, 48], bovine aorta [49–51], guinea pig aorta and vein [52], rabbit aorta [53], procine aorta [54], rat lung [55], and more recently from bovine and human capillaries [56]. These cells synthesize *in vitro* an extensive basement membrane-like structure which contains fibronectin [6, 50, 57], laminin [58] and type IV collagen [59, 60]. Bovine aortic endothelial cells also secrete type III pro-collagen as the major collagenous protein into the medium, but the cell pellet also contains types IV and V collagen [61, 62].

Confluent monolayers of endothelial cells develop both gap and tight junctions which are impervious to ruthenium red [63]. The apical surface of endothelial monolayers is non-adhesive for platelets [64] and endothelial cultures are active in the biosynthesis of prostacyclins [65] plasminogen activator [66, 67] and Factor VIII antigen [47, 68]. Endothelial monolayers therefore appear to express several of the properties expected for an endothelium *in vivo* and represent a reasonable model for extravasation studies.

However, endothelial cells have a marked tendency to undergrow the monolayer in a phenomenon called sprouting [51, 69]. The sprouting cells have been demonstrated to be of endothelial origin, but synthesize reduced amounts of fibronectin and a predominance of type I procollagen, rather than the types III and IV procollagens synthesized by monolayer cultures [70, 71]. Additionally, extracellular matrix proteins appear on the surface of sprouting cultures, and the upper surface becomes adhesive for platelets [71].

Although sprouting may also occur *in vivo* in the endothelium of regenerating or newly formed vessels [72], it is unlikely that these are sites of significant extravasation in the animal. Therefore, studies on the interactions of tumor and endothelial cells *in vitro* should be performed with non-sprouting endothelial cultures. Since sprouting can be prevented by suitable choice of endothelial cell strains [70], fibroblast growth factor [71] collagen gels [63] or the use of gelatin coated dishes (unpublished observations), this is not an insurmountable problem. Endothelial monolayers therefore represent a valuable experimental system in which to study the details of tumor cell extravasation.

The abilities of cultured tumor cells to exhibit their *in vivo* phenotype is not as easy to establish. The derivation of cell lines often involves the selection of cells endowed with specific properties which may be irrelevant to their survival in the animal or to their abilities to metastasize. In this regard, it should be remembered that cells within such lines are heterogeneous with respect to metastatic potential [30]. The relationship between experimental metastasis, in which cells are injected directly into the circulation, and spontaneous metastasis is also not clear [73] and this can complicate the description of the tumor cell phenotype. Caution is therefore needed in the extrapolation of results found in culture to the nature of spontaneous extravasation *in vivo*.

4. Tumor cell – endothelial cell interactions *in vitro*

The abilities of tumorigenic and non-tumorigenic cells to adhere to monolayers of bovine aortic and human umbilical vein endothelial cells and to cause retraction of the endothelial cells has been studied by Kramer and Nicolson [5]. In general, both tumorigenic and non-tumorigenic cells (such as fibroblasts) were able to adhere to, and cause the retraction of, endothelial cells. However, only invasive tumor cells, or normal cells with invasive potentials such as polymorphonuclear leukocytes and monocytes, were capable of invasion and migration under the re-sealed endothelial layer. Beesley et al. [74] have also shown that granulocytes are capable of the penetration of cultured endothelial layers.

The invasion of the cultured cell monolayers [5] appeared to be similar in some respects to penetration of the endothelium *in vivo* in that the predominant route appeared to be in the region of endothelial intercellular junctions. However, in contrast to some reports [37, 41] the tumor cells were never observed to penetrate directly through endothelial cytoplasms. Once the tumor cells had migrated under the endothelial cells, the continuity of the endothelium was restored so that the tumor cells were walled off in a similar manner to that reported by Ludatscher et al. [22] for hepatoma cells in rats.

In a subsequent study, Kramer et al. [6] examined the abilities of mouse B16-F1 and human Hs939 melanoma cells to adhere to confluent vascular endothelial cells and their isolated underlying matrix. The tumor cells adhered 5 to 8 times faster to the isolated subendothelial matrix than they did to the intact endothelial layer. Because fibronectin was the major constituent of the subendothelial matrix and was found on the basolateral but not the apical surfaces of endothelial cells *in vitro* [75] or *in vivo* [76], Kramer et al. [6] suggested that tumor cells might migrate to the subendothelial matrix by following an adhesive gradient. Indeed Carter [77] has shown that cells will migrate to the region with the greatest adhesive potential when presented with an adhesive gradient. These results may therefore explain why tumor cells rapidly penetrate endothelial layers *in vivo*.

The interaction of mouse mammary carcinoma cells with bovine aortic endothelial cells growing on collagen gels was studied by Zamora et al. [7]. The tumor cells were added in the form of multicellular spheroids (25–500 μm in diameter) and attached to the monolayer within 2 h, with nearly all the cell spheroids attached by 12 h. The attachment was often near the endothelial junctions and was followed by retraction of endothelial cells near the spheroid. Thereafter, tumor cells migrated away from the spheroids on top of the collagen gel, moved underneath the edges of the endothelial cells and sometimes invaded the collagen gel. The tumor cells were also observed to extend as cords of cells on top of the endothelium. The attachment of spheroids to the endothelium was inhibited by polyvalent compounds such as heparin and dextran sulfate, and since these compounds are known to influence metastatic incidence *in vivo* [78, 79], Zamora et al. [7] proposed that the system could be used to screen for substances

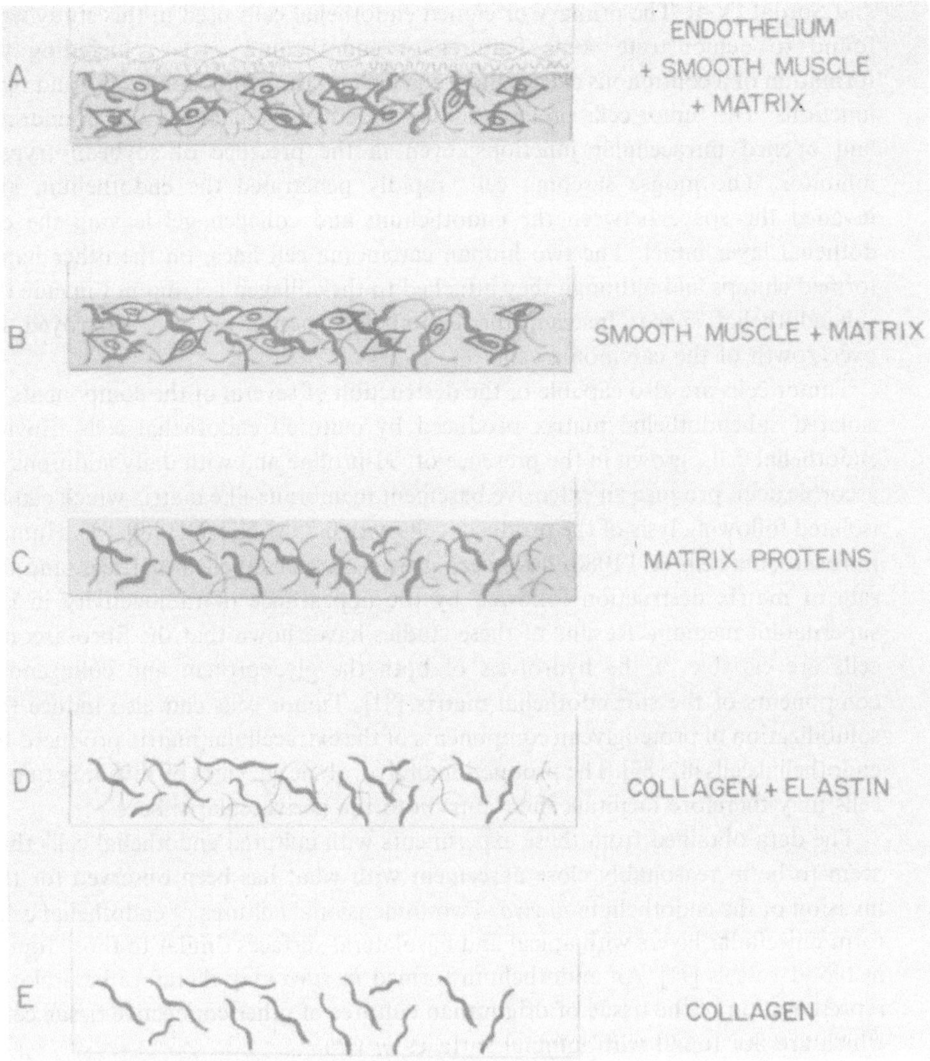

Figure 1. **Construction of an artificial blood vessel wall and its component parts *in vitro*. Rat smooth muscle cells cultured in the presence of ascorbic acid produce a cell multilayer containing large amounts of extracellular matrix proteins 1B. The extracellular matrix proteins may be prepared by cell lysis with 0.25M NH_4OH (1C). The matrix may be depleted of glycoproteins by trypsin treatment (1D) or depleted of elastin by elastase treatment to leave only matrix collagen on the dish (1E). When bovine endothelial cells are added to preformed multilayers of living rat smooth muscle cells, a structure with some of the morphological and biochemical characteristics of a blood vessel wall is formed (1A). All of these structures may be prepared in a consistent manner from cryopreserved cells and used as substrates for cells with invasive potentials.**

which might modify the metastatic process.

The interaction of human carcinoma cells and mouse sarcoma lines with bovine aortic endothelial cells grown on collagen gels was investigated by Bogenmann and Sordat [3, 4]. The primary or cloned endothelial cells used in this study were found to demonstrate some features of endothelium *in vivo* including the formation of a continuous extracellular matrix and the expression of gap and tight junctions. The tumor cells preferentially invaded endothelial cell-cell boundaries and opened intracellular junctions, even in the presence of soybean trypsin inhibitor. The mouse sarcoma cells rapidly penetrated the endothelium and invaded the space between the endothelium and collagen gel leaving the endothelial layer intact. The two human carcinoma cell lines, on the other hand, formed clumps and although they attached to the collagen gel, did not invade the subendothelial space. Instead, the endothelial monolayer was destroyed by overgrowth of the carcinoma cells.

Tumor cells are also capable of the destruction of several of the components of isolated subendothelial matrix produced by cultured endothelial cells. Bovine endothelial cells, grown in the presence of ^{3}H-proline and with daily additions of ascorbic acid, produce an extensive basement membrane-like matrix which can be isolated following lysis of the producer cells with 0.25M NH_4OH [80, 81]. Human fibrosarcoma cells (HT1080) have been grown on such labelled matrices, and the rate of matrix destruction followed by the appearance of radioactivity in the supernatant medium. Results of these studies have shown that the fibrosarcoma cells are capable of the hydrolysis of both the glycoprotein and collagenous components of the subendothelial matrix [81]. Tumor cells can also induce the solubilization of proteoglycan components of the extracellular matrix produced by endothelial cells [82, 83]. The production of hydrolytic enzymes by invading tumor cells may therefore facilitate their entry into the perivascular tissues.

The data obtained from these experiments with cultured endothelial cells thus seem to be in reasonably close agreement with what has been observed for the invasion of the endothelium *in vivo*. Two-dimensional cultures of endothelial cells form unicellular layers with apical and basolateral surfaces similar to those found in blood vessels [71]. An endothelium formed *in vitro* may therefore be a closer representation of the tissue of origin than cultures of other connective tissue cells which are not found with luminal surfaces *in vivo*.

In contrast, other attempts to study interactions between normal and tumor cell populations in monolayer culture [84, 85] have not been as successful possibly because these systems lacked this polarity. Thus, whereas two-dimensional heart cell monolayers are not destroyed by malignant mouse tumor cells, the cells in three-dimensional heart fragments are readily destroyed and completely replaced by the same tumor cells [86, 87]. Possible reasons for these marked differences in cell behavior are: 1) the loss of organotypic structure of the host tissue in monolayer culture, 2) phenotypic changes in cells spread on artificial substrates or 3) effects of the plastic or glass substrate which influence indirectly tumor cell normal cell interactions [86, 87].

5. Invasion of artificial vessel walls by tumor cells

Although endothelial cells growing on plastic or collagen gels form an 'endothelium' which has several of the characteristics of this structure *in vivo*, it still remains true that endothelial cells interact with other cells in blood vessels. Thus, pericytes which encircle capillaries, interdigitate extensively with endothelial cells [88] and this kind of interaction could, in turn, influence the process of extravasation. We have attempted to move closer to the *in vivo* situation by establishing an endothelial layer on top of preformed smooth muscle multilayers [89] to form a structure with some of the biochemical and morphological characteristics of a blood vessel wall (Figure 1).

Rat smooth muscle cells grown in the presence of ascorbic acid form 'tissues' *in vitro* in the sense that the cells grow as multilayers imbedded in extracellular matrix [90, 91; Figure 1B]. The extracellular matrix proteins may be labelled by the inclusion of ^{3}H-proline in the culture medium and isolated by the addition of 0.25M NH_4OH or 1% SDS (Figure 1C). The matrix contains glycoproteins, elastin and collagen and may be analysed by sequential enzyme digestion with trypsin, elastase and collagenase [91]. Alternatively, it can be depleted of glycoprotein components by trypsin treatment (Figure 1D), or the elastin can be removed by digestion with elastase to leave matrix collagen on the culture dish (Figure 1E). Artificial vessel walls are formed when bovine aortic endothelial cells are added to living rat smooth muscle multilayers (Figure 1A).

This system, as depicted in Figure 1, therefore allows one to investigate tumor cell degradation of blood vessel wall components at increasing levels of complexity. This is an important consideration since the components may interact in such a way as to modify their accessibility to, and degradation by, cells with hydrolytic potentials. Human fibrosarcoma cells of the HT1080 line [92] have been grown on all the structures diagramed in Figure 1, and the progress of degradation followed by the appearance of radioactivity in the culture medium.

HT1080 cells had the ability to hydrolyse all of the extracellular matrix proteins (Figure 1C) produced by cultured smooth muscle cells [93]. The degradation of the glycoprotein components was mediated by the generation of plasmin in the culture medium and the production by the HT1080 cells of plasminogen activator [94, 95], which converts the zymogen plasminogen to the active enzyme plasmin, therefore played an important part in matrix digestion. Glycoproteins are major constituents of most connective tissue matrices [96] and their prior degradation was necessary for the maximal rate of elastin and collagen hydrolysis by other HT1080 cell proteolytic activities [93]. Thus, while plasmin itself had no direct elastolytic or collagenolytic activity, its presence was necessary for the complete hydrolysis of the matrix, and it indirectly facilitated elastin and collagen degradation by the tumor cells. A similar role for plasmin was also found in our studies on the biodegradation of the matrix by stimulated mouse peritoneal macrophages

[97–99]. The extracellular matrix thus consists of a complex mixture of proteins whose complete breakdown by normal or tumor cells requires a battery of enzymes working together.

HT1080 cells were also found to be capable of destroying living smooth muscle cultures (Figure 1B), but the presence of an endothelial layer (Figure 1A) markedly inhibited the tumor cell degradative activity [100]. The inhibition was not due to a failure of the fibrosarcoma cells to penetrate the endothelium, since they were observed in the subendothelial zone 24 h after plating. The HT1080 cells continued to divide in the space between the endothelial and smooth muscle layers but their tissue degradative activity was considerably decreased.

More recently, we have shown that the degradative ability of these cells could be modulated by medium conditioned by bovine aortic endothelial cells [101], confirming our work with the artificial blood vessel walls. Such conditioned medium decreased either directly or indirectly the plasminogen activator activity in the HT1080 supernatant and this, in turn, limited the rate of matrix glycoprotein digestion. Endothelial cells and other normal connective tissue cells may therefore also influence tumor cell proteolytic activities *in vivo* and such influences may well be involved in tumor cell dormancy.

The use of artificial vessel walls therefore allows questions to be addressed to the importance of interactions between connective tissue cells, endothelial cells and extracellular matrix components in resisting invasion. It also allows for simultaneous morphological and biochemical observations so that more integrated studies should be possible. The chief disadvantages of the system are that it is constructed of cells from different species and these cells are derived from large vessels which are seldom invaded *in vivo* [1, 2].

6. Limitations of current experimental design

Recent advantages in the culture of endothelial cells have meant that the process of extravasation can now be studied in a far more controlled environment than was previously possible in whole animal experiments. However, it is extremely important that interactions between tumor and endothelial cells *in vitro* be compared critically to their behavior *in vivo* before general conclusions are drawn. In this regard it is pertinent to point out that just as there is no 'typical' tumor cell, endothelial cells from different organs and positions in the vasculature probably differ both functionally and biochemically. Therefore, the cell-cell interactions are likely to vary from one cell pair to another. Bearing these facts in mind, the main limitations of today's system are:

(i) Most metastasis occurs through capillaries yet most investigators have used endothelial cells derived from large vessels for invasion studies. This has largely been due to the easy availability of these cells, but since capillary endothelial cells have now been carried in long term culture [56], it should be possible to work with capillary-derived cells in the future.

(ii) Although endothelial cells appear to form a morphologically and biochemically differentiated 'endothelium' when growing on plastic, this substrate may introduce artifacts when studying the behavior of tumor cells once they have passed through the endothelial layer. The use of other substrates should therefore continue to be explored in the future.

(iii) Insoluble collagen is not deposited in the subendothelial matrix of endothelial cells growwing in the absence of ascorbic acid [80]. This is an important consideration since collagen is an important constituent of the subendothelial basement membrane *in vivo* and may have significant effects on the behavior of tumor cells and also act as a barrier to further invasion. Ascorbic acid should therefore be added routinely to endothelial cultures used for invasion studies.

(iv) Extravasation *in vivo* occurs in the presence of blood, whereas serum is used for *in vitro* experiments. There are several components present in blood which could play significant roles in tumor cell behavior but which are missing or present in reduced quantities in serum. Thus, lymphocytes, leukocytes, platelets, fibrinogen, clotting factors, plasminogen and protease inhibitors could all influence extravasation and these and other factors will require scrutiny in the future.

(v) The behavior of tumor and endothelial cells in the animal may be modulated by hormonal influences not present in culture. Since hormones, such as corticosteroids, are known to regulate protease production in some tumor cells [102], they could well influence extravasation.

(vi) Tumors are highly heterogeneous with regard to metastatic potential [30] and the use of subclones with defined metastatic abilities should be considered. However, it should be remembered that metastasis is a multistep process which requires the succesful completion of all of the steps necessary to establish a secondary tumor. Thus, failure to metastasize does not necessarily imply a deficiency in the ability to extravasate, and one cannot expect to draw simple correlations between metastatic ability and a single *in vitro* property of a tumor cell.

In spite of these reservations, the use of co-cultures of endothelial and tumor cells probably offers the only viable experimental approach to the detailed biochemical study of extravasation. Indeed, initial reports [3, 5, 7, 81, 100] have been encouraging in establishing the validity of the approach. Since none of the reservations above are insurmountable, these systems will continue to be refined so that we may gain a fuller understanding of this important step in the metastatic process.

References

1. Fidler IJ, Gersten DM, Hart IR: The biology of cancer invasion and metastasis. Adv Cancer Res 28:149–250, 1978.
2. Del Regato JA: Physiopathology of the metastasis. In: Pulmonary metastasis, Weiss L, Gilbert MA (eds), Boston: Hall, 1978, pp 104–113.
3. Bogenmann E, Sordat B: Interactions of tumor cells with endothelial cell monolayers grown on collagen gels. J Cell Biol 83(2):C293, 1979.
4. Bogenmann E, Sordat B: Cultured endothelial cells: a model system to study malignant cell invasion. Cancer Res (submitted).
5. Kramer RH, Nicolson GL: Interactions of tumor cells with vascular endothelial cell monolayers: a model for metastatic invasion. Proc Natl Acad Sci USA 76:5704–5708, 1979.
6. Kramer RH, Gonzalez R, Nicolson GL: Metastatic tumor cells adhere preferentially to the extracellular matrix underlying vascular endothelial cells. Int J Cancer 26:639–645, 1980.
7. Zamora PO, Danielson KG, Hosick HL: Invasion of endothelial cell monolayers on collagen gels by cells from mammary tumor spheroids. Cancer Res 40:4631–4639, 1980.
8. Blumenthal F: Über Erzeugung von Tumoren mit Blut Tumortieren. Z Krebsforsch 29:549–553, 1929.
9. Goldie H, Jeffries BR, Jones AM, Walker M: Detection of metastatic tumor cells by interperitoneal inoculation of organ brei from tumor-bearing mice. Cancer Res 13:566–572, 1953.
10. Pool EH, Dunlop GR: Cancer cells in the blood stream. Am J Cancer 21:99–102, 1934.
11. Sandberg AA, Moore GE: Examination of blood for tumor cells. J Natl Cancer Inst 19:1–11, 1957.
12. Willis RA: Spread of tumours in the human body, Ed 2, St. Louis: The C.V. Mosby Company, 1952.
13. Goldmann EE: Anatomische Untersuchungen über die Verbreitungswege bosartiger Geschwülste. Beitr Klin Chir 18:595–686, 1897.
14. Salsbury AJ: The significance of the circulating cancer cell. Cancer Treat Rev 2:55–72, 1975.
15. Fidler IJ: The relationship of emboli homogeneity, number, size and variability to the incidence of experimental metastasis. Eur J Cancer 9:223–227, 1973.
16. Liotta LA, Kleinerman J, Saidel GM: Quantitative relationships of intravascular tumor cells, tumor vessels and pulmonary metastases following tumor implantation. Cancer Res 34:997–1004, 1974.
17. Liotta LA, Kleinerman J, Saidel GM: The significance of hematogeneous tumor cell clumps in the metastatic process. Cancer Res 36:889–894, 1976.
18. Wood S: Pathogenesis of metastasis formation observed *in vivo* in the rabbit ear chamber. Arch Path 66:550–568, 1958.
19. Sherwin RP, Richters A: Pathobiologic nature of lymphocyte interactions with human breast cancer. J Natl Cancer Inst 48:1111–1115, 1972.
20. Sindelar WF, Tralka TS, Ketcham AS: Electron microscopic observations on formation of pulmonary metastases. J Surg Res 18:137–161, 1975.
21. Jones DS, Wallace AC, Fraser EE: Sequence of events in experimental metastases of Walker 256 tumor: light, immunofluorescent and electron microscopic observations. J Natl Cancer Inst 46:493–504, 1971.
22. Ludatscher RM, Luse SA, Suntzeff V: An electron microscopic study of pulmonary tumor emboli from transplantable Morris Hepatoma 5123. Cancer Res 27:1939–1952, 1967.
23. Marchesi VT, Florey HW: Electron microscopic observations on the emigration of leucocytes. Quart J Exp Physiol 45:343–348, 1960.
24. Carr I, McGinty F, Norris P: The fine structure of neoplastic invasion: invasion of liver, skeletal muscle and lymphatic vessels by the Rd/3 tumour. J Path 118:91–99, 1976.
25. Simionescu N, Simionescu M, Palade GE: Structural basis of permeability in sequential segments

of the microvasculature of the diaphragm. II Pathways followed by the microperoxidase across the endothelium. Microvascular Res 15:17–36, 1978.
26. Sugarbaker EV, Ketcham AS: Mechanisms and prevention of cancer dissemination: An overview. Semin Oncol 4:19–32, 1977.
27. Warren BA, Chauvin WJ, Phillips J: Blood-borne tumor emboli and their adherence to vessel walls. In: Cancer invasion and metastasis: biologic mechanisms and therapy, Day SB, et al. (eds), New York: Raven Press, 1977, pp 185–197.
28. Carr I, Underwood JCE: The ultrastructure of the local cellular response to neoplasia. Int Rev Cytol 37:329–347, 1974.
29. Warren BA: Environment of blood-borne tumor embolus adherent to vessel wall. J Med 4:150–177, 1973.
30. Poste G, Fidler IJ: The pathogenesis of cancer metastasis. Nature 283:139–146, 1980.
31. Fonck-Cussac Y, Delage J, Petit J: Observations ultrastructurales sur le mode d'implantation endovasculaire des métastases d'un carbronchique. Poumon 25:231–234, 1969.
32. Vlaeminck MN, Adenis L, Mouton Y, Demaille A: Etude expérimentale de la diffusion métastatique chez l'oeuf de poule embryonne, répartition, microscopie et ultrastructure des foyers tumoraux. Int J Cancer 10:619–631, 1972.
33. Wood S, Baker RR, Marzocchi B: Locomotion of cancer cells *in vivo* compared with normal cells. In: Mechanisms of invasion in cancer, Denoix P (ed). Berlin: Springer-Verlag, 1967, pp 26–30.
34. Baserga R, Saffiotti U: Experimental studies on histogenesis of blood-borne metastases. Arch Pathol 59:26–34, 1955.
35. Locker J, Goldblatt PJ, Leighton J: Ultrastructural features of invasion in chick embryo liver metastasis of Yoshida ascites hepatoma. Cancer Res 30:1632–1644, 1970.
36. Warren S, Gates O: The fate of intravenously injected tumor cells. Amer J Cancer 27:485–492, 1936.
37. Chew EC, Josephson RL, Wallace AC: Morphologic aspects of the arrest of circulating cancer cells. In: Fundamental aspects of metastasis, Weiss L (ed). Amsterdam: North-Holland, 1976, pp 121–150.
38. Spaet H, Stemerman MB: Platelet adhesion. Annals NY Acad Sci 201:13–21, 1972.
39. Nakamura K, Kawaguchi T, Asahina S, Sakurai T, Ebina Y, Yokoya S, Morita M: Electron microscopic studies on extravasation of tumor cells and early foci of hematogenous metastases. GANN Monograph on Cancer Res 20:57–72, 1977.
40. Dingemans KP: Invasion of liver tissue by blood-borne mammary carcinoma cells. J Natl Cancer Inst 53:1813–1824, 1974.
41. Dingemans KP, Roos E, van der Bergh Weerman MA, van de Pavert IV: Invasion of liver tissue by tumor cells and leukocytes: comparative ultrastructure. J Natl Cancer Inst 60:583–598, 1978.
42. DeBruyn PPH, Cho Y: Entry of metastatic malignant cells into the circulation from a subcutaneously growing myelogenous tumor. J Natl Cancer Inst 62:1221–1227, 1979.
43. Warren BA: Some aspects of blood borne tumour emboli associated with thrombosis. Z. Krebsforsch 87:1–15, 1976.
44. Stein O, Stein Y: Lipid synthesis and transport in the normal and atherosclerotic aorta. An autoradiographic study of rat and rabbit aortae incubated and perfused with choline-^{3}H and oleic acid-^{3}H. Lab Invest 23:556–566, 1970.
45. Zwillenberg HHL, Zwillenberg LO, Laszt L: Ultrastructural changes in organ cultures of bovine veins. Angiologica 9:292–300, 1972.
46. Poste G, Doll J, Hart IR, Fidler IJ: *In vitro* selection of murine B16 melanoma variants with enhanced tissue-invasive properties. Cancer Res 40:1636–1644, 1980.
47. Jaffe EA, Hoyer LW, Nachman RL: Synthesis of antihemophilic factor antigen by cultured human endothelial cells. J. Clin Invest 52:2757–2764, 1973.
48. Gimbrone MA, Cotran RS, Folkman J: Human vascular endothelial cells in culture, growth and DNA synthesis. J Cell Biol 60:673–684, 1974.

49. Booyse FM, Sedlak BJ, Rafelson ME: Culture of arterial endothelial cells: characterization and growth of bovine aortic cells. Thromb Diathes Hemorrh 34:825–839, 1975.
50. Gospodarowicz D, Greenburg G, Bialecki H, Zetter BR: Factors involved in the modulation of cell proliferation *in vivo* and *in vitro*: the role of fibroblast and epidermal growth factors in the proliferative response of mammalian cells. *In Vitro* 14:85–118, 1978.
51. Gospodarowicz D, Mecher AL: The control of cellular proliferation by the fibroblast and epidermal growth factors. Natl Cancer Inst Monogr 48:109–130, 1978.
52. Blose SH, Chacko S: *In vitro* behavior of guinea pig arterial and venous endothelial cells. Dev. Growth and Differentiation 17:153–165, 1975.
53. Buonassisi V, Venter JC: Hormone and neurotransmitter receptors in an established vascular endothelial cell line. Proc Natl Acad Sci USA 73:1612–1616, 1976.
54. Hayes LW, Goguen CA, Stevens AL, Magargal WW, Slakey LL: Enzyme activities in endothelial cells and smooth muscle cells from swine aorta. Proc Natl Acad Sci USA 76:2532–2535, 1979.
55. Parshley MS, Cerreta JM, Mandl I, Fierer JA, Turino GM: Characteristics of a clone of endothelial cells derived from a line of normal adult rat lung cells. *In Vitro* 15:709–722, 1979.
56. Folkman J, Haudenschild CC, Zetter BR: Long-term culture of capillary endothelial cells. Proc Natl Acad Sci USA 76:5217–5221, 1979.
57. Jaffe EA, Mosher DF: Synthesis of fibronectin by cultured human endothelial cells. J Exp Med 147:1779–1791, 1978.
58. Vlodavsky I, Gospodarowicz D: Respective roles of laminin and fibronectin in adhesion of human carcinoma and sarcoma cells. Nature 289:304–306, 1981.
59. Howard BV, Macarak EJ, Gunson D, Kefalides NA: Characterization of the collagen synthesized by endothelial cells in culture. Proc Natl Acad Sci USA 73:2361–2364, 1976.
60. Jaffe EA, Minick CR, Adelman B, Becker CG, Nachman R: Synthesis of basement membrane collagen by cultured human endothelial cells. J Exp Med 144:209–225, 1976.
61. Sage H, Crouch E, Bornstein P: Collagen synthesis by bovine aortic endothelial cells in culture. Biochemistry 18:5433–5441, 1979.
62. Sage H, Pritzl P, Bornstein P; Characterization of cell matrix associated collagens synthesized by aortic endothelial cells in culture. Biochemistry 20:436–442, 1981.
63. Bogenmann E, Sordat E: Characterization of primary and cloned bovine endothelial cells grown on collagen gels. In: Biology of the vascular endothelial cell, Cold Spring Harbor, NY, 1980, p 5.
64. Curwen KD, Gimbrone MA, Handin RI: *In vitro* studies of thromboresistance. The role of prostacyclin (PGI_2) in platelet adhesion to cultured normal and virally transformed human vascular endothelial cells. Lab Invest 42:366–374, 1980.
65. Weksler BB, Marcus AJ, Jaffe EA: Synthesis of prostaglandin I_2 (prostacyclin) by cultured human and bovine endothelial cells. Proc Natl Acad Sci USA 74:3922–3926, 1977.
66. Laug WE, Tokes Z, Benedict WF, Sorgente N: Anchorage-independent growth and plasminogen activator production by bovine endothelial cells. J Cell Biol 84:281–293, 1980.
67. Loskutoff DJ, Edgington TS: Synthesis of a fibrinolytic activator and inhibitor by endothelial cells. Proc Natl Acad Aci USA 74:3903–3907, 1977.
68. Jaffe EA, Nachman RL, Becker CG, Minick CR: Culture of human endothelial cells derived from umbilical veins. Identification by morphologic and immunologic criteria. J Clin Invest 52:2745–2756, 1973.
69. Schwartz S: Selection and characterization of bovine aortic endothelial cells. *In Vitro* 14:966–980, 1978.
70. Cotta-Pereiva G, Sage H, Bornstein P, Ross R, Schwartz S: Studies of morphological atypical ('sprouting') cultures of bovine aortic endothelial cells. Growth characteristics and connective tissue protein synthesis. J Cell Physiol 102:183–191, 1980.
71. Greenburg G, Vlodavsky I, Foidart JM, Gospodarowicz D: Conditioned medium from endothelial cell cultures can restore the normal phenotypic expression of vascular endothelium maintained *in vitro* in the absence of fibroblast growth factor. J Cell Physiol 103:333–347, 1980.

72. Ausprunk DH, Folkman J: Migration and proliferation of endothelial cells in preformed and newly formed blood vessels during tumor angiogenesis. J Microvasc Res 14:53–65, 1977.
73. Stackpole CW: Distinct lung-colonizing and lung metastasizing cell populations in B16 mouse melanoma. Nature 289:798–800, 1981.
74. Beesley JE, Pearson JD, Hutching SA, Carleton JS, Gordon JL: Granulocyte migration through endothelium in culture. J Cell Sci 38:237–248, 1979.
75. Birdwell CR, Gospodarowicz D, Nicolson GL: Identification, localization, and the role of fibronectin in cultured bivine endothelial cells. Proc Natl Acad Sci USA 75:3273–3277, 1978.
76. Linder E, Stenman S, Lehto V-P, Vaheri A: Distribution of fibronectin in human tissues and relationships to other connective tissue components. Ann NY Acad Sci 312:151–159, 1978.
77. Carter SB: Principles of cell mobility: the direction of cell movement and cancer invasion. Nature (London) 208:1183–1187, 1965.
78. Agostino D, Cliffton EE: Anticoagulants and the development of pulmonary metastasis. Arch Surg 84:449–453, 1962.
79. Hagmar B: Cell surface change and metastasis formation. A study on the effects of dextrans and heparin on tumour cells and experimental metastases in a syngeneic murine system. Acta Pathol Microbiol Scand Sect A Pathol 80:357–366, 1972.
80. DeClerck Y, Jones PA: The effect of ascorbic acid on the nature and production of collagen and elastin by rat smooth muscle cells. Biochem J 186:217–225, 1980.
81. Jones PA, Laug WE: Destruction by human tumor cells of basement membranes produced by cultured endothelial cells. Proc Am Assoc Cancer Res 21:210, 1980.
82. Kramer RH, Nicolson GL: Metastatic tumor cells induce the *in vitro* degradation of endothelial cells extracellular matrix. J Supramol Struct (Suppl 3): 181, 1979.
83. Kramer RH, Nicolson GL: Invasion of vascular endothelial cell monolayers and underlying matrix by metastatic human cancer cells. In: International cell biology, Schweiger HG (ed). Heidelberg: Springer-Verlag, 1981, pp 794–799.
84. Abercrombie M, Heaysman JEM: Invasive behavior between sarcoma and fibroblast populations in cell culture. J Natl Cancer Inst 56:561–570, 1976.
85. Knyrim K, Paweletz N: Cell interactions in a 'bilayer' of tumor cells: a scanning electron microscope study. Virchows Arch B Cell Pathol 25:309–325, 1977.
86. Mareel MMK: Is invasiveness *in vitro* characteristic of malignant cells? Cell Biol Int Rep 3:627–640, 1979.
87. Mareel M, Kint J, Meyvisch C: Methods of study of the invasion of malignant C3H-mouse fibroblasts into embryonic chick heart *in vitro*. Virchows Arch B Cell Pathol 30:95–111, 1979.
88. Tilton RG, Kilo C, Williamson JR, Murch DW: Differences in pericyte contractile function in rat cardiac and skeletal muscle microvasculatures. Microvasc Res 18:336–352, 1979.
89. Jones PA: Construction of an artificial blood vessel wall from cultured endothelial and smooth muscle cells. Proc Natl Acad Sci USA 76:1882–1886, 1979.
90. Bierman EL, Stein O, Stein Y: Lipoprotein uptake and metabolism by rat aortic smooth muscle cells in tissue culture. Circ Res 35:136–150, 1974.
91. Jones PA, Scott-Burden T, Gevers W: Glycoprotein, elastin and collagen secretion by rat smooth muscle cells. Proc Natl Acad Sci USA 76:353–357, 1979.
92. Rasheed S, Nelson-Rees WA, Toth EM, Arnstein P, Gardner MB: Characterization of a newly derived human sarcoma cell line (HT-1080). Cancer 33:1027–1033, 1974.
93. Jones PA, DeClerck Y: Destruction of extracellular matrices containing glycoproteins, elastin and collagen by metastatic human tumor cells. Cancer Res 40:3222–3227, 1980.
94. Laug WE, Jones PA, Benedict WF: Studies on the relationship between fibrinolysis of cultured cells and malignancy. J Natl Cancer Inst 54:173–179, 1975.
95. Jones PA, Laug WE, Benedict WF: Fibrinolytic activity in a human fibrosarcoma cell line and evidence for the induction of plasminogen activator secretion during tumor formation. Cell 6:245–252, 1975.

96. Anderson JC: Glycoproteins of the connective tissue matrix. Intl Rev Connect Tissue Res 7:251–322, 1976.
97. Werb Z, Banda MJ, Jones PA: Degradation of connective tissue matrices by macrophages. I. Proteolysis of elastin, glycoproteins and collagen by proteinases isolated from macrophages. J Exp Med 152:1340–1357, 1980.
98. Jones PA, Werb Z: Degradation of connective tissue matrices by macrophages. II. Influence of matrix composition on proteolysis of glycoproteins, elastin and collagen by macrophages in culture. J Exp Med 152:1527–1536, 1980.
99. Werb Z, Bainton DF, Jones PA: Degradation of connective tissue matrices by macrophages. III. Morphological and biochemical studies on extracellular, pericellular, and intracellular events in matrix proteolysis by macrophages in culture. J Exp Med 152:1537–1553, 1980.
100. Jones PA, Neustein H, Gonzales F, Bogenmann E: Invasion of an artificial blood vessel wall by human fibrosarcoma cells. Cancer Res 41:4613–4620, 1981.
101. Heisel MA, Jones PA, Laug WE: Modulation of the degradative properties of human fibrosarcoma cells by endothelial cells. Proc Amer Assoc Cancer Res 22:248, 1981.
102. Wigler M, Ford JP, Weinstein IB: Glucocorticoid inhibition of the fibrinolytic activity of tumor cells. In: Proteases and biological control. Reich E, Rifkin DB, Shaw E (eds), Cold Spring Harbor Laboratory, 1975, pp 849–856.

16. The regulation of invasion by a cartilage-derived anti-invasion factor

B.U. PAULI and K.E. KUETTNER

1. Introduction

The ability to invade normal tissues which surround primary tumors and to subsequently metastasize to distant sites are the distinguishing features of malignant neoplasms [1–5]. In order to invade and metastasize, tumor cells must overcome several structural barriers presented by host tissues [2, 3, 5]. In most mammalian tissues, structural barriers consist of a meshwork of tightly packed and highly cross-linked collagen fibrils. These fibrils are embedded in a viscoelastic ground substance whose major components are structural macromolecular complexes, i.e. proteoglycans, glycoproteins, and elastin [6–11]. The normal packing of these macromolecules may leave little or no space for the free movement of tumor cells. Cleavage by proteinases may therefore provide a mechanism by which tumor cells invade [12–20]. Numerous reports of increased proteolytic (collagenolytic) activity associated with various tumors, obtained either by extraction or tissue culture techniques, have strengthened the concept of a primary involvement of proteinases in tumor invasion [16–36]. Considerable progress has since been achieved in analyzing the role of matrix-degrading enzymes in the invasion of tumors. Despite this, the cellular origin and the local regulation (synthesis, secretion, activation, inhibition) of most of these enzymes remain in doubt, mainly because of the heterogeneity of tumor specimens used by the various investigators [16–36].

Assuming that the concept of proteinase involvement in tumor invasion is correct, proteinase inhibitors derived from host tissues and serum, may be efficient in impeding invasion of malignant tumors [20, 37–41]. Such proteinase inhibitors may already be responsible for the classical observation that connective tissues are unequally susceptible to invasive processes, even though these tissues are composed of similar structural macromolecules and thus, are cleaved by identical proteinases [39, 41–44]. We have provided evidence to support the hypothesis that a selective resistance of connective tissues exists, and that it may be determined by tissue-specific anti-invasion factors which express themselves as inhibitors of matrix-degrading proteinases, inhibitors of cell proliferation, and/or inhibitors of cell migration [37–39, 41, 44–54]. This hypothesis was originally derived from our analysis of human osteosarcoma patients in whom bone was readily penetrated by the rapidly expanding tumor mass, whereas uncalcified cartilage of the epiphyseal growth plate resisted penetration by this malignancy [39, 41, 44].

L.A. Liotta and I.R. Hart (eds.), Tumor Invasion and Metastasis. ISBN-13: 978-94-009-7513-2.
© 1982 Martinus Nijhoff Publishers, The Hague/Boston/London.

2. Resistance of normal cartilage to invasion

2.1. In vivo observations

Osteosarcomas are malignant tumors which almost always arise singly in the metaphyseal ends of long bones, particularly in the lower end of the femur, and the upper ends of the tibia and humerus [42, 43, 55]. In an extensive series of osteosarcoma cases, McKenna et al. [56] reported a peak incidence for this malignancy in patients of approximately twenty years of age. Only rarely was osteosarcoma encountered in patients over the age of 40. Males were affected about twice as often as females. The tumor mass generally filled the marrow cavity at its primary site, destroyed the metaphyseal cancellous bone, and extended along a broad front against the epiphyseal growth plate. In young, growing patients in whom growth plates consisted of uncalcified hyaline cartilage, this tissue abruptly stopped the extension of the tumor. Tumor cells reached as far as the vascular loops extended, namely to the area of the last hypertrophic chondrocyte and its calcified matrix. Osteosarcoma cells were unable to penetrate the matrix of viable hyaline cartilage [39, 41, 44, 57]. In advanced stages of the disease, osteosarcoma had frequently eroded, penetrated, and replaced the metaphyseal compact bone. Tumor masses had characteristically lifted the periosteum, producing Codman's triangle [55]. The epiphyseal bone in young patients was generally occupied by tumor masses only after tumor cells had reached and penetrated the epiphyseal compact bone, by migrating along the cleavage plane between perichondrium and epiphyseal cartilage. Rarely, we could observe a direct extension of osteosarcoma from the metaphysis to the epiphysis. In patients in whom such a direct extension was observed, tumor cells invaded through pre-existing, nutrative vascular channels which had been reported to occur in the human growth plate. In advanced cases of the disease, direct extension of osteosarcoma through the growth plate was encouraged by microfractures, ischemic necrosis, or local inflammatory processes, secondary to the loss of structural support of underlying bone [47, 57–59]. In patients above age 18, in whom the growth plate consisted of calcified cartilage or was already ossified, osteosarcoma extended without restriction up to the calcified matrix of the articular cartilage. The matrix of the viable articular cartilage was not penetrated by osteosarcoma cells.

This phenomenon of cartilage resisting invasion by osteosarcoma cells is not unique, and can be observed in other cartilagenous tissues with other primary or metastatic tumors [15]. For example, bronchial cartilage was found to be relatively resistant to invasion by bronchogenic carcinoma, laryngeal cartilage to laryngeal squamous cell carcinoma, and intervertebral cartilage to metastatic mammary and prostatic carcinomas.

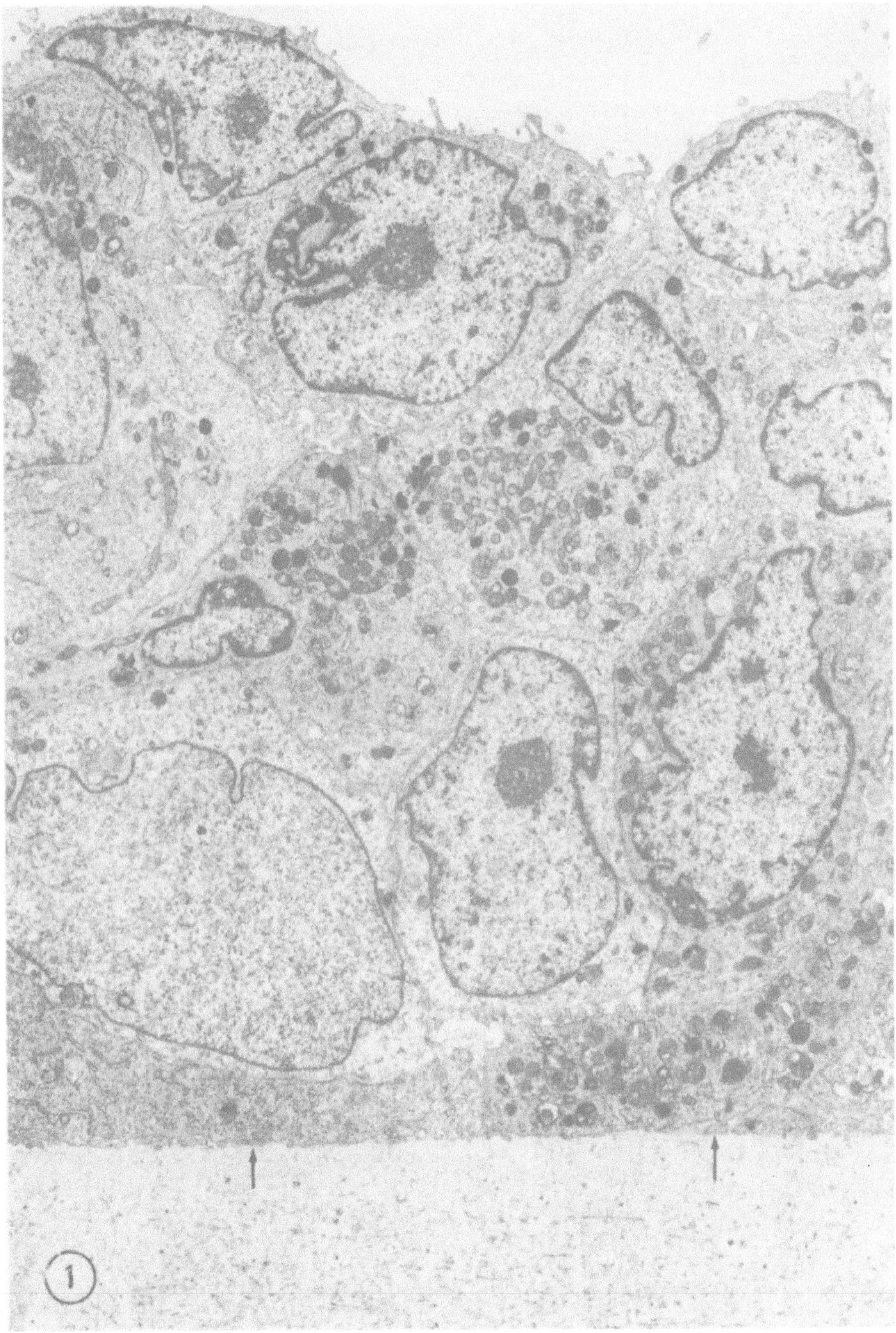

Figure 1. Human TE-85 osteosarcoma cells grown on articular phalangeal cartilage are unable to penetrate the cartilagenous matrix. Microvilli of basal tumor cells extend parallel to the cartilage growth surface (arrow). × 5 100.

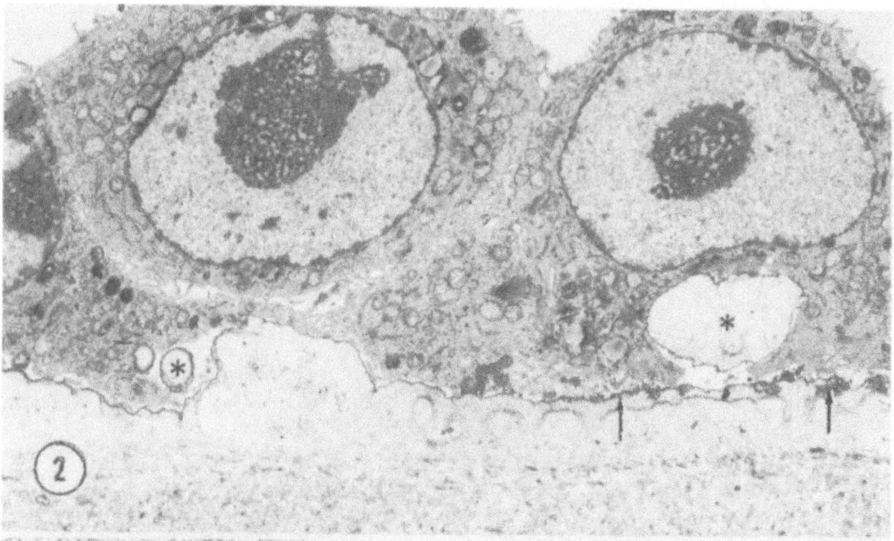
2

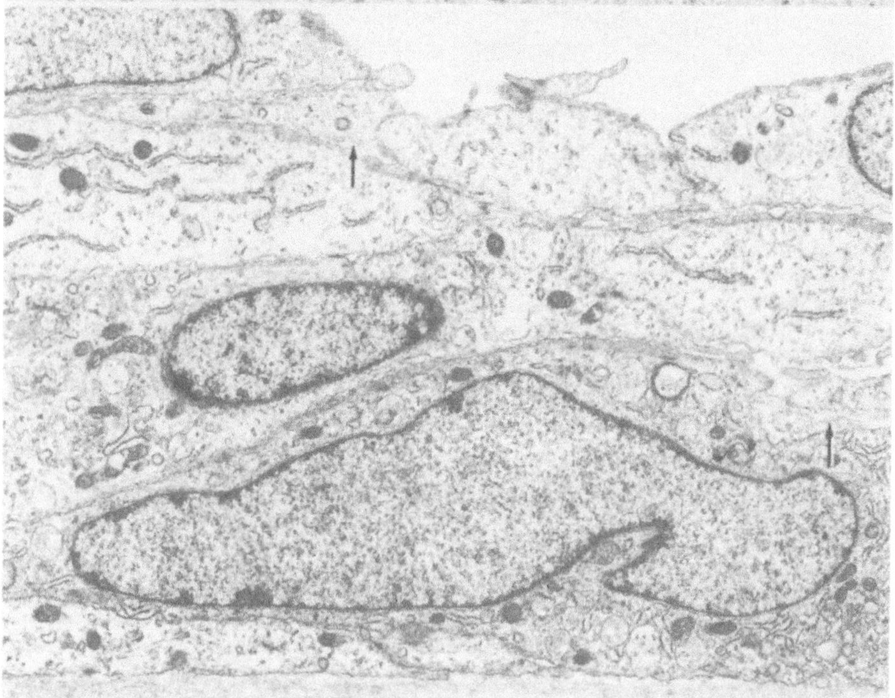
3

2.2. In vitro observations

The interaction of human osteosarcoma cells with mammalian hyaline cartilage was studied by utilizing a modification [39, 44] of the culture system described by Fell and Thomas [60]. Cartilage-bone explants obtained from human ribs (costochondral junction) and phalanges of 11- to 13-year-old children, were placed onto Millipore membranes. Membranes with explants were elevated above the bottom of the culture dish by Falcon stainless-steel grids. Medium was added until the fluid level wetted the Millipore membrane. After an initial culture period of two days, human TE-85 osteosarcoma cells [61] were seeded onto the explanted tissues and incubated under standard conditions. On the bone side of the explant, tumor cells readily attached to the bone spicules, rapidly multiplied, and enveloped entire spicules within seven days of incubation. Lacunar invaginations into the bone spicules contained osteosarcoma cells and were interpreted to be caused by erosive and destructive (collagenolytic) activities of tumor cells on the bony matrices [39, 44]. Collagenolytic activity was previously detected in serum-free medium of TE-85 osteosarcoma cells [37] and was responsible for the degradation of extracellular (collagenous) matrices *in vitro* [62].

In contrast to bone, a few tumor cells were able to attach to the cartilage tissue. They formed only solitary cell clusters and were unable to penetrate the cartilagenous matrix (Figure 1) [44]. At the cartilage-bone interface, tumor cells extended as far into the cartilagenous matrix as the blood vessels, namely to the area of the last hypertrophic chondrocyte and its calcified matrix [39, 41, 44]. Mesenchyme and blood vessels of nutrative cartilage canals were consistently penetrated and replaced by osteosarcoma cells. Similar observations were made when human mammary carcinoma cells or rat bladder carcinoma cells were grown on cartilage-bone explants (Figure 2) [39, 41, 53, 54]. Human foreskin fibroblasts, which were used as control cells in these experiments, covered bone and cartilage equally with one to several cell layers. There was no evidence of matrix erosion and cell invasion (Figure 3) [44].

After explants were removed, it was observed that osteosarcoma cells (or carcinoma cells) had grown underneath the bone but not beneath the cartilage. This zone of no growth beneath the cartilage usually resisted invasion by osteosarcoma cells for 3 to 4 days, after which time the tumor cells started to overgrow even these areas [41, 44]. By 7 days this zone was covered with tumor cells and was indistinguishable

---

Figure 2. Invasive carcinoma cells derived from carcinogen-induced rat urinary bladder tumors are grown on bone explant. Accumulations of electron-dense, fibrillar material at the lumenal-bone interface (arrow) and ongoing phagocytosis of bony sequesters (asterisk) are evidence of matrix destruction by tumor cells. × 4900.

Figure 3. Human foreskin fibroblasts do not invade normal hyaline cartilage. There is some matrix deposited between individual fibroblasts (arrow). × 5200.

from the remaining surface of the millipore membrane, where osteosarcoma cells grew up to 4 cell layers thick. No such effect was observed in control cultures with human foreskin fiboblasts, even though the migratory activity of these cells was similar to that of osteosarcoma cells. Fibroblasts either grew under the cartilage explant or immediately covered the growth surface of the explant after its removal from the millipore membrane [44].

These experiments support our initial *in vivo* observations that viable hyaline cartilage is highly resistant to invasion by malignant tumor cells [39, 41, 44]. The limited growth of tumor cells on the cartilage surfaces and, more significantly, the inhibition of tumor cell growth underneath the cartilage explants, even after the explants had been removed from the growth supporting millipore surfaces, suggested that cartilage may have released a factor which was deposited onto the membranes and influenced growth and proliferation of tumor cells. Such a diffusable inhibitory factor was shown previously to be responsible for the inhibition of cartilage neovascularization, when viable cartilage explants were grown on the chick chorioallantoic membrane (CAM) [39, 48, 49, 63]. The resistance to vascular penetration was lost when cartilage was depleted of this diffusable factor by salt extraction (i.e. at concentrations higher than 1 M NaCl) prior to its explantation on the CAM [39, 48, 49]. Since tumor cells may invade connective tissues by the same mechanisms as vascular endothelial cells penetrate tissues during histogenesis or wound healing, it seemed logical to examine whether extracted cartilage might show a similar behavior toward malignant tumor cells as toward vascular endothelial cells. In such experiments, salt extraction of hyaline cartilage was performed under identical conditions without causing denaturation or dissolution of the collagenous network in the cartilagenous matrix.

3. Susceptability of extracted cartilage to invasion

In order to avoid the complexity of the CAM assay system, the behavior of salt-extracted cartilage towards tumor cell invasion has been studied utilizing a novel *in vitro* culture system (Figure 4) [53, 54]. The main constituent of this system was a hollow, stainless-steel cylinder (inner diameter; 4 mm). The edge of the cylinder was sharpened at one end so that a disk could be cut from a cartilage slice. This manipulation, which was performed under aseptic conditions, closed the hollow cylinder on its sharpened end with a 1 mm thick cartilage disk. Thus, the disks which had been obtained from fresh metacarpophalangeal joints of pre-adult bovines, and had been extracted with 1 M or 3 M NaCl or guanidine hydrochloride (GuHCl) for 36 h at 4° C, could be used as growth surfaces for TE-85 osteosarcoma cells or control human foreskin fibroblasts. This novel culture system had the advantage over the previously described one [44] in that tumor cells or control cells could be grown in defined numbers and in intimate contact with the cartilage surfaces.

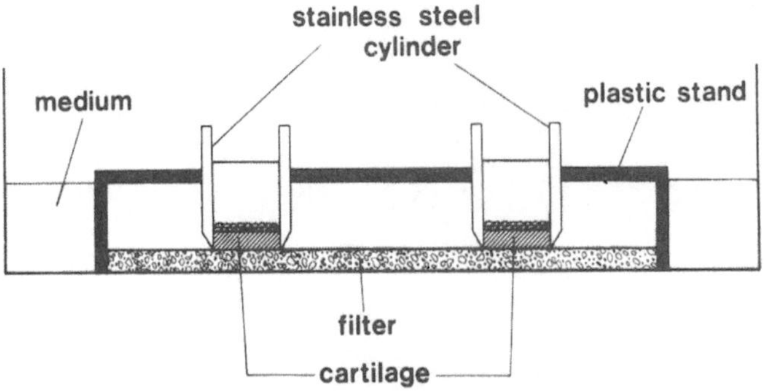

Figure 4. In vitro organ cell culture system consists of a hollow, stainless steel cylinder which has been closed on its sharpened end with a 1 mm thick cartilage disk. Cylinders with cartilage disks are placed vertically onto a filter support that lays on the bottom of the culture dish. They are held in position by a plastic stand. Thirty thousand cells, suspended in 100 μl growth medium are plated through the opening of the cylinder onto the cartilage disk. Fresh growth medium (50 μl) is added daily.

The treatment of fresh articular cartilage with 1 M and 3 M GuHC1 depleted the tissue of the soluble proteoglycan pool and the factor which inhibited neovascularization in the CAM [39, 48, 49]. One molar GuHC1 removed approximately one third of the total macromolecular proteoglycans from the cartilage disks, 3 M GuHCl removed approximately one half, as determined from the uronic acid content of the extract and the tissue [53]. This depletion was most prominent in the marginal zones of the extracted cartilage, as evidenced by morphologic examination after ruthenium red staining of the extraced cartilage discs. GuHCl-extraction did not yield detectable amounts of collagen and did not denature the collagenous fibers, as shown by the preservation of the normal cross-banding pattern of these macromolecules [53, 54].

In this organ-cell culture system, tumor cells or control cells were plated such that the cartilage discs were covered by one to three cell layers. Osteosarcoma cells growing in contact with the devitalized, extracted cartilage immediately began to penetrate the cartilagenous matrix. Early indications of cell penetration were characterized by the appearance of numerous microvilli which extended perpendicularly from the basal tumor cell membranes to force their way into the matrix between intact collagen fibers. After a culture period of 14 days, deep invasion was observed only in 3M GuHCl-extracted cartilage disks (Figure 5) [41, 53]. Single tumor cells or tumor cell clusters penetrated as far as 300 μm into the extracted, 1 mm thick cartilagenous disk. Penetration of cells was frequently associated with rarefaction of the matrix and widening of interfibrillar spaces in the collagenous network (Figure 5). Adjacent to tumor cell membranes, collagen fibers were fragmented and had lost the characteristic cross-banding pattern. Entire fibers were depolymerized into thin fibrils and amorphous, electron-dense material had occasionally accumulated [53]. Penetration of tumor cells through the entire cartilage disk was not observed during the time course of the experiment.

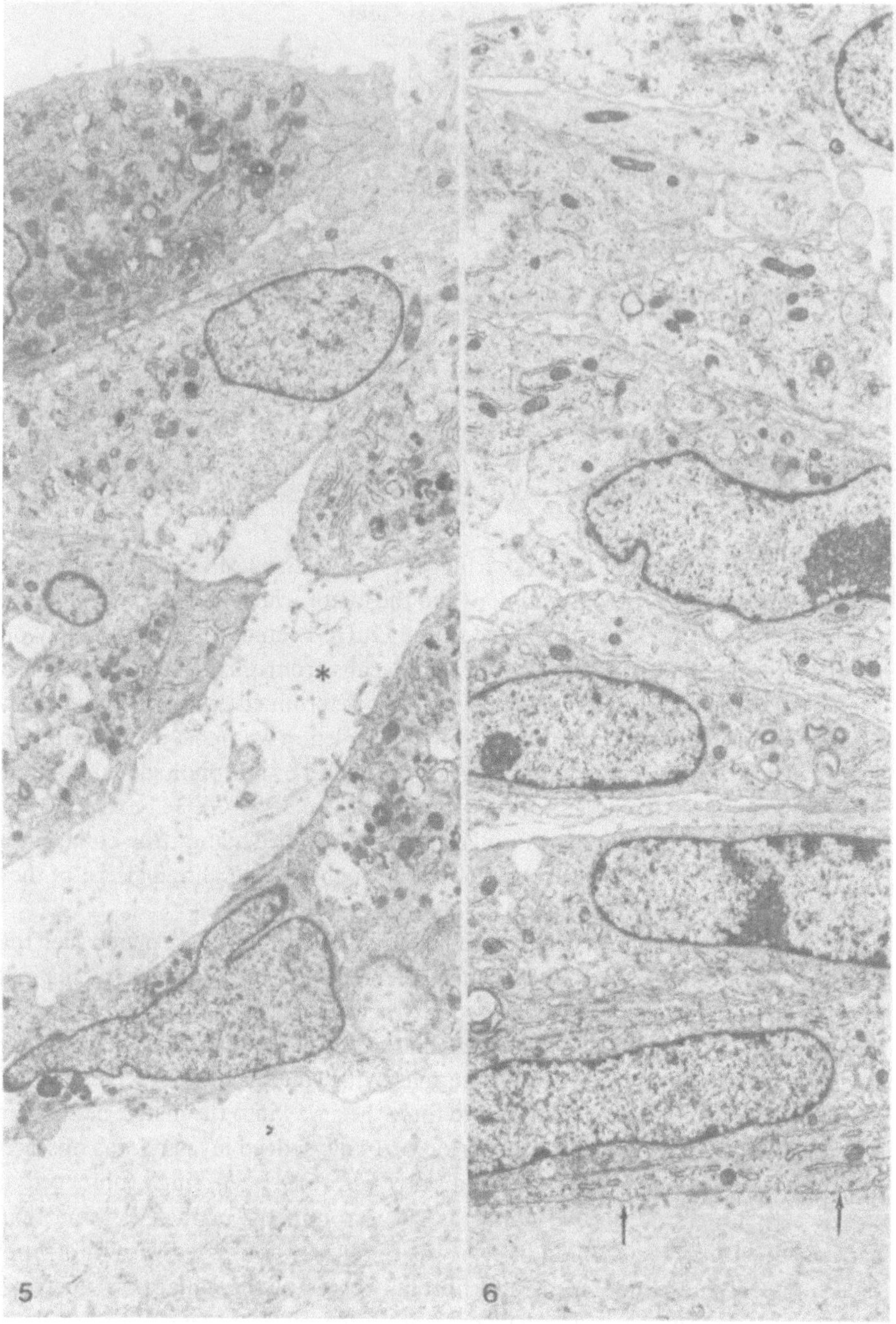

Figure 5. TE-85 osteosarcoma cells grown on 3M GuHCl-extracted articular cartilage penetrate deeply into the carilagenous matrix. Penetration of cells is associated with rarefaction (asterisk) of the matrix and widening of the interfibrillar space of the cartilagenous network. × 3 700.

Figure 6. Foreskin fibroblasts are unable to penetrate the 3 M GuHCl-extracted cartilage. × 5 200.

Fibroblasts behaved as non-invasive cells on both 1 M and 3 M GuHCl-extracted cartilage. They covered the surface irregularities of the disks without showing any signs of penetration into the tissue (Figure 6). Similar observations were made when tumor cells or control cells were cultured on normal, viable hyaline articular cartilage, or devitalized, unextracted cartilage. Although cells grew in large numbers in intimate contact with the cartilage matrix, there was no evidence of matrix destruction and invasion, as determined by electron microscopy of random samples (Figure 1).

The observation that salt-extracted, devitalized cartilage could be penetrated by malignant tumor cells, yet was non-permissive to fibroblastic ingrowth led us to postulate that hyaline cartilage contained extractable matrix components that inhibited invasion in an experimental system [39, 41, 44, 53, 54]. Large scale extractions of hyaline cartilage, were therefore performed in order to analyze the extractable substances for their effect on the invasive apparatus of malignant tumor cells.

4. Cartilage-derived anti-invasive factor

4.1. Isolation and biochemical characterization

The isolation proceedures for anti-invasion factor (AIF) is standard and has been described in detail elsewhere [37, 38, 49, 50, 64]. Slices of fresh hyaline cartilage prepared from the nasal septa of 18-month-old bovines were extracted with 1 M NaCl (0.05 M sodium acetate, pH 5.8; 24 h; 4° C). The extract was decanted from the tissue and adjusted to 3 M NaCl by adding solid NaCl, in order to minimize non-specific protein-protein interactions. Ultrafiltration of the crude cartilage extracts yielded two fractions (Figure 7): (1) The XM-50 retentate (MW $>$50 000), and after dialysis and concentration, (2) The UM-2 retentate, designated as anti-invasion factor (AIF) (1 000 $<$MW $<$50 000). The XM-50 retentate contained the majority of the proteins as indicated by standard biochemical analyses (uronic acid, hexose, and hydroxyproline). In contrast, AIF contained only about 40 μg protein per gram tissue, with mininal amounts of uronic acid, hexose, and hydroxyproline. SDS-PAGE revealed that the AIF consisted of seven major protein bands (Figure 8). The protein with the highest molecular weight comigrated with serum albumin (MW 69 000). Immunologically identified albumin was present in this preparation due to its incomplete rejection by the XM-50 membrane, as indicated by the manufacturer (Amicon Corp.). The protein with the lowest molecular weight migrated between Trasylol^{R} (MW 6 500) and insulin (MW 5 700).

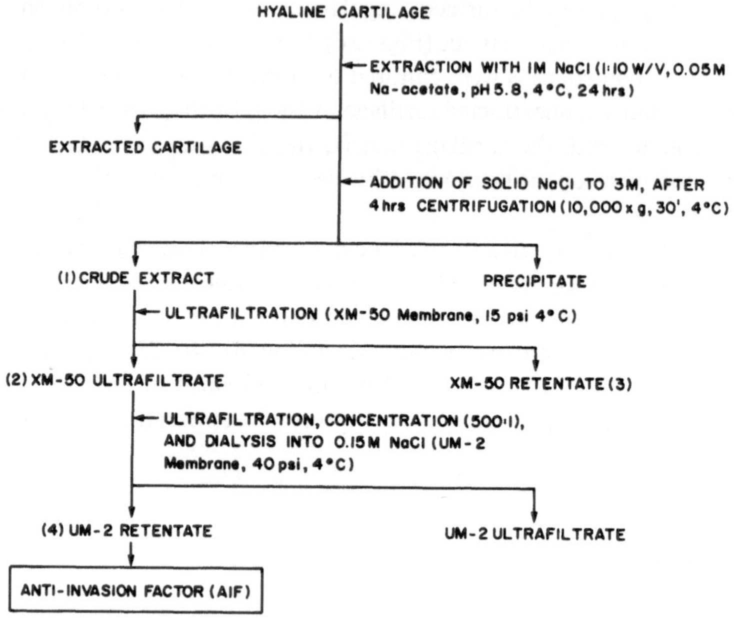

Figure 7. Flow-chart for the isolation of anti-invasion factor (AIF) from hyaline cartilage (for details see text).

4.2. Inhibition by AIF of invasion into extracted cartilage

Treatment of hyaline cartilage with 1 M and 3 M GuHCl depleted the matrix of AIF and the extractable proteoglycan pool and caused the loss of the natural resistance to invasion [39, 41, 53, 54]. If, as we had postulated, AIF and not some altered physical condition was the responsible factor for this behavior, the addition of AIF to the extracted cartilage would theoretically restore resistance to invasion. In a series of experiments, TE-85 osteosarcoma cells were plated onto 3 M GuHCl-extracted, devitalized cartilage discs as described above, and AIF (100 μg/ml) was added [41, 53]. Morphology and growth behavior of TE-85 osteosarcoma cells and human foreskin fibroblasts were indistinguishable from those of the corresponding cells grown on viable, unextracted articular cartilage in the absence of AIF (Figure 9). Tumor cells grew in one to three cell layers on the surfaces of the extracted cartilage. They were characterized by abundant rough endoplasmic reticulum, prominent Golgi zones, and numerous, randomly dispersed polyribosomes. Tumor cells growing in contact with the cartilage surfaces only occasionally contained microvilli which penetrated into the cartilage matrix. There was no morphologic evidence of matrix destruction or tumor cell invasion [53]. Fibroblasts showed no signs of invasion, yet were stimulated by AIF to produce large amounts of extracellular matrix (Figure 10). These data provide strong evidence that the resistance

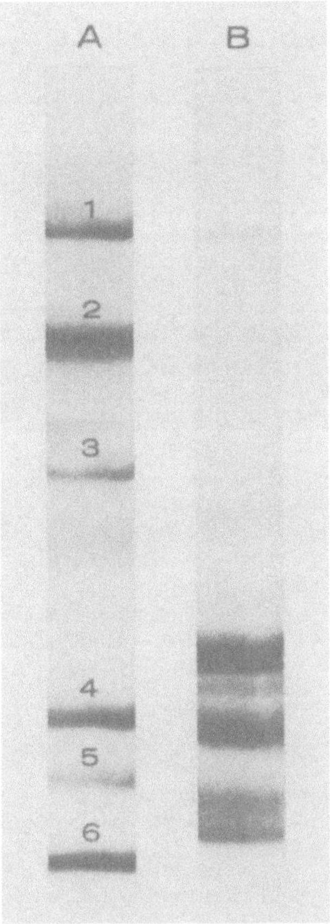

Figure 8. SDS-PAGE shows the following protein standards (column A): (1) albumin, MW 69 000; (2) ovalbumin, MW 43 000; (3) chymotrypsinogen A, MW 25 000; (4) lysozyme, MW 14 400; (5) Trasylol^{R}, MW 6 500; (6) insulin, MW 5 700; and AIF (column B). AIF consists of 7 major protein bands. The protein with the highest MW comigrates with serum albumin [1]. The protein with the lowest MW migrates between Trasylol^{R} [5] and insulin [6].

of cartilage to tumor invasion is regulated by an extractable, low molecular weight factor which specifically inhibits the degradation of matrix macromolecules and thus prevents penetration of tumor cells into cartilagenous matrices, even in the absence of potential masking effects provided by the extracted proteoglycans.

4.3. *Proteinase inhibitory activity*

The anti-invasion factor derived from bovine hyaline cartilage expresses inhibitory activity against a variety of proteinases. Kuettner et al. [37, 45, 52] and Sorgente et al. [46] have shown that AIF contained cationic protein fractions which possessed

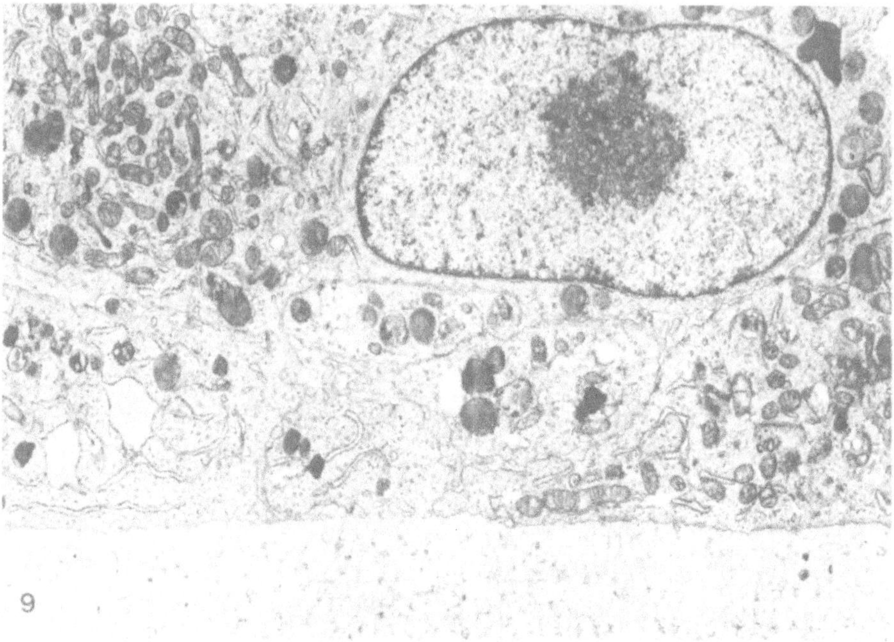
9

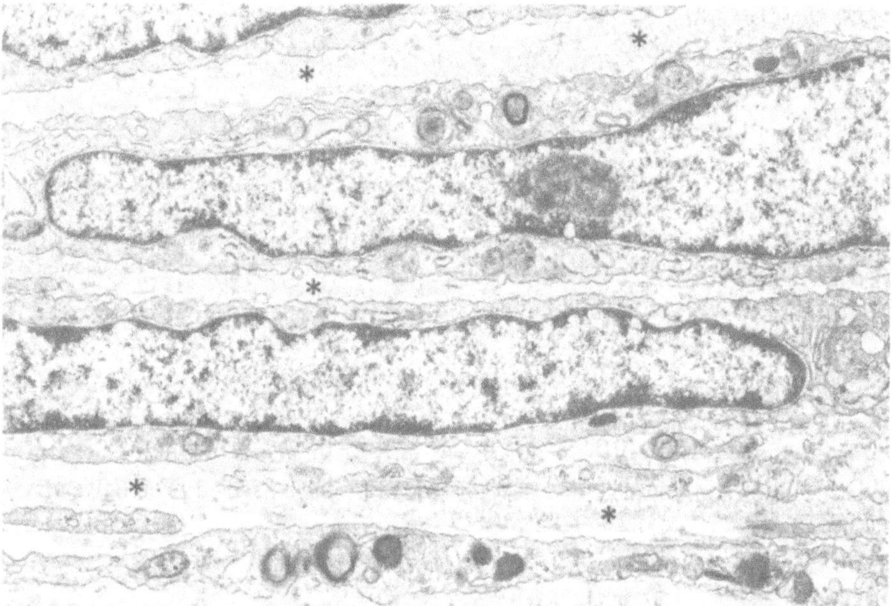
10

inhibitory activities directed against both commercially supplied trypsin and mammalian collagenases which had been derived from human skin or conditioned media of TE-85 osteosarcoma cells or human mammary carcinoma cells. At a concentration of 100 μg/ml, AIF inhibited trypsin activity in a manner similar to that observed for 250 μg/ml of the Trasylol^R standard, as determined by a fibrin agar diffusion method [45, 46]. Collagenase inhibitory activity was measured with a standard fibril assay, utilizing thermally reconstituted, trypsin-resistant fibrils of (^{14}C)-glycine labelled skin collagen derived from guinea pigs. Concentrated conditioned media (50:1) of TE-85 osteosarcoma cells were used as sources of tumor collagenase [37]. A proteinase inhibitory fraction of AIF significantly inhibited this collagenolytic activity. It was suggested that the inhibitory activities against both trypsin and collagenase were due to a single protein that had a molecular weight of approximately 11 000 dalton. Roughley et al. [65] subsequently showed that the inhibitors of trypsin and mammalian collagenase resided in distinct molecules, and that bovine nasal cartilage also contained a third inhibitor directed against the thiol proteinases cathepsin B and papain. By gel chromatography, the inhibitors of collagenases, thiol proteinases, and trypsin were eluted as though they had molecular weights of approximately 20 000, 13 000, and 7 000 dalton, respectively. A trypsin inhibitor appeared at the same elution volume as the commercially supplied basic pancreatic trypsin inhibitor (Trasylol^R). It resembled Trasylol^R with respect to molecular weight [65–67], amino acid composition [66], antigenicity [66], and range of susceptible proteinases [45, 46, 65–68]. Susceptible proteinases were trypsin [45, 46, 65–67], chymotrypsin [45, 46, 65–67], plasmin [66], proteoglycans-degrading enzymes derived from human leucocyte extracts [47, 67], and tumor cell surface-associated neutral proteinases [68]. The similarity between the cartilage-derived trypsin inhibitor and Trasylol^R motivated these investigators to postulate that Trasylol^R and the cartilage-derived trypsin inhibitor were identical, and that the presence of Trasylol^R in cartilage could be due to synthesis by chondrocytes, or to uptake from the blood plasma [65]. The latter hypothesis seemed especially intriguing given the fact that highly anionic molecules of the cartilage matrix (i.e. the glycosaminoglycans-containing proteoglycan [10] may act as a sponge for the low-molecular-weight, highly cationic molecules which naturally occur in small quantities in the blood plasma. By this mechanism Trasylol^R could be continuously removed from the blood plasma and accumulated in hyaline cartilage as this tissue

---

Figure 9. TE-85 osteosarcoma cells grown on 3 M GuHCl-extracted cartilage in AIF-containing medium are unable to penetrate the cartilagenous matrix. There is no morphologic evidence of matrix destruction. × 7 500.

Figure 10. Human foreskin fibroblasts exposed to AIF do not penetrate the 3 M GuHCl-extracted articular cartilage, yet are stimulated to produce enormous quantities of extracellular matrix (asterisk). × 12 000.

Table 1

A. Inhibition of type IV collagenolytic activity by AIF.

Treatment	Radioactivity in supernate	
	cpm	% Inhibition
Tumor type IV collagenolytic activity	1507 ± 40	0
Tumor type IV collagenolytic activity + AIF (40 μg/ml)	314 ± 38	79
Tumor type IV collagenolytic activity + EDTA (30 mM)	156 ± 24	90
Bacterial collagenase	1950 ± 80	

B. Inhibition of type V collagenolytic activity by AIF.

Treatment	Radioactivity in supernate	
	cpm	% Inhibition
Tumor type V collagenolytic activity	1894 ± 66	0
Tumor type V collagenolytic activity + AIF (40 μg/ml)	392 ± 28	79
Tumor type V collagenolytic activity + EDTA (30 mM)	75 ± 12	96
Bacterial collagenase	2008 ± 70	

For the standard assay of collagenase activity, 400 μl of the enzyme solution was activated with 100 μl of trypsin (100 μl/ml; 3 times crystallized, Sigma) at 37° C for 4 min, followed by addition of 100 μl of soybean trypsin inhibitor (500 μg/ml, Sigma). The substrate (^{14}C-proline labeled type IV collagen derived from metastatic murine PMT sarcoma or type V collagen derived from murine M-5076 reticulum cell sarcoma; 2000 cpm) was added in 50 μl of 0.05 M Tris-HCl, pH 7.6, containing 0.2 M NaCl and 5 mM $CaCl_2$. The final volume was 650 μl. The reaction was carried out for 4 h at 37° C and stopped by addition of 20 μl of bovine serum albumin (1 mg/ml) and 100 μl of a solution of 10% trichloroacetic acid (TCA), and 0.5% tannic acid (TA) to a final concentration of 2% TCA and 0.1% TA. The mixture was incubated for 30 min at 4° C and centrifuged at 5000 xg for 15 min at 4° C to remove undigested material. Aliquots of 400 μl of the supernatent, containing digested products, were dissolved in 10 ml of Aquasol (Amersham) and counted for radioactivity in a Beckman scintillation counter [81, 82].

AIF was added to the enzyme assay at a concentration of 40 μg/ml. Control experiments included type IV collagenolytic activity with EDTA (30 mM), and bacterial collagenase.

ages. However, preliminary data obtained in our laboratory indicate that Trasylol^{R} is synthesized by bovine articular chondrocytes in culture.

The cartilage-derived thiol proteinase inhibitor described by Roughley et al. [65]

corresponds to the thiol proteinase inhibitors isolated from chick egg-white [69], rabbit skin [70, 71], and rat skin [72, 73]. These inhibitors were reported to have similar thermal stabilities and molecular weights, and thus might be identical. Inhibitory activities were detected against both cathepsin B and papain. In each case the degree of inhibition increased linearly with the concentration of the inhibitor to complete inhibition.

The collagenase inhibitory activity has been shown to produce a single chromatographic fraction with a molecular weight of about 22 000 dalton on Ultragel AcA54 [65]. Its electrophoretic mobility and molecular weight appeared different from those of the collagenase inhibitors in serum [19, 20, 75] and polymorphonuclear leukocytes [76], and from that of the collagenase inhibitors synthesized in cultures by various explants from animal tissues [77–79]. In contrast to these collagenase inhibitors, the cartilage-derived collagenase inhibitory activity resists thiol binding reagents, and inhibits leukocyte-specific collagenase [80].

In collaboration with Dr. L.A. Liotta, we have recently shown that the cartilage-derived anti-invasion factor also expressed strong inhibitory activities against the neutral metalloproteinases which cleave basement membrane collagens of types IV and V [81, 82]. In a pilot experiment using AIF at a concentration of 40 μg/ml type IV collagenolytic activity derived from metastatic murine PMT sarcomas was inhibited by approximately 80%. A similar degree of inhibition was observed for type V collagenolytic activity derived from metastatic murine M-5076 reticulum cell sarcoma (Table 1).

The spectrum of proteinase inhibitors which is present in extracts of bovine hyaline cartilage may play a significant role in the regulation of tumor invasiveness. The inhibition of major classes of matrix-degrading enzymes may prevent destruction and penetration of host connective tissue barriers by malignant tumor cells, i.e. epithelial and endothelial basement membranes. On the basis of their small molecular size, cartilage-derived proteinase inhibitors may have relatively free access to most tissue sites from which the potent, serum-derived proteinase inhibitor α2-macroglobulin is excluded due to its large molecular size [20].

4.4. Anti-proliferative activity

The cartilage-derived anti-invasion factor (AIF) possesses a strong anti-proliferative activity which is directed against bovine aortic endothelial cells in culture [39, 41, 50, 51, 83]. AIF inhibits the proliferation of these cells in a dose-dependent manner as evidenced by both cell counts and ^{3}H-thymidine incorporation (Figure 11). At a concentration of 100 μg AIF/1 ml culture medium, the anti-proliferative activity inhibits cell proliferation by 80–90%. Sorgente and Dorey [83] have recently isolated and partially purified the endothelial cell growth inhibitor from the AIF of bovine scapular hyaline cartilage by ion exchange chromatography on CM-Sephadex C-25. They observed two peaks of endothelial cell inhibitory activity. Each was eluted

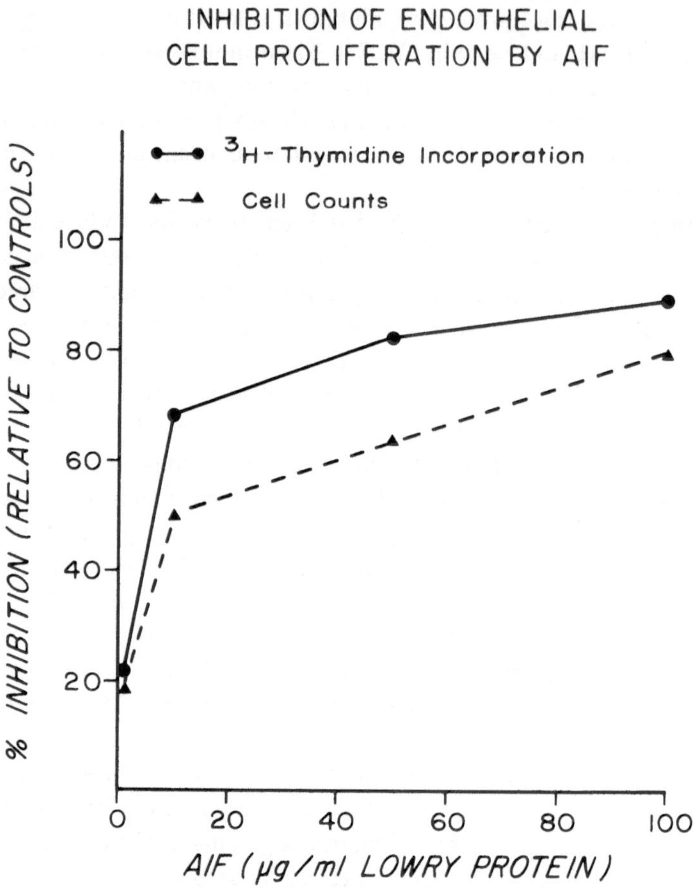

Figure 11. AIF inhibits the proliferation of bovine aortic endothelial cells in a dose-dependent manner, as determined by ^{3}H-thymidine incorporation and cell counts of triplicate cultures.

in a position separated from a peak of trypsin inhibitory activity. The first peak, which was reported to contain about 90% of the total inhibitory activity, appeared immediately before the trypsin inhibitor, while the second peak appeared after the trypsin inhibitor. The endothelial cell growth inhibitor (2 μg/ml) is non-toxic. It increased the doubling time of endothelial cell cultures from 24 h to 40 h. Their findings suggested that the anti-proliferative activity arrested endothelial cells in Gl phase. AIF had no anti-proliferative effects against adult fibroblasts or smooth muscle cells [41, 50, 53].

4.5. Anti-angiogenic activity

Using the rabbit cornea as an assay system, Folkman and his associates showed that neovascularization of tumors could be inhibited when a small piece of viable hyaline cartilage was positioned between the tumor implant and the corneoscleral junction [84–86]. Vessels which normally grew rapidly towards the corneal tumor implant, proliferated at extremely show rates. At the end of the second week, they had only reached half of the distance which they had reached during the first week in the control experiments [85, 86]. A diffusable factor, isolated from a 1 M GuHCl-extract of bovine scapular cartilage, was recognized to be responsible for the inhibition of the tumor-induced vascular proliferation [85]. This factor is probably identical to the anti-invasion factor (AIF) previously described by Kuettner and associates [39, 41, 48, 49, 50, 51]. Biochemical data and studies with endothelial cell cultures inidicate that the anti-proliferative activity in AIF may correspond to the anti-angiogenic activity described by Folkman et al. [41]. This factor appears to have a direct effect on the cell cycle of endothelial cells, and may therefore be an antagonist to tumor angiogenesis factor [83].

4.6. *Morphologic changes of AIF-exposed tumor cells in vitro*

The effect of cartilage-derived AIF on human osteosarcoma cells *in vitro* was studied by scanning electron microscopy, according to the methods of Pauli et al. [87]. Osteosarcoma cells (5×10^4 cells) were plated on Thermanox^R plastic cover slips (24 × 36 mm) and preincubated for 6 h in RPMI-1640 culture medium containing 10% fetal bovine serum and antibiotics. After washing the cells, some cultures were exposed for 24 or 48 h to 100 μg/ml of AIF in the culture medium, others were cultured for identical periods in medium without AIF. In unexposed cultures, osteosarcoma cells were flat, fully spread, and showed several lamellae (Figure 12). In cultures exposed for 24 h to AIF, some osteosarcoma cells appeared retracted and resumed a spindly or stellate shape, with numerous, delicate, thread-like cytoplasmic processes extending to the area these cells had occupied before exposure to AIF (Figure 13) [41]. Both unexposed and exposed cells were covered by pleomorphic microvilli. After 48 h of exposure to AIF, more osteosarcoma cells had undergone this shape transformation. Migration was greatly inhibited in shape-transformed cells. Microvilli of a few cells appeared clumped, and there were occasional cytoplasmic blebs. Cell lysis was not observed. These changes were reversible when AIF was removed from the growth medium. These observations suggested that AIF inhibited spreading and locomotion on the plastic growth surface.

4.7. *Inhibition of tumor growth in vivo*

Pilot experiments show that cartilage-derived AIF significantly inhibits the growth of transplantable tumors in rats when injected systemically [38]. Six weanling rats

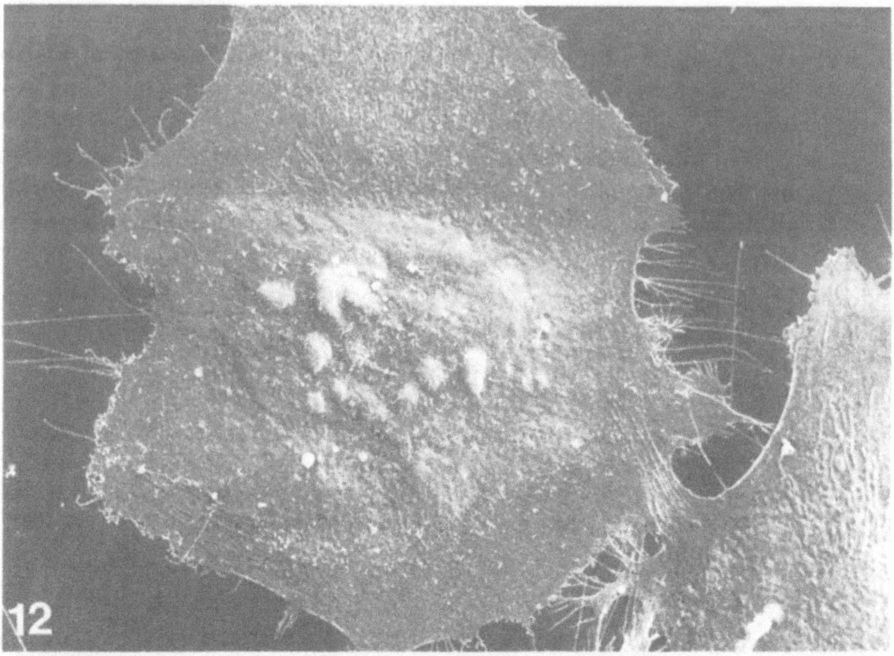

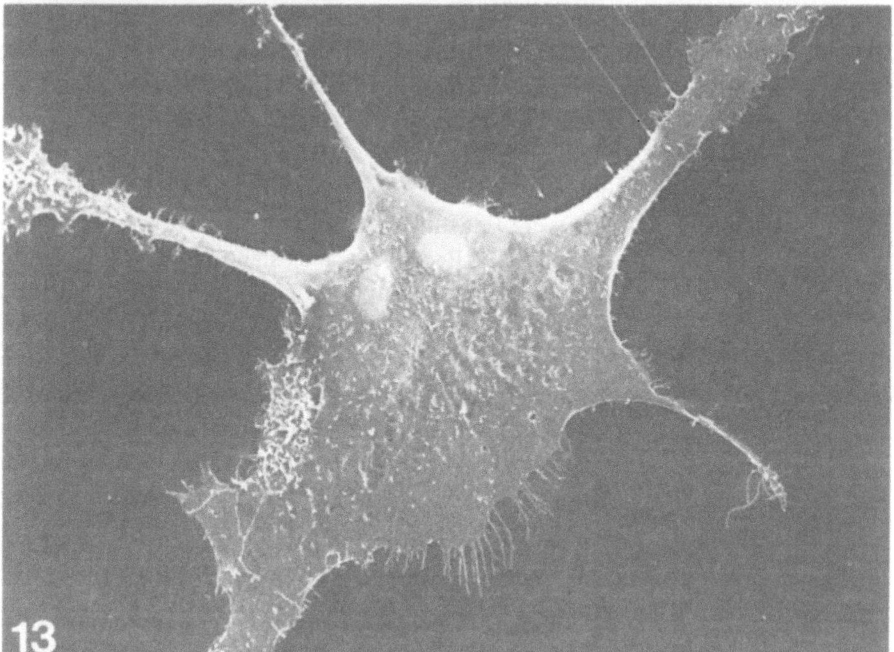

Figure 12. TE-85 osteosarcoma cell spreads extensively on plastic coverslip and shows several lamellae. SEM. × 1 100.

Figure 13. TE-85 osteosarcoma cell exposed for 24 h to 100 μg/ml of AIF appears stellar and displays delicate cytoplasmic processes. Migration is greatly diminished. SEM. × 1 300.

were injected with 1×10^5 herpes simplex virus-transformed rat fibroblasts. Three of the six rats were treated by intraperitoneal injections of 1 mg of AIF in 1 ml of a 0.9% NaCl solution. The remaining three rats received an equal volume of a 0.9% saline solution without AIF. After 3 weeks, AIF-treated and control rats were sacrificed, and tumors were excised and weighed. In the AIF-treated animals, tumors weighed 1.97 ± 0.52 ($\pm$ S.E.) g. In contrast, tumors in control rats weighed 7.37 ± 1.69 g ($p < 0.05$). Histologically, tumors of AIF-treated rats were surrounded by significantly thicker fibrous capsules than those of control rats. This finding may correspond to the observation that fibroblasts exposed to AIF *in vitro* are surrounded by excessive extracellular matrix. In AIF-treated rats, greater numbers of tumor cells showed severe nuclear abnormalities (i.e. chromatin clumping, karyorrhexis, karyolysis), and there were fewer mitotic figures. Non-tumorous host tissues showed no evidence of cytotoxic reactions to AIF. Epithelia with rapid cell turnover, such as those of the intestinal tract, appeared unaffected (Pauli and Kuettner, unpublished data).

The presumed effector molecules in these experiments reside in the anti-proteolytic activity and the anti-proliferative activity of AIF [38]. The anti-angiogenic activity of AIF was difficult to assess by the routine histologic techniques applied in these pilot experiments. It appeared however, that tumors in both animal groups were equally well vascularized.

4.8. Anti-invasion factor derived from other connective tissues

By adapting the proceedures established in our work on cartilage-derived AIF, similar low-molecular-weight factors were prepared from extracts of other tissues (i.e. bovine aorta, bovine heart valves, and bovine urinary bladder mucosa and submucosa). The aortic factor has been characterized in several publications by Eisenstein and his associates [38, 46, 88]. These investigators reported that the aortic factor inhibited (a) the growth of bovine aortic endothelial cells and embryonic fibroblasts *in vitro*; (b) tryptic as well as chymotryptic activities, as demonstrated in a fibrin-agar diffusion assay; (c) collagenases prepared from tadpole or human skin; and (d) tumor growth in culture, as well as in animal hosts after systemic injection [38].

A low-molecular-weight factor with similar biological activities has recently been isolated from extracts of bovine urinary bladder mucosa and submucosa [89]. This factor expresses strong proteinase inhibitory activity against trypsin, and to a lesser extent against chymotrypsin. The trypsin-inhibitory activity co-migrated electrophoretically with that of Trasylol^R, but not with bovine serum proteinase inhibitory activities. The bladder-derived factor caused inhibition of bovine aortic endothelial cells, as determined by cell counts and ^{3}H-thymidine incorporation. Similar to the cartilage-derived AIF, it had no effect on normal adult fibroblasts derived from human or rat skin.

5. Conclusions

In this experimental series, we have provided evidence that the resistance of cartilage to tumor invasion may be due to an extractable, low-molecular-weight factor, functionally defined as anti-invasion factor (AIF) [39, 41]. This factor contains the following anti-invasive activities: (1) proteinase (collagenase) inhibitory activity; (2) anti-proliferative and anti-migratory activities directed against endothelial cells (anti-angiogenic activity); and (3) tumor growth inhibitory activity. These activities occur in the low-molecular-weight ($1\,000 < MW < 50\,000$) protein fraction of a 1 M NaCl-extract of hyaline cartilage or, as shown only recently, in chondrocyte cultures established from bovine articular cartilage (Kuettner and Pauli, unpublished data). They may well act as local regulators for some of the major mechanistic pathways by which tumor cells are thought to invade host tissues and metastasize to distant sites, namely by matrix-degrading enzymes and increased locomotion [2, 3, 5, 39, 41]. In addition, they may inhibit tumor neovascularization [84] and control local tumor growth [38]. On the basis of their small molecular size, they are proposed to have relatively free access to most tissue sites, thus increasing their efficacy [20]. The various protein fractions found in cartilage-derived AIF are currently purified and biochemically characterized in our laboratories.

Acknowledgements

Appreciation is expressed to the research assistants who are presently involved with the research concerning the cartilage-derived, anti-invasion factor: Mr. S. Anderson, Mrs. Shu-Yuan Chi, Mr. R. Croxen, Mr. G. Gall, Mr. L. Madsen, Ms. C. Sanes-Miller, and Mrs. N. Wrobel. The authors wish to thank Drs. R.S. Weinstein, J.O. Galante, and J.C. Daniel for helpful discussions and advice during the investigations, and Ms. C. Sanes-Miller for preparing and reviewing the manuscript.

This work was supported by NIH grants CA-21566 and CA-25034, and in part by grants AM-09132 and R-1206 from the Council for Tobacco Reserach-USA, Inc.

References

1. Fidler IJ: Tumor heterogeneity and the biology of cancer invasion and metastasis. Cancer Res 38:2651–2660, 1978.
2. Fidler IJ, Gersten DM, Hart IR: The biology of cancer invasion and metastasis. Adv Cancer Res 28:149–250, 1978.
3. Hart IR, Fidler IJ: Cancer invasion and metastasis. Q Rev Biol 55:121–142, 1980.
4. Poste G, Fidler IJ: The pathogenesis of cancer metastasis. Nature 283:139–146, 1980.
5. Sträuli P: A concept of tumor invasion. In: Proteinases and tumor invasion, Strauli P, Barrett AJ, Baici A (eds). New York: Raven Press, 1980, pp 1–13.
6. Miller EJ: Biochemical characteristics and biological significance of the genetically distinct collagen. Mol Cell Biochem 13:165–192, 1976.
7. Kefalides NA, Alper R, Clark CC: Biochemistry and metabolism of basement membranes. Int Rev Cytol 61:167–228, 1979.

8. Prokop DJ, Kivirikko KI, Tuderman L, Guzman NA: The biosynthesis of collagen and its disorders. N Engl J Med 301:13–23, 1979.
9. Bornstein P, Sage H: Structurally distinct collagen types. Annu Rev Biochem 49:957–1003, 1980.
10. Hascall VC: Interaction of cartilage proteoglycans with hyaluronic acid. J Supramol Struct 7:101–120, 1977.
11. Sandberg LB: Elastin structure in health and disease. In: International review of connective tissue research, Vol 7, Hall DA, Jackson DS (eds). New York: Academic Press, 1976, pp 160–210.
12. Birbeck MSC, Wheatley DN: An electron microscopic study of the invasion of ascites tumor cells into the abdominal wall. Cancer Res 25:490–497, 1965.
13. Hashimoto K, Yamanishi Y, Dabbous MK: Electron microscopic observations of collagenolytic activity of basal cell epithelioma of the skin *in vivo* and *in vitro*. Cancer Res 32:2561–2567, 1972.
14. Strauch L: The role of collagenases in tumor invasion. In: Tissue interactions in carcinogenesis, Tarin D (ed). New York: Academic Press, 1972, pp 399–433.
15. Willis RA: The spread of tumors in the human body. Third ed. London: Butterworths, 1973.
16. Harris ED, Jr, Krane SM: Collagenases. N Engl J Med 291:557–563, 605–652, 1974.
17. Gross J: Aspects of animal collagenases. In: Biochemistry of collagen, Ramachandran GN, Reddi AH (eds). New York: Plenum Press, 1976, pp 275–317.
18. Bauer EA, Gordon JM, Reddick ME, Eisen AZ: Quantitation and immunocytochemical localization of human skin collagenase in basal cell carcinoma. J Invest Dermatol 69:363–367, 1977.
19. Wooley DE, Tetlow LC, Evanson JM: Collagenase immunolocalization studies of rheumatoid and malignant tissues. In: Collagenase in normal and pathological connective tissues. Woolley DE, Evanson JM (eds). Chichester: Wileys, 1980, pp 105–125.
20. Woolley DE, Tetlow LC, Mooney CJ, Evanson JM: Human collagenase and its extracellular inhibitors in relation to tumor invasiveness. In: Proteinases and tumor invasion, Sträuli P, Barrett AJ, Baici A (eds). New York: Raven Press, 1980, pp 97–113.
21. Robertson DM, Williams DC: *In vitro* evidence of neutral collagense activity in an invasive mammalian tumor. Nature 221:259–260, 1969.
22. Fiszer-Szafarz B, Gullino PM: Hyaluronidase activity of normal and neoplastic interstitial fluid. Proc Soc Exp Biol Med 133:805–807, 1970.
23. Taylor AC, Levy BM, Simpson JW: Collagenolytic activity of sarcoma tissue in culture. Nature 228:366–367, 1970.
24. Dresden MH, Heilman SA, Schmidt JD: Collagenolytic enzymes in human neoplasms. Cancer Res 32:993–996, 1972.
25. Harris ED, Jr, Faulkner CS, Wood S, Jr: Collagenase in carcinoma cells. Biochem Biophys Res Commun 48:1247–1253, 1972.
26. Hashimoto K, Yamanishi Y, Maeyens E, Dabbous MK, Kanzaki T: Collagenolytic activities of squamous-cell carcinoma of skin. Cancer Res 33:2790–2801, 1973.
27. Yamanishi Y, Maeyens E, Dabbous MK, Ohyama H, Hashimoto K: Collagenolytic activity in malignant melanoma: physicochemical studies. Cancer Res 33:2507–2512, 1973.
28. Abramson M, Schilling RW, Huang CC, Salome RG: Collagenase activity in epidermoid carcinoma of the oral cavity and larynx. Ann Otol Rhinol Laryngol 84:158–163, 1975.
29. McCroskery PA, Richards JF, Harris ED, Jr: Purification and characterization of collagenase extracted from rabbit tumors. Biochem J 152:131–142, 1975.
30. Hatcher VB, Wertheim MS, Rhee CY, Tsien G, Burk PG: Relationship between cell surface protease activity and doubling time in various normal and transformed cells. Biochim Biophys Acta 451:499–510, 1976.
31. Liotta LA, Kleinerman J, Catanzaro P, Rynbrandt D: Degradation of basement membrane collagen by murine tumor cells. J Natl Cancer Inst 58:1427–1431, 1977.
32. Biswas C, Moran WP, Bloch KJ, Gross J: Collagenolytic activity of rabbit V_2-carcinoma growing at multiple sites. Biochem Biophys Res Commun 80:33–38, 1978.
33. Poole AR, Tiltman KJ, Recklies AD, Stoker TAM: Differences in secretion of the proteinase

cathepsin B at the edges of human breast carcinomas and fibroadenomas. Nature 273:545–547, 1978.
34. Wirl G, Frick J: Collagenase-A marker enzyme in human bladder cancer? Urol Res 7;103–108, 1979.
35. Gross J, Highberger JH, Johnson-Wint B, Biswas C: Mode of action and regulation of tissue collagenases. In: Collagenase in normal and pathological connective tissues, Wooley DE, Evanson JM (eds). Chichester: Wiley, 1980, pp 11–35.
36. Liotta LA, Tryggvason K, Garbisa S, Hart I, Foltz CM, Shafie S: Metastatic potential correlates with enzymic degradation of basement membrane collagen. Nature 284:67–68, 1980.
37. Kuettner KE, Soble L, Croxen RL, Marczynska B, Hiti J, Harper E: Tumor cell collagenase and its inhibition by cartilage-derived protease inhibitor. Science 196:653–654, 1977.
38. Eisenstein R, Schumacher B, Meineke C, Matijevitch B, Kuettner KE: Growth regulators in connective tissue. Systematic administration of an aortic extract inhibits tumor growth in mice. Am J Pathol 91:1–10, 1978.
39. Kuettner KE, Pauli BU: Resistance of cartilage to normal and neoplastic invasion. In: Proceedings, mechanisms of localized bone loss. Horton JE, Tarpley TM, Davis WF (eds). Special Supplement to Calcified Tissue Abstracts, 1978, pp 251–278.
40. Baugh RJ, Schnebli HP: Role and potential therapeutic value of proteinase inhibitors in tissue destruction. In: Proteinases and tumor invasion, Sträuli P, Barrett AJ, Baici A (eds). New York: Raven Press, 1980, pp 157–179.
41. Kuettner KE, Pauli BU: Resistance of cartilage to invasion. In: Bone metastasis, Weiss L, Gilbert HA (eds). Boston: G.K. Hall, 1981, pp 131–165.
42. Spjut HJ, Fechner RE, Ackerman LV: Tumors of the bone and cartilage, Washington D.C., Armed Forces Institute of Pathology, 1971.
43. Del Regato JA, Spjut HJ: Ackerman and del Regato's cancer, diagnosis, treatment, and prognosis. St. Louis: C.V. Mosby, 1977.
44. Kuettner KE, Pauli BU, Soble L: Morphological studies on the resistance of cartilage to invasion by osteosarcoma cells *in vitro* and *in vivo*. Cancer Res 38:277–287, 1978.
45. Kuettner KE, Croxen RL, Eisenstein R, Sorgente N: Proteinase inhibitor activity in connective tissues. Experientia 30:595–597, 1974.
46. Sorgente N, Kuettner KE, Eisenstein R: The isolation, purification and partial characterization of proteinase inhibitors from bovine cartilage and aorta. In: Proceedings of the 23rd colloquium on protides of the biological fluids, Peeters H (ed). Oxford: Pergamon Press, 1976, pp 227–230.
47. Kuettner KE, Harper EJ, Eisenstein R: Protease inhibitors in cartilage. Arthritis Rheum 20 (supplement):S124–S129, 1977.
48. Eisenstein R, Sorgente N, Soble LW, Miller A, Kuettner KE: The resistance of certain tissues to invasion: I. Penetrability of explanted tissues by vascularized mesenchyme. Am J Pathol 73:765–774, 1973.
49. Sorgente N, Kuettner KE, Soble LW, Eisenstein R: The resistance of certain tissues to invasion. II. Evidence for extractable factors in cartilage which inhibit invasion by vascularized mesenchyme. Lab Invest 32:217–222, 1975.
50. Eisenstein R, Kuettner KE, Neapolitan C, Soble LW, Sorgente N: The resistance of certain tissues to invasion. III. Cartilage extracts inhibit the growth of fibroblasts and endothelial cells in culture. Am J Pathol 81:337–348, 1975.
51. Eisenstein R, Kuettner KE, Soble LW, Sorgente N: Tissue inhibitors are cell growth regulators. In: Proceedings of the 23rd colloquium on protides of the biological fluids, Peeters H (ed). Oxford: Pergamon Press, 1976, pp 217–219.
52. Kuettner KE, Hiti J, Eisenstein R, Harper E: Collagenase inhibition by cationic proteins derived from cartilage and aorta. Biochem Biophys Res Commun 72:40–46, 1976.
53. Pauli BU, Memoli VA, Kuettner KE: Regulation of tumor invasion by cartilage-derived anti-invasion factor *in vitro*. J Natl Cancer Inst 67:65–73, 1981.
54. Pauli BU, Memoli VA, Kuettner KE: *In vitro* determination of tumor invasiveness using extracted

hyaline cartillage. Cancer Res 41:2084–2091, 1981.
55. Robbins SL, Cotran RS: Pathologic basis of disease. Philadelphia: W.B. Saunders, 1979, pp 1501–1505.
56. McKenna RJ, Schwinn CP, Soong KY, Higinbotham NL: Sarcomata of the oesteogenic series (osteosarcoma, fibrosarcoma, chondrosarcoma, parosteal osteogenic sarcoma and sarcomata arising in abnormal bone). An analysis of 552 cases. J Bone Joint Surg 48A:1–26, 1966.
57. Enneking WF, Kagan A: Transepiphyseal extension of osteosarcoma: incidence, mechanism and implications. Cancer 41:1526–1537, 1978.
58. Young MH: Changes in the growth cartilage resulting from ischemic necrosis of the metaphysis. J Pathol Bacteriol 85:481–488, 1963.
59. Spira E, Farin I: The vascular supply to the epiphyseal plate under normal and pathologic conditions. Acta Orthop Scand 38:1–22, 1967.
60. Fell HB, Thomas L: The influence of hydrocortisone on the action of excess vitamin A on limb bone rudiments in culture. J Exp Med 114:343–361, 1961.
61. McAllister RM, Gardner MB, Greene AE, Bradt C, Nichols WW, Landing BH: Cultivation *in vitro* of cells derived from a human osteosarcoma. Cancer 27:397–402, 1971.
62. Jones PA, DeClerck YA: Destruction of extracellular matrices containing glycoproteins, elastin, and collagen by metastatic human tumor cells. Cancer Res 40:3222–3227, 1980.
63. Kuettner KE, Soble LW, Sorgente N, Eisenstein R: The possible role of protease inhibitors in cartilage metabloism. In: Proceedings of the 23rd colloquim on protides of the biological fluids, Peeters H (ed). Oxford: Pergamon Press, 1976, pp 221–225.
64. Horton JE, Wezeman FN, Kuettner KE: Inhibition of bone resorption *in vitro* by a cartilage-derived anti-collagenase factor. Science 199:1342–1345, 1978.
65. Roughley PJ, Murphy G, Barrett AJ: Proteinase inhibitors of bovine nasal cartilage. Biochem J 169:721–724, 1978.
66. Rifkin DR, Crowe RM: Isolation of a proteinase inhibitor from tissues resistant to tumor invasion. Hoppe-Seyler's Z Physiol Chem 358:1525–1531, 1977.
67 Knight JA, Stephens RW, Bushell GR, Ghosh P, Taylor TKF: Neutral protease inhibitors from human intervertebral disc and femoral head articular cartilage. Biochim Biophys Acta 584:304–310, 1979.
68. Hatcher VB, Tsien G, Oberman MS, Burk PG: Inhibition of cell proliferation and protease activity by cartilage factors and heparin. J Supramol Struct 14:33–46, 1980.
69. Sen LC, Whitaker JR: Some properties of a ficin-papain inhibitor from avian egg white. Arch Biochim Biophys 158:623–632, 1973.
70. Udaka K, Hayashi H: Further purification of a protease inhibitor from rabbit skin with healing inflammation. Biochim Biophys Acta 97:251–261, 1965.
71. Udaka K, Hayashi H: Molecular-weight determination of a protease inhibitor from rabbit skin with healing inflammation. Biochim Biophys Acta 104:600–603, 1965.
72. Järvinen M, Hopsu-Havu VK: Alpha-N-benzoylarginine-2-naphthylamide hydrolase (cathepsin B_1?) from rat skin. II. Purification of the enzyme and demonstration of two inhibitors in the skin. Acta Chem Scand B 29:772–780, 1975.
73. Järvinen M: Purification and properties of two protease inhibitors from rat skin inhibiting papain and other SH-proteases. Acta Chem Scand B 30:933–940, 1976.
74. Wooley DE, Roberts DR, Evanson JM: Small molecular weight B_1 serum protein which specifically inhibits human collagenases. Nature 261:325–327, 1976.
75. Murphy G, Sellers A: The extracellular regulation of collagenase activity. In: Collagenase in normal and pathological connective tissues, Woolley DE, Evanson JM (eds). Chichester: Wiley, 1980, pp 65–81.
76. Kopitar M, Lebez D: Intracellular distribution of neutral proteinases and inhibitors in pig leucocytes. Eur J Biochem 56:571–581, 1975.
77. Murphy G, Cartwright EC, Sellers A, Reynolds JJ: The detection and characterization of collagen-

ase inhibitors from rabbit tissues in culture. Biochim Biophys Acta 483:493–498, 1977.
78. Sellers A, Reynolds JJ: Identification and partial characterization of an inhibitor of collagenase from rabbit bone. Biochem J 167:353–360, 1977.
79. Sellers A, Reynolds JJ, Meikle MC: Neutral metallo-proteinases of rabbit bone. Biochem J 171: 493–496, 1978.
80. Sellers A, Cartwright EC, Murphy G, Reynolds JJ: Evidence that latent collagenases are enzyme-inhibitor complexes. Biochem J 163:303–307, 1977.
81. Liotta LA, Tryggvason K, Garbisa S, Gehron-Robey P, Abe S: Partial purification and characterization of a neutral protease which cleaves type IV collagen. Biochemistry 20:100–104, 1981.
82. Liotta LA, Lanzer WL, Garbisa S: Identification of a type V collagenolytic enzyme. Biochem Biophys Res Comm 98:184–190, 1981.
83. Sorgente N, Dorey CK: Inhibition of endothelial cell growth by a factor isolated from cartilage. Exp Cell Res 128:63–71, 1980.
84. Brem H, Arensman R, Folkman J: Inhibition of tumor angiogenesis by a diffusable factor from cartilage. In: Extracellular matrix influences on gene expression, Slavkin HC, Greulich RC (eds). New York: Academic Press, 1975, pp 767–772.
85. Brem H, Folkman J: Inhibition of tumor angiogenesis mediated by cartilage. J Exp Med 141: 427–439, 1975.
86. Folkman J: Vascularization of tumors. Sci Am 234:59–73, 1976.
87. Pauli BU, Kuettner KE, Weinstein RS: Intercellular junctions in FANFT-induced carcinomas of rat urinary bladder in tissue culture: *in situ* thin-section, freeze-fracture, and scanning electron microscopy studies. J Microscopy 115:271–282, 1978.
88. Eisenstein R, Harper E, Kuettner KE, Schumacher B, Matijevitch B: Growth regulators in connective tissues. II. Evidence for the presence of several growth inhibitors in aortic extracts. Paroi Arterielle 5:163–170, 1979.
89. Waxler B, Kuettner KE, Memoli VA, Pauli BU: Anti-invasive factor(s) derived from bovine urinary bladder. J Cell Biol 87:116a, 1980.

17. Role of cell attachment proteins in defining cell-matrix interactions

H. K. KLEINMAN

Introduction

Recent studies indicate that most normal cells require an extracellular matrix for survival, proliferation, differentiation, and migration [for review see 1]. The components of a given matrix contain unique constituents including one or more genetically distinct collagens (Table 1) and proteoglycans (Table 2). In addition, cell- and matrix-specific glycoproteins such as fibronectin, laminin, and chondronectin (Table 3) are present as attachment factors to bind cells into the matrix. The matrix provides the structural support for the tissue, and the ability of a cell to adhere to the matrix determines which cells will be found in a tissue and controls how and when the cells will synthesize matrix, differentiate, and migrate.

In addition, matrix components, either alone or in concert, regulate the migration and state of differentiation of tumor cells. Transformed, tumorigenic, and metastatic cells have different characteristics from normal cells. Transformed cells are usually less adherent than normal cells, produce less collagen, and contain smaller amounts of attachment proteins on their surfaces [2–9]. The matrix surrounding tumor cells is often deranged [10], possibly because tumor cells often contain abnormally high collagenase activity and degrade excessive amounts of collagen [11]. In addition, metastatic cells produce a unique collagenase able to degrade basement membranes [12] and this may facilitate their ability to move from one site to another. Tumor cells often show a preference for attachment to type IV collagen and basement membranes [13, 14]. This chapter will outline our current knowledge of extracellular matrices with particular emphasis on the attachment proteins. Since the activity of these attachment factors is dependent on collagens and proteoglycans, these topics will be covered briefly.

Table 1. The collagens.

Type	Composition	Tissue location
I	$[\alpha1(I)]_2\alpha2(I)$	Skin, bone, tendon, dermis, cornea
II	$[\alpha1(II)]_3$	Cartilage, cornea, vitreous body
III	$[\alpha1(III)]_3$	Fetal skin, blood vessels, organs
IV	$[\alpha1(IV)]_3$	Basement membrane
	$[\alpha2(IV)]_3$	
V	$[\alpha1(V)]_2\alpha2V$	Blood vessels, smooth muscle

L.A. Liotta and I.R. Hart (eds.), Tumor Invasion and Metastasis. ISBN-13: 978-94-009-7513-2.
© 1982 Martinus Nijhoff Publishers, The Hague/Boston/London.

1. Attachment proteins

At present, three attachment glycoproteins [1], fibronectin [4–8], laminin [14, 15], and chondronectin [16, 17] have been isolated (Table 3) and others probably exist. These factors promote the adhesion of cells to their tissue-specific collagenous substrates *in vitro* (Table 4). Such interactions presumably contribute in part to cell sorting during embryogenesis and tissue formation.

1.1. Fibronectin

Fibronectin is a large glycoprotein found in abundance in serum (300 μg/ml), on

Table 2. The proteoglycans.

	Proteoglycan structure (or composition)			
Tissue	MW	Protein content	GAG type	GAG MW
Cartilage	1 500 000	10%	chondroitin	25 000
			keratan	10 000
Aorta	1 500 000	18%	chondroitin, dermatan	40 000
Basement membrane	750 000	40%	heparan	70 000
Corneal stroma	150 000	70%	chondroitin, dermatan	55 000
	75 000	70%	keratan	10 000
Mast cells	1 000 000	<10%	heparin	60–100 000

Table 3. The attachment proteins.

	Fibronectin	Laminin	Chondronectin
Molecular weight	450 000 ↓ reduction 220 000	1 000 000 ↓ reduction 220 000 ± 440 000	180 000 ↓ reduction 80 000
Amount required for cell attachment	1–5 μg	1–5 μg	5–50 ng
Amount in serum	~300 μg/ml	<1 μg/ml	<20 μg/ml
Heat lability	57°	49°	52°
Tissue location	Dermis, some basement membranes	Basement membranes	Cartilage, vitreous body
Collagen binding	III > I, II, IV > V	IV	II (cofactor required)
Proteoglycan binding	Heparin > hyaluronic acid	Heparin, heparan sulfate	Heparin, chondroitin sulfate

Table 4. Adhesion characteristics of cells.

Adhesion factor	Fibronectin	Laminin	Chondronectin
Collagen substrate	I, II, III, IV	IV	II
Cells	established cells such as CHO, 3T3, BHK etc. primary fibroblasts hepatocytes periosteal cells myoblasts smooth muscle cells osteosarcoma cells PMT (highly metastatic pulmonary tumor) cells	breast epithelial cells guinea pig epidermal cells pigmented epithelial cells vascular endothelial cells lens epithelial cells choroid epithelial cells parietal yolk sac cells EHS sarcoma cells TERA (transformed epidermal) cells PAM 212 (transformed epidermal) cells PMT (highly metastatic pulmonary tumor) cells	chondrocytes

cell surfaces, and in the extracellular matrix of connective tissues [4–8]. It constitutes approximately 1% of the total serum protein and can be isolated by collagen-Sepharose affinity chromatography [18] followed by a second purification procedure such as DEAE-cellulose column chromatography or by heparin-Sepharose affinity chromatography. Cell surface fibronectin, which can be extracted from cultured cells with urea [19], differs in some physical properties and biological activities from serum fibronectin [20]. Although the presence of fibronectin in a variety of tissues has been demonstrated by indirect immunofluorescence [21], few investigators have been successful in obtaining tissue-derived material in quantity, presumably because it is crosslinked to the matrix [22].

Fibronectin is composed of two 220 000 dalton chains linked by disulfide bonds near the carboxyl terminus (Figure 1). Peptide mapping techniques indicate that the chains are identical [23], although some minor differences in the rate of migration in SDS gels have been reported for the chains from plasma fibronectin [24]. Physical studies have shown that there are various globular domains in the molecule connected by flexible regions [25]. Oligosaccharides comprising 6–10% of the molecule are located near the amino terminus.

Fibronectin has been found to aggregate and to bind to a variety of other molecules (Table 5). These interactions are related to the biological functions of fibronectin (Tables 4–6). The interaction of fibronectin with collagen and its crosslinking by Factor XIII_a involve specific amino acid sequences on both molecules [26, 27]. In wound healing, the binding of fibronectin to fibrin and fibrinogen may help to stabilize the clot [28] and provide a surface on which

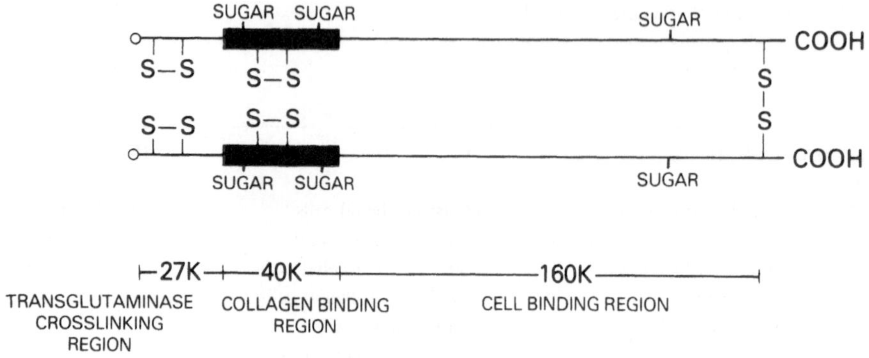

Figure 1. Schematic model for the fibronectin molecule. The location of various biologically active domains was assigned according to references [3–6].

macrophages and fibroblasts can adhere [29]. Its presence in the clot may also recruit and activate macrophages at a wound since fibronectin is chemotactic [30] and opsonic [7]. Fibronectin is also a chemotactic factor for fibroblasts [30] which may be important in wound repair. Increased levels of fibronectin have been found in the lung fluids of patients with fibrotic lung disease suggesting that elevated fibronectin may cause fibrosis by recruiting an excess of fibroblasts [31].

Fibronectin binds to various proteoglycans, including heparin, hyaluronic acid and heparan sulfate [32–37]. A specific heparin-binding site on fibronectin has been identified [33]. Fibronectin is present in the 'heparin-precipitable fraction' of plasma and heparin appears to be required for some of its opsonic activities [7]. Heparin also enhances the binding of fibronectin to native collagen and appears to stabilize the fibronectin-collagen interaction [35–37]. Although heparin is not generally present in extracellular matrices, a closely related proteoglycan, heparan sulfate, is present on the cell surface and in the matrix deposited by many cultured cells [32, 38]. Laminin [39] and chondronectin [17] also bind to heparin. In addition, certain complex gangliosides, which are also present on the cell surface, bind to fibronectin [40]. Unlike heparan sulfate, gangliosides compete with the cell surface receptor for the binding of fibronectin suggesting that they could be receptors for fibronectin. Further studies are needed, however, to establish the nature of the cellular fibronectin receptor.

1.2. Laminin

Laminin is a high molecular weight (1 000 000 dalton) glycoprotein found in all basement membranes [41, 42]. Laminin, which was originally prepared from the EHS tumor by salt extraction followed by ion exchange chromatography [15], can also be prepared from a variety of endothelial and epithelial cell cultures. It can be isolated from the conditioned culture medium by heparin-Sepharose affinity chromatography after first removing fibronectin by gelatin-Sepharose affinity chromatography. Laminin is composed of two types of chains (400 000 and 200 000 dalton) linked by disulfide bonds (Figures 2 and 3). Peptide maps indicate that the component chains are not identical [41].

Laminin has been shown to bind preferentially to type IV (basement membrane) collagen where it promotes the adhesion of various epithelial and endothelial cells [14]. Cells which can adhere via laminin can also synthesize sufficient laminin for adhesion [14]. Heparan sulfate, a proteoglycan which is chemically related to heparin, is present in basement membranes at the interface of the lamina lucida and lamina densa [43, 44]. It is possible that laminin in basement membranes binds to the heparan sulfate proteoglycan and to type IV collagen to form the basic unit of this extracellular matrix.

Laminin may have functions other than mediating cell-matrix adhesion. In the

Table 5. Molecules known to interact with fibronectin.

Molecule known to bind	Function of interaction
Heparin	Enhances opsonization reaction
Heparan sulfate	Promotes stable collagen binding
Hyaluronic acid	?
Fibrin (ogen)	Strengthens the hemostatic clot
Factor XIII_a	Strengthens clot and possibly extracellular matrix by crosslinking fibronectin to itself, collagen and fibrin
Collagen	Forms extracellular matrix; binding causes conformational change so fibronectin can now bind to cell surfaces
Gangliosides (GD_{1a} and GT_1)	Cell surface receptor for fibronectin?
Actin	promotes opsonization of these materials
DNA	
Staphylococci	

Table 6. Biological activities of fibronectin.

Promotes opsonization reactions
Promotes cell-substrate adhesion* ↓
Promotes cell-cell aggregation
Agglutinates formalinized red blood cells*
Promotes cell spreading*
Promotes random and directed cell migration*
Inhibits myoblast fusion
Inhibits chondrocyte differentiation
Binds to type I collagen and delays fibril formation

*Laminin is known to have similar activities.
↓ Chondronectin is known to have similar activities.

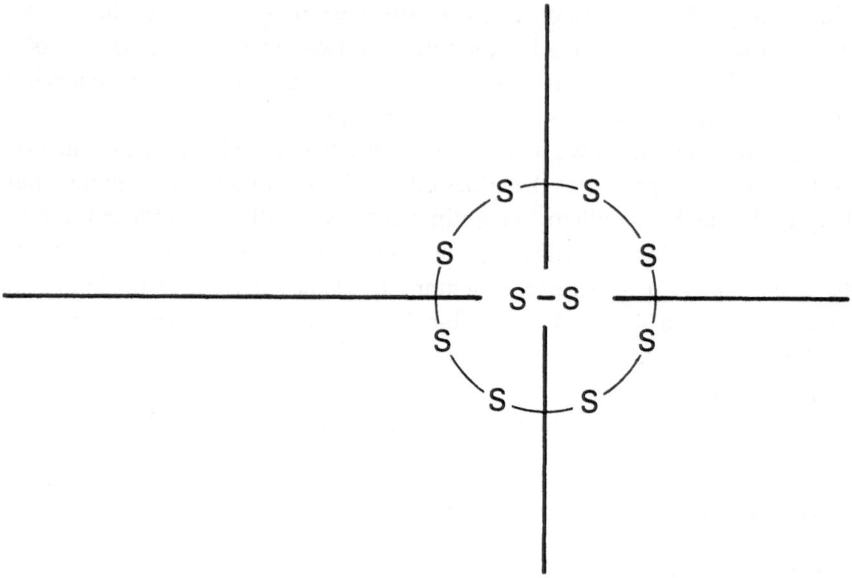

Figure 2. Schematic model for the laminin molecule. The location of the chains is based on reference [41].

developing embryo, laminin may be important in morphogenesis since it is present earlier than collagen type IV [44]. Preliminary studies suggest it may also promote the migration of certain epithelial cells *in vitro* (H.E.J. Seppä and V.P. Terranova, personal communication).

1.3. Chondronectin

Chondronectin is a chondrocyte-specific glycoprotein present in serum, extracts of cartilage, chondrocyte-conditioned medium and the vitreous body [16, 17]. It can be isolated from these sources by ion exchange chromatography, followed by lectin and dye affinity chromatography [17]. Chondronectin has a molecular weight of 180 000 dalton, and, upon reduction yields chains of ~80 000 dalton.

Although chondronectin promotes the adhesion of chondrocytes to type II (cartilage) collagen, its own binding to collagen is negligible. Experiments with proteoglycan monomer and with xylosides (Hewitt, unpublished observations), which inhibit proteoglycan synthesis, and with cycloheximide, which inhibits protein synthesis, demonstrate that factors such as proteoglycans are also required to stabilize the chondronectin-collagen complex and allow chondrocytes to adhere to matrix. Chondronectin has been found to bind to heparin-Sepharose columns [17] and to chondroitin sulfate-Sepharose affinity columns (A.T. Hewitt, personal communication).

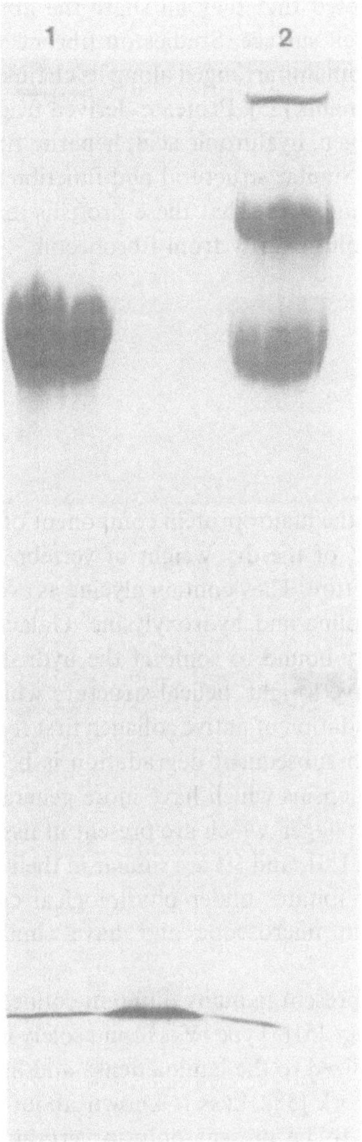

Figure 3. SDS (5%) polyacrylamide gel of fibronectin [1] and laminin [2].

1.4. Comparative properties of the cell attachment proteins

Fibronectin, laminin, and chondronectin are chemically and immunologically distinct and are present in different tissues [1]. Particularly notable are the differences in the size of these proteins, in their binding to various collagens and to different cell types, and in their distinct tissue distributions (Table 3). On the other hand, it should be noted that they all share the ability to bind to collagen, to heparin, and to the cell surface. Studies on fibronectin indicate that it contains different functional domains arranged along its chains separated by more exposed, protease-sensitive domains [25]. Protease-derived fragments of fibronectin which react with either collagen, hyaluronic acid, heparin, fibrin, or the cell surface have been described [4–6]. Similar structural and functional domains exist for laminin and chondronectin, suggesting that these proteins may have had similar origins but have diverged evolutionarily from fibronectin.

2. Collagen

2.1. Structure

Collagens [45–49] are the major protein component of most extracellular matrices and represent 20–35% of the dry weight of vertebrates. Collagens have unique composition and structure. They contain glycine as every third amino acid residue as well as hydroxyproline and hydroxylysine. Galactosyl or glucosyl-galactosyl residues are covalently bound to some of the hydroxylysine side chains. Native collagen molecules have a tight, helical structure which makes them resistant to most proteases. Degradation of native collagen first requires the activity of specific collagenases, although subsequent degradation is believed to be carried out by proteases such as cathepsins which have more general activity [50]. There are at least five isotypes of collagen which are present in tissue-specific locations (Table 1) [46]. Collagen types I, II, and III are similar in their dimensions (300 by 1.5 nm) and form fibrous precipitates under physiological conditions. These fibers are visible in the electron microscope and have similar but characteristic fine structures [45].

Types I and III are present in many different connective tissues, while type II is found mainly in cartilage [51]. Type IV is found solely in basement membranes [41] where it has been localized to the lamina densa and has been described as a non-fibrillar, felt-like network [52]. Less is known about the distribution of type V collagen which seems to be present only in certain basement membranes and connective tissues [53, 54]. Collagen is produced by many types of cultured cells, and the particular isotype(s) produced depends on the origin of the cells. For example, fibroblasts synthesize types I and III [55], chondrocytes synthesize type II [56], and endothelial cells synthesize type IV [57]. Under certain culture conditions when chondrocytes lose their cartilage phenotype, they begin synthesizing type I collagen [58].

2.2. Cellular Functions

Collagen *in vitro* has been shown to enhance the adhesion and growth of many cells [59] and to prolong the life span of cultures of chick embryo fibroblasts [60]. Although most cells also require fibronectin to adhere to collagen [1], it appears that hepatocytes isolated in the absence of proteases and platelets adhere directly to collagen substrates [61, 62]. Collagen also promotes the differentiation of various cells such as myoblasts [63], corneal epithelial cells [64], and guinea pig epidermal cells [65]. It can promote migration by serving as a substrate over which the cells migrate [66] and/or as an attractant [67].

3. Proteoglycans

3.1. Structure

Proteoglycans comprise a considerable but variable proportion (up to 30%) of the dry weight of extracellular matrices. Proteoglycans are a diverse group of macromolecules which consist of glycosaminoglycan chains covalently bound to a protein core [68]. Seven types of glycosaminoglycan side chains have been described, and each has a characteristic disaccharide repeating unit [69] as well as small amounts (~ 3%) of other sugars which are usually located near the region linking the glycosaminoglycan to the protein core. The chains vary in size from 10^7 dalton for hyaluronic acid to 10^4 dalton for heparin. Proteoglycans from different tissues often contain immunologically distinct protein cores and vary in the amount and type of glycosaminoglycan chain present (Table 2). For example, the cartilage proteoglycan contains both chondroitin and keratan sulfate glycosaminoglycan side chains each linked covalently to the same protein core. The corneal stroma proteoglycans, in contrast, have chondroitin and keratan sulfate side chains attached to two different protein cores, resulting in two separate proteoglycan species [70].

The proteoglycans of cartilage and aorta each interact with hyaluronic acid to produce large aggregate structures [71]. The interaction between the hyaluronic acid and the proteoglycan is stabilized by a low molecular weight (42 000 dalton) glycoprotein known as link protein. The resulting aggregates can bind to collagen and are visible by electron microscopy [72].

3.2. Functions

The polyanionic nature of proteoglycans may allow them to control the water and ion content of tissues. As cartilages age, for example, both the water content and elasticity decrease with the decrease in the size of the proteoglycan [73]. Hyaluronic acid is particularly viscous and may serve as a lubricant for joints. Proteoglycans such as heparan sulfate in the glomerular basement membrane may act to restrict the passage of certain materials and thus provide selective filtration [41]. In addition, corneal proteoglycans are interspersed among the highly ordered collagen fibrils of the cornea [74], and the resulting structure may be essential for transparency of the cornea.

Heparan sulfate and hyaluronic acid are both present on the surfaces of cells and in the extracellular matrix deposited by cells, suggesting that they may have a role in cell adhesion [32]. Both heparan sulfate and hyaluronic acid can bind to fibronectin [33], whereas a related proteoglycan, heparin, binds to fibronectin, laminin, and chondronectin [1]. In addition, heparin promotes [36] and strengthens the binding of fibronectin to collagen [35]. Thus, it appears that for certain extracellular matrices the attachment factors not only link the cell to the matrix but also interact with and stabilize the other matrix components.

4. Changes in Matrix Molecules and Adhesion Factors with Cell Transformation and Malignancy

4.1. Cell transformation

Transformed cells are generally more rounded and less adherent to the substrate than their untransformed counterparts. It is therefore not surprising that decreases in the synthesis of various matrix components including fibronectin [75, 76], laminin [9], collagen [2], and sulfated glycosaminoglycans [77–81] following the transformation of cells have been reported. Changes in chondronectin levels following transformation have not been studied, but the tumor promotor phorbol-12-myristate-13-acetate causes chondrocytes to dedifferentiate and to reduce chondronectin synthesis [82]. The decreased synthesis of fibronectin and collagen by fibroblasts is due to decreased levels of mRNA coding for these macromolecules [3]. The proline analogue *cis*-hydroxyproline, which selectively blocks collagen synthesis, prevents the growth of normal but not of transformed cells [83]. This indicates that in culture normal cells are dependent on a collagenous substrate, whereas transformed cells do not need a collagen matrix to survive.

Interestingly, excess exogenous fibronectin can restore a normal morphology to transformed cells [84], but the growth rate and other transformed characteristics are unaffected. Treatment of cells either with butyrate [85] or with dexamethasone [86] increases the amount of exogenous fibronectin which is deposited on the surface of transformed cells possibly by increasing the number of fibronectin receptors on the membrane. The effects of exogenous laminin, collagen and/or proteoglycans on transformed cells have not yet been tested. Dexamethasone increases collagen synthesis by transformed cells [86] without affecting other characteristics of transformation. Changes have also been reported in the structure of the extracellular matrix components after transformation. The type of collagen synthesized by BALB 3T3 cells changes after transformation [87]. Also an increase in the level of phosphorylation of fibronectin [88] and an alteration of the sulfate content of heparan sulfate have been reported after transformation [89]. Such changes are relatively minor, however, and could be secondary effects.

4.2. Malignancy

The possibility that the presence or absence of adhesion proteins can determine the tumorigenicity and metastatic potential of transformed cells has been of considerable interest. Most of the work in this area has been carried out with fibronectin. Preliminary studies suggested that the degree of tumorigenicity of cells transformed in culture correlated with a lack of cell surface fibronectin [90]. However, subsequent studies have not confirmed this relationship [91]. Conversely, while many tumors do not contain fibronectin, it appears that cells from the tumors can synthesize it in culture [92]. Cells isolated from primary tumors synthesize more fibronectin *in vitro* than do cells isolated from its metastases [92]. On the other hand, certain invasive carcinomas have been shown to contain decreased levels of fibronectin [93]. Elevated levels of fibronectin in urine [94] and serum [95, 96] have been suggested as a marker for prostatic and other cancers. However, patients with certain tumors have decreased serum fibronectin levels, particularly in the late stage [97]. Such studies demonstrate that no generalizations about the relationship between fibronectin levels and tumors cells can be made.

Unlike some differentiated cells, tumor cells can adhere to various substrates including collagen types I and IV. Studies with cells from a limited number of tumors suggest that type I collagen (interstitial) and fibronectin comprise an adhesive substrate for tumor cells *in vitro* [13]. Laminin, but not fibronectin, is required for tumor cell adhesion to type IV (basement membrane) collagen. Since most malignancies are derived from epithelial cells, it is not surprising that many tumorigenic cells, such as transformed adult mouse connective tissue cells (TACT), bind to type IV collagen [13]. This interaction could be important in attachment of the metastatic cell to the basement membrane. Terranova et al. [98] have shown that the ability of B16 melanoma cells to bind to type IV collagen via laminin can be used to select for more highly metastatic cells than were present in the original population. Such studies suggest the importance of the cell-laminin interaction in certain types of malignancy, but more investigations are needed. Tumor cells may adhere and survive in different tissues as a result of their ability to utilize more than one adhesion mechanism. Although it is not clear whether fibronectin and laminin have a role in the adhesion of tumor cells *in vivo*, its degradation may be a step in the invasion process. Fibronectin is protease-sensitive and likely to be degraded by the invading cells [99].

Chondrocytes from normal cartilage do not contain fibronectin and adhere exclusively via chondronectin. In contrast, chondrocytes from a chondrosarcoma use both fibronectin and chondronectin to adhere to collagen [100]. This chondrosarcoma also contains both fibronectin and chondronectin in the extracellular matrix. Thus, it may be that specific changes in the recognition by the cell surface receptors or in the production of áttachment factors are associated with tumorigenicity.

Transformed cells often yield tumors *in vivo* which are rich in collagen [101–103] and proteoglycans [104–107]. For example, fibrosarcomas are rich in type I collagen [101] while chondrosarcomas contain type II collagen [102] and chondroitin sulfate proteoglycan [105]. Although qualitative differences have not been found between the collagens synthesized by tumors and by their normal cellular counterparts, there is considerable evidence to suggest that the structure and the relative amounts of the proteoglycans differ between normal and malignant tissues. For example, the proteoglycan made by a rat chondrosarcoma has been shown to lack keratan sulfate side chains found in normal cartilage proteoglycan [108] and the heparan sulfate in cancerous livers has an altered charge density probably due to a decrease in sulfate content [107].

The type of collagen or proteoglycan produced by tumors may be diagnostic of their origin. For example, osteogenic sarcoma and Ewing's sarcoma are often difficult to distinguish from each other based on clinical evidence, but cultured Ewings's cells make type I and III collagens while those from osteogenic sarcoma produce only type I collagen [103]. Also, it has recently been proposed that metastases from breast cancer can be detected by the presence of type IV collagen in lymph nodes [109]. Malignant glial cells [78] and many other transformed cells [80, 110, 111] synthesize increased levels of hyaluronic acid, and there is an increased amount of hyaluronic acid in the pleural and peritoneal fluids of patients with mesothelioma [112].

5. Summary

The cells of the body are held within their respective tissues by their interactions with extracellular matrices. These matrices contain proteoglycans and collagenous components unique for each tissue. Specific attachment factors such as fibronectin [1, 4–7], laminin [15], and chondronectin [16, 17] have recently been characterized for various tissues, but other factors probably exist. The extracellular matrix components not only contribute to mechanical properties of tissues, such as resistance to compression and selective filtration, but also promote cell adhesion and play a regulatory role in such cellular activities as migration [30, 66, 67], proliferation [59, 60], and differentiation [1, 63–65]. Recently, it has been shown that some cells do not require growth factors if the appropriate extracellular matrix is present [113].

Tumors are rich in extracellular matrix components which are often characteristic of the tissue from which the cells have been derived [78–80, 100–106]. In fact, it has been suggested that metastases of breast (epithelial) carcinoma can be identified in lymph nodes by the presence of type IV (basement membrane) collagen [109]. Although no defect in the structure of collagen or of the attachment factors derived from tumors has been detected, alterations in the structure of the proteoglycan of chondrosarcoma have been reported [105, 108]. However, the absence of keratan sulfate from the chondrosarcoma proteoglycan is not unique since proteoglycan from prechondrogenic mesenchyme also lacks this glycosaminoglycan [114], suggesting that tumor cells synthesize a proteoglycan characteristic of a less differentiated precursor.

How the extracellular matrix influences tumor growth and spread is unclear. Tumor cells interact with, penetrate through, grow in, and synthesize extracellular matrix components. Studies on these interactions may help to elucidate the mechanisms of tumor growth and metastases.

References

1. Kleinman HK, Klebe RJ, Martin GR: Role of collagenous matrices in the adhesion and growth of cells. J Cell Biol 88:473–485, 1981.
2. Arbogast BW, Yoshimura M, Kefalides N, Holtzer H, Koji A: Failure of cultured chick embryo fibroblasts to incorporate collagen into their extracellular matrix when transformed by Rous sarcoma virus. J Biol Chem 252:8863–8868, 1977.
3. Adams SL, Sobel ME, Howard BH, Olden K, Yamada KM, DeCrombrugghe B, Pastan I: Levels of translatable mRNAs for cell surface protein, collagen precursors, and two membrane proteins are altered in Rous sarcoma virus transformed chick embryo fibroblasts. Proc Natl Acad Sci USA 74:3399–3403, 1977.
4. Mosher DF: Fibronectin. Prog Hemostasis Thromb 5:111–151, 1980.
5. Ruoslahti E, Engvall E, Hayman EG: Fibronectin: current concepts of its structure and functions. Coll Res 1:95–128, 1981.
6. Pearlstein E, Gold LI, Garcia-Pardo A: Fibronectin: a review of its structure and biological activity. Mol Cell Biochem 29:103–128, 1980.
7. Vaheri A, Ruoslahti E, Mosher DF: Fibroblast surface protein. Ann NY Acad Sci 321:1–456, 1978.
8. Grinnell F: Cellular adhesiveness and extracellular substrata. Int Rev Cytol 53:65–144, 1978.
9. Hayman EG, Engvall E, Ruoslahti E: Concomitant loss of cell surface fibronectin and laminin from transformed rat kidney cells. J Cell Biol 88:352–357, 1981.
10. Spjut HJ, Dorfman HD, Fechner RE, Ackerman LV (eds), Atlas of tumor pathology fascicle 5. Tumors of bone and cartilage. Armed Forces Institute of Pathology, 1975, pp 117–244.
11. Gullino PM, Grantham FH: The influence of the host and the neoplastic cell population on the collagen content of a tumor mass. Cancer Res, 23:648–655, 1963.
12. Liotta LA, Abe S, Robey PG, Martin GR: Preferential digestion of basement membrane collagen by an enzyme derived from a metastatic murine tumor. Proc Natl Acad Sci USA, 76:2268–2272.
13. Murray JC, Liotta LA, Rennard SI, Martin GR: Collagen adhesion characterization of murine metastatic and nonmetastatic tumor cells *in vitro*. Cancer Res 40:347–351, 1980.

14. Terranova VP, Rohrbach DH, Martin GR: Role of laminin in the attachment of PAM 212 (epithelial) cells to basement membrane collagen. Cell 22:719–728, 1980.
15. Timpl R, Rohde H, Gehron Robey P, Rennard SI, Foidart JM, Martin GR: Laminin – a glycoprotein from basement membrane. J Biol Chem 254:9933–9937, 1979.
16. Hewitt AT, Kleinman HK, Pennypacker JP, Martin GR: Identification of an adhesion factor for chondrocytes. Proc Natl Acad Sci USA 77:385–388, 1980.
17. Hewitt AT, Varner HH, Martin GR: Isolation of chondronectin. In: Immunochemistry of Collagen Vol. I, Furthmayr H (ed). Boca Raton, Florida: CRC Press (in press).
18. Hopper KE, Adelmann BC, Gentner G, Gay S: Recognition by guinea pig peritoneal exudate cells of conformationally different states of the collagen molecule. Immunology 30:249–259, 1976.
19. Yamada KM, Yamada SS, Pastan I: Cell surface protein partially restores morphology, adhesiveness and contact inhibition of movement to transformed fibroblasts. Proc Natl Acad Sci USA 73:1211–1221, 1976.
20. Yamada KM, Kennedy DW: Fibroblast cellular and plasma fibronectin are similar but not identical. J Cell Biol 80:492–497, 1979.
21. Linder E, Vaheri A, Ruoslahti E, Wartiovaara J: Distribution of fibroblast surface antigen in the developing chick embryo. J Exp Med 142:41–49, 1975.
22. Bray BA: Cold-insoluble globulin (fibronectin) in connective tissue of adult human lung and in trophoblast basement membrane. J Clin Invest 62:745–752, 1978.
23. Kurkinen M, Vartio T, Vaheri A: Polypeptides of human plasma fibronectin are similar but not identical. Biochim Biophys Acta 624:490–498, 1980.
24. Chen AB, Armani DL, Mosesson MW: Heterogenity of the cold-insoluble globulin of human plasma (CIg), a circulating cell surface protein. Biochim Biophys Acta 493:310–322, 1977.
25. Alexander SS, Colonna G, Yamada KM, Pastan I, Edelhoch H: Molecular properties of a major cell surface protein from chick embryo fibroblasts. J Biol Chem 253:5820–5824, 1978.
26. Kleinman HK, McGoodwin EB, Martin GR, Klebe RJ, Fietzek PP, Woolley DE: Localization of the binding site for cell attachment in the $\alpha 1$(I) chain of collagen. J Biol Chem 253:5642–5646, 1978.
27. Mosher DF, Schad PE, Vann JW: Cross-linking of collagen and fibronectin by factor XIII_a: Localization of participating glutaminyl residues to a tryptic fragment of fibronectin. J Biol Chem 255:1181–1188, 1980.
28. Engvall E, Ruoslahti E, Miller EJ: Affinity of fibronectin to collagen of different genetic types and to fibrinogen. J Exp Med 147:1584–1595, 1978.
29. Klebe RJ: The isolation of a collagen-dependent cell attachment factor. Nature 250:248–251, 1974.
30. Gauss-Müller V, Kleinman HK, Martin GR, Schiffmann E: Role of attachment factors and attractants in fibroblast chemotaxis. J Lab Clin Med 96:1071–1080, 1980.
31. Rennard SI, Crystal RG: Broncheoalveolar lavage fibronectin: elevation in patients with interstitial lung disease. J Clin Invest 69:113–122, 1982.
32. Culp LA, Murray BA, Rollins BJ: Fibronectin and proteoglycans as determinants of cell-substratum adhesion. J Supramol Struct 11:401–427, 1979.
33. Yamada KM, Kennedy DW, Kimata K, Pratt RM: Characterization of fibronectin interactions with glycosaminoglycans and identification of active proteolytic fragment. J Biol Chem 255:6055–6063, 1980.
34. Hayashi M, Schlesinger DH, Kennedy DW, Yamada KM: Isolation and charaterization of a heparin-binding domain of cellular fibronectin. J Biol Chem 255:10017–10020, 1980.
35. Ruoslahti E, Engvall E: Complexing of fibronectin, glycosaminoglycans and collagen. Biochim Biophys Acta 631:350–358, 1980.
36. Johansson S, Höök M: Heparin enhances the binding of fibronectin to collagen. Biochemical J 187:521524, 1980.

37. Jilek F, Hörmann H: Fibronectin (cold-insoluble globulin). VI. Influence of heparin and hyaluronic acid on the binding of native collagen. Hoppe-Seyler's Z Physiol Chem 360:597–603, 1979.
38. Kraemer PM, Heparan sulfate of cultured cells. II Acid-soluble and -precipitable species of different cell lines. Biochemistry 10:1445–1451, 1971.
39. Sakashita S, Engvall E, Ruoslahti E: Basement membrane glycoprotein laminin binds to heparin. FEBS Lett 116:243–246, 1980.
40. Kleinman HK, Martin GR, Fishman PH: Ganglioside inhibition of fibronectin-mediated cell adhesion to collagen. Proc Natl Acad Sci USA 76:3367–3371, 1979.
41. Timpl R, Martin GR: Components of basement membrane. In: Immunochemistry of collagen, Vol. II, Furthmayr H (ed). Boca Raton, Florida: CRC Press (in press).
42. Chung AE, Jaffe R, Freeman IL, Vergnes J-P, Braguiski JE, Carlin B: Properties of a basement membrane related glycoprotein synthesized in culture by a mouse embryonal carcinoma-derived line. Cell 16:277–281, 1979.
43. Hassell JR, Gehron Robey P, Barrach HJ, Wilczek J, Rennard SI, Martin GR: Isolation of a heparan sulfate-containing proteoglycan from basement membrane. Proc Natl Acad Sci USA 77:4494–4498, 1980.
44. Ekblom P, Alitalo K, Vaheri A, Timpl R, Saxen L: Induction of a basement membrane glycoprotein in embryonic kidney: possible role of laminin in morphogenesis. Proc Natl Acad Sci USA 77:482–485, 1980.
45. Gay S, Miller EJ: Collagen in the physiology and pathology of connective tissue. Stuttgart: Gustav-Fischer Verlag, 1978.
46. Bornstein P, Sage H: Structurally distinct collagen types. Annu Rev Biochem 49:957–1003, 1980.
47. Ramachandran GN, Reddi AH: Biochemistry of collagen. New York: Plenum Press, 1976.
48. Prockop DJ, Kivirikko KI, Tuderman L, Guzman NA: The biosynthesis of collagen and its disorders. N Engl J Med 301:13–23, 77–85, 1979.
49. Eyre D: Collagen: Molecular diversity in the body's protein. Science (Wash D.C.) 207:1315–1322, 1980.
50. Gross J: Collagen biology: structure, degradation, and disease. Harvey Lect 68:351–432, 1974.
51. Miller EJ, Matukas VJ: Biosynthesis of collagen: the biochemist's view. Fed Proc 33:1197–1201, 1974.
52. Yaoita H, Foidart J-M, Katz SI: Localization of the collagenous components in skin basement membrane. J Invest Dermatol 70:191–193, 1978.
53. Burgeson RE, El Adli FA, Kaitila II, Hollister DW: Fetal membrane collagens: identification of two new alpha chains. Proc Natl Acad Sci USA 73:2579–2583, 1976.
54. Chung ER, Rhodes K, Miller EJ: Isolation of three collagenous components of probable basement membrane origin. Biochem Biophys Res Commun 71:1167–1174, 1976.
55. Gay S, Martin GR, Müller PK, Timpl R, Kühn K: Simultaneous synthesis of types I and III collagen by fibroblasts in culture. Proc Natl Acad Sci USA 73:4037–4040, 1976.
56. Uitto J: Biosynthesis of type II collagen. Removal of amino- and carboxyl-terminal extensions from procollagen synthesized by chick embryo cartilage cells. Biochemistry 15:3421–3429, 1977.
57. Howard BV, Macarak EJ, Gunson D, Kefalides NA: Characterization of the collagen synthesized by endothelial cells in culture. Proc Natl Acad Sci USA 73:2361–2364, 1976.
58. von der Mark K, Gauss V, von der Mark H, Müller P: Relationships between cell shape and type of collagen synthesized as cells lose their cartilage phenotype in culture. Nature (London) 267:531–532, 1977.
59. Erhmann RL, Gey GO: The growth of cells on a transparent gel of reconstituted rat tail collagen. J Natl Cancer Inst 16:1375–1403, 1956.
60. Gey GO, Svotelis M, Foard M, Bareg FB: Long-term growth of chicken fibroblasts on a collagen substrate. Exp Cell Res 84:63–71, 1974.
61. Santoro SA, Cunningham LW: Fibronectin and the multiple interaction model for platelet-

collagen adhesion. Proc Natl Acad Sci USA 76:2644–2648.
62. Johansson S, Kjellen L, Höök M: Substrate adhesion of rat hepatocytes. A comparison of laminin and fibronectin as attachment proteins. J Cell Biol 90:260–264, 1981.
63. Hauschka SD, Konigsberg IR: The influence of collagen on the development of muscle colonies. Proc Natl Acad Sci USA 55:119–126, 1966.
64. Meier S, Hay ED: Control of corneal differentiation by extracellular materials. Collagen as a promoter and stabilizes of epithelial stroma production. Develop Biol 38:249–270, 1974.
65. Murray JC, Stingl G, Kleinman HK, Martin GR, Katz SI: Epidermal cells adhere preferentially to type IV (basement membrane) collagen. J Cell Biol 80:197–201, 1978.
66. Greenberg JH, Seppä S, Seppä H, Hewitt AT: Role of collagen and fibronectin in neural crest cell adhesion and migration. Develop Biol 87:259–266, 1981.
67. Postlethwaite AE, Seyer JM, Kang AH: Chemotactic attraction of human fibroblasts to type I, II and III collagens and collagen-derived peptides. Proc Natl Acad Sci USA 75:871–875, 1978.
68. Hascall VC: Interaction of cartilage proteoglycan with hyaluronic acid. J Supramol Struct 7:101–120, 1977.
69. Stoolmiller AC, Dorfman A: The metabolism of glycosaminoglycans. Comp Biochem 17:241–274, 1969.
70. Hassell JR, Newsome DA, Hascall VC: Characterization and biosynthesis of proteoglycans of corneal stroma from rhesus monkey. J Biol Chem 254:12346–12354, 1979.
71. Hascall VC, Heinegård D: Aggregation of cartilage proteoglycan I. The role of hyaluronic acid. J Biol Chem 249:4232–4241, 1974.
72. Oegema TR, Laidlaw J, Hascall VC, Dziewictkowski DD: The effect of proteoglycans on the formation of fibrils from collagen solution. Arch Biochem Biophys 170:698–709, 1975.
73. Inerot S, Heinegård D, Audell L, Olsson S-E: Articular-cartilage proteoglycans in aging and osteoarthritis. Biochem J 169:143–156, 1978.
74. Hassell JR, Newsome DA, Krachmer JH, Rodrigues MM: Macular corneal dystrophy: failure to synthesize a mature keratan sulfate proteoglycan. Proc Natl Acad Sci USA 77:3705–3709, 1980.
75. Hynes RO: Cell surface protein and malignant transformation. Biochim Biophys Acta 458:73–107, 1976.
76. Vaheri A, Mosher DF: High molecular weight cell surface glycoprotein (fibronectin) lost in malignant transformation. Biochem Biophys Acta 516:1–25, 1978.
77. Cohn RH, Caissman J-J, Bernfield MR: Relationship of transformation, cell density, and growth control to the cellular distribution of newly synthesized glycosaminoglycan. J Cell Biol 71:280–294, 1974.
78. Glimelius B, Norling B, Westermark B, Wasteson Å: A comparative study of glycosaminoglycans in cultures of human, normal and malignant glial cells. J Cell Physiol 98:527–538, 1979.
79. Chiarigi VP, Vannuchi S, Urbano P: Exposure of trypsin-removable polyanions on the surface of normal and virally transformed BHK21/C13 cells. Biochim Biophys Acta 345:283–293, 1974.
80. Muto M, Yoshimura M, Okayama M, Koji A: Cellular transformation and differentiation. Effect of Rous sarcoma virus transformation on sulfated proteoglycan synthesis by chicken chondrocytes. Proc Natl Acad Sci USA 74:4173–4177, 1977.
81. Underhill CB, Keller JM: Density-dependent changes in the amount of sulfated glycosaminoglycans associated with mouse 3T3 cells. J Cell Physiol 89:53–64, 1976.
82. Lowe ME, Pacifici M, Holtzer H: Effects of phorbol-12-myristate-13-acetate on the phenotypic program of cultured chondroblasts and fibroblasts. Cancer Res 38:2350–2355, 1978.
83. Liotta LA, Vembu D, Kleinman HK, Martin GR, Boone C: Collagen required for proliferation of cultured connective tissue cells but not their transformed counterparts. Nature (London) 272:622–624, 1978.
84. Ali IU, Mautner VM, Lanza R, Hynes RO: Restoration of normal morphology, adhesion and cytoskeleton in transformed cells by addition of a transformation-sensitive surface protein. Cell 11:115–126, 1977.

85. Hayman EG, Engvall E, Ruoslahti E: Butyrate restores fibronectin at cell surface of transformed cells. Exp Cell Res 127:478–481, 1980.
86. Furcht LT, Mosher DF, Wendelschaefer-Crabb, Foidart JM: Reversal by glucocorticoid hormones of the loss of a fibronectin and procollagen matrix around transformed human cells. Cancer Res 39:2077–2083, 1979.
87. Hata RI, Peterkofsky B: Specific changes in collagen phenotype of BALB 3T3 cells: result of transformation by sarcoma viruses or a chemical carcinogen. Proc Natl Acad Sci USA 74:2933–2937, 1977.
88. Ali IU, Hunter T: Structural comparison of fibronectin from normal and transformed cells. J Biol Chem 256:7671–7677, 1981.
89. Underhill CB, Keller JM: A transformation-dependent difference in the heparan sulfate associated with the cell surface. Biochem Biophys Res Commun 63:448–454, 1975.
90. Chen LB, Gallimore PH, McDougall JK: Correlation between tumor induction and the large external transformation-sensitive protein on the cell surface. Proc Natl Acad Sci USA 73:3570–3574, 1976.
91. Kahn P, Shin SI: Cellular tumorigenicity in nude mice: test of associations among loss of cell surface fibronectin, anchorage independence, and tumor forming ability. J Cell Biol 82:1–16, 1979.
92. Chen LB, Summerhayes I, Hsieh P, Gallimore PH: Possible role of fibronectin in malignancy. J Supramol Struct 12:139–150, 1979.
93. Smith HS, Riggs JL, Mosesson MW: Production of fibronectin by human epithelial cells in culture. Cancer Res 39:4138–4144, 1979.
94. Webb KS, Lin GH: Urinary fibronectin. Potential as a marker in prostatic cancer. Invest Urol 17:401–404, 1980.
95. Todd HD, Coffee MS, Waalkes TP, Abeloff MD, Parsons RG: Serum levels of fibronectin and a fibronectin-like DNA-binding protein in patients with various diseases. J Natl Cancer Inst 65:901–904, 1980.
96. Zardi L, Cecconi C, Barbieri O, Carnemolla B, Picca M, Santi L: Concentration of fibronectin in plasma of tumor-bearing mice and synthesis by Ehrlich ascites tumor cells. Cancer Res 39:3774–3779, 1979.
97. Mosher DF, Williams EM: Fibronectin concentration is decreased in plasma of severely ill patients with disseminated intravascular coagulation. J Lab Clin Med 91:729–735, 1978.
98. Terranova VP, Liotta LA, Russo R, Martin GR: Laminin-mediated selection of metastatic tumor cells. Cancer Res, in press, 1982.
99. Vartio T, Seppä H, Vaheri A: Susceptibility of soluble and matrix fibronectins to degradation by tissue proteinases, mast cell chymase and cathepsin G. J Biol Chem 256:471–477, 1981.
100. Kimata K, Foidart JM, Pennypacker JP, Kleinman HK, Martin GR, Hewitt AT: Fibronectin in tumor cartilage matrix. Cancer Res, in press, 1982.
101. Moro L, Smith BD: Identification of collagen $\alpha 1(I)$ trimer and normal type I collagen in a polyoma virus induced mouse tumor. Arch Biochem Biophys 182:33–41, 1977.
102. Smith BD, Martin GR, Miller EJ, Dorfman A, Swarm R: Nature of the collagen synthesized by a transplantable chondrosarcoma. Arch Biochem Biophys 166:181–186, 1975.
103. Stern R, Wilczek J, Thorpe WP, Rosenberg SA, Cannon G: Procollagens as markers for the cell of origin of human bone tumors. Cancer Res 40:325–328, 1980.
104. Sweet MBE, Thonar EJMA, Berson SD, Skikne MI, Immelman AR, Kerr WA: Biochemical studies of the matrix of craniovertebral chordoma and a metastasis. Cancer 44:652–660, 1979.
105. Pal S, Strider W, Margolis R, Gallo G, Lee-Huang S, Rosenberg, L: Isolation and characterization of proteoglycans from human chondrosarcomas. J Biol Chem 253:1279–1289, 1978.
106. Brunish R, Asbol-Hansen G: Acid mucopolysaccharides in the Rask-Nielsen transplantable mouse mastocytoma. Acta Pathol Microbiol Scand 65:185–191, 1965.
107. Nakamura N, Kojima J: Changes in charge density of heparan sulfate isolated from cancerous

human liver tissues. Cancer Res 41:278–288, 1981.
108. Oegema TR, Hascall VC, Dziewiatkowski DD: Isolation and characterization of proteoglycans from the Swarm rat chondrosarcoma. J Biol Chem 250:6151–6159, 1975.
109. Liotta LA, Foidart JM, Robey PG, Martin GR, Gullino PM: Identification of micrometastases of breast carcinomas by presence of basement membrane collagen. Lancet 2:146–147, 1979.
110. Satoh C, Duff R, Rapp F, Davidson EA: Production of mucopolysaccharide by normal and transformed cells. Proc Natl Acad Sci USA 70:54–56, 1973.
111. Hopwood JJ, Dorfman A: Glycosaminoglycan synthesis by cultured human skin fibroblasts after transformation with simian virus 40. J Biol Chem 252:4777–4785, 1977.
112. Waxler B, Eisenstein R, Battifora H: Electrophoresis of tissue glycosaminoglycans as an aid in the diagnosis of mesothaliomas. Cancer 44:221–227, 1977.
113. Gospodarowicz D, Vlodovsky I, Savion N: The extracellular matrix and the control of proliferation of vascular endothelial and vascular smooth muscle cells. J Supramol Struct 13:339–372, 1980.
114. DeLuca S, Heinegård D, Hascall VC, Kimura JH, Caplan AI: Chemical and physical changes in proteoglycans during development of chick limb bud chondrocytes grown *in vitro*. J Biol Chem 252:6600–6608, 1977.

18. Attachment of metastatic tumor cells to collagen

J.C. MURRAY, L.A. LIOTTA and V.P. TERRANOVA

1. Introduction

It has recently been demonstrated that a great degree of specificity exists in the interaction of cells with their extracellular matrices [1, 2, 3]. Collagen, a major component of extracellular matrix, exists in at least five genetically distinct forms; type I and type III collagens are found in the stroma of many tissues [4], type II in cartilage [5] and type IV in basement membranes [6]. While mesenchymal cells adhere to stromal collagens *in vitro* [1], epithelial cells show a specificity for type IV (basement membrane) collagen [2, 7]; that is, cells appear to adhere to the types of collagen with which they are normally in contact *in vivo*. *In vitro* these interactions are mediated by high molecular weight glycoproteins; mesenchymal cells utilize fibronectin to bind to all collagens [2], whereas epithelial cells adhere preferentially to type IV basement membrane collagen using laminin. *In vivo*, fibronectin appears as a major component of mesenchymal extracellular matrices [7], whereas laminin is a major component of basement membranes and is absent from other tissues [8, 9].

Fibronectin is frequently either absent from, or present in reduced amounts on the cell surface after viral transformation and in cells cultured from certain tumors [7, 10, 11]. A similar phenomenon has also been observed with laminin in normal and transformed rat kidney cells [12]. Like fibronectin, collagen production is frequently diminished after transformation [13, 14, 15]. These findings have led various investigators to speculate that malignancy may be related to alterations in the synthesis of extracellular matrix components or alterations in the interactions between tumor cells and these components [16, 17].

It is the aim of this chapter to consider the interaction of tumour cells with collagenous substrates *in vitro* and how such interactions may relate to one or more steps in the metastatic process. In the following pages we describe the use of a simple cell adhesion assay, originally described by Klebe [18], to study the interaction of cultured transformed cells and cloned cells of known metastatic potential, with different types of collagen and adhesion factors.

L.A. Liotta and I.R. Hart (eds.), Tumor Invasion and Metastasis. ISBN-13: 978-94-009-7513-2.
© 1982 Martinus Nijhoff Publishers, The Hague/Boston/London.

2. Materials and methods

2.1. Preparation of collagen substrates

Type I collagen was prepared from lathyritic rat skin [19], Type II collagen from a rat chondrosarcoma [20], Type III collagen from fetal calf skin [21], Type IV collagen from the EHS sarcoma, a transplantable murine tumour producing a basement membrane-like matrix [22].

The various collagens were dissolved in 0.5 N acetic acid and diluted to a concentration of 10 μg/ml. 1 ml of the dilute collagen solution was added to 35 mm bacteriological plastic dishes and allowed to air dry at room temperature. These dishes can be sterilized under u.v. light overnight if necessary.

2.2. Preparation of fibronectin

Fibronectin was prepared from normal human serum by adsorption to a column of denatured type I collagen covalently bound to Sepharose 4B [23, 24] equilibrated in minimal essential medium (MEM). An excess of serum was left on the column for 18 h at 4° C, after which the column was washed with MEM. Fibronectin was eluted from the column with 1 M KBr-0.05 M Tris-HCl, pH 5.3, subsequently dialysed against MEM in the cold and stored at 20° C. Fibronectin prepared in this manner consisted of a major protein component of 400 000 dalton on SDS-gel electrophoresis. After reduction with marcaptoethanol, the major band had a mobility of approximately 200 000 dalton, characteristic of fibronectin [8].

2.3. Preparation of laminin

Laminin was extracted from the EHS sarcoma using neutral 0.5 M NaCl-extraction [9] followed by 1.7 M NaCl precipitation to remove type IV collagen. This extract was chromatographed on DEAE cellulose equilibrated in 2 M urea, 0.05 M Tris-HCl, pH 8.6, followed by chromatography on Agarose A5M equilibrated with 0.4 M NaCl, 0.05 M Tris, pH 7.4. On SDS gel electrophoresis, laminin consists after reduction of two major protein components of 400 000 dalton and 200 000 dalton.

2.4. Cells attachment assays

Cell attachment assays were carried out using a modification of the assay described by Klebe [18]. Collagen-coated dishes were preincubated with MEM containing 200 μg/ml bovine serum albumin to inhibit nonspecific cell binding for 1 h (room temperature). Freshly trypsinized cells from culture dishes were then added along with the attachment factor to be tested to the dishes, and the incubation continued at 37° C for various times. To assess the amount of attachment, dishes were rinsed three times with PBS to remove unattached cells. Attached cells were removed with 0.1% trypsin EDTA in PBS and counted electronically. Where indicated, cells were preincubated with growth medium plus 25 μg/ml cycloheximide to inheibit protein synthesis. For attachment studies cells were then trypsinized and the assay continued as above, in the presence of 25 μg/ml cycloheximide

2.5. Collagen analysis

In some experiments the amount of collagen production by various cell lines was measured. Total collagen synthesis was estimated by bacterial collagenase digestion of [^{3}H] proline containing collagenous proteins [25].

2.6. Cells

Cell strains ACT (adult connective tissue) and TACT (transformed adult connective tissue) are normal and spontaneously transformed mouse connective tissue cells, respectively [26]. TACT cells are tumorigenic in syngeneic hosts, but non-metastatic. PMT was selected from a pulmonary metastasis of the T241 fibrosarcoma [27].

Cell lines F1 and F10 are variants of the B16 mouse melanoma, selected *in vitro* by Dr. I. Fidler, and exhibit a ten-fold difference in metastatic efficiency by the tail vein injection assay [28, 29]. Line B16-B1 6 is a variant with increased invasive capacity *in vitro* and *in vivo*, selected from B16 F10 by Dr. I. Hart.

3. Results

3.1. ACT, TACT and PMT: A simple model for malignancy in mesenchymal cells

Previous observations of specificity in the adhesion of normal cells to different types of collagen led us to carry out preliminary experiments on the interaction of tumorigenic cells with collagenous substrates. In view of the evidence that malignant cells have altered interactions with the extracellular matrix [30], we chose to examine the difference between a cell line which was highly metastatic and its putative cell of origin: that is, a dermal fibroblast. The PMT cell line produces multiple pulmonary metastases in the syngeneic host (C57/BL6 mouse) both spontaneously and after i.v. injection through the tail vein. A suitable benign control was TACT, a cell line which arose spontaneously in cultures of murine dermal fibroblasts and which on subcutaneous injection produces fibrosarcomas which never

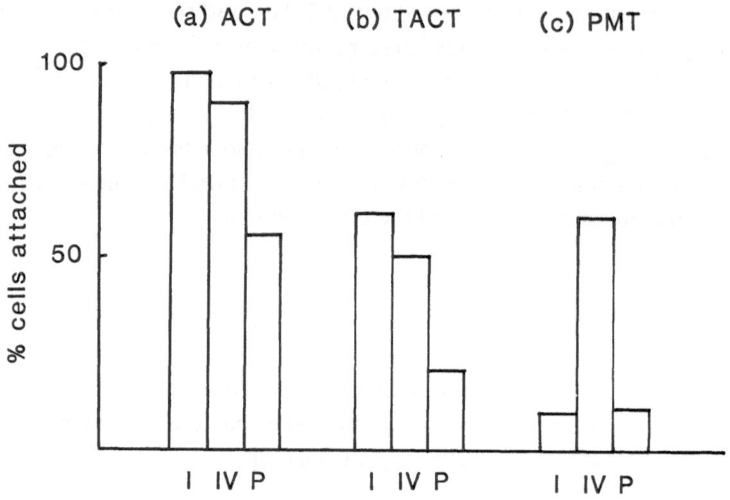

Figure 1. Attachment of ACT, TACT and PMT cells to type I and type IV collagen-coated dishes and plastic (P), after 3 h at 37° C in the absence of serum.

metastasize. Together with the primary culture of dermal fibroblasts from C57/BL6 mice these represented a series of cells of increasing malignancy and of similar origin.

Cell adhesion assays, in the absence of serum or any additional factor, indicated that whereas the ACT and TACT cells show no specificity for adhesion to different types of collagen, PMT cells attached preferentially to type IV (basement membrane) collagen (Figure 1). ACT cells, as other normal mesenchymal cells we have studied [1], adhere rapidly to all types of collagen, as well as to plastic substrates (Types II and III not shown).

TACT cells also adhere to all types of collagen, although less rapidly than ACT and in small numbers. These cells do not however adhere to plastic. These differences may be due to differences in levels of collagen synthesis between these cells; ACT produces five times more collagen than TACT [17], and therefore the normal cell may be able to synthesize a matrix upon which it rests. The metastatic PMT cells which adhere rapidly to type IV (basement membrane) collagen, are unable to adhere spontaneously to type I collagen or plastic. These results suggested that the mechanisms by which cells adhere to type I collagen was defective in the metastatic PMT cell. As this function is generally attributed to fibronectin [1], we investigated the effect of fibronectin on the adhesion of these cells to collagen (Figure 2). These attachments assays showed that both normal and malignant (TACT not shown) cell types responded to fibronectin and adhered more rapidly to collagen, suggesting that all three cell types retain receptors for fibronectin. In addition, experiments with cycloheximide which blocked binding to type IV indicates that the PMT binding factor for type IV collagen was the product of de novo protein synthesis.

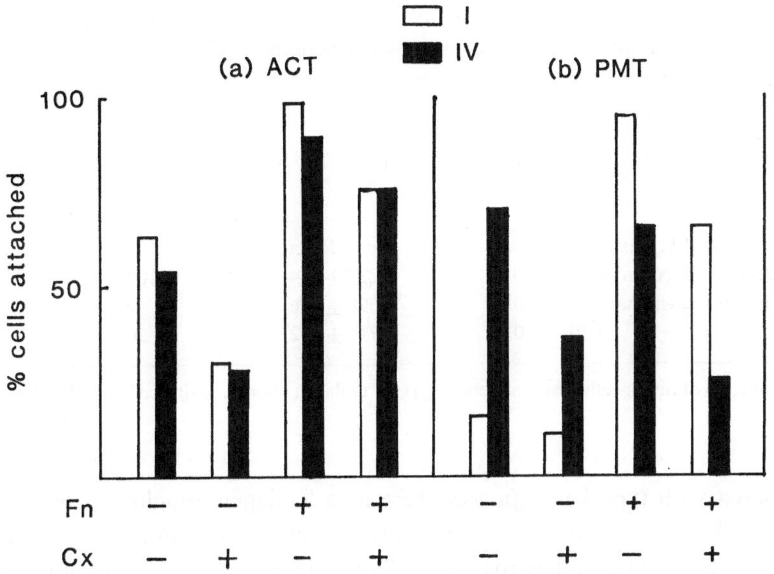

Figure 2. Attachment of ACT and PMT cells to type I and type IV collagen-coated dishes in the presence and absence of fibronectin, with and without pretreatment with cycloheximide to inhibit protein synthesis.

Fibronectin did not restore adhesion of PMT to type IV. Fidler [28] has proposed that tumors consist of heterogeneous cell populations and that several subpopulations can be selected out *in vivo* by their ability to form pulmonary metastases, suggesting that potentially metastatic cells may have specific properties which are not expressed in the non-metastatic population.

Warren and Vales [31] have shown that bloodborne tumor cells adhere to exposed areas of the basement membrane in the subendothelium.

We therefore designed further experiments to investigate whether the interaction between malignant cells and type IV collagen may be related to metastatic propensity.

3.2. Adhesion to type IV collagen and metastatic potential

Further experiments were carried out to determine whether the interaction between PMT cells and type IV collagen correlated to metastatic potential. For these experiments we used variants of the B16 mouse melanoma and the UV2237 mouse fibrosarcoma. These tumor systems were established by I. Fidler, and have been selected *in vivo* for their ability to grow as lung colonies in mice after injection through the tail-vein. This assay is thought to give reasonable correlation with the metastatic potential of these cells *in vivo* [32]. In Table 1, we give the data for two variants of the B16 melanoma. The differential adhesion to type IV collagen as

Table 1. Correlation of adhesion to type IV collagen substrates, type IV degrading activity, and incidence of spontaneous metastases among several tumorigenic cell lines.

Cell type	Collagen attachment index*	Type IV degrading activity (cpm / 2 × 10^5 cells)	Mice bearing pulmonary mets. 18 days after i.m. injection (%)
Mouse dermal fibroblast	0.00	none detected	0
PMT (murine fibrosarcoma)	0.30	8230 ± 214	100
B16 (murine melanoma) F1	0.05	398 ± 36	0
F10	0.23	,714 ± 62	30

* Proportion of tumor cells which adhere to type IV collagen after removing cells which adhere to type I collagen.

compared with type I is expressed here as a 'collagen attachment index' and is calculated as the proportion of cells which spontaneously adhere to type IV after removing cells which adhere to type I collagen. These data are shown along with the number of spontaneous metastases produced after i.m. injection. In addition we have included levels of type IV collagenase activity, which has recently been shown to be a characteristic of metastasizing tumor cells [32]. Taken together, these data suggest a significant correlation between the interaction of the cells with a type IV collagen substrate, their ability to degrade that substrate, and the metastatic potential of the cells *in vivo*.

We further attempted to select out cells of increased metastatic potential by using their ability to adhere to type IV collagen. Table 2 shows the data for the numbers of lung colonies in mice injected with PMT cells previously allowed to attach to type I or type IV substrates. These data suggest that the cells of greater metastatic potential adhere preferentially to type IV collagen compared to type I collagen substrates.

Table 2. Number of experimental metastases in C57/BL6 mice after i.v. injection of 10^5 cells pre-selected on type I and type IV collagen-coated dishes.

Substrate	Metastases/lung 18 days after i.v. injection
Type I collagen:	
adherent	2.0 ± 1.5
non-adherent	9.4 ± 1.6
Type IV collagen:	
adherent	12.5 ± 2.0
non-adherent	4.2 ± 0.5

Trypsinized cultured PMT cells were allowed to attach for 3 h to collagen-coated dishes. Adherent cells were removed with a rubber policeman and suspensions of adherent and non-adherent cells injected into 6 mice in each group.

In the case of the sarcoma cells we demonstrated that fibronectin synthesis is diminished, thus possibly accounting for their defective adhesion to type I collagen substrates, but that the adhesion mechanism for type IV collagen is apparently intact. Metastatic melanoma cells also appear to have preferential binding to type IV collagen. Therefore we may speculate that the inability to bind to stromal collagen combined with the ability to bind to type IV collagen is related, in the case of melanoma and sarcoma cells, to metastatic potential.

3.3. Laminin as a cell attachment factor

Considering the recent work [9] on the ability of laminin to bind epithelial cells to basement membrane type IV collagen, we looked at the ability of laminin to act as the adhesive factor for metastatic tumor cells. Recently it has been shown [33, 34] that laminin is the attachment factor for the metastatic population of cells. Both the B16 and PMT-2 cell lines were examined using the nonmetastatic tumorigenic C3H fibrosarcoma as a control. Following laminin attachment to type IV collagen, cells were injected intravenously into C57/BL6 mice and the number of pulmonary metastatic colonies were counted. Table 3 shows that the laminin-type IV collagen attached cells produced significantly more metastases per injection of viable cells compared to the unattached cells. Furthermore, the laminin type IV attached cells showed a higher metastatic potential than did the fibronectin-type IV attached or unattached population. The subpopulation of B16 or PM 2 cells that were selected by their ability to attach to type IV collagen in the presence of laminin showed 10 times the metastatic activity of unattached cells or of cells attached in the presence of fibronectin. In addition, incubation of cells with anti-laminin antibody prior to injection into mice markedly reduced the number of pulmonary metastases.

Table 3. Pulmonary metastases mean po/mouse produced by subpopulations of adherent tumor cells (2×10^5 cells).

Cell type	Parent	ALM Ab	LM ATT	FN ATT
PM2	90	5	102	30
Bl6	110	16	160	22

Parent: Parent tumor cell population. ALM Ab: treatment with antilaminin antibodies.
LM ATT: Tumor cells attached to type IV collagen in the presence of laminin.
FN ATT: Tumor cells attached to type IV collagen in the presence of fibronectin.

4. Conclusions

The malignant behavior of tumor cells is thought to be closely related to abnormalities in their adhesive properties [30]. Many recent studies have focused attention on the role of collagen as a natural substrate for the growth and differentiation of normal cells, and demonstrated that, *in vivo*, collagenous matrices may aid in the maintenance and expression of normal phenotypic characteristics (for review see [3]). Extending these findings, we have examined the behavior of tumorigenic cells on collagenous substrates in order to determine whether malignancy can be correlated *in vitro* with the adhesive behavior of the cells.

Using a simple collagen adhesion assay, we have demonstrated difference in adhesive properties of cells of clearly differing malignant potential. These differences were shown to be correlated in the case of the PMT sarcoma system at least, with the ability of these cells to elaborate the major structural components of the extracellular matrix: fibronectin and collagen. Furthermore we have shown that laminin is the attachment factor for some types of highly metastatic tumor cells.

These characteristics are postulated to be related to the tumorigenic potential of the cells. In addition, these studies have revealed that changes in the specificity of adhesion to different types of collagen may arise which appear to be related to the ability of the cells to metastasize. The retention of the laminin attachment mechanism whereby the sarcoma cells adhere strongly to type IV (basement membrane) collagen may be responsible for the ability of the cells to adhere to basement membrane *in vivo* and ultimately establish successful metastatic colonies. This hypothesis is supported by the observation that cells of greater metastatic potential *in vivo* can be selected by their ability to bind preferentially to type IV collagen using laminin as the attachment factor.

References

1. Kleinman HK, Murray JC, McGoodwin EB, Martin GR: Connective tissue structure: cell binding to collagen. J Invest Dermatol 71:9–11, 1978.
2. Murray JC, Stingl GS, Kleinman HK, Martin GR, Katz SI: Epidermal cells adhere preferentially to type IV (Basement membrane) collagen. J Cell Biol 80:197–202, 1979.
3. Kleinman HK, Klebe RJ, Martin GR: Role of collagenous matrices in the adhesion and growth of cells. J Cell Biol 88:473–485, 1981.
4. Miller EJ, Epstein EH, Jr, Piez KA: Identification of three genetically distinct collagens by cyanogen bromide cleavage of insoluble skin and cartilage collagen. Biochem Biophys Res Commun 42:1024–1029, 1971.
5. Miller EJ, Matukas VJ: Chick cartilage collagen: a new type of α1 chain not present in bone skin of the species. Proc Natl Acad Sci USA 64:1264–1268, 1969.
6. Kefalides NA: Structure and biosynthesis of basement membranes. Int Rev Connect Tissue Res 6:63–104, 1973.
7. Yamada KM, Olden K: Fibronectins-adhesive glycoproteins of cell surface and blood. Nature (London), 275:179–184, 1978.

8. Timpl R, Rohde H, Robey PG, Rennard SI, Foidart JM, Martin GR: Laminin-a glycoprotein from basement membranes. J Biol Chem 254:9933–9937, 1979.
9. Terranova VP, Rohrbach DH, Martin GR: Role of Laminin in the attachment of PAM 212 (Epithelial) cells to basement membrane collagen. Cel 22:719–726, 1980.
10. Hynes RO: Cell surface protein and malignant transformation. Biochim Biophys Acta 458:73–107, 1976.
11. Vaheri A, Mosher D: Fibroblast surface antigen produced but not retained by virus-transformed human cells. J Exp Med 142:530–535, 1975.
12. Hayman EG, Engrall E, Ruoslahti: Concomitant loss of cell surface fibronectin and laminin from transformed rat kidney cells. J Cell Biol 88:352–357, 1981.
13. Levison W, Bhatnagar RS, Liu TZ: Loss of the ability to synthesize collagen in fibroblasts transformed by Rous Sarcoma virus. J Natl Cancer Inst 55:807–810, 1975.
14. Kamine J, Rubin H: Coordinate control of collagen synthesis and cell growth in chick embryo fibroblasts and the effect of viral transformation on collagen synthesis. J Cell Physiol 92:1–12, 1977.
15. Green H, Todaro GJ, Goldberg B: Collagen synthesis in fibroblasts transformed by oncogenic viruses. Nature (London) 209:916–917, 1966.
16. Chen LB, Burridge K, Murray A, Walsh ML, Copple CD, Bushness A, McDougall JK, Gallimore PH: Modulation of cell surface glycocalyx: studies on large external, transformation sensitive protein. Ann N.Y. Acad Sci 312:366–381, 1978.
17. Murray JC, Liotta L, Rennard SI, Martin GR: Adhesion characteristics of murine metastatic and nonmetastatic tumor cells *in vitro*. Cancer Res 40:347–351, 1980.
18. Klebe RJ: Isolation of a collagen-dependent cell attachment factor. Nature (London) 250:248–251, 1974.
19. Bornstein P, Piez K: The nature of the intramolecular cross-links on collagen. The separation and characterization of peptides from the cross-link region of rat-skin collagen. Biochemistry 5: 1966.
20. Smith BD, Martin GR, Miller EJ, Dorfman A, Smith R: Nature of the collagen synthesized by a transplantable chondrosarcoma. Arch Biochem Biophys 166:181–186, 1975.
21. Epstein E: $\alpha 1(III)_3$ human skin collagen released by pepsin digestion and preponderance in fetal life. J Biol Chem 249:3225–3231, 1974.
22. Orkin RW, Gehron P, McGoodwin EB, Martin GR, Valentine T, Swarm R: A unique tumor producing a matrix of basement membrane. J Exp Med 145:209–219, 1977.
23. Hopper DE, Adelman BC, Genter G, Gay S: Recognition by guinea pig peritoneal exudate cells of conformationally different states of the collagen molecule. Immunology 30:249–259, 1976.
24. Engvall E, Ruoslahti E: Binding of soluble form of fibroblast surface protein, fibronactin, to collagen. Int J Cancer 20:1–5, 1977.
25. Green H, Goldberg B: Synthesis of collagen by mammalian cell lines of fibroblastic and non-fibroblastic origin. Proc Natl Acad Sci USA 53:1360 1365, 1965.
26. Liotta L, Vembu D, Kleinman HK, Martin GR, Boone C: Collagen required for proliferation of cultured connective tissue cells but no their transformed counter-part. Nature (London) 272:622–624, 1978.
27. Liotta L, Veimbu D, Saini RK, Boone C: *In Vivo* monitoring of the death rate of artificial murine pulmonary metastases. Cancer Res 38:1231–1236.
28. Fidler IJ: Selection of successive tumor lines for metastasis. Nature New Biol 242:148–149, 1973.
29. Fidler IJ, Kripke ML: Metastasis results from preexisting variant cells within a malignant tumor. Science 197:893–895, 1977.
30. Coman DR: Cellular adhesiveness in relation to the invasiveness of cancer. Cancer Res 14:519–531, 1954.
31. Warren BA, Vales O: The adhesion of thromboplastic tumor emboli to vessel walls *in vivo*: Br J Exp Pathol 53;301–313, 1972.
32. Liotta LA, Tryggvason K, Garbisa S, Hart I, Foltz CM: Nature (London) 284:67–68, 1980.
33. Terranova VP, Liotta LA, Russo R, Martin GR: Role of laminin in the attachment of metastatic

tumor cells. Cancer Res, in press.
34. Liotta LA, Terranova VP, Lanzer W, Russo R, Siegal G, Garbisa S: Basement membrane attachment and degradation by metastatic tumor cells. In: New trends in basement membrane research, Schone HH (ed). Munich: S. Karger, in press.

19. Biochemical mechanisms involved in tumor cell penetration of the basement membrane

L.A. LIOTTA, S. GARBISA and K. TRYGGVASON

Cancer invasion and metastases is such a highly complex process that it is difficult to study the specific biochemical mechanisms involved. One way to circumvent this problem is to break the process down into a series of defined tumor-host interactions, and then to focus on one type of interaction. For example, past investigators have focused on the interaction of metastatic tumor cells with isolated populations of host cells such as lymphocytes, macrophages, or endothelial cells [1–3]. Those types of experiments were made feasible by technical advances which enabled investigators to obtain pure populations of host cells. With recent advances in the understanding of connective tissue biochemistry [4–7], it is now possible to purify specific components of the host extracellular matrix for use in experiments related to tumor invasion.

Table 1. Examples of extracellular matrix elements penetrated by metastasizing tumor cells.

Host tissue	Structural element	Biochemical components
epithelium, endothelium, mesothelium	desmosomes, tight junctions, anchoring fibrils	disulfide-bonded proteins
interface between organ parenchyma and supporting connective tissue	basement membranes	fibronectin, laminin, proteoglycans, type IV collagen, type V collagen
interstitial connective tissue stroma	anchoring fibers, collagen fibers elastic fibers	type I collagen, type III collagen type V collagen, elastin, proteoglycans glycoproteins, fibronectin
cartilage, bone	gbound substance, mineralized matrix	proteoglycans, glycosaminoglycans, hydroxyapatite, type II collagen, type I collagen, elastin.

L.A. Liotta and I.R. Hart (eds.), Tumor Invasion and Metastasis. ISBN-13: 978-94-009-7513-2.
© 1982 Martinus Nijhoff Publishers, The Hague/Boston/London.

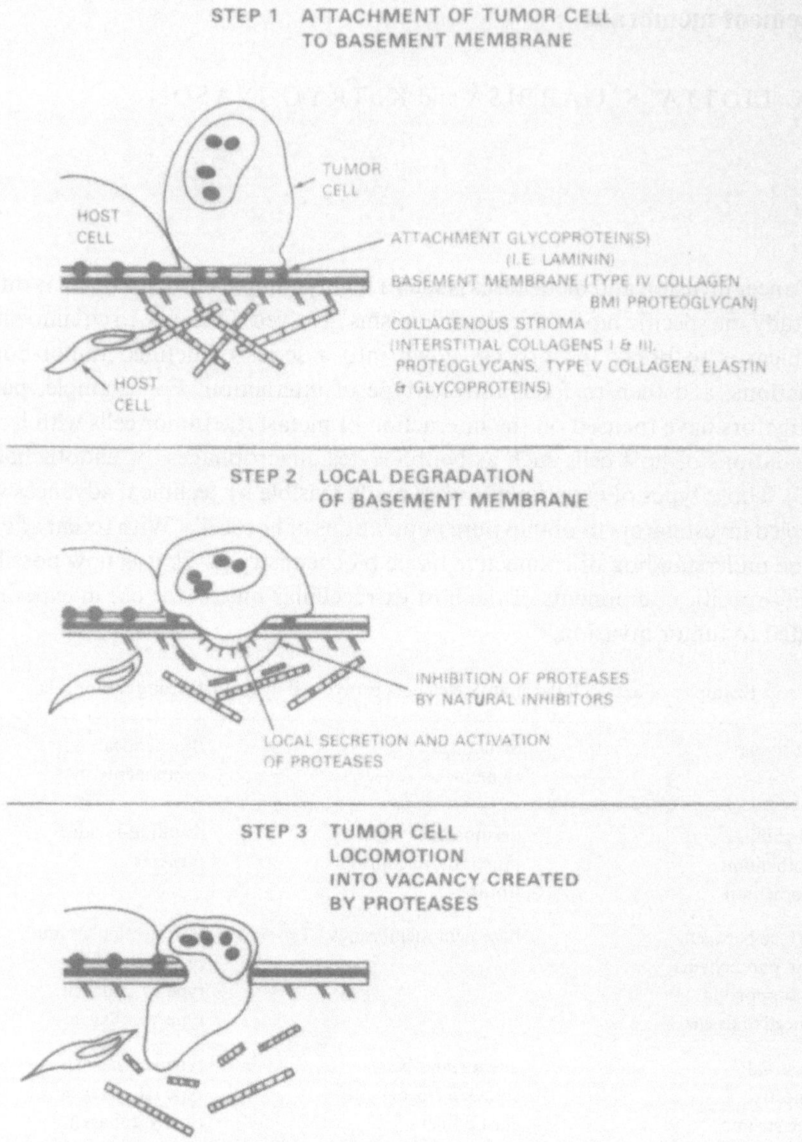

Figure 1. Three step hypothesis for tumor cell penetration of the basement membrane (BM). The first step is tumor cell attachment to exposed BM which may occur via attachment factors such as laminin, fibronectin or proteoglycans. The second step is local proteolytic degradation of the BM. More than one type of protease may be involved. Degradation occurs in a localized region where the concentrations of the enzyme are enough to overcome surrounding host tissue protease inhibitors. The third step is tumor cell locomotion into the zone of lysis.

Metastasizing tumor cells encounter a number of different host extracellular connective tissue barriers as they disseminate from the primary tumor and finally grow as a metastatic colony (Table 1). The basement membrane (BM) is one type of extracellular matrix which tumor cells encounter at more than one step in the metastatic process. The continuous BM forms a scaffolding supporting organ parenchyma cells, and also delineates the boundaries of tissue compartments [8–10]. Tumor cells must penetrate the BM when they cross from one tissue to another, or as they enter and exist blood vessels. In this chapter we will review experimental studies which attempt to probe the biochemical mechanism by which tumor cells penetrate the BM. The evidence to date indicates that BM penetration occurs in three steps (Figure 1). The first step is tumor cell attachment to the BM [11]. Tumor cells preferentially bind to the exposed BM compared to the surface of the endothelium or endothelium resting on the BM [3, 12, 13]. The second step is local dissolution of the BM which occurs at the point of tumor cell contact, and can result in the protrusion of a tumor cell pseudopodia through the BM [11, 14–16]. The third step is tumor cell locomotion through the BM defect. The direction of locomotion may be influenced by chemotactic factors derived from connective tissue, serum, or host cells [17, 18]. During the attachment and locomotion steps the invading tumor cell may utilize one or more specific attachment glycoproteins such as laminin or fibronectin [19]. Proteolytic degradation of the BM may be necessary for step two (Figure 1). The evidence for this hypothesis is as follows: a) The BM is a tough resilient barrier [9, 20] which excludes the passage of colloidal carbon [21], and therefore does not normally contain pores large enough for tumor cells to passively move through. b) Tumor cells *in vitro* can actively degrade whole BM [22, 23], extracellular matrix produced by cultured cells [3, 24], or isolated BM structural proteins [25, 26]. Tumor cell derived proteases can be purified which degrade BM collagen [27, 28]. c) Protease inhibitors block tumor cell penetration of extracellular matrix *in vitro* [29].

We will now review the structure and chemical composition of the BM, and the properties of tumor cell associated proteases which degrade BM components.

1. Basement membrane composition

The BM is a complex tissue supporting element and selective permeability barrier composed of collagenous, glycoprotein, and proteoglycan building blocks. The BM is organized into three major layered units [9, 30]:

a) The lamina lucida externa is an electron lucent region, 200–400 Å wide, located on the side of the BM facing the organ parenchyma cells.

b) The lamina densa (also called basal lamina) is the middle layer, 200–1000 Å wide, which is electron dense and amorphous.

c) The lamina lucida externa is an electron lucent region of variable width at the interface of the BM with the connective tissue stroma.

Within epithelial BM, anchoring filaments (20–80 Å thick) form a bridge between the epithelial tonofilament-desmosome complex and the lamina densa. On the opposite side of the BM, anchoring fibers with a periodic banding pattern, smaller anchoring fibrils, and tubular microfilaments run between the lamina densa and the interstitial collagen of the connective tissue stroma [30].

The lamina lucida externa contains attachment glycoproteins such as laminin [31] and fibronectin [32, 33], as well as proteoglycans [34–36]. The latter constituent may regulate the BM permeability [35]. The lamina densa zone is the structural member of the BM and contains Type IV collagen [4–7]. Type V collagen is another type of BM associated collagen found adjacent to the lamina densa on the stromal side [36–38]. Type IV collagen is uniquely localized in the BM, whereas type V collagen is also found outside of the BM zone (Table 1).

2. Proteolyc degradation of the BM

The BM is a highly stable crosslinked with a slow turnover rate in normal adult tissues [9, 10]. Nevertheless, during certain developmental and pathologic states, such as mammary gland involution and tumor invasion, histological studies have demonstated rapid local breakdown of the BM. We have used two approaches to characterize the proteases responsible for BM degradation under normal physiologic conditions.

The first is to study the effect of known purified proteases on preparations of whole BM *in vitro*, or isolated purified basement membrane components [51, 62]. The second approach is to identify, purify, and characterize proteases secreted by metastatic tumor cells which degrade BM components [26–28]. A large number of proteolytic enzymes have been identified which can potentially degrade at least some of the proteins found in the BM.

Proteases can be grouped (Table 2) according to their catalytic sites, specific susceptibility to inhibitors, optimum pH, and cation requirements [40]. For example, a proteolytic activity that is optimum at pH 8, inactive at pH 5 and inhibited by PMSF (phenylmethylsulfonilfluoride) is a neutral serine protease. A proteolytic activity which has neutral pH requirements, is not inhibited by PMSF and is inhibited by specific metal ion chelators (EDTA) is a neutral metal protease.

Two proteases which are likely to play a role in the degradation of BM are special types of collagenolytic enzymes, and plasmin (generated through plasminogen activator).

Classic mammalian collagenase is a metal protease first described by Gross and co-workers [42]. This enzyme makes a single cleavage within the triple helix of the collagen molecule, producing a 3/4 and a 1/4 length product [42]. Prior to collagenase cleavage the collagen molecule is relatively protease resistant [42]. However, the collagenase cleavage products rapidly denature at 37° C and become highly susceptible to proteases which will not normally cleave native collagen [43].

Table 2. Example proteases.

Class	Inhibitor	Characteristic	Examples	Possible functions
Serine protease	Fluorophosphates	'active' serine group	Trypsin	Digestion
			Thrombin	Coagulation
			Plasmin	Fibrinolysis
			Plasminogen activator	Plasmin generation
			Elastase	Digestion
Sulphydryl protease	Iodoacetate N-ethylmaleimide	CySH	Papain	Digestion: extracellular
			Cathepsin B Cathepsin D	Digestion: intracellular
Acid protease	Diazoketones	Acid pH optimum	Pepsin	Protein Digestion
Metal-dependent protease	Metal chelators	Zn^{++}, Ca^{++} dependent Neutral pH optimum	Collagenase	Collagen digestion

Animal and human neoplasms have been studied for the production of collagenolytic activity (see other chapters in this book). Gullino et al. [44] were the first to show that the tumor could influence the metabolism of associated host collagen. Yamanishi [45] used a variety of assay methods to show that basal cell carcinoma and squamous cell carcinoma contain markedly increased collagenase compared to normal skin. Dresden et al. [46] proposed that human tumors cause overproduction of the normal type of collagenase enzyme . Abramson [47] has correlated aggressive *in vivo* growth in carcinomas of the head and neck with collagenase activity. Kuettner et al. [48] have postulated that collagenase inhibitors may prevent tumors from invading cartilage. Biswas et al. [49] showed that the site of carcinoma transplantation influenced the level of associated collagenase.

In all of the above studies the substrate used was type I collagen. Since the major structural protein of the BM is type IV collagen, the measured collagenolytic activity did not necessarily relate to BM degradation. Furthermore, the work of Woolley et al. [50] indicated that type IV collagen was resistant to classic collagenase. Therefore, we studied the substrate specificity of a metastatic tumor cell collagenase and of human skin collagenase for the degradation of collagens types I, II, III, IV and V [51].

Human skin collagenase failed to degrade collagen types IV and V under conditions where collagens I, II and II were cleaved completely. The metastatic tumor collagenase preferentially degraded type IV basement membrane collagen [27, 28, 51]. A separate metastatic tumor metal protease was identified which preferentially degraded type V collagen [28]. These findings along with the protease studies of others indicate that the genetically distinct collagens vary markedly in their protease susceptibility (Table 3). A family of metal proteases may exist with different collagen substrate specificities. Interstitial collagens type I, II and III are cleaved at a specific locus by the 'classic' mammalian collagenase obtained from such sources as skin, rheumatoid synovium and leukocytes, under conditions where type IV (base-

Table 3. Collagen type differences in protease susceptibility.*

Collagen substrate	Interstitial** collagenase	Substrate specific*** metal proteases	Leucocyte**** elastase	Plasmin*****	Mast cell serine protease******
Type I	+	—	—	—	—
Type II	+	—	—	—	—
Type III	+	—	+	—	—
Type IV	—	+	+	—	+
Type V	—	+	—	—	—

* + sign indicates degradation of native collagen at an enzyme tosubstrate ratio of 1/100.
** Woolley et al. [50], Stricklin et al. [55], Gross [42], Liotta et al. [51], Bornstein and Sage [6].
*** Liotta et al. [51, 26–28], Maindardi et al. [57], Reynolds et al. [41], Uitto et al. [56].
**** Gadek et al. [58], Mainardi et al. [59, 60], Uitto et al. [56], Tryggvason et al. [63].
***** Liotta et al. [62].
****** Sage and Bornstein [61].

ment membrane) and type V collagen are not cleaved. Leucocyte collagenase degrades type I but not type III collagen [53]. Human skin collagenase degrades type III collagen at a faster rate than types I or II [54, 55]. A leucocyte metal protease degrades type IV but not type V collagen, while alveolar macrophage metal proteases have been identified which degrade type V and type IV collagen [56, 57].

Certain types of serine proteases also have collagenolytic activity. Leucocyte elastase degrades pepsinized type IV collagen and type III collagen but not the other types of collagen [58–60]. Mast cell serine protease degrades pepsinized type IV collagen [61]. These results suggested that other serine proteases associated with tumor cells such as plasminogen activator, plasmin, and thrombin (these enzymes are reviewed elsewhere in this book) should be checked for collagenolytic activity. Therefore, we incubated highly purified urokinase, plasmin and alpha thrombin with each type of collagen. Both pepsinized and acid soluble type IV collagen was used as a substrate [62]. None of these enzymes produced a major cleavage of any type of collagen when digestion was performed under native substrate conditions (25° C, 18 h, enzyme to substrate ratio 1/100) (Table 2). By electron microscopy and immunohistology none of these serine proteases significantly degraded the basement membrane lamina densa [62].

3. Properties of tumor cell type IV collagenolytic activity

Type IV collagenolytic activity associated with cultured metastatic tumor cells is found in an active form associated with the cell layer [25] and a latent form secreted into the culture media [26–28]. The latent form can be activated with trypsin or plasmin. The enzyme is a metal protease which is inhibited by EDTA, alpha 2 macroglobulin, and cartilage derived natural collagenase inhibitors, but not by PMSF, N-ethyl maleimide or DFP. Type IV collagenolytic enzyme purified from human tumor cells migrates as a doublet on get electrophoresis with an apparent molecular weight of approximately 70KD (Figure 1).

Type IV collagenolytic activity is assayed using ^{14}C or ^{3}H biosynthetically labeled acid extracted type IV collagen substrate purified from organ cultures of the EHS sarcoma [7, 27]. This tumor of unknown cellular origin is benign, encapsulated, and produces a copious BM matrix [7]. The assay is performed by growing the cells on dishes coated with labeled substrate or by incubating serum free conditioned media with soluble substrate. After incubation, the undigested substrate is precipitated and the radioactivity in the supernate fraction is counted. At 37° C the enzyme cleaves the substrate into multiple fragments. However, at temperatures lower than 35° C specific large cleavage products are produced [27]. The enzyme apparently produces a specific cleavage of within a major pepsin resistant region of the type IV collagen molecule (Figure 2) under conditions where the other collagen types are not degraded. Whether or not other non-collagenous substrates exist for this enzyme remains to be determined.

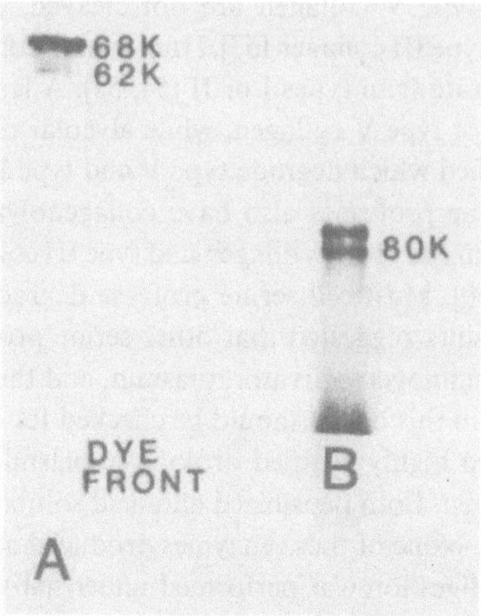

Figure 2. Polyacrylamide gel electrophoresis of purified tumor cell derived metal proteases which degrade type IV and type V collagen. Samples are run with reduction of disulfide bonds. Approximate molecular weights are indicated.

IA: Type IV collagenase affinity purified from human tumor cells [63]. The enzyme migrates as a doublet. 7.5% polyacrylamide gel.

IB: Type V collagenase [28] purified from murine reticulum cell sarcoma [64] by high pressure liquid chromatography and DEAE cellulose chromatography. The enzyme migrates as a doublet. 5.0% polyacrylamide gel.

4. Correlation of type IV collagenolytic activity with metastatic propensity

The ability of tumor cells to proteolytically degrade the BM structural component type IV collagen may be necessary but not sufficient for metastasis formation [22, 26]. For at least one group of metastatic murine tumors the type IV collagenolytic activity correlated with their ability to produce spontaneous metastases [26]. However, it is unlikely that a strict quantitative relationship between type IV collagenolysis and metastatic ability exists for all types of tumors. It is also possible that in some cases non-enzymatic mecahnisms exist for BM penetration such as rupture by mechanical pressure, migration of tumor cells through defects in abnormally formed host BM, or BM damaged by inflammatory cells. Nevertheless, all the highly metastatic tumor cells tested to date (fibrosarcomas, carcinomas, hepatomas, melanomas and a reticulum cells sarcoma) have consistently elevated type IV collagenolytic activity, compared to benign control cells. A group of six melanoma clones all derived from pulmonary metastases (kindly supplied by Dr. J. Fidler) all had significant type IV collagenolytic activity even though they differed in degree of melanin pigmentation. High metastatic tumor cells may be switched toward catabolism rather than synthesis of matrix components. The protease activity responsible for the catabolism is not unique to tumor cells but is also elevated

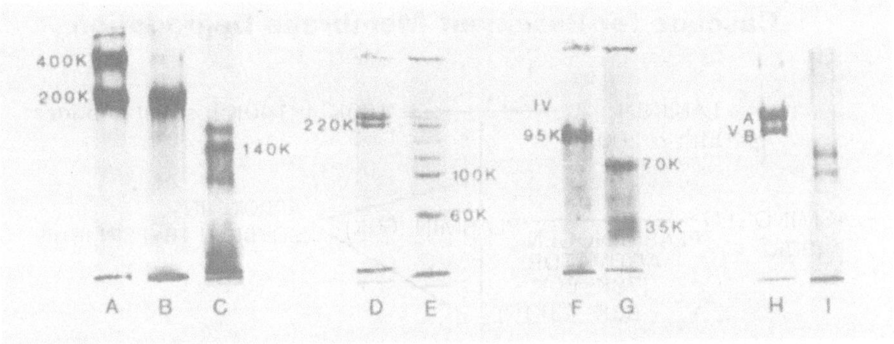

Figure 3. Polyacrylamide gel electrophoresis of purified basement membrane associated proteins degraded with tumor cell associated proteases [62]. Samples in lanes A-E are run with reduction of disulfide bonds. Laminin (50 μg) alone; 200 κ and 400 κ chains have a ratio of 1/1.8 (A). Laminin (50 μg) plus alpha thrombin (0.5 μg) 25° C, 4 h. The 400 κ chain is preferentially degraded (B). Laminin (50 μg) plus human plasmin (0.5 μg), 20° C, 4 h. Both chains are degraded (C). Human serum fibronectin (30 μg) alone (D). Fibronectin (30 μg) plus human plasmin (0.3 μg) 20° C, 4 h. Specific cleavage products are produced (E). Pepsinized murine type IV collagen 95 κ alpha chain alone (30 μg) (F). Cleavage of type IV collagen by tumor type IV collagenase [27] (0.3 μg) 18° C, 40 h. The cleavage produces two specific products (G). Pepsinized placenta type V collagen (50 μg) alone (H). Type V collagen (50 μg) plus tumor cell type V collagenase [28] (0.1 μg) 25° C, 40 h (1).

in normal cells under conditions where the matrix is being turned over during developmental remodeling [65].

5. Degradation of basement membrane non-collagenous components

At least two specific types of glycoproteins have been identified in the BM. These are laminin and fibronectin (see chapter by H, Kleinman). Laminin is not found outside the BM, whereas fibronectin is found in serum and interstitial matrix. Laminin is a disulfide bonded molecule which (under reducing conditions) migrates as two chains (400κD and 200κD) on polyacrylamide gell electrophoresis [31], Fibronectin migrates to a molecular weight of 220 κ [32, 33]. Both glycoproteins are degraded by plasmin and alpha thrombin (Figure 3) but not by highly purified plasminogen activator (urokinase) [62, 64]. At physiologic concentration, plasmin cleaves both chains of laminin producing specific products. Alpha thrombin selectively digests the 400κD beta chain of laminin. Both of these enzymes may therefore play a significant *in vivo* role in the degradation of non-collagenous components of the BM.

We also studied the ability of a variety of cell types to elaborate protease activities which could directly degrade laminin. ^{14}C biosynthetically labeled laminin was used in a new protease assay which demonstrates appropriate linearity and saturation kinetics [62]. Leucocytes, macrophages, and highly metastatic tumor

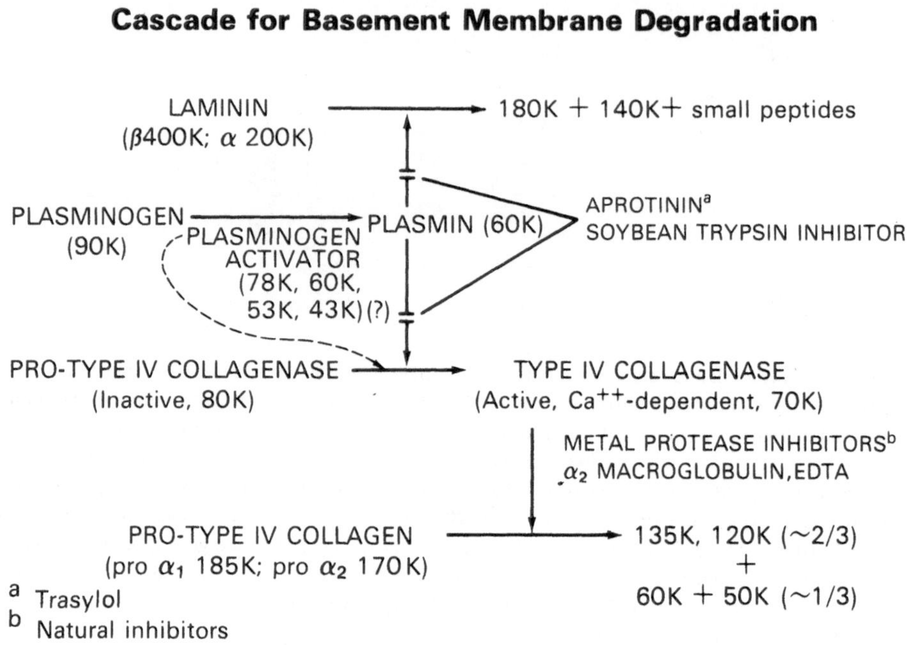

Figure 4. Schematic diagram of cascade for tumor cell degradation of the basement membrane laminin and type IV collagen. Plasminogen activator secreted by the tumor cell activates plasminogen to form plasmin. Plasmin directly degrades laminin and fibronectin (not shown) and also activates latent type IV collagenase to degrade type IV collagen. This proces may occur in a localized region adjacent to the tumor cell (see Figure 1).

cells were found to secrete laminin degrading proteases. The addition of plasminogen to the serum free conditioned media enhanced the laminin degrading activity significantly. Such a response supports a plasmin-mediated degradation of laminin. However, since degradation also occurred in the absence of plasminogen, other neutral proteases different from plasmin must be involved in the degradation of laminin as well.

6. Cascade for basement membrane degradation

Plasminogen activator and collagenolytic metal proteases, both produced by metastasizing tumor cells, may act in concert to degrade the whole BM (Figure 4). Plasminogen activator can generate plasmin from plasminogen (see other chapters in this book for reviews on plasminogen activator). The plasmin produced by this reaction can directly degrade non-collagenous BM components such as laminin and fibronectin. In addition, plasmin can activate latent metal proteases which would degrade BM collagenous and proteoglycan components. The actual cascade of BM degradation *in vivo* probably occurs adjacent to the tumor cell surface where the

Table 4. Susceptibility of basement membrane components to selected tumor cell associated serine proteases.*

Substrate	Plasminogen activator	Plasmin**	Alpha** thrombin
Whole crosslinked*** basal lamina (lamina densa)	—	—	—
Native type IV*** collagen	—	—	—
Laminin	—	+ +	+
Fibronectin	—	+ + +	+ + +

* The + sign indicates degradation by the purified enzyme as judged by electron microscopy or polyacrylamide gel electrophoresis [62].

** These enzymes are generated through by activators elaborated by tumor cells.

*** These substrates are degraded by tumor cell derived metal proteases [26, 27, 62].

local concentration of enzymes is enough to override natural protease inhibitors (Figure 1). Such inhibitors are ubiquitous throughout the extracellular matrix and are present in serum [68]. At any point in time only a small proportion of the total tumor cell population may be expressing BM degrading protease activity.

7. Conclusions

1. Tumor cell penetration of the extracellular matrix is the result of a complex interplay with host biochemical and cellular factors. The process may involve intrinsic tumor cell properties, attachment glycoproteins, latent and active connective tissue matrix degrading proteases, protease activators and inhibitors, and special properties of host connective tissue components.

2. Current evidence indicates that tumor cell penetration of the basement membrane (BM) matrix barrier is necessary for hematogenous metastases to occur. Such penetration may involve proteolytic destruction of the BM. Cultured highly metastatic tumor cells can be shown to actively damage whole BM *in vitro*, and *in vivo* zones of BM damage are noted adjacent to invading tumor cells. It would also seem logical that degradation of stroma and bone collagenous matrices would make room for invading tumor cells. Proteases which play a role in invasion may be elaborated directly by tumor cells or may be produced by host cells such as endothelium, stromal cells and immune cells.

3. The BM is composed of collagenous and non-collagenous elements. Degradation of the collagenous element (type IV collagen) is necessary for proteolytic destruction of the whole BM. Classic collagenase fails to degrade type IV collagen.

Separate proteases have been identified which degrade this type of collagen. In general the different collagen types vary markedly in their protease susceptibility. A family of metal proteases exists (of which classic interstitial collagenase is a subgroup) with selective specificities for the different collagen types.

4. Plasminogen activator (urokinase) alone fails to degrade the following components of the BM zone: fibronectin, laminin, type IV collagen, or type V collagen. Among these BM components, plasmin and alpha thrombin can degrade fibronectin and laminin.

5. At least some strains of cultured tumor cells can elaborate proteases which degrade one or more of the genetically distinct types of collagen. All the highly metastatic tumor cells tested to date exhibit a consistently elevated production of metal proteases which can degrade the basement membrane. It is unlikely that a quantitative difference in these proteases would correlate with metastatic propensity in all types of tumors, but some minimal ability to degrade basement membranes would seem necessary for hematogenous metastases. If proteases play a role *in vivo* their action is probably restricted to a local pericellular region controlled by the balance between enzyme and tissue protease inhibitors. Whether this balance can be therapeutically altered in favor of the host remains to be determined.

References

1. Wood GW, Gillespie GY: Studies on the role of macrophages in regulation of growth and metastasis of murine chemically induced fibrosarcomas. Int J Cancer 16:1022–1029, 1975.
2. Fidler IJ, Gersten DM, Hart IR: The biology of cancer invasion and metastasis. Adv Cancer Res 28:149–250, 1978.
3. Kramer RH, Nicolson GL: Interactions of tumor cells with vascular endothelial cell monolayers: a model for metastatic invasion. Proc Natl Acad Sci 76:5704–5708, 1979.
4. Kefalides NA (ed): Biology and chemistry of basement membranes. New York: Academic Press, 1978.
5. Miller EJ: Biochemical characteristics and biologic significance of the genetically distinct collagens. Mol Cell Biochem 13:165–192, 1976.
6. Bornstein P, Sage H: Structurally distinct collagen types. Ann Rev Biochem 49:957–1003, 1980.
7. Timpl R, Martin GR, Bruckner P, Wick G, Wiedemann H: Nature of the collagenous protein in tumor basement membrane. Eur J Biochem 84:43, 1978.
8. Pierce GB: Epithelial basement membrane. Origin, development and role in disease. In: Balazs chemistry and molecular biology of the intercellular matrix. London: Academic Press, 1970.
9. Vracko R: Basal lamina scaffold – Anatomy and significance for maintenance of orderly tissue structure. Am J Pathol 77:314, 1974.
10. Robert AM, Robert L, Boniface R: Frontiers of matrix biology. Vol. 7. Biochemistry and pathology of basement membranes. Basel: S. Karger, 1979.
11. Babai F: Etude ultrastructural sur la pathogénie de l'invasion du muscle strié par des tumeurs transplantables. J Ultrastr Res 56:287–303, 1976.
12. Warren BA, Vales O. The adhesion of thromboplastic tumour emboli to vessel walls *in vivo*. Br J Exp Pathol 53:301–311, 1972.
13. Poste G, Doll J, Hart IR, Fidler IJ: *In vitro* selection of murine B16 melanoma variants with enhanced tissue invasive properties. Cancer Res 40:1636–1644, 1980.

14. Vlaeminck MN, Adenis L, Mouton Y, Demaille A: Etude expérimentale de la diffusion métastatique chez l'oeuf de poule embryonne. Répartition, microscopie et ultrastructure des foyers tumoraux. Int J Cancer 10:619–631, 1972.
15. Wallace AC, Chew E, Jones DS: The arrest and extravasation of cancer cells in the lung. In: Pulmonary metastasis, Vol. 3, Weiss L, Gilbert HA (eds). Boston: G.K. Hall, 1978, pp 26–42.
16. McKinney R, Singh B: Basement membrane changes under neoplastic oral mucous membrane. Oral Surg 44:875–888, 1977.
17. Orr W, Varani J, Ward PA: Characteristics of the chemotactic response of neoplastic cells to a factor derived from the fifth component of complement. Am J Path 93:405–422, 1978.
18. Orr W, Varani J, Gondek MD, Ward PA, Mundy GR: Chemotactic responses of tumor cells to products of resorbing bone. Science 203:176–179, 1979.
19. Kleinman HK, Klebe RJ, Martin GR: Role of collagenous matrices in the adhesion and growth of cells. J Cell Biol 88:473–485, 1981.
20. Murphy ME, Johnson PC: Possible contribution of basement membrane to the structural rigidity of blood capillaries. Microvasc Res 9:242–245, 1975.
21. Marchesi VT: Ultrastructural aspects of acute inflammation. Pathol Ann 5:343–353, 1970.
22. Liotta LA, Kleinerman J, Catanzaro P, Rynbrandt D: Degradation of basement membrane by murine tumor cells. J Natl Cancer Inst 58:1427–1431, 1977.
23. Liotta LA, Lee C, Morakis DJ: New method for preparing whole intact surfaces of human basement for tumor invasion studies. Cancer Lett 11;141–152, 1980.
24. Jones PA, DeClerk YA: Destruction of extracellular matrices containing glycoproteins, elastin, and collagen by metastatic human tumor cells. Cancer Res 40:3222–3227, 1980.
25. Garbisa S, Kniska K, Tryggavason K, Foltz C, Liotta L: Quantitation of basement membrane collagen degradation by living tumor cells *in vitro*. Cancer Lett 9:359–366, 1980.
26. Liotta LA, Tryggvason K, Garbisa S, Hart I, Foltz CM, Shafie S: Metastatic potential correlates with enzymaic degradation of membrane collagen. Nature 284:67–68, 1980.
27. Liotta LA, Tryggvason K, Garbisa S, Gehron-Robey P, Abe S: Partial purification and characterization of a neutral protease which cleaves type IV collagen. Biochemistry 20:100–104, 1981.
28. Liotta LA, Lanzer WL, Garbisa S: Identification of a type V collagenolytic enzyme. Biochem Biophys Res Commun 98:184–190, 1981.
29. Pauli BU, Memoli VA, Kuettner KE: *In vitro* determination of tumor invasiveness using extracted hyaline cartilage. Cancer Res 41:2084–2091, 1981.
30. Daroczy J, Feldmann J, Kiraly K: Human epidermal basal lamina: its structure connections and functions. In: Front Matrix Biol, Vol. 7. Basel: Karger, 1979, pp 208–234.
31. Timpl R, Rohde H, Gehron-Robey P, Rennard S, Foidart JM, Martin GR: Laminin – a glycoprotein of basement membranes. J Biol Chem 254:9933–9937, 1979.
32. Chen LB (ed): Selected abstracts on fibronectin and related transformation-sensitive cell surface proteins. ICRDB, Oncology Overviews, 1981.
33. Linder E, Vaheri A, Ruoslahti E, Wartiovaara J: Distribution of fibroblast surface antigen in the developing chick embryo. J Exp Med 142:41–49, 1975.
34. Bernfield MR, Cohn RH, Banerjee SD: Glycosaminoglycans and epithelial organ formation. Am Zool 13:1067–1083, 1973.
35. Caulfield JP, Farquhar MG: The permeability of glomerular capillaries to graded dextrans. J Cell Biol 63:883–903, 1974.
36. Hassell J, Gehron-Robey R, Barrach H, Wilczek J, Rennard S, Martin GR: Isolation of a heparin-sulfate containing proteoglycan from basement membrane. Proc Natl Acad Sci 77:4494–4498, 1981.
37. Burgeson RE, El Adli FA, Kaitila II, Hollister DW: Fetal membrane collagens: identification of two new collagen alpha chains. Proc Natl Acad Sci USA 73:2579–2580, 1976.
38. Madri JA, Furtmayr H: Isolation and tissue localization of Type AB_2 collagen from normal lung parenchyma. Amer J Path 94:323–331, 1980.
39. Gay S, Rhodes R, Gay R, Miller E: Collagen molecules comprised of l(v) chains: an apparent

localization in the exocytoskeleton. Collagen Rel Res 1:53–58, 1981.
40. Neurath H, Walsh K: Role of proteolytic enzymes in biological regulation (a review). Proc Natl Acad Sci 73:3825–3832, 1976.
41. Reynolds JJ, Murphy G, Sellers A: A new factor that may control collagen resorption. Lancet II: 333–335, 1977.
42. Gross J, Highberger JH, Johnson-Wint B, Biswas C: Mode of action and regulation of tissue collagenases. In: Collagenases in normal and pathologic connective tissues, Woolley & Evanson (eds). John Wiley, 1980.
43. Sakai T, Gross J: Some properties of the products of the reactions of tadpole collagenase with collagen. Biochem 6:518–528, 1967.
44. Gullino PM, Grantham FH: The influence of the host and the neoplastic cell population on the collagen content of a tumor mass. Cancer Res 23:648–653, 1963.
45. Yamanishi Y, Maeyens E, Dabbons MK, Ohyama H, Hashimoto K: Collagenolytic activity in malignant melanoma; physiochemical studies. Cancer Res 33:2507–2512, 1973.
46. Dresden MH, Heilman SA, Schmidt JD: Collagenolytic enzymes in human neoplasms. Cancer Res 32:993–996, 1972.
47. Abramson M, Scholling RW, Huang CC, Salome RG: Collagenase activity in epidermoid carcinoma of the oral cavity and larynx. Ann Otal Rhinol Laryngol 84:158, 1975.
48. Kuettner KE, Soble L, Croxen RL, Marcqynska B, Hiti J, Harper E: Tumor cell collagenase and its inhibition by a cartilage derived protease inhibitor. Science 196:643–654, 1977.
49. Biswas C, Moran W, Bloch K, Gross J: Collagenolytic activity of rabbit V_2 carcinoma growing at multiple sites. Biochem Biophys Res Commun 80:33–38, 1978.
50. Woolley DE, Glanville RW, Roberts DR, Evanson JM: Purification characterization and inhibition of human skin collagenase. Biochem J 169:265–276, 1978.
51. Liotta LA, Abe S, Gehron-Robey P, Martin GR: Preferential digestion of basement membrane collagen by an enzyme derived from a metastatic murine tumor. Proc Natl Acad Sci USA 76:2268, 1979.
52. Woolley D, Evanson J: Collagenases in normal and pathologic connective tissue. London: John Wiley, 1980.
53. Horwitz AL, Hance AJ, Crystal RG: Granulocyte collagenase: selective digestion of type I relative to type III collagen. Proc Natl Acad Sci USA 74:897–901, 1977.
54. Eisen AZ, Jeffrey JJ, Gross J: Human skin collagenase. isolation and mechanisms of attack on the collagen molecules. Biochim Biophys Acta 151:637–645, 1968.
55. Stricklin GP, Bauer EA, Jeffrey JJ, Eisen AZ: Purification of skin collagenase. Biochemistry 16:1607–1615, 1977.
56. Uitto VJ, Schwarts D, Veis A: Degradation of basement membrane collagen by neutral proteases from human granulocytes. Eur J Biochem 105:409–417, 1980.
57. Mainardi CL, Seyer JM, Kang AH: Type-Specific Collagenolysis: A type V collagen degrading enzyme from macrophages. Biochem Biophys Res Comm 97:1108–1115, 1980.
58. Gadek JE, Fells GA, Wright DG, Crystal RG: Human neutrophil elastase functions as a type III collagen 'Collagenase'. Biochem Biophys Res Com 95:1815–1822, 1980.
59. Mainardi CL, Hasty DL, Seyer JM, Kang A: Specific cleavage of human type III collagen by human polymorphonuclear leukocyte elastase. J Biol Chem, 1980.
60. Mainardi CL, Dixit SN, Kang AH: Degradation of (type IV) basement membrane collagen by a proteinase isolated from human polymorphonuclear leucocyte granules. J Biol Chem 255:5435–5441, 1980.
61. Sage H, Bornstein P: Characterization of a novel collagen chain in human placenta and its relation to AB collagen. Biochemistry 18:3815–3822, 1979.
62. Liotta LA, Goldfarb R, Brundage R, Siegal G, Terranova V, Garbisa S: Effect of plasminogen activator, plasmin and thrombin or glycoprotein and collagenous components of basement membrane. Cancer Res 41:4629–4636, 1981.

63. Tryggvason K, Pihlajaniemi T, Liotta LA, Salo T: Biosynthesis and turnover of basement membrane collagen. In: New trends in basement membrane research, Schone (ed). Munich: S. Karger (in press).
64. Liotta LA, Goldfarb RH, Terranova VP: Cleavage of laminin by thrombin and plasmin: Alpha thrombin selectively cleaves the beta chain of laminin. Thrombosis Res 21:663–673, 1981.
65. Hart I, Talmadge J, Fidler IJ: Metastatic behavior of a murine reticulum cell sarcoma organ specific growth. Cancer Res 41:1281–1287, 1981.
66. Salomon D, Liotta LA, Kidwell WR: Differential growth factor responsiveness of rat mammary epithelium pated on different collagen substratum in serum free medium. Proc Natl Acad Sci 78:382–386, 1981.
67. Salomon D, Liotta L, Foidart J, Yaar M: Synthesis and turnover of basement membrane components in cultured teratocarcinoma cells. Coll Res. In press.
68. Sellers A, Murphy G, Meikle M, Reynolds JJ: Rabbit bone collagenase inhibitor blocks the activity of other neutralmetalloproteinases. Biochem Biophys Res Comm 87:581–587, 1979.

20. Tumor formation and malignant invasion: role of basal lamina

D. E. INGBER and J. D. JAMIESON

1. Introduction

Carcinoma is by far the most commonly occurring form of cancer and is a neoplasm of epithelial cell origin. In any neoplasm, local invasion and metastasis are the two most reliable criteria that designate the tumor as malignant. Direct invasion is the first and most crucial step in the malignant process and is defined in carcinomata by local disruption of basal lamina with tumor cell infiltration into the underlying connective tissue space (Figure 1).

Classically, basal lamina has been viewed as a host barrier through which a malignant tumor must gain the ability to invade and its dissolution has been commonly accepted as an end result of the neoplastic disorganization process. Over the past decade, basal lamina has been shown to be a product of epithelial cells [1–3] which serves to stabilize epithelial cell differentiation and orientation during organogenesis [1, 4]. In addition, this structure is most likely an architectural foundation for cell anchorage *in vivo* and so may play a central role in cell growth regulation. As the early stages of oncogenesis are characterized by a deregulation of cell differentiation, orientation, and proliferation, it is possible that the gradual loss of basal lamina integrity that precedes its complete disruption may be involved in neoplastic disorganization prior to the onset of malignant invasion. Thus, the main goal of this discussion is to present the biology of invasion in perspective of the entire neoplastic process and to hopefully raise some new questions regarding the role of basal lamina in the development of invasive carcinomata.

Neoplasia is commonly viewed at a cellular level as a disease which results from loss of control of cell proliferation and differentiation. Cancer is essentially a disease of 'self', as it results from a deregulation of the finely coordinated symbiotic processes by which independent cells are integrated into tissues, tissues into organs, and organs into a functional living organism. Discussion of the biology of malignant invasion in the past relied heavily upon alterations of such general cellular characteristics as intercellular adhesion, motility, proliferative capacity, and production of lytic products. We believe that examination of the malignant process at a tissue level will serve to more accurately place these isolated cellular qualities in perspective of the biologic mechanism that underlies neoplastic invasion *in vivo*.

L.A. Liotta and I.R. Hart (eds.), Tumor Invasion and Metastasis. ISBN-13: 978-94-009-7513-2.
© 1982 Martinus Nijhoff Publishers, The Hague/Boston/London.

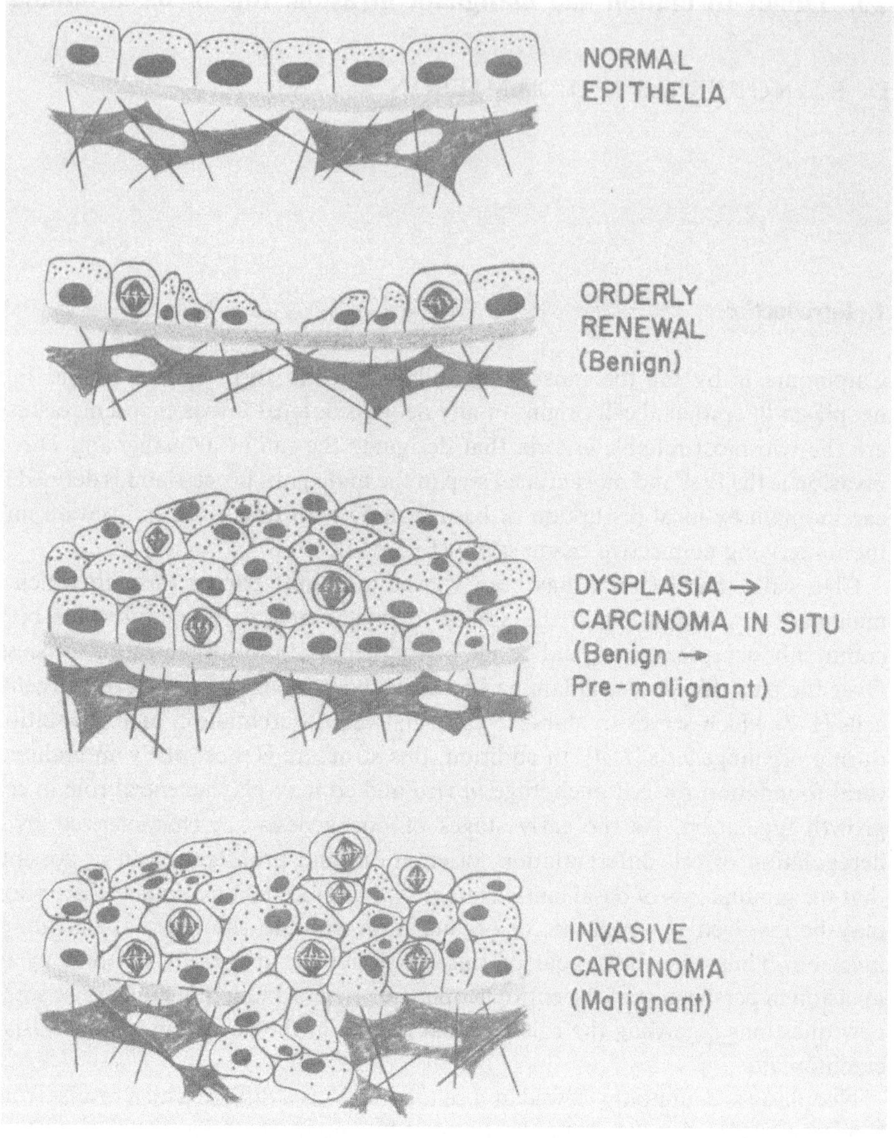

Figure 1. Schematic diagram of the process by which normal epithelial architecture becomes disorganized during the development of invasive carcinomata. The solid line represents the basal lamina beneath the epithelium.

All tissues exhibit characteristic patterns of structural and functional organization which are determined during embryologic development and are normally maintained throughout adult life. Thus, understanding of the principles which underlie morphogenetic organization facilitates analysis of neoplastic disorganization of adult tissue morphology. We will review the biology of normal histogenesis and malignant oncogenesis with special emphasis on the role of basal lamina. We will also present data from our own laboratory which supports the concept that basal lamina serves to stabilize epithelial cell orientation and that loss of this architectural foundation may also be involved in the process of neoplastic disorganization. A hypothetical model for the role of basal lamina in the maintenance of normal epithelial tissue architecture is presented.

2. Basal lamina structure and composition

Basal lamina is commonly recognized by electron microscopists as a continuous sheet of amorphous electron dense material that consistently appears at the base of epithelial cells along their interface with connective tissue. This extracellular scaffolding is actually a complex of different macromolecules. At this time, there are at least two different known basal lamina collagens, named type IV collagen [5] and type V collagen [6], which differ from interstitial collagens in that they retain their non-triple helical ends and do not organize into a periodic array. Laminin [7] and fibronectin [8] are two different large glycoproteins that have been found within basal lamina although localization of fibronectin to all basal laminae is not clear at this time [9]. Proteoglycans such as heparan sulfate and chondroitin sulfate, as well as the glycosaminoglycan (GAG), hyaluronic acid, have also been demonstrated within basal lamina [10–12]. We must emphasize that this list is most likely incomplete and that we are only at the beginning of understanding the macromolecular organization of this structure.

3. Developmental systems

(Epithelial-mesenchymal interactions)

In the embryo, genesis of a tissue's characteristic form (e.g., acinar vs. tubular) and deposition of basal lamina are both determined by complex interactions between adjacent epithelial and mesenchymal societies. While the light microscopic basement membrane (i.e., basal lamina plus adjacent connective tissue matrix) may be of both epithelial and mesenchymal origin, basal lamina is actually a product of the epithelial cells [1, 2]. However, it appears that it is the basal lamina scaffolding that serves to physically stabilize the tissue's characteristic three-dimensional configuration. For example, maintenance of the organized morphology of the salivary gland rudiment is dependent upon the continued presence of its basal lamina [1]. Similarly, basal lamina has been shown to stabilize corneal epithelial cell form and differentiation in the chick embryo [2, 4].

Localized differentials in basal lamina turnover may be integrally involved in directing the histogenetic organization process. While the epithelium appears to impose some degree of morphologic stability through production of its basal lamina in the developing salivary gland, the mesenchyme apparently induces histogenetic changes by basal lamina degradation or dissolution at selective sites [13]. It is interesting to note that an increased rate of cell division is observed in areas associated with accelerated basal lamina turnover (e.g., tips of growing lobules) [14]. On the other hand, the mesenchyme may also serve to induce accumulation of basal lamina by the epithelium through its secretion of fibrillar collagen. For instance, clefts between growing lobules display an increased amount of fibrillar collagen as well as a decreased rate of both basal lamina turnover and cell division. Similarly, both basal lamina and extracellular GAGs accumulate under mammary epithelia when grown on native collagen gels [3, 15], although collagenous stroma promotes only GAG accumulation in cultured embryonic chick corneal epithelia [4]. Production of new basal lamina in this system requires the added presence of live mesenchymally-derived fibroblasts within the stroma [16]. Thus, the upkeep of normal basal lamina and so the stabilization of the specific form of an organized epithelial structure may require the continued interaction of epithelial and mesenchymally-derived societies and products.

4. Cell-substratum interactions

(Control of cell growth and form)

Ordered and controlled cell growth is essential for the development and maintenance of organized tissue structures. Some aspects of growth control may be observed and studied in cell culture, although the magnitude of the effect of the tissue culture environment, particularly the planar surface of the substrate, upon cell activity is not clear. The principles of mammalian cell growth controls and *in vitro* behavior were established with embryonic cell strains and 'fibroblast-like' cell lines but can be extended with some variations and exceptions to most other cultured cell lines.

One of the first *in vitro* cell behaviors described was 'contact inhibition' or the arrest of locomotion that results when animal cells come in contact with one another [17]. Another commonly described growth characteristic is 'density dependent inhibition of growth' (DDIG) which refers to the tendency of most cultured cells to form monolayers or to grow to a certain 'saturation density' and then become quiescent despite the continuing abundance of nutrients in the medium [18]. Most normal cell lines will also only grow if attached to and spread on a solid substrate [19, 20]. For instance, deoxyribonucleic acid (DNA), ribonucleic acid (RNA), and protein synthesis are all inhibited when anchorage-dependent fibroblasts are placed in suspension culture [20]. Recovery of protein synthesis rapidly follows reattachment while nuclear events such as DNA synthesis require extensive cell spreading and are tightly coupled to cell shape both in the fibroblast system and in a variety of other non-transformed cell lines including epithelial cells [20–23]. Cell form, in turn, appears to be determined by the physical conformation and adhesiveness of the substratum in combination with crowding by neighboring cells.

While these growth phenomena are not well understood, *in vitro* growth criteria are commonly used to define the 'transformed' state. Transformed tissue culture cells commonly display a decreased serum requirement for growth, decreased anchorage requirements, and loss of contact inhibition, DDIG, and shape regulation relative to their normal counterparts [23, 24]. It must be noted that these parameters may not be directly related to growth regulation and oncogenesis *in vivo*.

All of the basal lamina constituents appear to be involved in normal cell-substratum interactions *in vitro*, especially in the process of cell anchorage. Fibronectin is a well-known adhesion molecule for connective tissue cells [25] and laminin has recently been shown to be a specific attachment protein for certain epithelial cell lines to type IV collagen *in vitro* [26]. Thus, it is highly likely that some or all of these molecules may function in a similar anchoring capacity *in vivo*. It is interesting to note that addition of fibronectin to some transformed fibroblast lines partially restores morphology, adhesiveness, and contact inhibition [27]. This morphologic reversion, however, is not accompanied by an alteration in growth properties. Changes in cell surface GAGs also appear to correlate with DDIG [28, 29] as well as transformation [30] in certain experimental systems. However, while viral transformation has been shown to inhibit deposition of fibronectin and laminin into an insoluble matrix at the surface of cultured kidney epithelial cells [31], the roles of laminin and type IV collagen in the growth control of transformed epithelial cells still remain to be determined.

Studies in embryonic systems also support the concept that substratum interactions may be involved in the regulation of epithelial cell growth. Normal epidermal growth and differentiation is characterized by the presence of mitotic figures only in the basal cell layer in contact with basal lamina. Enzymatic separation of the epidermis from its dermis removes basal lamina and results in loss of normal basal cell form and proliferative activity [32, 33]. Maintenance or recovery of orientation and active DNA synthesis can occur *in vitro* in the presence of embryo extract, but is effective only if the epidermis touches a suitable substrate such as a Millipore filter. The basal layer will synthesize DNA only where it is in contact with the Millipore substrate while cells flatten and cease dividing over holes in the filter. A morphologic basal lamina is not seen in either region [32]. On the other hand, both basal lamina continuity and proliferative activity are restored by culturing the epithelium with mesenchymally-derived tissue [34]. Thus, epithelial organization may require a substrate or scaffolding in addition to the presence of specific molecular factors which may serve to coordinate those molecules into an ordered architectural array.

In support of this hypothesis, it has been recently observed that while fibroblasts may readily attach to a substrate containing adsorbed monovalent lectins, cell spreading requires the presence of a tetravalent lectin [35]. The spatial distribution of multiple binding sites in close proximity may act to functionally 'cross-link' or organize cell surface adhesive molecules into a threshold configuration that triggers cell spreading and initiation of new DNA and RNA synthesis. It is possible that the structural organization of adhesive and/or supportive molecules such as laminin and type IV collagen within basal lamina serves a similar 'valency' function for epithelial cells *in vivo*.

Recently, the introduction of native collagen gels as culture substrata [36, 37] has enabled a variety of normal adult epithelial cell lines to be grown and studied *in vitro*. While some epithelia lose their characteristic epithelial shape and differentiated cell products after brief periods of culture on plastic substrata, various cell lines will retain their specialized qualities for extended periods of time when grown on native collagen gels [3, 37, 38]. In addition, if the gels are floated on media, cells interact with the substratum (i.e., adhere and create their own tension) and form higher order tissue structures such as acini in association with production of morphologic basal lamina [3, 39].

It appears that adult epithelial cells may have to interact with the underlying substratum in order to grow and form organized tissue structures *in vivo* as well. Adult mammary gland development in the rat requires the presence of basal lamina. Inhibition of new collagen deposition by treatment with cis-hydroxyproline results in dissolution of basal lamina and involution-like structural alterations of the tissue [40]. The observation that DNA synthesis and cell division do not commonly occur in areas free of contact with basal lamina [41] in most normal epithelial tissues may also be significant.

5. Neoplastic disorganization of tissue architecture

A normal epithelium is a dynamic structure [42] and its basal lamina serves as a scaffolding for orderly cell replacement in that it retains the tissue's original architectural form and assures for accurate regeneration of pre-existing structures [43]. While orderly renewal is characterized by increased proliferative activity and cell migration, it is a benign process because it is highly organized and reversible. On the other hand, an epithelium may come to escape its normally tight growth constraints and result in loss of normal cell to cell relationships with a piling up of atypical epithelial cells. This pathologic state is termed dysplasia and represents one point on a spectrum of loss of growth regulation. The epithelium progresses further down the spectrum as the degree of tissue disorganization increases until it reaches the subjective point when it is termed neoplastic. This state is considered irreversible and is associated with a relative increase in the number of mitotic figures as well as their abnormal presence outside of the basal cell layer (Figure 1).

The loss of cell orientation and disorganization of tissue morphology observed during oncogenesis may be in part due to tumor cells gaining the ability to survive and proliferate free of normal contact with either morphologic basal lamina or specific basal lamina components. Normal rat mammary epithelial cell viability appears to be dependent upon contact with an intact basal lamina *in vivo* [40] and *in vitro* studies have shown that the attachment and proliferation of some normal epithelia [44, 45] and connective tissue cells [46, 47] requires *de novo* collagen synthesis and secretion. In the case of normal mammary epithelia, this *in vitro* requirement can be circumvented by plating the cells on a layer of type IV collagen but not type I collagen [44]. Growth of various tumorigenic cell lines is, however, independent of both deposition of extracellular collagen [46, 47] and, as discussed previously, anchorage to a substratum suggesting a direct correlation between loss of substratum dependence, growth autonomy, and subsequent tissue disorganization.

6. Neoplasia as a disease of tissue genesis

(Epithelial-mesenchymal interactions)

While the notion that neoplastic transformation involves various degrees of 'dedifferentiation' during carcinogenesis is common, it appears that a tumor is most likely 'a caricature of its tissue of origin in both appearance and mode of development' [48]. Neoplastic cells *in vivo* are part of an organized tumor structure consisting of at least three compartments — the tumor cell parenchyma, the vascular system and the interstitial space. If the oncogenetic process is an 'analog of normal tissue genesis with proliferation outweighing the differentiative and organizational capacity of the component cells' [48], then the propagation of an epithelial neoplasm may be controlled or regulated, in part, through interactions between the epithelial tumor cells and mesenchymally-derived connective tissue.

Heterologous tissue interactions may continue to play a fundamental role in the maintenance of normal epithelial tissue morphology throughout adult life. For example, adult mouse mammary gland epithelium retains the capacity to undergo morphogenesis when mixed with embryonic mesenchyme [49] and the histologic form of normal epidermal grafts is determined by the location of host dermis in a variety of experimental systems [50]. Thus, it is not surprising that examination of the microscopic anatomy of various neoplasms suggests that epithelial-stromal interactions may be important in the propagation of carcinomata as well [51]. For instance, while collagen was shown to be a product of host fibroblasts in a variety of tumor systems, the amount of collagen produced was apparently regulated and determined by neoplastic cell populations [52]. The colonial architecture of Hela cells when grown with fibroblasts also varies in accordance with the source of the connective tissue [53]. Furthermore, chemical carcinogenesis of epidermis can not be entirely explained in terms of a direct carcinogen-epithelial cell reaction as epidermal tumor formation appears to require the presence of closely apposed carcinogen-treated dermis [54]. It is interesting to note that tumor cells also elicit a factor which induces tumor vascularization by stimulating host endothelial proliferation and migration [55].

More in-depth study of the role of the epithelial-mesenchymal interaction in the oncogenetic process has been made possible through the use of embryonic systems. Malignant transformation of embryonic mouse submandibular gland by polyoma virus can occur *in vitro* in intact or reconstituted submandibular rudiments but not in either isolated submandibular epithelium or mesenchyme [56]. However, chromosomal studies indicate that the *resultant* tumor is epithelial in origin [57]. It is interesting to note that these tumor cells can then substitute for normal mesenchyme in supporting either normal epithelial morphogenesis in salivary glands or in the malignant transformation by virus of normal isolated embryonic epithelia [58]. Similarly, certain tumors have been found competent to induce proliferation in adjacent normal tissues [59] while, in other systems, peritumoral stroma has been shown to exhibit mitogenic qualities of its own [60]. Recently, grafted human epithelial tumors have also been shown to be able to recruit normal murine stromal cells to become tumorigenic in nude mice [61]. On the other hand, combination of various disorganized epithelial tumors with normal embryonic mesenchyme results in normal epithelial organization and histodifferentiation [62–64]. These findings bring the simple monoclonal origin of cancer into question and emphasize the importance of continued epithelial-mesenchymal interactions in the neoplastic process.

7. Malignant invasion

The pathogenesis of tumor invasion may also involve interactions between different tissues. Studies of the invasive growth of non-malignant epithelium show that proliferation of underlying connective tissue and local dissolution of basement membrane occur before epithelial growth begins [65]. Ultrastructural changes in the epidermal-dermal junction also precede tumor formation during skin carcinogenesis [66] and, as mentioned earlier, successful epidermal cell transformation appears to require the presence of carcinogen-treated dermis [54].

While all irritative chemicals induce focal breaks in basal lamina which may be due to associated epithelial cell proliferation [67] and local inflammatory response [68], only carcinogens result in pathologic epithelial penetration of adjacent tissues. Early stages of skin carcinogenesis are characterized by basal lamina gaps, thickening, and reduplication as well as loosening of basal cells from one another and underlying connective tissue [66]. These alterations probably represent repeated stages of breakdown and attempted repair of basal lamina. It is interesting to note that *in vitro* studies indicate that normal migrating epidermal cells deposit type V collagen (i.e., basal lamina collagen) and that cell movement ceases upon pharmacologic inhibition of new collagen deposition [45]. However, in the later stages of carcinogenesis normal repair mechanisms are overcome or do not function fully and eventually epithelial tumor cells appear which are able to divide and migrate independent of anchorage to basal lamina.

Furthermore, fibrillar connective tissue may also play a major role in the invasive process. In sponge matrix culture, infiltration by tumor cells was found to be dependent upon the alignment of connective tissue fibers at the margin of the growing tumor [69]. Invasion was least where fibrillar connective tissue was parallel and greatest when perpendicular to the surface of the growing tumor mass. Thus, if the connective tissue around the tumor is not invaded by tumor elements and rather fibroblasts and their collagenous products come to orient so as to maintain or limit tissue boundaries, then a capsule may form around the tumor nodule and to some extent counteract the spread of malignant cells. On the other hand, aberrant regulation of both the epithelial and connective tissue cell populations could result in a complete breakdown of tissue boundaries.

As described prèviously, a direct correlation exists between epithelial tumor invasion and local basal lamina disruption as well as a correlation of non-invasion with the presence of continuous basal lamina [70–72]. However, basal lamina discontinuities are extremely rare in a virally induced murine mammary tumor which is spontaneously metastatic [73], although the smallest metastatic tumor focus studied in this system differed from all others in displaying frequent breaks in its basal lamina. This observation must be considered in light of the dynamic nature of epithelial architecture and heterogeneity of cell populations [48, 74] within different microenvironments of rapidly or sporadically growing neoplasms. The possibility of local environmental changes causing intermittent basal lamina dissolution and resynthesis can not be ruled out. For example, while basal lamina was absent from a primary murine squamous cell carcinoma, a perfectly formed one appeared along most of the epithelial tumor boundary at a secondary site [66]. The use of only morphologic criteria for the determination of the functional and structural integrity of basal lamina must also be questioned. Preliminary investigations using the pancreatic rudiment system in our laboratory indicate that incubation with cis-hydroxyproline results in a complete loss of type IV collagen but not of laminin from basal lamina as detected by immunofluorescence microscopy, while a continuous basal lamina is still observed by electron microscopy (manuscript in preparation).

In conclusion, malignant transformation of a benign neoplasm may result either from incomplete maintenance of basal lamina or through the acquisition of some new transformed cell product which compromises its structural integrity. As both embryonic basal lamina production and tumor propagation appear to involve epithelial-mesenchymal interactions, different local connective tissue microenvironments may significantly affect adjacent epithelial tumor architecture. It is interesting to note that while studies in the past were unsuccessful in finding any consistent correlation between general proteolytic or collagenolytic activity and invasive behavior [75], a direct correlation has recently been shown between the

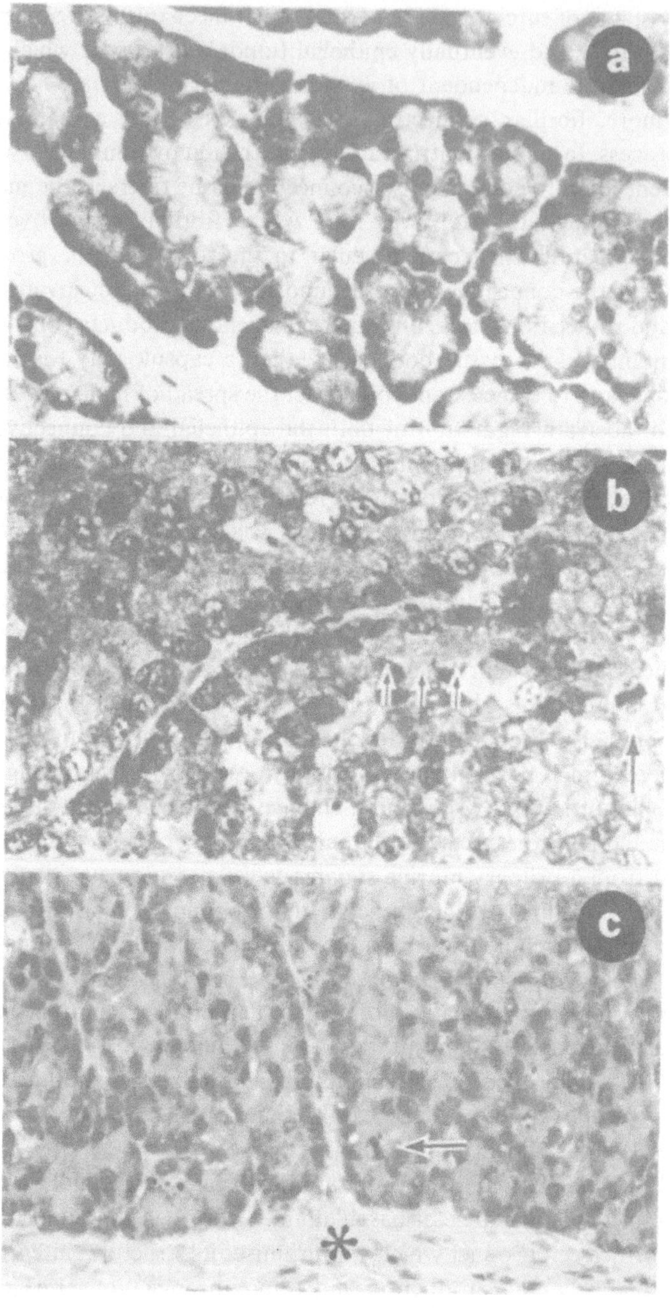

Figure 2. Light micrographs of normal pancreas and acinar cell tumor stained with hematoxylin and eosin. Tips of triple arrows abut on apical poles of three neighboring reoriented tumor cells that are palisading along the adjacent vessel; larger arrows indicate mitotic figures within the disorganized tumor parenchyma;*, tumor capsule. a) Pancreas (× 460). b) Tumor (× 460). c) Tumor (× 300).

enzymatic degradation of type IV collagen and metastatic potential in a variety of tumor systems [76]. The observation that tumor vascularization also involves intermittent breakdown and redeposition of capillary basal lamina by host endothelia has also often been overlooked in relation to the mechanism by which metastatic tumor cells enter the vasculature.

8. Current laboratory investigations

We are currently using a transplantable carcinoma of the rat exocrine pancreas as a model system in order to investigate the role of basal lamina in the maintenance of organized tissue structures as well as neoplastic disorganization [77]. The tumor was discovered with associated metastatic foci in nafenopin-treated rats in the laboratory of Reddy and Rao [78] and was kindly provided to us for study. This epithelial cell tumor is extremely interesting in that it is comprised of cytologically differentiated acinar cells that do not form acini and have lost their normal epithelial organization. However, as will be described later, our investigations indicate that the tumor cells reorganize and display normal epithelial orientation within particular microenvironments of subcutaneous and intraperitoneal implants. Thus, this epithelial tumor is an excellent system for studying the process by which epithelial organization is determined and stabilized and may provide some insight into the way in which loss of basal lamina is involved in the neoplastic disorganization of epithelial structures.

Normal rat exocrine pancreas is characterized by a classic acinar pattern of epithelial cell organization (Figure 2a). Nuclei are located within the basal portions of cells at the periphery of each acinus, while the apical poles are filled with zymogen granules and abut on the centroacinar lumen. On the other hand, the parenchyma of the acinar cell tumor is distinguished by a complete absence of obvious epithelial organization as well as frequent mitotic figures (Figures 2b, c). However, consistent palisading and reorientation of the epithelial tumor cells can be seen in areas of direct contact with both the vasculature (Figure 2b) and the connective tissue capsule (Figure 2c) with nuclei and zymogen granules relocating within the basal and apical cytoplasm, respectively.

This bizarre mixture of epithelial organization and disorganization within the same tumor can be seen more clearly by electron microscopy (Figure 3). While basal lamina does not appear between cells within the parenchyma of the tumor (see Figure 4 in ref. 79), a basal lamina with characteristic morphology appears to underlie the basal portions of reoriented tumor cells adjacent to vascular adventitia (Figure 4) and capsular stroma (Figure 5). The basal lamina of the tumor and that of the vessel are physically separated from each other by a connective tissue matrix and both display occasional discontinuities. Basal lamina breaks may be related to the greatly increased growth activity associated with the epithelial tumor cells as well as host endothelia and fibroblasts.

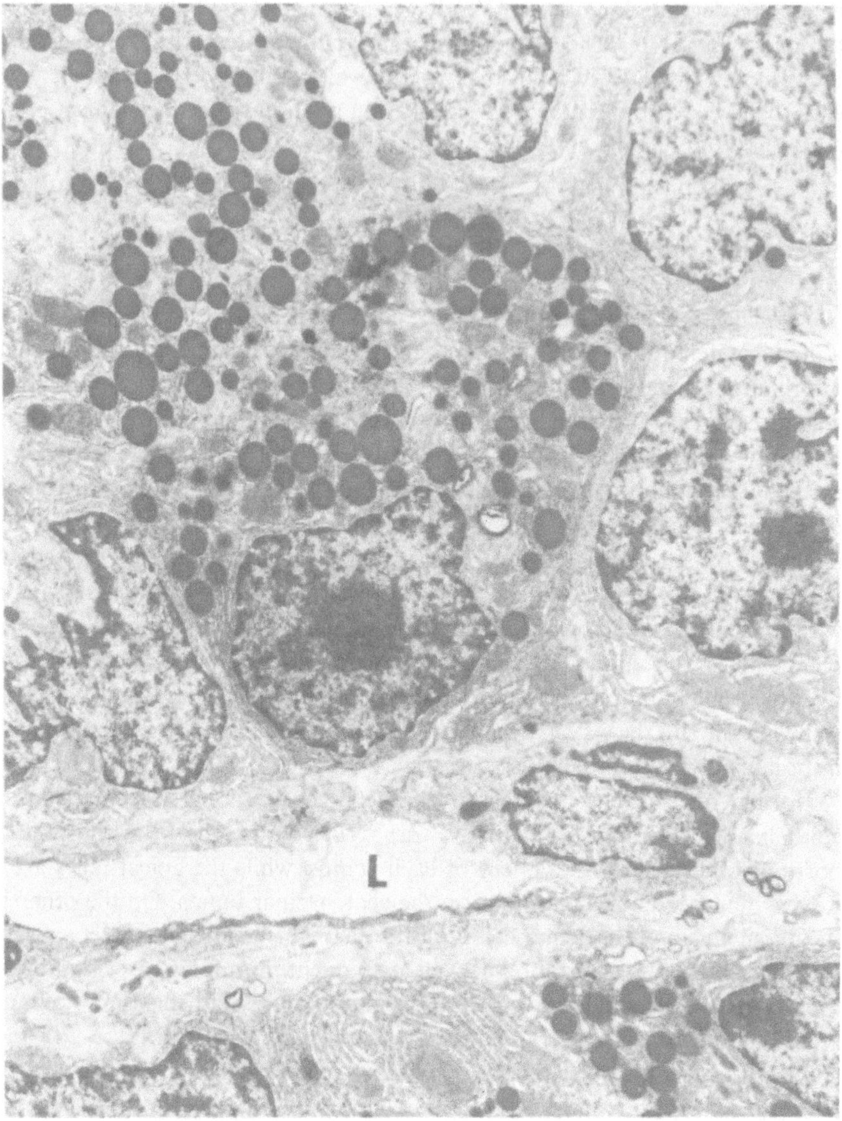

Figure 3. Electron micrograph of tumor containing a small blood vessel. Stained with uranyl acetate and lead citrate; L, lumen of vessel (× 10 500).

As basal lamina is a complex of different macromolecules, the *in vivo* distribution of laminin and type IV collagen was studied by indirect immunofluorescence (antibodies were provided by Dr. J.A. Madri, Dept. of Pathology, Yale University School of Medicine). These immunofluorescence studies reveal linear type IV collagen and laminin staining within all acinar and vascular basal laminae in normal rat pancreas (Figures 6a, b). However, similar investigations indicate that type IV collagen staining is completely absent from the parenchyma

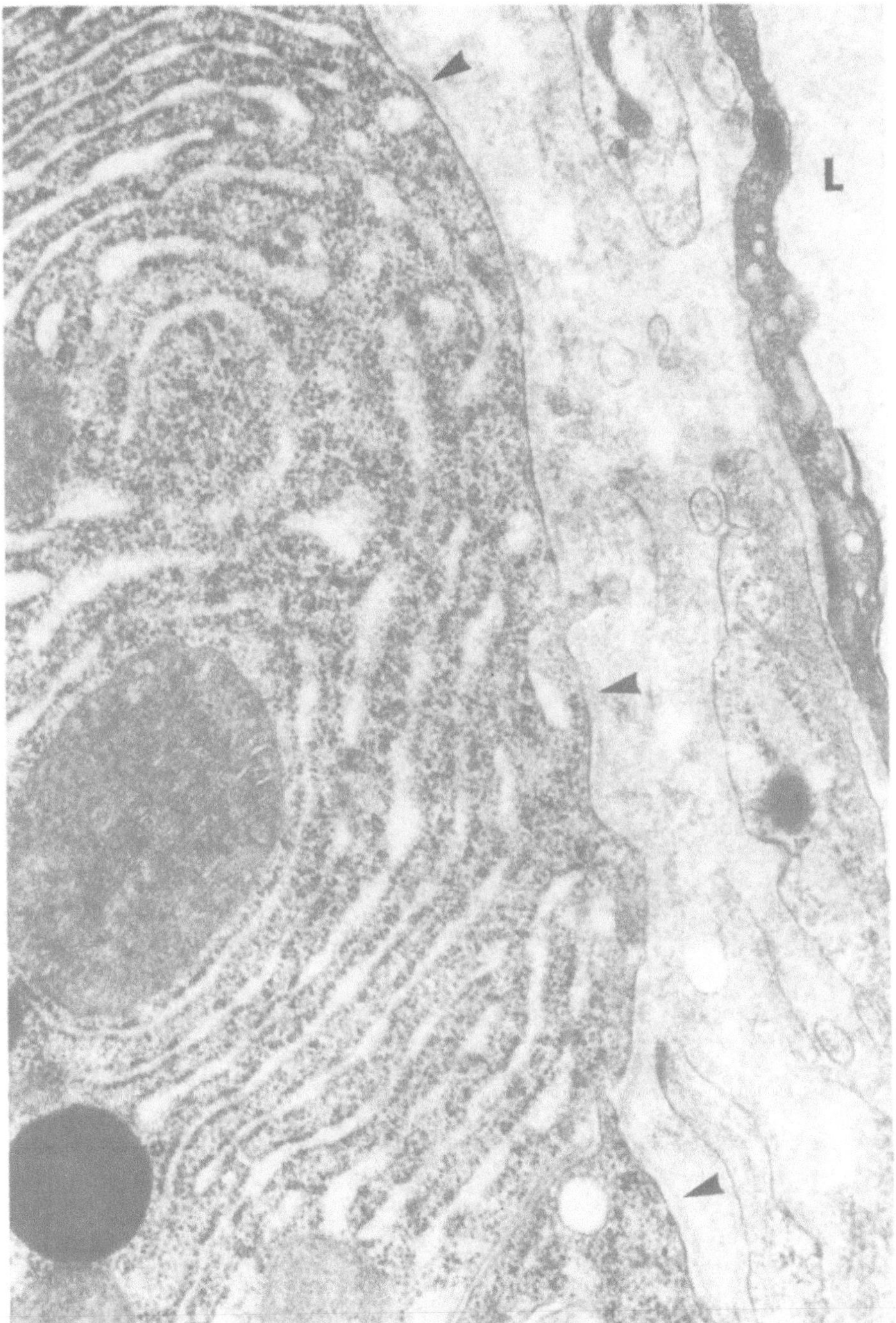

Figure 4. Electron micrograph of tumor-vessel interface. Stained with uranyl acetate and lead citrate. Tips of arrowheads abut on tumor basal lamina which is separate from that of the vessel; L, lumen of vessel (× 48 500).

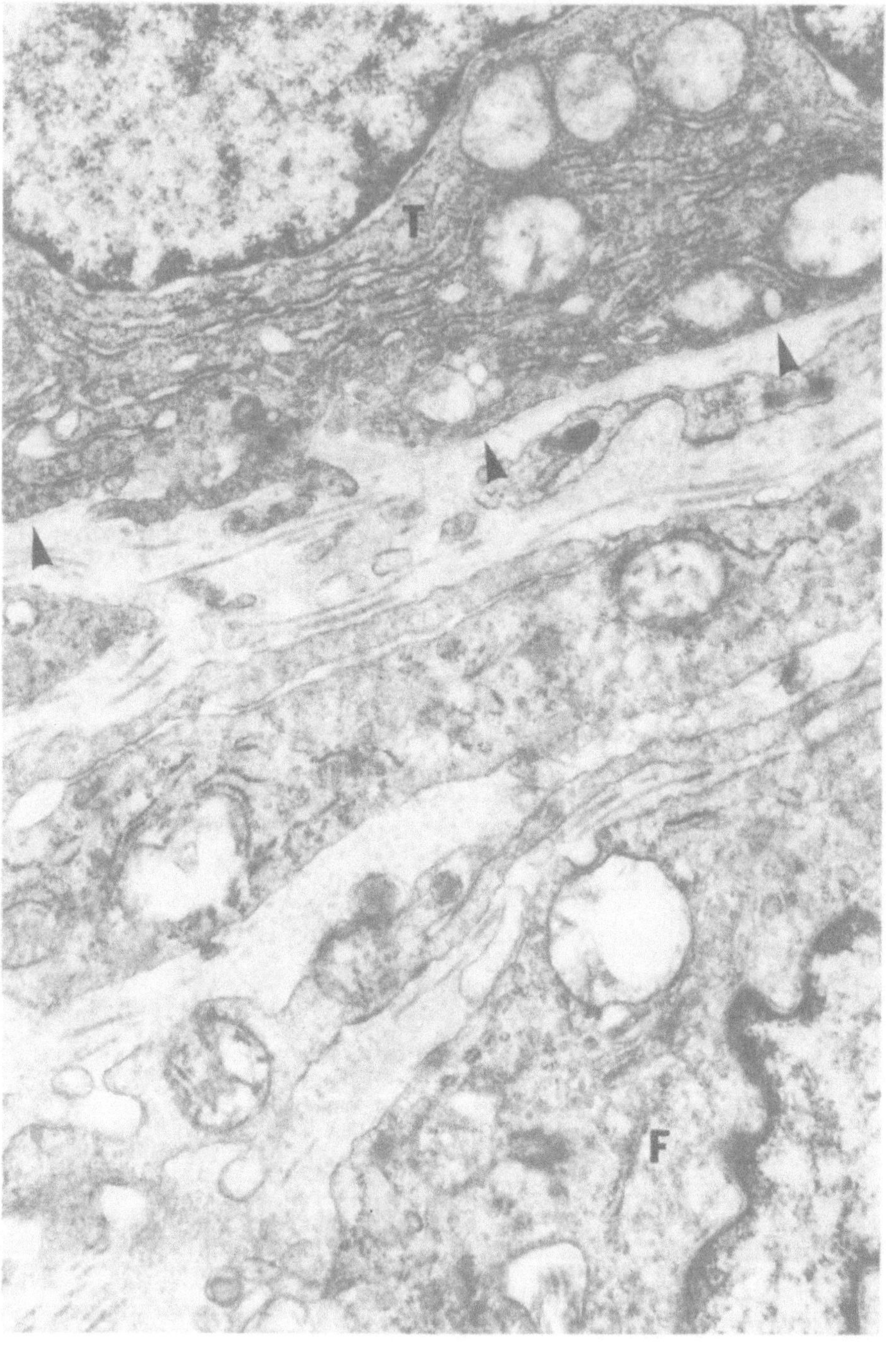

Figure 5. Electron micrograph of tumor-connective tissue capsule interface. Stained with uranyl acetate and lead citrate. Tips of arrowheads abut on tumor basal lamina; T, tumor cell; F, fibroblast within capsular stroma (× 33 000).

of the pancreatic tumor (Figure 6c) while laminin appears in a punctate distribution outlining the tumor cells (Figure 6d). On the other hand, a normal linear distribution of both laminin and type IV collagen appears along the vasculature in areas of tumor cell reorganization.

It is interesting to note that preliminary investigations in our laboratory using antibodies to fibronectin and to types I, III, and V collagens indicate that fibronectin and type V collagen are deposited in a linear manner with a distribution similar to that of type IV collagen in both tumor and normal pancreas. While types I and III collagens also only appear surrounding acini and vessels in normal pancreas and along vessels in the tumor, they are limited to the interstitial space and display a more fibrillar deposition pattern. Immunofluorescent localization studies on tissue obtained from the capsular regions of the tumor are currently under way.

9. Discussion

These data indicate that this pancreatic acinar cell tumor has lost the ability to produce or maintain a complete and organized basal lamina within its parenchyma and this correlates directly with loss of epithelial cell orientation. A degradative enzyme has been isolated from the media of cultured metastatic tumor cells that is specific for type IV collagen and is normally produced in a latent form which requires tryptic activation [80]. The presence of type IV collagenase activity or of its potential activators within the different microenvironments of this pancreatic acinar cell tumor may in part explain local differences in type IV collagen distribution while laminin is retained. It is possible that loss of type IV collagen from the parenchyma may play some role in the release of other basal lamina constituents such as laminin from a normally organized basal lamina as well as in the associated loss of epithelial organization. For instance, the punctate intercellular distribution of laminin seen in the tumor parenchyma is not unlike that seen within certain embryonic cell populations prior to their orientation into organized epithelial layers in association with deposition of type IV collagen and the organization of both molecules into linear basal lamina [81, 82].

On the other hand, epithelial tumor cell reorientation does occur and is consistently seen in association with a normal linear distribution of laminin and type IV collagen as well as morphological basal lamina in areas of contact with vascular adventitia. The observation that tumor reorganization and basal lamina also appear along capsular stroma suggests that epithelial tumor cell reorientation is not due to some vessel-specific quality such as nutrient availability but, rather is related to the juxtaposition of epithelially and mesenchymally-derived tissues. This is once again analogous to the social interactions discussed earlier in relation to normal histogenesis (Figure 7).

Thus, it appears that this epithelial tumor may be on the fulcrum of net

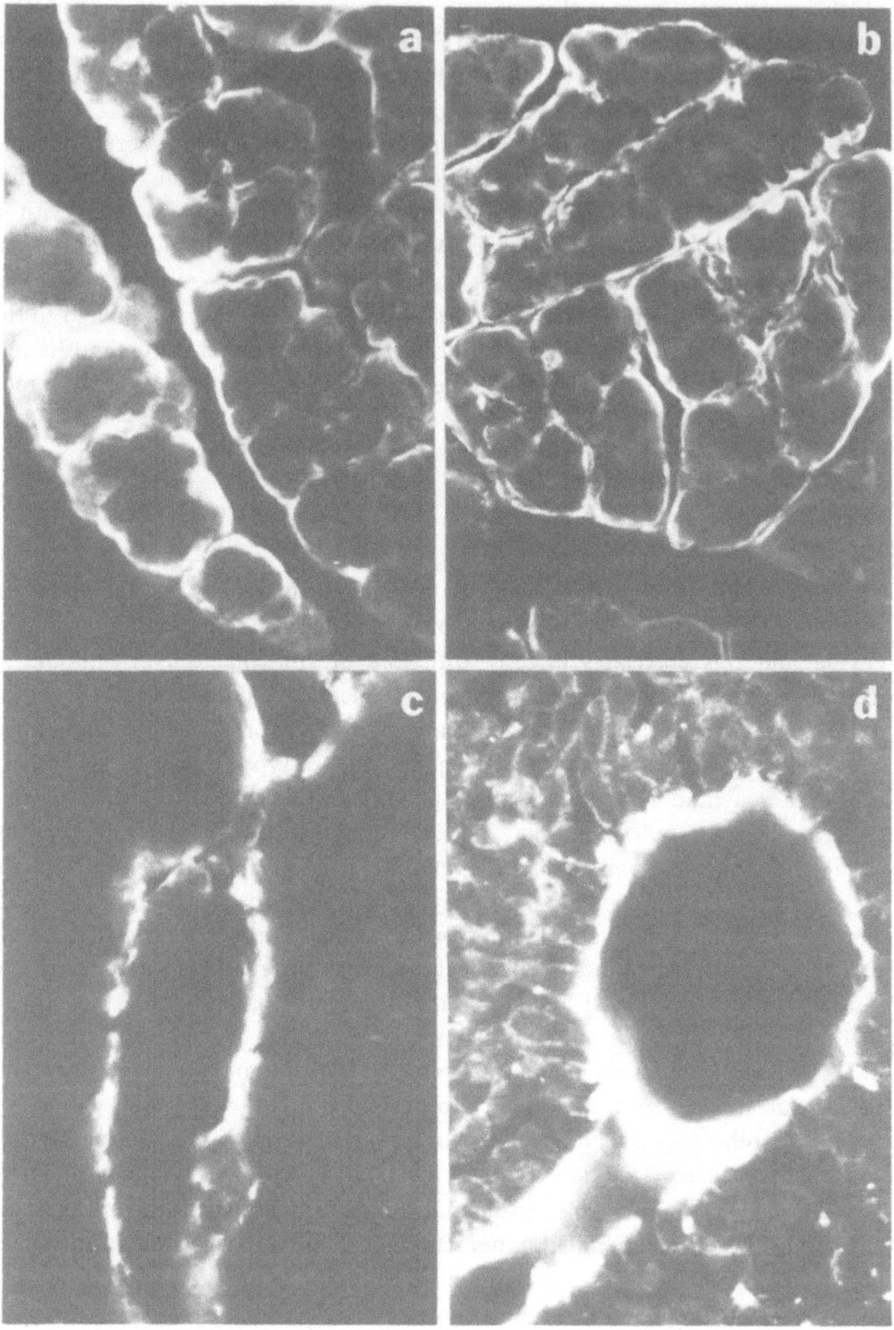

Figure 6. Immunofluorescence micrographs of standard cryostat sections of pancreas and tumor (× 300). a) Pancreas stained for type IV collagen. b) Pancreas stained for laminin. c) Tumor stained for type IV collagen. d) Tumor stained for laminin. (See ref. 77 for methods.)

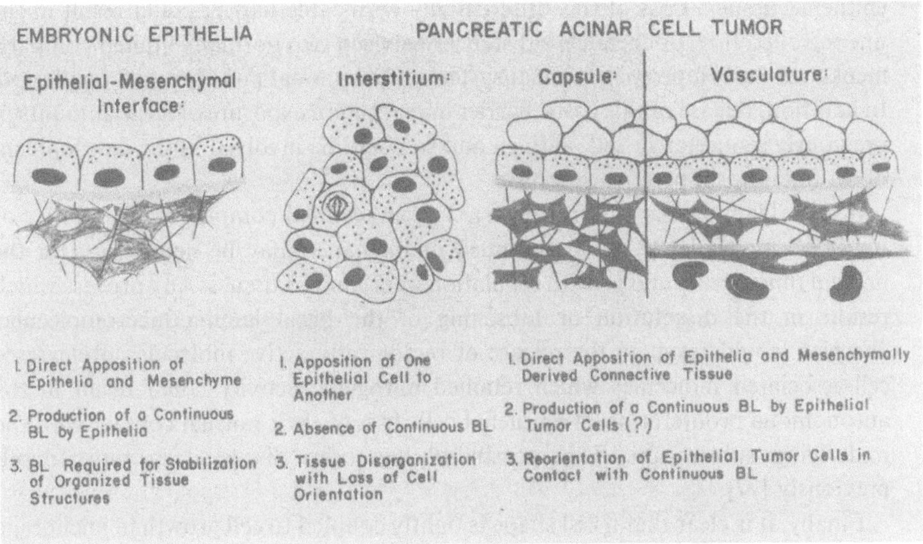

Figure 7. Schematic summary of the epithelial organization process within embryonic tissues and the pancreatic acinar cell tumor. The solid line represents basal lamina beneath the epithelium.

synthesis or net breakdown of its own basal lamina. The pancreatic acinar tumor cells do not seem to be able to maintain an intact basal lamina or epithelial orientation within the tumor parenchyma. However, in the correct microenvironment, these tumor cells appear to be able to interact with mesenchymally-derived connective tissue and, in a manner reminiscent of the embryonic state, organize and concurrently lay down a basal lamina of their own stabilizing this epithelial reorientation. Resultant cell polarization might redirect potential degradative activity away from the tumor cell base further promoting basal lamina accumulation at the tumor boundary. Failure to maintain basal lamina at the tumor margin (e.g., additional loss of type IV collagen) may occur in other tumor systems which display invasive behavior in addition to uncontrolled cell proliferation and tissue disorganization. Thus, incomplete maintenance of basal lamina may be involved in neoplastic disorganization as well as in the breakdown of tissue boundaries during the progression from a normal epithelium to an invasive carcinoma.

10. Theoretical considerations

As basal lamina has been shown to have many functions, dissolution of this ubiquitous structure may have profound and varied effects upon associated epithelia. For instance, basal lamina serves as a filtration barrier in the kidney glomerulus [83] and it may have an analogous but less specialized role in other epithelial tissues. Loss of this differentially permeable barrier could result in the uncontrolled flow of chemical substances between two normally limited compartments and so compromise normal systems of hormonal and chemical regulation. In addition, release of this tissue barrier may result in exposure of large amounts of previously sequestered 'self' antigen and so could be involved in the development of an immunosuppressive response.

As basal lamina may also function as an extracellular complex of informative or inductive molecules [84], its continued maintenance may be mandatory for the normal functioning and growth regulation of organized tissues. Any process which results in the dissolution or loosening of the basal lamina macromolecular complex, could result in the release of biologically active molecules. Release of cell-associated molecules which retained mitogenic activity could result in the autonomous proliferation of epithelial cells free of their normal contact with the underlying substratum. This possibility has been discussed in more depth previously [77].

Finally, it is clear that if cell shape is tightly coupled to cell growth in anchorage dependent cells [20–23], efficient control of cell proliferation within an epithelium may require a stable tissue morphology *in vivo* and thus, a well maintained basal lamina. The architectural form of a tissue may itself serve to regulate the shape, orientation, and growth of its cells through transmission of the physical forces of tension and compression characteristic for a given three-dimensional configuration [77]. This system might function in a manner analogous to the way in which the cellular society inhabiting bone is able to recognize and respond to physical loads and, in turn, grow and lay down their bone matrix directly along lines of tension and compression [85]. Similarly, Thompson relates the structural forms and growth patterns of a great variety of organisms to physical forces and spatial constraints in his classic book on growth and form [86].

An epithelial structure can be regarded as a tensile or tensegrity system, that is, an architectural unit of the highest efficiency which consists of *discontinuous* compression-resistant members (e.g., microtubules, cytoskeletal microfilaments, fibrillar collagen) interconnected directly or indirectly by a *continuous* series of tension elements (e.g., plasmalemma, contractile microfilaments, basal lamina) [87–89]. The term, 'tensegrity,' derives from the concept of 'tensional integrity' and is a most efficient and economical architectural system in which all loads are distributed equally over all elements. As dynamic tensile structures, cells alter their shape until an equilibrium configuration is attained which most efficiently and evenly distributes the load given the characteristic architectural distribution of anchors within the substratum. Thus, cells within a tissue might respond to physical alterations in their environment as a coordinated unit due to the equal and simultaneous distribution of forces to all of the elements of this organic tensegrity system.

In this manner, the structural coordination, homogeneity of cell form, and effective systems of intercellular communication required for successful tissue function (e.g., polarized secretion) are facilitated and maintained by normally constant architectural relationships. Alteration of the physical forces within the structural framework of the epithelium (e.g., cell death or removal, basal lamina dissolution) results in a change in cell form and a subsequent increase in local cell division until the original state of compression in regained [21]. It is interesting to note that cell flattening is a stimulus to DNA synthesis in cultured lens epithelial cells [22] and, as described previously, that an accelerated rate of basal lamina turnover is associated with increased proliferative activity within the developing salivary gland [14].

Continued stress or a protracted release of spatial constraints might result in increased proliferative activity with an associated loss of normal epithelial cell arrangements. Neoplastic transformation would be prohibited as long as cell viability and proliferative capacity remained dependent upon continued anchorage to basal lamina and thus, this dysplastic state would be reversible. This hypothesis is supported by investigations in our own laboratory in which partial dissolution of basal lamina within developing pancreatic rudiments by pharmacologic inhibition of collagen deposition inhibits morphogenesis and produces pancreatic tubules that display a piling up of epithelial cells as well as a large increase in the number of mitotic figures. All of these effects are readily reversed upon removal of the drug.

In any case, release of tensile constraints with sustained proliferative activity over an extended period of time could lead to selection of an anchorage-independent subpopulation of autonomously proliferating epithelial cells. In this manner, chronic stimulation of cell division and migration may lead to spontaneous cell 'transformation' *in vivo* just as continued culturing may do *in vitro*. As this neoplasm grew in size, autonomous epithelial cells would become separated from neighboring connective tissue by many cell diameters and so would be less susceptible to the regulatory influences of associated connective tissue. Thus, a positive feedback system develops which could eventually result in malignant invasion through either loss of basal lamina synthetic capacity, increased degradative potential, or through the acquisition of some new transformed cell product which in some way further compromises basal lamina integrity.

Thus, if stable tissue morphology is determined and regulated through transmission of the forces of tension and compression through a specific architectural arrangement (e.g., tensegrity), then any physical or functional interruption of transmission of these forces in the connection from substratum to cell anchor to plasmalemma to intracellular cytoskeletal assembly might produce a cell which is effectively blind to the informative forces that normally limits its growth and orientation. Similarly, a break at any other point in the transduction of these forces or shape changes into a biochemical response could result in a similar state of autonomy. While gradual basal lamina dissolution may be directly involved in the early stages of oncogenesis of certain neoplasms, other tumors may enter this positive feedback system at a later stage after gaining the ability to proliferate autonomously by some other pathologic mechanism (e.g., viral transformation, chemical mutagenesis).

In conclusion, we would like to propose that basal lamina may be integrally involved in the regulation of epithelial cell shape and growth as both a tension element of an organic tensegrity system and as a foundation or substratum consisting of a complex of different anchoring and supportive macromolecules.

Acknowledgment

We wish to acknowledge the technical assistance of Ms. Amy Hsu and Ms. Rosalie Manzi and the excellent assistance of Ms. Marybeth Hicks in preparing the manuscript. This work was supported by Medical Scientist Training Program grant GM-07205 (D.E.I.) and U.S. Public Health Service grant AM-17389 (J.D.J.).

References

1. Banerjee SD, Cohn RH, Bernfield MR: Basal lamina of embryonic salivary epithelia. Production by the epithelium and role in maintaining lobular morphology. J Cell Biol 73:445–463, 1977.
2. Dodson JW, Hay ED: Secretion of collagenous stroma by isolated epithelium grown *in vitro*. Exp Cell Res 65:215–220, 1971.
3. Emerman JT, Pitelka DR: Maintenance and induction of morphological differentiation in dissociated mammary epithelium on floating collagen membranes. *In Vitro* 13:316–328, 1977.
4. Meier S, Hay E: Control of corneal differentiation by extracellular materials. Collagen as promoter and stabilizer of epithelial stroma production. Dev Biol 38:249–270, 1974.
5. Timpl R, Martin GR, Bruckner P, Wick G, Wiedeman H: Nature of the collagenous protein in a tumor basement membrane. Eur J Biochem 84:43–52, 1978.
6. Burgeson RE, El Adli EA, Kaitila II, Hollister DW: Fetal membrane collagens: identification of two new collagen alpha chains. Proc Natl Acad Sci USA 73:2579–2583, 1976.
7. Timpl R, Rohde H, Robey PG, Rennard SI, Foidart J-M, Martin GR: Laminin – A glycoprotein from basement membrane. J Biol Chem 254:9933–9937, 1979.
8. Vaheri A, Ruoslahti E, Mosher DF (eds): Fibroblast surface protein. Ann NY Acad Sci 312:1–456, 1978.
9. Madri JA, Roll FJ, Furthmayr H, Foidart J-M: Ultrastructural localization of fibronectin and laminin in the basement membranes of the murine kidney. J Cell Biol 86:682–687, 1980.
10. Kanwar YS, Farquhar MG: Presence of heparan sulfate in the glomerular basement membranes of the murine kidney. Proc Natl Acad Sci USA 76:1303–1307, 1979.
11. Lemkin MC, Farquhar MG: Sulfated and nonsulfated glycosaminoglycans and glycopeptides are synthesized by kidney *in vivo* and incorporated into glomerular basement membranes. Proc Natl Acad Sci USA 78:1726–1730, 1981.
12. Cohn RH, Banerjee SD, Bernfield MR: Basal lamina of embryonic salivary epithelia. Nature of glycosaminoglycan and organization of extracellular materials. J Cell Biol 73:464–478, 1977.
13. Bernfield MR, Banerjee SD: The basal lamina in epithelial-mesenchymal interactions. In: Biology and chemistry of basement membranes, Kefalides N (ed). New York: Academic Press, 1978, pp 137–148.
14. Bernfield MR, Banerjee SD, Cohn RH: Dependence of salivary epithelial morphology and

branching morphogenesis upon acid mucopolysaccharide-protein proteoglycan at the epithelial surface. J Cell Biol 52:674–689, 1972.
15. David G, Bernfield MR: Collagen reduces glycosaminoglycan degradation by cultured mammary epithelial cells: possible mechanism for basal lamina formation. Proc Natl Acad Sci USA 76:786–790, 1979.
16. Dodson JW, Hay ED: Secretion of collagen by corneal epithelium. J Exp Zool 189:51–72, 1974.
17. Abercrombie M: Contact inhibition: the phenomenon and its biological implications. Natl Cancer Inst Monogr 26:249–277, 1967.
18. Stoker MGP, Rubin H: Density dependent inhibition of cell growth in culture. Nature 215:171–172, 1967.
19. Iwig M, Lasch J, Glaesser D: Growth regulation of lens epithelial cells. Chemically-modified sepharose as a suitable substratum for studying cell-substratum interactions. Cell Diff 9:1–12, 1980.
20. Ben-Zeev A, Farmer SR, Penman S: Protein synthesis requires cell-surface contact while nuclear events respond to cell shape in anchorage-dependent fibroblasts. Cell 21:365–372, 1980.
21. Folkman J, Moscona A: Role of cell shape in growth control. Nature 273:345–349, 1978.
22. Iwig M, Glaesser D, Bethge M: Cell shape-mediated growth control of lens epithelial cells grown in culture. Exp Cell Res 131:47–56, 1981.
23. Folkman J, Greenspan HP: Influence of geometry on control of cell growth. Biochim Biophys Acta 417:211–236, 1975.
24. Holley RW: Control of growth of mammalian cells in cell culture. Nature 258:487–490, 1975.
25. Kleinman HK, Klebe RJ, Martin GR: Role of collagenous matrices in the adhesion and growth of cells. J Cell Biol 88:473–485, 1981.
26. Terranova VP, Rohrbach DH, Martin GR: Role of laminin in the attachment of PAM 212 epithelial cells to basement membrane collagen. Cell 22:719–726, 1980.
27. Yamada KM, Yamada SS, Pastan I: Cell surface protein partially restores morphology, adhesiveness, and contact inhibition of movement to transformed fibroblasts. Proc Natl Acad Sci USA 73:1217–1221, 1976.
28. Roblin R, Albert SO, Gelb NA, Black PH: Cell surface changes correlated with density-dependent growth inhibition. Glycosaminoglycan metabolism in 3T3, SV3T3, and Con A selected revertant cells. Biochemistry 14:347–357, 1975.
29. Underhill CB, Keller JM: Density-dependent changes in the amount of sulfated glycosaminoglycans associated with mouse 3T3 cells. J Cell Physiol 89:53–64, 1976.
30. Underhill CB, Keller JM: A transformation-dependent difference in the heparan sulfate associated with the cell surface. Biochem Biophys Res Comm 63:448–454, 1975.
31. Hayman EG, Engvall E, Ruoslahti E: Concomitant loss of cell surface fibronectin and laminin from transformed rat kidney cells. J Cell Biol 88:352–357, 1981.
32. Wessels NK: Substrate and nutrient effects upon epidermal basal cell orientation and proliferation. Proc Natl Acad Sci USA 52:252 259, 1964.
33. Kallman F, Evans J, Wessells NK: Normal epidermal basal cell behavior in the absence of basement membrane. J Cell Biol 32:231–236, 1967.
34. Jensen H, Mottet N: Ultrastructural changes in keratinizing epithelium following trypsinization, epidermal detachment and apposition to mesenchymes. J Cell Sci 6:511–535, 1970.
35. Carter WG, Rauvala H, Hakomori SI: Studies on cell adhesion on surfaces coated with carbohydrate-reactive proteins (glycosidases and lectins) and fibronectin. J Cell Biol 88:138–148, 1981.
36. Elsdale T, Bard J: Collagen substrata for studies on cell behavior. J Cell Biol 54:626–637, 1972.
37. Michalopoulos G, Pitot HC: Primary culture of parenchymal liver cells on collagen membranes. Exp Cell Res 94:70–78,1975.
38. Yang J, Guzman R, Richards J, Nandi S: Primary cultures of mouse mammary tumor epithelial cells embedded in collagen gels. *In Vitro* 16:502–506, 1980.

39. Yang J, Richards J, Bowman P, Guzman R, Enami J, McCormick K, Hamamoto S, Pitelka D, Nandi S: Sustained growth and three-dimensional organization of primary mammary tumor epithelial cells embedded on collagen gels. Proc Natl Acad Sci USA 76:3401–3405, 1979.
40. Wicha MS, Liotta LA, Vonderhaar BK, Kidwell WR: Effects of inhibition of basement membrane collagen deposition on rat mammary gland development. Dev Biol 80:253–266, 1980.
41. Potten CS: The epidermal proliferative unit: the possible role of the central basal cell. Cell Tissue Kinet 7:77–88, 1974.
42. Walker F: Basement-membrane turnover in the rat. J Pathol 107:119–121, 1972.
43. Vracko R: Basal lamina scaffold-anatomy and significance for maintenance of orderly tissue structures. Am J Pathol 77:314–346, 1974.
44. Wicha MS, Liotta LA, Garbisa G, Kidwell WR: Basement membrane collagen requirements for attachment and growth of mammary epithelium. Exp Cell Res 124:181–190, 1979.
45. Stenn KS, Madri JA, Roll FJ: Migrating epidermis produces AB2 collagen and requires continual collagen synthesis for movement. Nature 277:229–232, 1979.
46. Liotta LA, Vembu D, Kleinman HK, Martin GR, Boone C: Collagen required for proliferation of cultured connective tissue cells but not their transformed counterparts. Nature 272:622–624, 1978.
47. Vembu D, Liotta LA, Paranjpe M, Boone CW: Correlation of tumorigenicity with resistance to growth inhibition by cishydroxyproline. Exp Cell Res 124:247–252, 1979.
48. Pierce GB, Shikes R, Fink LM: Cancer: a problem of development biology. Englewood Cliffs, NJ: Prentice Hall, 1978.
49. Sakakura T, Sakagami Y, Nishizura Y: Persistence of responsiveness of adult mouse mammary gland to induction by embryonic mesenchyme. Dev Biol 72:201–210, 1979.
50. Tarin D: Tissue interactions and the maintenance of histological structure in adults. In: Tissue interactions in carcinogenesis, Tarin D (ed). New York: Academic Press, 1972, pp 81–94.
51. Leighton J: Propagation of cancer: target for future chemotherapy. Cancer Res 29:2457–2465, 1969.
52. Gullino PM: The internal milieu of tumors. Prog Exp Tumor Res 8:1–25, 1966.
53. Foley JF, Aftonomos B-Th, Heidrick ML: Influence of fibroblast collagen and mucopolysaccharides on HeLa cell colonial morphology. Life Sci 7:1003–1008, 1968.
54. Orr JW, Spencer AT: Transplantation studies on the mechanism of carcinogenesis. In: Tissue interactions in carcinogenesis, Tarin D (ed). New York: Academic Press, 1972, pp 291–304.
55. Folkman J: Tumor Angiogenesis. Adv Canc Res 19:331–358, 1974.
56. Dawe CJ, Morgan WD, Slatick MS: Influence of epithelio-mesenchymal interactions on tumor induction by polyoma virus. Int J Cancer 1:419–450, 1966.
57. Dawe CJ, Whang-Peng J, Morgan WD, Hearon EC, Knutsen T: Epithelial origin of polyoma salivary tumors in mice: evidence based on chromosome-marked cells. Science 171:394–397, 1971.
58. Dawe CJ, Morgan WD, Slatick MS: Salivary gland neoplasms in the role of normal mesenchyme during salivary gland morphogenesis. In: Epithelial-mesenchymal interactions, Fleischmajer R, Billingham RE (eds). Baltimore: Williams & Wilkins, 1968, pp 293–312.
59. Argyris TS, Argyris BF: Differential response of skin epithelium to growth-promoting effects of subcutaneous transplanted tumor. Cancer Res 22:73–77, 1962.
60. Redler P, Lustig ES: Differences in the growth-promoting effect of normal and peritumoral dermis on epidermis *in vitro*. Dev Biol 17:679–691, 1968.
61. Goldenberg DM, Pavia RA: Malignant potential of murine stroma cells after transplantation of human tumors into nude mice. Science 212:65–67, 1981.
62. Lakshmi MS, Sherbet GV: Embryonic and tumour cell interactions. In: Neoplasia and cell differentiation, Sherbet GV (ed). New York: S. Karger, 1974, pp 380–396.
63. DeCosse JJ, Gossens CL, Kuzma JF: Breast cancer: induction of differentiation by embryonic tissue. Science 181:1057–1058, 1973.
64. Ellison ML, Ambrose EJ, Easty GC: Differentiation in a transplantable rat tumour maintained in organ culture. Exp Cell Res 55:198–204, 1969.

65. Vasiliev JVM: The role of connective tissue proliferation in invasive growth of normal and malignant tissues: a review. Br J Cancer 12:524–536, 1958.
66. Tarin D: 1972 Morphological studies on the mechanism of carcinogenesis. In: Tissue interactions in carcinogenesis, Tarin D (ed). New York: Academic Press, 1972, pp 227–290.
67. Sugar J: Ultrastructural and histochemical changes during the development of cancer in various human organs. In: Tissue interactions in carcinogenesis Tarin D (ed). New York: Academic Press, 1972, pp 127–160.
68. Mainardi CL, Dixit SN, Kang AH: Degradation of type IV basement membrane collagen by a proteinase isolated from human polymorphonuclear leukocyte granules. J Biol Chem 255:5435–5441, 1980.
69. Leighton J, Kalla RL, Kline I, Belkin M: Pathogenesis of tumor invasion. I. Interactions between normal tissues and 'transformed' cells in tissue culture. Cancer Res 19:23–27, 1959.
70. Luibel FJ, Sanders E, Ashworth CT: An electron microscopic study of carcinoma in situ and invasive carcinoma of the cervix uteri. Cancer Res 20:357–361, 1960.
71. Ozzello L: The behavior of basement membranes in intraductal carcinoma of the breast. Am J Pathol 35:887–895, 1959.
72. Rubio CA, Biberfeld P: The basement membrane in experimental induced atypias and carcinoma of the uterine cervix in mice. Virchows Arch A Path Anat Histol 381:205–209, 1979.
73. Pitelka DR, Hamamoto ST, Taggart BN: Basal lamina and tissue recognition in malignant mammary tumors. Cancer Res 40:1600–1611, 1980.
74. Fidler IJ: Tumor heterogeneity and the biology of cancer invasion and metastasis. Cancer Res 38:2651–2660, 1978.
75. Gould V, Battifora H: Origin and significance of the basal lamina and some interstitial fibrillar components in epithelial neoplasms. Pathol Ann 11:353–386, 1976.
76. Liotta LA, Tryggvason K, Garbisa S, Hart I, Foltz CM, Shafie S: Metastatic potential correlates with enzymatic degradation of basement membrane collagen. Nature 284:67–68, 1980.
77. Ingber DE, Madri JA, Jamieson JD: Role of basal lamina in neoplastic disorganization of tissue architecture. Proc Natl Acad Sci USA 78:3901–3905, 1981.
78. Reddy JK, Rao MS: Transplantable pancreatic carcinoma of the rat. Science 198:78–80, 1977.
79. Jamieson JD, Ingber DE, Muresan V, Sarras MP Jr, Maylie-Pfenninger M-F, Iwanij V: Cell surface properties of normal, differentiating, and neoplastic pancreatic acinar cells. Cancer 47:1516–1525, 1981.
80. Liotta LA, Tryggvason K, Garbisa S, Robey PG, Abe SG: Partial purification and characterization of a neutral protease which cleaves type IV collagen. Biochemistry 20:100–104, 1981.
81. Leivo I, Vaheri A, Timpl R, Wartiovaara J: Appearance and distribution of collagens and laminin in the early mouse embryo. Dev Biol 76:100–114, 1980.
82. Ekblom P, Alitalo K, Vaheri A, Timpl R, Saxen L: Induction of a basement membrane glycoprotein in embryonic kidney: possible role of laminin in morphogenesis. Proc Natl Acad Sci USA 77:485–489, 1980.
83. Farquhar MG: Structure and function in glomerular capillaries: role of the basement membrane in glomerular filtration. In: Biology and chemistry of basement membranes, Kefalides NA (ed). New York: Academic Press, 1978, pp 43–80.
84. Grobstein C: Mechanisms of organogenetic tissue interaction. Natl Cancer Inst Monogr 26:279–299, 1967.
85. Koch JC: The laws of bone architecture. Am J Anat 21:177–298, 1917.
86. Thompson DW: On growth and form, New York: Cambridge University Press, 1977.
87. Buckminster Fuller R: Synergetics, New York: Macmillan, 1975, p 372.
88. Otto F: Pneumatic structures. In: Tensile structures, Otto F (ed). Cambridge, Mass: M.I.T. Press, 1973, p 148.
89. Kenner H: Geodesic Math, Berkeley, Calif.: University of California Press, 1976, pp 3–7.

21. Plasminogen activator in metastasis

J.C. BARRETT and S. SHEELA

1. Introduction

Proteases play a key role in the regulation of many biological processes [1]. They can serve to create rapid and permanent changes which can either turn on (e.g., zymogen activation) or turn off (e.g., protein degradation) physiological reactions. Protease activation of consecutive zymogen reaction (e.g. enzyme cascades) can also amplify regulated processes. Furthermore, the presence or absence of protease inhibitors provides an additional level for control mechanisms of cellular processes. For a complex biological process, like tumor cell metastasis, proteases undoubtedly play some role. It is the purpose of this chapter to discuss possible roles proteases may have in regulating metastasis formation.

Malignant cells exhibit three important phenotypes: loss of growth regulation, invasiveness, and metastasis formation. Each of these cellular phenotypes possibly results from a number of molecular changes, which may occur by more than one mechanism in different cells. For a normal cell to progress to a malignant cell, it must undergo a number of different qualitative as well as quantitative changes [2, 3]. Furthermore, cellular heterogeneity is a common characteristic of malignant cells [4]. Even with highly invasive, malignant tumors, metastasis formation is a rare event and only a small percentage of the tumor cells actually succeed in this process [4]. Tumor cell heterogeneity is thought to be essential for the generation of cells that can survive and achieve all the steps required for metastasis [4].

Proteases are likely to be involved in some and possibly many of the cellular changes required for malignancy. This is *not* to say that proteases are the cause of malignant transformation. Rather, it is our hypothesis that proteases will cause or facilitate cellular changes, including heterogeneity, and that these changes will increase the probability that a normal cell will progress to malignancy or that a tumor cell will have an increased capacity to metastasize. Malignant cells may arise without involvement of proteolytic enzymes; however, if during neoplastic development cells acquire increased proteolytic activity, the rate of malignant progression will increase by any one of several possible mechanisms. These mechanisms will be discussed later in consideration of the possible roles of proteases in controlling the malignant phenotype of cells.

Previous studies with plasminogen activator, a protease commonly found associated with many different tumor cells, will be used to illustrate how proteases can

L.A. Liotta and I.R. Hart (eds.), Tumor Invasion and Metastasis. ISBN-13: 978-94-009-7513-2.
© 1982 Martinus Nijhoff Publishers, The Hague/Boston/London.

modulate the malignant properties of tumor cells. A description of the properties of plasminogen activator and the evidence for an association of the enzyme with tumor cells are discussed in the next section.

1.1. Characterization of plasminogen activators

Plasminogen activator is a serine protease which catalyzes the conversion of plasminogen, a serum component, into an active protease, plasmin, by limited proteolysis. Plasminogen activators are glycoproteins [5] and exist in multiple forms ranging in molecular weight from 28 000 to 165 000 dalton.

Vertebrate plasminogen activators can be divided into at least three groups: urinary plasminogen activators (e.g., urokinase), tissue plasminogen activators, and circulating plasminogen activators. More recently plasminogen activators from cells in culture have been described. These latter enzymes may belong to any or all of the three types mentioned above.

The most well characterized form of plasminogen activator is urokinase, which is purified from urine. It has been demonstrated that both human urine and the medium collected from kidney cells in organ or tissue culture contain two forms of plasminogen activator with molecular weights of either 30 000 or 55 000 dalton [6]. Monospecific antibodies to highly purified preparations of either form of urokinase cross-react with the urokinase of differing molecular weight [7, 8].

Astrup in 1947 [9] demonstrated the presence of plasminogen activator in tissue and defined it as an acid stable, plasminogen dependent protease extracted from tissues at high salt concentrations [10]. Tissue plasminogen activators have been isolated from human myometrium [11], polymorphonuclear monocytes [12], vascular tissue [13] and adrenal tissue [14]. These enzymes have molecular weights ranging form 65–85 000 dalton and antibodies to urokinase generally do not precipitate these tissue plasminogen activators although there are some exceptions [15]. These enzymes are stable to both acid treatment and heating in contrast to urokinase [16]. These results indicate a structural difference between some of the tissue plasminogen activators and urokinase.

Circulating or 'physiological' plasminogen activators in human blood, which exist commonly as zymogens or as activator-inhibitor complexes, have molecular weights ranging from 98–165 000 dalton and are not inhibited by antisera specific for urokinase. Intrinsic plasminogen activators of plasma can be distinguished from extrinsic plasminogen activators of blood (which probably have their origin in tissues) by their specific inhibition by Cl-inhibitor which inhibits most of the fibrinolytic activity in plasma [17]. At least two extrinsic plasminogen activators of blood have been purified having molecular weights of 60 000 and 10 000 dalton; the former is acid stable and the latter acid labile and both resemble tissue plasminogen activators from human uterine tissue immunologically and in molecular weight characteristics [11]. Antibodies against tissue activator from porcine ovaries inhibit both human uterine tissue plasminogen activator and extrinsic plasma plasminogen activators, while antibodies to urokinase fail to inhibit either of them [11]. This indicates that these enzymes are also distinct serine proteases, different from urokinase.

Many cells types grown in culture produce plasminogen activators which are either identical or closely related to urokinase in their molecular weight and sensitivity to antibodies [18]. The first definitive observation of the presence of plasminogen activator in cell culture was made by Barnett and Baron who demonstrated that human epidermoid carcinoma cells and primary cultures of rhesus monkey kidney cells produce a plasminogen activator in serum-free medium [19]. However, this enzyme was not released into the medium. Human kidney cells produce at least two low molecular weight and one high molecular weight form of plasminogen activator and these enzymes cross-react with antibodies to urokinase [6]. Also, plasminogen activators released by human lung, osteosarcoma, pancreatic carcinoma [20], spleen, and thyroid [21] cells exist as 30000 and 60000 molecular weight forms and cross-react with antibodies to urinary urokinase [22]. In contrast, a number plasminogen activators of cells from brain tumors or cerebral melanomas do not cross-react with antibodies to urokinase. Thus, even though a majority of human cells in culture produce plasminogen activators identical to urokinase, there are cells which produce plasminogen activators of entirely different immunological reactivity.

Immunological comparisons of activators produced in cultures of normal and transformed cells showed that plasminogen activators released by viral-transformed hamster embryo cells (SV-40 transformed) are antigenically identical to activators produced by normal hamster lungs but different from the plasminogen activator produced by hamster kidney cells [22]. Human fetal kidney cells in culture produce a plasminogen activator immunologically identical to human urokinase and to an activator released in cultures of ovarian carcinoma [23]. Antibodies to plasminogen activator from virus transformed hamster cells or human urokinase were highly species specific with the former having apparently no activity against human or mouse plasminogen activators [22] and vice versa [14].

1.2. Association of plasminogen activator with tumor cells

Several studies indicate that tumor cell invasion is accompanied by proteolysis [23]. There are a large number of reports describing high levels of different classes of proteinases associated with a variety of malignant neoplasms [24–28]. It is beyond the scope of this review to discuss all these reports. We will focus our remarks on plasminogen activator.

Fischer [29] noted in 1925 that primary explants of viral sarcomas of chickens grown on plasma clots possessed enhanced fibrinolytic activity when compared to explants of normal tissues. This observation was not fully appreciated until after

1973 when Reich and his colleagues published a series of important papers [30–33] which demonstrated the enhanced fibrinolytic activity of many types of tumor cells. Furthermore, these authors proposed a role for this activity in a number of phenotypes displayed by malignant cells including morphological changes [34, 35], cell migration [36], decreased cellular adhesion [37], disorganization of intracellular actin containing cables [38] and loss of growth control [39]. Quigley et al. [40] demonstrated that the enhanced fibrinolytic activity of tumor cells in culture is due to the cellular synthesis of plasminogen activator and the subsequent conversion of serum plasminogen to plasmin, which is reponsible for the observed fibrinolytic activity. Although some malignant cells in culture produce plasminogen independent proteases [41], plasminogen activator is by far the most ubiquitous protease associated with malignant transformation.

A variety of normal cells [42] synthesize plasminogen activators *in vitro* and *in vivo* (e.g., macrophages, granulocytes, mammary epithelium, keratinizing epithelium, parietal endoderm, trophoblasts, kidney, lung, etc.). This implies that plasminogen activator is important for a number of normal physiological processes. Furthermore, this indicates that plasminogen activator production is not sufficient for neoplastic transformation. These results do not however preclude a role for plasminogen activator in malignancy. It is possible that this or some other protease is necessary, but not sufficient, for malignant transformation. Also, it is our hypothesis that proteases are not necessarily required for malignancy but that these enzymes can facilitate the expression of a number of cellular phenotypes required for malignancy or the rate of malignant progression of a cell by increasing epigenetic and/or genetic instability. In analogy to the behavior of malignant cells, many of the normal physiological cellular reactions with which plasminogen activator synthesis

Table 1. Possible roles of proteases in controlling malignant properties of tumor cells.

Malignant phenotype	Possible function of proteases
I. Loss of growth regulation	1. Modulation of cell surface
	2. Disruption of membrane-nucleus communication
	3. Stimulation of DNA synthesis
	4. Stimulation of hormone production
	5. Alteration of gene expression
	6. Modulation of differentiation
II. Invasiveness	1. Destruction of extracellular matrix
	2. Activation of proteases/collagenases
	3. Increased cell motility/migration
III. Metastasis formation	1. Cleavage of membrane proteins
	2. Activation of gene expression
	3. Decreased cell attachment
	4. Stimulation of angiogenesis
	5. Formation and dissolution of fibrin capsule
	6. Increased tumor hetereogeneity

is correlated involve tissue remodeling with cellular invasion or migration (e.g. involution of mammary epithelium [43], ovulation [44], and stimulated macrophages [45]. This supports a role for plasminogen activator in cellular invasion due to either a normal or pathological process.

Enhanced plasminogen activator synthesis has been observed with certain non-tumorigenic cell lines grown in culture of mouse (e.g., 3T3) or hamster (e.g., BHK and FOL) origin [46, 47]. Since these cells are not malignant, these results have been cited as evidence against a role of plasminogen activator production in neoplasia. However, these aneuploid cell lines are not 'normal' since they have an increased propensity to progress to neoplasia when compared to diploid cells. For this reason we have termed these cells preneoplastic [47]. Following exposure of normal diploid cells to chemical carcinogens, enhanced fibrinolytic activity is observed within two weeks after treatment whereas neoplastic progression of these cells requires 6–15 weeks [3, 48]. Furthermore, cells with enhanced fibrinolytic activity have a much greater probability to progress to malignancy than cells without this activity [3]. These results support our hypothesis that acquisition of fibrinolytic activity (i.e., plasminogen activator), while perhaps not a cause of neoplastic transformation, may reflect a loss of control of the normal function of the cellular genetic apparatus during the process of neoplastic transformation [48, 49].

2. Role of proteases in controlling malignant properties of tumor cells

As mentioned earlier we have considered loss of growth regulation, invasiveness, and metastasis formation as three essential features of malignant cells. The possible roles of proteases in controlling and facilitating the expression of these malignant phenotypes are listed in Table 1.

2.1. Loss of growth regulation

There are several mechanisms by which proteases may affect growth control (Table 1). A direct stimulation of cell growth by exogeneous proteases has been demonstrated with several different types of cells grown in culture. Burger [50] first reported that trypsin, pronase, and ficin stimulate cell division of mouse 3T3 cells at confluence. Most of the cells treated with protease escape contact inhibition of cell growth and undergo one cell division. However, this result was not reproduced in a number of other studies with 3T3 cells [51, 52, 53] and this may be related to differences in the serum requirements of various 3T3 lines which will affect whether or not protease stimulation of growth occurs [53].

Protease stimulation of growth with other cell types can be reproducibly demonstated [23]. Confluent chick embryo fibroblasts are particularly sensitive to low concentrations of trypsin [52, 54, 55] and thrombin [56, 57]. Thrombin, at concentrations as low as 5×10^{-9} M, can stimulate DNA synthesis in these cells in the absence of serum [56–58], providing an excellent experimental system to study the effects of proteases on growth stimulation.

The mechanism by which exogeneous proteases stimulate cell division is unknown. One possibility is that the protease affects the cell surface, which results in the activation of cell growth. Exogeneous addition of proteases can result in cleavage of cell surface proteins [59] including growth factor receptors [60]. Furthermore, exogeneous proteases stimulate glucose transport [56, 61–63], lower cellular cAMP levels [64], and increase the number of microvilli on the cell surface [65], all of which may be related to stimulation of DNA synthesis.

It is also possible that the action of the proteases occurs intracellularly. Zetter et al. [66] and Martin and Quigley [57, 58] have demonstrated that thrombin binds to cells and is internalized prior to stimulation of DNA synthesis. Chymotrypsin, which is not mitogenic under the same conditions as thrombin, is not internalized [57, 58]. Several intracellular functions of proteases may be involved in altering cellular growth regulation. Exogeneous protease can induce the disorganization of intracellular actin cables in nontumorigenic cells [67]. Alternations in actin-containing cables are found in many tumorigenic cells [38] and this is correlated with the production of plasminogen activator by these cells [38, 67]. Morphological alterations of transformed cells may be related to protease mediated changes in cell surface protein and/or intracellular actin organization [34, 59]. Whether the alteration in intracellular organization occurs as a result of extracellular or intercellular proteolytic action is unclear. An alteration of intercellular organization may disrupt membrane-nucleus communication which in turn would affect the control of cell growth regulation.

Another function of protease production which may affect cellular growth control is the stimulation of active growth hormones. Proteolytic control of hormone production, for example, proinsulin, is a well-established normal physiological reaction [1]. Recently, production of growth factors (e.g., sarcoma growth factor) by neoplastic cells has been demonstrated [68]. The role of proteases in this process has not been studied, but is potentially an important mechanism for proteolytic modulation of cellular growth control.

In addition to affecting membrane and cytoplasmic proteins, proteases may play a role in initiating DNA synthesis directly. Stubblefield and Brown [69] have proposed three roles for proteases in control of DNA replication: (1) proteases may release DNA polymerase bound to chromatin or membranes (2) protease molecules may be an essential part of the replication complex, and (3) proteases may activate zymogen forms of DNA polymerase or other proteins required in the replication complex. The results of Brown et al. [70] are consistent with these possibilities. They have demonstrated an alteration in the sedimentation coefficient of DNA polymerase activity in trypsin treated cells and have shown that nuclei from G_1 cells can be stimulated to synthesize DNA by treatment with trypsin. Furthermore, Moise and Hosoda [71] have shown that cleavage of the gene 32 product of bacteriophage

T4 results in three products, two of which have affinity for native DNA not observed with uncleaved gene 32 protein. They propose a model for the unwinding of DNA in advance of the replication fork with proteolytic control of the attachment and release of the gene 32 protein. Stubblefield and Brown [69] have proposed a theory of cancer based on the notion of protease mediated initiation of DNA synthesis.

Loss of growth control in neoplastic cells is illustrated by the ability of tumorigenic, but not nontumorigenic cells, to grow when suspended in a semisolid media such as agar or methocel. This phenomenon is also called anchorage independent growth because the cells do not require attachment to a substrate for growth. Growth of cells in semisolid media correlates with tumorigenicity for a number of different cell types from different species, although exceptions to this correlation exist [49]. Still, for many cell types this phenotypic marker correlates very well with neoplastic potential and is the most reliable *in vitro* index of tumorigenicity.

Ossowski et al. [34] Pollack et al. [39] suggested that enhanced fibrinolytic activity of cells, which results from increased secretion of plasminogen activator [72], is causally related to the ability of cells to grow in semisolid media. This is an important hypothesis considering the relationship between growth in agar and tumorigenicity and suggests a direct function for this protease in the loss of growth control of malignant cells. For this reason it is important to critically evaluate the evidence for a role of plasminogen activator in anchorage independent growth of tumor cells. There are four types of experiments which produce supportive findings for this relationship: correlative studies [39, 72], experiments with plasminogen depleted serum [34, 39, 72], experiments with sera which contain elevated levels of plasminogen [39, 72] and studies with cells transformed by temperature sensitive mutants of tumor viruses [33, 34].

We have recently re-examined the relationship between plasminogen dependent fibrinolytic activity and anchorage independent growth of chemically transformed hamster cells [49]. Malignant cell lines derived from Syrian hamster embryo fibroblasts display not only a qualitative correlation between growth in semisolid media and tumorigenicity *in vivo*, but also a quantitative correlation between the efficiency of growth in agar and the number of cells required to produce a tumor in 50% of the animals injected. The high degree of correlation between growth in agar and tumorigenicity of Syrian hamster cell lines makes this an attractive cellular system to study the molecular basis for growth in agar and hopefully, tumorigenicity. In our study, we examined the relationship between plasminogen activator production and anchorage independent growth by the four approaches mentioned above and concluded that there is no evidence to support a role of plasminogen activator production in this alteration of growth control.

Cell lines isolated on the basis of varying levels of fibrinolytic activity did not display a correlation between the level of fibrinolytic activity and cloning efficiency in semisolid agar. Plasminogen depletion of serum by lysine sepharose affinity chromatography reduced the ability of the serum to support growth of the cells in agar. Part of this reduction was ascribed to a general decrease in the ability of plasminogen depleted serum to support anchorage dependent cell growth in liquid media. The ability of plasminogen depleted serum to support anchorage dependent and independent cell growth could not be restored by exogeneous plasminogen, suggesting that the process of plasminogen depletion removed factors, other than plasminogen, which are responsible for the reduction in growth support by this depleted serum. Addition of plasminogen to fetal bovine serum did not enhance the ability of cells to grow in agar. Mutants of hamster cells temperature sensitive for growth in agar were not temperature sensitive for production of plasminogen activator. Thus, the results with hamster cells do not support a direct role of plasminogen activator production for growth in semisolid media of these cells. The results presented previously to support the relationship between growth in agar and enhanced fibrinolytic activity can be explained by other variables in the experiments. Of course, enhanced fibrinolytic activity may be necessary but not sufficient for anchorage independent growth. There is no evidence at present to conclusively demonstrate a role of plasminogen activator or any other protease in controlling cell growth.

In addition to acting directly to cause loss of growth control or possibly neoplastic transformation, proteases may function in facilitating these changes. That is, enhanced levels of proteases may increase the cell's capacity for epigenetic or genetic changes, which may increase the rate of neoplastic progression of altered cells.

For example, regulation of the bacterial error prone DNA repair enzymes is under proteolytic control. In response to certain types of DNA damage, eg. UV light, bacterial cells produce a protease, the rec A gene product, which cleaves the λ repressor and initiates lysogenic induction and the synthesis of repressed error prone DNA repair enzymes ('SOS' functions). This repair system differs from the non-induced repair processes of the cells in that repair of DNA damage leads to the production of gene mutations. Thus, proteolytic control of gene expression and genetic instability is evident in this system.

Miskin and Reich [73] have recently reported that following exposure to UV and other DNA damaging agents chicken, hamster, rat, mouse, and human fibroblasts increase synthesis of plasminogen activator by eight- to fifteen-fold. This enzyme induction requires genetic transcription and translation. The correlation between DNA damage and synthesis of plasminogen activator suggests an analogy to the production of the rec A gene product, a protease, in *E. coli* and the subsequent induction of error prone DNA repair enzymes. The validity of this analogy remains to be determined. However, if the synthesis of plasminogen activator by carcinogen treated cells does lead to the induction of gene expression at other loci and possibly error prone DNA repair function, then this protease could play a key role facilitating neoplastic progression.

In this light it is interesting to note that we have reported that increased plasminogen activator production is an early event in the neoplastic progression of carcinogen treated Syrian hamster embryo cells [3, 48]. This phenotypic change did not correlate with any other specific phenotypic transformation of the cells (for example, morphological transformation occurred in the absence of enhanced fibrinolytic activity and anchorage independent growth and neoplastic transformation occurred many cell generations after enhanced fibrinolytic activity was observed) [48]. However, cells with increased plasminogen activator synthesis had a much greater propensity to progress and become tumorigenic than cells which lacked this protease [3]. We suggested that the production of this enzyme may reflect a loss of genetic control during the process of neoplastic progression. The results of Miskin and Reich are in accord with this notion.

Finally, it should be noted that loss of growth regulation may occur without any stimulation of cell proliferation. Growth control is maintained by a balance of cell proliferation and differentiation. If cellular differentiation is modulated by proteases by any of the mechanisms discussed above (e.g., membrane alterations or changes in gene expression), then control of cell growth can be disrupted without a stimulation of cell proliferation. It is possible that tumor promoters exert their influence on carcinogenesis by such a mechanism. It has been demonstrated by several investigators that tumor promoters inhibit or alter cellular differentiation and this is proposed as a theory for their mechanism of action. The observations that protease inhibitors inhibit tumor promotion and that tumor promoters stimulate plasminogen activator synthesis provide evidence that proteases may be involved in these processes [23].

2.2. Invasiveness

Destruction of the extracellular matrix, thereby permitting cellular invasion, is an obvious function for proteases in malignant cell behavior. However, the evidence that proteases are important in this function is limited. Jones and DeClerck [74] recently reported that tumor cells can degrade the collagen, elastin, and glycoprotein components of an extracellular matrix produced by heart smooth muscle cells *in vitro*. They presented evidence that plasminogen activator production by the cells mediated the degradation of the glycoproteins in this matrix. Several studies have also demonstrated that tumor cells secrete high levels of collagenases [75].

Basement membrane, the amorphous extracellular lining material of epithelial and endothelial cells, is of primary importance in the invasion phase of metastasis by malignant cells. For blood borne metastasis, tumor cells must penetrate the endothelial basement membrane to enter the blood vessel. Furthermore, since basement membranes separate epithelial cells from their mesenchymal components, the basement membrane is the first barrier encountered by invasive carcinomas. The primary characteristic which distinguishes invasive carcinomas from carcinoma *in situ* is the disruption of the basement membrane [76, 77, 78].

Ultrastructural studies have shown that invasive tumor cells disrupt and destroy basement membranes in the vicinity of the tumor cells. Luibel et al. [77] and

Ashworth et al. [76], based on electron microscopic studies of human cervix, observed that there is a marked disruption of basement membrane in invasive carcinoma with no change in normal epithelium or carcinoma *in situ.* Studies of Frithiof [79] revealed that there is either an extremely thin or multilayered basement membrane alternating with absence of such a membrane in invasive squamous carcinoma of the oral cavity. Studies of Birbeck and Wheatley [80] indicated that tumor cells preferentially attach to the basement membrane leading to local disruption through which the tumor cells can penetrate the connective tissue. Whether the disruption of the basement membrane in these studies is the result of physical forces or enzymic processes is unknown. We are interested in isolating pure basement membrane for studies on the degradation of basement membrane by tumor cells as a model for one step in neoplastic invasion. We have chosen to study pulmonary basement membrane since the lung is an important site of invasion for metastatic cells [81].

Most studies on the ultrastructural and biochemical properties of basement membranes have employed lens capsuse and renal glomerular basement membranes, because they are located in anatomically advantageous regions in addition to being large (1200–2000 Å) and readily isolated in pure form [82, 83, 84]. The isolation and purification of basement membranes from other tissues poses serious technical problems because of the presence of other insoluble extracellular proteins such as fibrillar collagen and elastin in most tissues. This is especially evident in basement membranes of the lung alveoli. The most common procedure for the isolation and purification of basement membranes from various tissues involves an initial sonication of a tissue to disrupt the cells and free the basement membrane [84]. This method has the disadvantage of disrupting and fragmenting the basement membrane. This results in basement membrane preparations which are morphologically altered and sometimes contaminated with cell membrane fragments [85, 86].

In our attempt to obtain pure basement membrane from hamster lungs, we have tried a number of isolation procedures developed by others including sonication [82] and extraction with acetic acid [84] or various detergents like sodium deoxycholate [85] and N-lauroyl sarcosine [87]. We have compared the purity of the resulting basement membrane by these methods and none of the above procedures were satisfactory for the isolation of pulmonary basement membrane from hamster lung. Taking into account the fact that detergents solubilize cell membranes, intracellular proteins, and plasma proteins and that acetic acid extraction removes interstitial collagen effectively, we have developed a method for the isolation of pure pulmonary basement membrane. This method involves an initial extraction of the minced lung tissues with acetic acid followed by extraction with the anionic detergent, N-lauroyl sarcosine. Since this method does not require sonication, it yields an apparently intact basement membrane. Reductive alkylation of the isolated basement membrane with ^{3}H-$NaBH_4$ results in the preparation of radiolabeled basement membrane. The tritium label is predominantly in the glycoproteins.

Basement membranes are composed of both collagen and glycoprotein components and the complex of these components results in an insoluble amorphous matrix [86]. Disruption of basement membrane may involve the degradation of either or both of these components. Hence, for tumor cells to invade through basement membrane, they may need both a protease to degrade the glycoproteins and a collagenase to degrade the collagen. Liotta and coworkers have shown recently that tumor cells have a collagenase specific for the type IV collagen of basement membrane and have proposed that this enzyme plays an important role in tumor cell invasion [88]. However, since collagen in basement membrane is complexed with glycoproteins, it is possible that degradation of the glycoprotein component of basement membranes is a critical step in invasion by either directly leading to basement membrane destruction or by exposing in type IV collagen in the glycoprotein matrix and permitting its degradation by collagenase(s).

We have recently demonstrated that tumor cells can degrade the glycoprotein portion of isolated, intact pulmonary basement membrane [89]. Our results further indicate that tumor cell degradation of the basement membrane is mediated by cellular plasminogen activator. The evidence for this is that the ability to degrade basement membrane correlated with the enhanced fibrinolytic activity of the cell lines studied; that the ability of the tumor cells to degrade basement membrane is lost in the absence of plasminogen but is restored if plasminogen is added to plasminogen depleted serum; and that inhibitors of plasmin are inhibitory for degradation of basement membrane. These results indicate a role for the secretion of plasminogen activator in the pathogenesis of invasive tumor cells. Recent studies by Ossowski and Reich [90] and by Wang et al. [91] have indicated a correlation between plasminogen activator and tumor metastasis suggesting that this enzyme is important in at least some steps in the development of metastasis.

Since many proteases and collagenases are synthesized in an inactive zymogen form, proteases may play a role in the activation of these enzymes. Proteases may also play a role in invasion by increasing cellular motility and migration.

2.3. Metastasis formation

As mentioned earlier metastasis is a complex phenomenon requiring several steps. Various roles for proteases in these steps can be expected (Table 1). In addition to the effects discussed earlier, cleavage of membrane proteins by proteases may change the antigenic properties of the cells or influence cell-cell aggregation and cell attachment. Also proteolytic activation of zymogens or gene transcription may facilitate malignant cell behavior. Formation of a fibrin capsule around a micrometastasis may aid in preventing immunological recognition. In this case increased proteolytic activity may be a disadvantage for the tumor, whereas the same cell may have required proteases for cellular invasion prior to the micrometastasis formation. Thus, it can be seen that the generation of tumor heterogeneity is an important aspect of malignant progression and the possible role of protease mediated modulation of gene expression may be important.

It is also possible that proteases are important in angiogenesis. Endothelial cells, which invade and migrate through normal tissue in response to angiogenesis factor, contain high levels of proteases particularly plasminogen activator. However, the role of proteases in this process is unknown.

3. Conclusion

From the above discussions it should be clear that proteases are versatile enzymes that can affect many cellular processes. We are quite convinced that these enzymes are important in tumor cell invasion and metastasis, although their exact roles require further research. It is unlikely, in our view, that proteases are *the* cause of malignant transformation. Rather it is our hypothesis that proteases serve a role in connection with other cellular changes in expressing the malignant phenotype. An intriguing possibility is that proteases increase the rate of genetic or epigenetic change in a cell population. This could be extremely important in facilitating malignant progression or tumor cell heterogeneity.

References

1. Neurath H, Walsh KA: Role of proteolytic enzymes in biological regulation (a review). Proc Natl Acad Sci USA 73:3825–3832, 1976.
2. Foulds L: Neoplastic development, Vol. 1. London: Academic Press, 1969.
3. Barrett JC, Ts'o POP: Evidence for the progressive nature of neoplastic transformation. Proc Natl Acad Sci USA 75:3761–3765, 1978.
4. Fidler IJ: Tumor heterogeneity and the biology of cancer invasion and metastasis. Cancer Res 38:2651–2660, 1978.
5. McLellan WL, Vetterlein D, Roblin R: The glycoprotein nature of human plasminogen activators. FEBS Lett 115:181–184, 1980.
6. Christman JK: Multiple forms of plasminogen activator. In: Biological markers of neoplasia: basic and applied aspects. Ruddon RW (ed). New York: Elsevier, 1978, pp 433–449.
7. Holmberg L, Bladh B, Åstedt B: Purification of urokinase by affinity chromatography. Biochim Biophys Acta 445:215–222, 1976.
8. Åstedt B, Bladh B, Holmberg L: Some characteristics of urokinase released in organ culture of human kidney. Experientia 33:589–591, 1976.
9. Astrup T, Permin PM; Fibrinolysis in the animal organism. Nature 159:681–682, 1947.
10. Astrup T: Tissue activators of plasminogen. Fed Proc 25:42–51, 1966.
11. Rijken DC, Wijngaards G, Welbergen J: Relationship between tissue plasminogen activator and the activators in blood and vascular wall. Thrombos Res 18:815–830, 1980.
12. Granelli-Piperno A, Vassalli JD: Secretion of plasminogen activator by human polymorphonuclear leukocytes. Modulation by glucocorticoids and other effectors. J Exp Med 146:1693–1706, 1977.
13. Aoki N, Von Kaulla KN: Dissimilarity of human vascular plasminogen activator and human urokinase. J Lab Clin Med 78:354–362, 1971.
14. Kucinski CS, Fletcher AP, Sherry S: Effect of urokinase antiserum on plasminogen activators.

Demonstration of immunological dissimilarity between plasma plasminogen activator and urokinase. J Clin Invest 47:1238–1253, 1968.
15. Bernik MB, White WF, Oller EP, Kwaan HC: Immunologic identity of plasminogen activator in human urine, heart and blood vessels and tissue culture. J Lab Clin Med 84:546–558, 1974.
16. Kok P: Separation of plasminogen activators from human plasma and a comparison with activators from human tissues and urine. Thrombos Haemostas 41:734–744, 1979.
17. Kluft C: Levels of plasminogen activators in human plasma, new methods to study the intrinsic and extrinsic activators. In: Progress in chemical fibrinolysis and thrombolysis, Vol. 3, Davidson JW, Rowan RM, Samana MM, Desnoyers PC (eds). New York: Raven Press, 1978, p 141.
18. Åstedt B: Immunological detection of tumor plasminogen activator *in vitro* and *in vivo*. In: Biological markers of neoplasia: basic and applied aspects, Ruddon RW (ed). New York: Elsevier, 1978, pp 481–489.
19. Barnett EV, Baron S: An activator of plasminogen produced by cell culture. Proc Soc Exp Biol Med 102:308–311, 1959.
20. Wu M, Arimura G, Yunis A: Purification and characterization of a plasminogen activator secreted by cultured human pancreatic carcinoma cells. Biochemistry 16:1908–1913, 1977.
21. Granelli-Piperno A, Reich E: A study of proteases and protease inhibitor complexes in biological fluids. J Exp Med 148:223–234, 1978.
22. Christman JK, Silverstein SC, Acs G: Immunological analysis of plasminogen activators from normal and transformed cells. Evidence that the plasminogen activators produced by SV-40 virus-transformed hamster embryo cells and normal hamster lung cells are antigenically identical. J Exp Med 142:419–434, 1975.
23. Quigley JP: Proteolytic enzymes of normal and malignant cells. In: Surfaces of normal and malignant cells, Hynes RO (ed). Sussex, England: Willy, 1979, pp 247–285.
24. Dresden MH, Hellamn SA, Schmidt JD: Collagenolytic enzymes in human neoplasms. Cancer Res 32:993–996, 1972.
25. Robertson DM, Williams DC: *In vitro* evidence of neutral collagenase activity in an invasive mammalian tumor. Nature 221:259–260, 1969.
26. Bosmann HB, Hall TC: Enzymic activity in invasive tumors of human breast and colon. Proc Natl Acad Sci USA 71:1833–1837, 1974.
27. Hashimoto K, Yamanishi Y, Maeyens E, Dabbous MK, Kanzaki T: Collagenolytic activities of squamous cell carcinoma of the skin. Cancer Res 33:2790–2801, 1973.
28. Kazakova OV, Orekkovich VN, Pourchot L, Schuck JM: Effect of cathepsins from normal and malignant tissues on synthetic peptides. J Biol Chem 247:4224–4225, 1972.
29. Fisher A: Bertrog Zur Biologie der Gewebezellen. Eine vergleichend biologische Studie der normalen and malignen Gewebezellen *in vitro*. Arch Entwicklungsmech Org 104:210, 1925.
30. Reich E: Tumor-associated fibrinolysis. Fed Proc 32:2174–2175, 1973.
31. Rifkin DB, Loeb JN, Moore G, Reich E: Properties of plasminogen activators formed by neoplastic human cell cultures. J Exp Med 139:1317–1328, 1974.
32. Ossowski L, Unkeless JC, Tobia A, Quigley JP, Rifkin DB, Reich E: An enzymatic function associated with transformation of fibroblasts by oncogenic viruses II. Mammalian fibroblast cultures transformed by DNA and RNA tumor viruses. L Exp Med 137:112–126, 1973.
33. Unkeless JC, Tobia A, Ossowski L, Quigley JP, Rifkin DB, Reich E: An enzymatic function associated with transformation of fibroblasts by oncogenic viruses. I. Chick embryo fibroblast cultures transformed by avian RNA tumor viruses. J Exp Med 137:85–111, 1973.
34. Ossowski L, Quigley JP, Kellerman GM, Reich E: Fibrinolysis associated with oncogenic transformation. Requirement of plasminogen for correlated changes in cellular morphology, colony formation in agar and cell migration. J Exp Med 138:1056–1064, 1973.
35. Ossowski L, Quigley JP, Reich E: Fibrinolysis associated with oncogenic transformation: morphological correlates. J Biol Chem 249:4312–4320, 1974.
36. Ossowski L, Quigley JP, Reich E: Plasminogen, a necessary factor for cell migration *in vitro*. In:

Proteases and biological control, Reich E, Rifkin DB, Shaw E (eds). Cold Spring Harbor Laboratory, Cold Spring Harbor. New York, 1975, pp 901–913.
37. Weber MJ: Inhibition of protease activity in cultures of Rous sarcoma virus-transformed cells: effect on the transformed phenotype. Cell 5:253–261, 1975.
38. Pollack R, Rifkin DB: Actin-containing cables within anchorage-dependent rat embryo cells are dissociated by plasmin and trypsin. Cell 6:495–506, 1975.
39. Pollack R, Risser R, Conlon S, Rifkin DB: Plasminogen activator production accompanies loss of anchorage regulation in transformation of primary rat embryo cells by simian virus 40. Proc Natl Acad Sci USA 71:4792–4796, 1974.
40. Quigley JP, Ossowski L, Reich E: Plasminogen, the serum proenzyme activated by factors from cells transformed by oncogenic viruses. J Biol Chem 249:4306–4311, 1974.
41. Chen LB, Buchanan JM: Plasminogen-independent fibrinolysis by proteases produced by transformed chick embryo fibroblasts. Proc Natl Acad Sci USA 72:1132–1136, 1975.
42. Reich E: Activation of plasminogen: a widespread mechanism for generating localized extracellular proteolysis. In: Biological markers of neoplasia: basic and applied aspects. Ruddon RW (ed). Elsevier North Holland, 1978, pp 491–500.
43. Ossowski L, Biegel D, Reich E: Mammary plasminogen activator. Correlation with involution, hormonal modulation and comparison between normal and neoplastic tissue. Cell 16:929–940, 1979.
44. Beers WH, Strickland S, Reich E: Ovarian plasminogen activator: relationship to ovulation and hormonal regulation. Cell 6:387–394, 1975.
45. Unkeless JC, Gordon S, Reich E: Secretion of plasminogen activator by stimulated macrophages. J Exp Med 139:834–850, 1974.
46. Rifkin DB, Pollack R: Production of plasminogen activator by established cell lines of mouse origin. J Cell Biol 73:47–55, 1977.
47. Barrett JC: A preneoplastic stage in the spontaneous neoplastic transformation of Syrian hamster embryo cells in culture. Cancer Res 40:91–94, 1980.
48. Barrett JC, Crawford BD, Grady DL, Hester LD, Jones PA, Benedict WF, Ts'o POP: The temporal acquisition of enhanced fibrinolytic activity by Syrian hamster embryo cells following treatment with benzo(a)pyrene. Cancer Res 37:3815–3823, 1977.
49. Barrett JC, Sheela S, Ohki K, Kakunaga T: Reexamination of the role of plasminogen activator production for growth in semisolid agar of neoplastic hamster cells. Cancer Res 40:1438–1442, 1980.
50. Burger MM: Proteolytic enzymes initiating cell division and escape from contract inhibition of growth. Nature 227:170–171, 1970.
51. Holley RW: Factors that control the growth of 3T3 cells and transformed 3T3 cells. In: Proteases and biological control, Reich E, Rifkins DB, Shaw E (eds). Cold Spring Harbor, New York, 1975, pp 779–784.
52. Cunningham DD: Effect of proteases on Con A specific agglutinability and proliferation of density-inhibited fibroblasts. In: Proteases and biological control, Reich E, Rifkin DB, Shaw E (eds). Cold Spring Harbor, New York, 1975, pp 795–806.
53. Noonan KD: Role of serum in proteases-induced stimulation of 3T3 cell division past the monolayer stage. Nature 259:573–576, 1976.
54. Sefton BM, Rubin H: Release from density dependent growth inhibition by proteolytic enzymes. Nature 227:843–845, 1970.
55. Rubin H: Overgrowth stimulating factor released from Rous sarcoma cells. Science 167:1271–1272, 1970.
56. Chen LB, Buchanan JM: Mitogenic activity of blood components. I. Thrombin and prothrombin. Proc Natl Acad Sci USA 72:131–135, 1975.
57. Martin BM, Quigley JP: Binding and uptake of thrombin: possible role in the thrombin-induced mitogenesis of chick embryo fibroblasts. In: Chemistry and biology of thrombin, Lundblad RL, Fenton JW, Mann KG (eds). Michigan, USA: Ann Arbor Science, 1977.

58. Martin BM, Quidley JP: Binding and internalisation of ^{125}I thrombin in chick embryo fibroblasts: possible role in mitogenesis. J Cell Physiol 96:155–164, 1978.
59. Hynes RO: Alteration of cell surface proteins by viral transformation and by proteolysis. Proc Natl Acad Sci USA 11:3170–3174, 1973.
60. Hollenberg MD, Fishman PH, Bennet V, Cuatrecasas P: Cholera toxin and cell growth: role of membrane gangliosides. Proc Natl Acad Sci USA 71:3976–3978, 1974.
61. Hale AH, Weber M: Hydrolase and serum treatment of normal chick embryo cells: effects on hexose transport. Cell 5:245–252, 1975.
62. Sefton BM, Rubin H: Stimulation of glucose transport in cultures of density-inhibited chick embryo cells. Proc Natl Acad Sci USA 68:3154–3157, 1971.
63. Blumberg PM, Robbins RW: Effects of proteases on activation of resting chick embryo fibroblasts and on cell surface proteins. Cell 6:137–147, 1975.
64. Sheppard JR: Difference in the cyclic adenosine 3′,5′-monophosphate levels in normal and transformed cells. Nature (New Biol) 236:14–16, 1972.
65. Willingham MC, Pastan I: Cyclic AMP modulates microvillus formation and agglutinability in transformed and normal mouse fibroblasts. Proc Natl Acad Sci USA 72:1263–1267, 1975.
66. Zetter BR, Chen LB, Buchanan JM: Binding and internalisation of thrombin by normal and transformed chick cells. Proc Natl Acad Sci USA 75:750–753, 1977.
67. Pollack R, Osborn M, Weber K: Patterns of organization of actin and myosin in normal and transformed cultured cells. Proc Natl Acad Sci USA 72:994–998, 1975.
68. Todaro GJ, Delarco JE, Cohen S: Transformation by murine and feline factor to cells. Nature 264:26–31, 1976.
69. Stubblefield E, Brown RL: The role of proteases in the initiation of the DNA synthesis phase of the cell cycle: a cancer theory. In: Growth kinetics and biochemical regulation of normal and malignant cells: a collection of papers presented at the 29th Annual Symposium on Fundamental Cancer Research, Drewinko B, Humphrey RM (eds), 1976.
70. Brown F, Freedman ML, Troll W: Sensitive fluorescent determination of trypsin-like proteases. Biochem Biophys Res Commun 53:75–81, 1973.
71. Moise H, Hosoda J: T_4 gene 32 protein model for control of activity at replication fork. Nature 259:455–458, 1976.
72. Pollack R, Risser R, Conlon S, Freedman V, Shin S, Rifkin DB: Production of plasminogen activator and colonial growth in semi-solid medium are *in vitro* correlates, tumorigenicity in the immune-deficient nude mouse. In: Proteases and biological Control, Reich E, Rifkin DB, Shaw E (eds). Cold Spring Harbor, New York 1975, pp 885–899.
73. Miskin R, Reich E: Plasminogen activator: Induction of synthesis by DNA damage. Cell 19:217–224, 1980.
74. Jones PA, DeClerck YA: Destruction of extracellular matrices containing glycoproteins, elastin and collagen by metastatic human tumor cells. Cancer Res 40:3222–3227, 1980.
75. Strauch L: The role of collagenases in tumor invasion. In: Tissue interactions in carcinogenesis, Tarin D (ed). 1972, pp 399–433.
76. Ashworth CT, Stembridge VA, Luibel FJ: A study of basement membranes of normal epithelium, carcinoma *in situ* and invasive carcinoma of uterine cervix utilizing electron microscopy and histochemical methods. Acta Cytol 5:369–381, 1961.
77. Luibel FJ, Sanders E, Ashworth CT: An electron microscopic study of carcinoma *in situ* and invasive carcinoma of the cervix uteri. Cancer Res 20:357–361, 1960.
78. Rubio CA, Biberfeld P: The basement membrane in experimentally induced atypias and carcinoma of the uterine cervix in mice. Virchows Arch A Path Anat Histol 381:205–209, 1979.
79. Frithiof L: Electron microscopic observation on structures related to the epithelial basement membrane in squamous cell carcinoma. Acta Otolaryng 73:323–334, 1972.
80. Birbeck MSC, Wheatley DN: An electron microscopic study of the invasion of ascites tumor cells into the abdominal wall. Cancer Res 25:490–497, 1965.

81. Poste G, Fidler IJ: The pathogenesis of cancer metastasis. Nature 283:139–146, 1980.
82. Fukushi S, Spiro RG: The lens capsule: sugar and amino acid composition. J Biol Chem 244:2041–2048, 1969.
83. Spiro RG: Studies on the renal glomerular basement membrane: preparation and chemical composition. J Biol Chem 242:1915–1922, 1967.
84. Kefalides NA, Denduchis B: Structural components of epithelial and endothelial basement membranes. Biochemistry 8:4631–4621, 1969.
85. Meezan E, Hjelle JT, Brendel K, Carlson EC: A simple versatile, nondisruptive method for he isolation of morphologically and chemically pure basement membranes from several tissues. Life Sci 17:1721–1732, 1975.
86. Kefalides NA, Winzler RJ: The chemistry of glomerular basement membrane and its relation to collagen. Biochemistry 5:702–713, 1966.
87. Ligler FS, Robinson GB: A method for the isolation of renal basement membranes. Biochim Biophys. Acta 468:327–340, 1977.
88. Liotta LA, Abe S, Robey PG, Martin GR: Preferential digestion of basement membrane collagen by an enzyme derived from a metastatic murine tumor. Proc Natl Acad Sci USA 76:2268–2272, 1979.
89. Sheela S, Barrett JC: Degradation of basement membrane mediated by cellular plasminogen activator. Carcinogenesis, in press, 1982.
90. Ossowski L, Reich E: Loss of malignancy during serial passage of human carcinoma in culture and óscordance between malignancy and transformation parameters. Cancer Res 40:2310–2315, 1980.
91. Wang BS, McLoughlin GA, Richle JP, Mannick JA: Correlation of the production of plasminogen activator with tumor metastasis in B16 mouse melanoma cell lines. Cancer Res 40:288–292, 1980.

22. Proteases in tumor invasion and metastasis

R.H. GOLDFARB

1. Introduction

1.1. Metastasis and invasion

Metastatic cells comprise only a small, particular sub-populatation of highly malignant cells which pre-exist with a primary tumor [1–3]. The metastatic spread of cancer appears to be a selective process which is dependent upon complex interactions between metastatic cells and host properties [1, 4] including, for example, either effective or compromised anti-metastatic immune reactivity. Discrete sequential steps contribute to the mechanism of metastatic tumor growth, and cells with metastatic potential must survive and complete each step in order to successfully establish secondary tumor foci [1].

Following molecular and cellular events that lead to malignant transformation, the tumor cells that comprise a primary neoplasm no longer respond to normal regulatory mechanism that control cellular migration and proliferation. Following progressive growth of the primary tumor, angiogenesis takes place whereby a new blood supply is generated which allows for tumor expansion [5]. Following progressive growth and vascularization of the primary neoplasm, metastatic cells invade surrounding tissue and penetrate through blood and/or lymph node vessels. Subsequent to invasive penetration of vessel walls, metastatic cells detach, are released into the circulation, and a portion of the cells form emboli. The metastatic cells must survive obstacles in the circulation, including the lytic capacity of immune killer cells, and then arrest in small vascular vessels of secondary organs. Following these events, metastatic cells must invasively extravasate through the wall of the arresting vessel, penetrate and infiltrate surrounding tissue, and undergo proliferation. During these events the hosts immune response as well as other host defenses appear to be evaded or overcome. Metastatic cells that survive these steps progressively grow into a secondary tumor mass, and the entire process may then be repeated.

The host-metastatic cell interaction is influenced by a multitude of biophysical, biochemical, cellular, and immunological properties, which have as of now not been completely described in molecular terms. Nevertheless, metastatic cells are highly invasive, and invasiveness appears to play a major role in metastatic tumor growth; the invasive properties of metastatic cells are indeed critical for the degradative

L.A. Liotta and I.R. Hart (eds.), Tumor Invasion and Metastasis. ISBN-13: 978-94-009-7513-2.
© 1982 Martinus Nijhoff Publishers, The Hague/Boston/London.

penetration of mechanical obstacles, such as blood vessel walls and the stroma of organs, which must be overcome during the metastatic process [6].

1.2. Proteolytic enzymes, invasion, and metastasis

It has been suggested that invasive growth of metastatic cells is either a mechanical process or may be a consequence of degradative enzymes [6]. It seems unlikely that non-degradative properties of tumor cells, such as decreased cellular adhesion, are sufficient to account for such invasive behavior [6]. It instead appears that an active mechanism is operative in metastatic invasion and that degradative proteolytic enzymes, generated by highly malignant cells, play a major role in this process. Indeed, microscopic studies have shown local dissolution of normal cellular basement membrane at its point of physical contact with invading tumor cells, suggesting an enzymatic mechanism in metastatic invasion [6].

Proteolytic enzymes have therefore been extensively studied for their invasive abilities and for their potential to degrade cellular, structural components, including the basement membrane. In addition to their ability to modify cellular and extracellular protein components, proteases also have the ability to enhance cellular migration and induce cellular growth. Proteases may therefore function as regulatory molecules that are responsible for several phenotypic characteristics of malignant cells [7]. Proteolytic enzymes may play an important direct role in tumor cell migration, proliferation, and invasion. In addition, proteases may interact with additional molecules involved with proliferation and motility and thereby indirectly enhance tumor cell invasion [8].

This chapter will focus on the role of proteases in tumor invasion and metastasis and review various classes of tumor associated enzymes that have been extensively studied in this regard. In particular, this chapter will concentrate on the role of plasminogen activator and type IV collagenase in tumor invasion and discuss the role of these enzymes in degradation of the basement membrane and specific basement membrane components. In addition, the role of tumor associated proteases in tumor angiogenesis, regulation of tumor cell proliferation, and tumor immunology will be discussed with respect to tumor invasion and metastasis.

2. Historical background

2.1. Fibrinolysis and malignant tumors: early studies

For many years investigators suggested or provided evidence that proteolytic enzymes are associated with malignant tumors and may play an active role in tumor invasion. Fibrinolytic activity of malignant cells was first reported between 1915 and 1935 [9]. A number of investigators subsequently examined the association between fibrinolysis and tumor growth and considered the possible role of proteolytic enzymes in the spread of cancer. Early studies demonstrated that 'proplasmin' was activated into plasmin by a plasminogen activator under physiologic conditions [10], and it was argued that such activation accounted for fibrinolysis in various disease states [11]. It was reported that a number of human malignant tumors displayed spontaneous fibrinolytic activity [12, 13], and it was noted that tumor explants produced neutral proteases including plasminogen activator. Fibrinolytic activity in human breast carcinoma samples, based on tumor cell production of plasminogen activator, was correlated with increased invasive growth and lymph node metastases [14, 15]; tumor cell fibrinolytic activity was considered to have a promoting effect on tumor spread [9, 16]. These early reports, therefore, strongly suggested a role for fibrinolytic activity, mediated in part by plasminogen activator, in tumor spread and invasion. Quantitative approaches in cell culture have more recently confirmed and extended the role of plasminogen activator and plasmin generation in the malignant phenotype and will be discussed in detail below. Before concluding this section it should be pointed out that this early interest in fibrinolytic activity and pathological conditions led to a quantitative assay for both proteolytic activity [17] and inhibitors of proteases [18] that utilized iodinated fibrin as a substrate.

3. Peptidases and proteases of tumors and their interstitial spaces.

A role for proteases in the spread of cancer was also suggested by studies with peptidases and proteinases associated with tumor interstitial fluids. It was reported that various catheptic enzymes and polypeptidases showed increased activity in interstitial tumor fluids and, within tumor cells, relative to normal intraperitoneal fluids [19]. It was argued that these fluids have the potential to mediate the enzymatic attack of various substrates at both neutral and alkaline pH [20]. Collagenases and proteinases active at physiologic pH were not observed, and it was concluded that such activities were either lacking, or effectively inhibited. In subsequent studies it was reported that cathepsin B is a protease which plays a role in the destructive capacity of malignant tumors and is, to some extent, responsible for cellular detachment, invasiveness, and formation of metastasis [21]. More contemporary work [22, 23] has demonstrated that cathepsin B secretion was higher for malignant than non-malignant tissue, thereby suggesting that the secretion and extracellular action of cathepsin B, or a thiol proteinase which resembles cathepsin B, might play a role in tumor infiltration and metastasis. Recently, it was reported that cathepsin B is significantly enhanced in a B 16 melanoma variant of high metastatic potential and is localized to the lysozomes of the tumor cells [24]. It is of interest that cathepsin D levels have also been found to be elevated in tumor interstitial fluids [25].

Glycosyl transferases, glycosidases, and proteases were also shown to be elevated relative to normal tissue [26] and suggested a role for enhanced enzymatic activity in both tumor invasiveness and maintenance of the neoplastic state. A number of other groups have also studied various other proteases in relationship to malignancy, and the reader is referred to a recent review [27] for descriptions which are beyond the scope of the present chapter.

4. Correlation of malignant transformation with protease activity

4.1. Cell culture studies

The advent of quantitative cell culture systems allows for a critical, well-controlled evaluation of the role of proteases in malignant transformation. Normal, non-transformed cell cultures, upon exposure to proteolytic enzymes, display phenotypic characteristics of malignantly transformed cells. It was found that protease treatment of normal cultures: converted them to a lectin agglutinable form; caused initiation of cellular division; released cells from density dependent inhibition of growth; caused microvilli typical of the morphology of transformed cells; led to the loss of specific cell-surface proteins; decreased levels of cellular cyclic AMP; and enhanced glucose transport [reviewed in 27].

If limited proteolysis plays a role in the establishment or promotion of the malignant phenotype, then it is expected that the selective inhibition of proteolytic activity should cause malignantly transformed cells to express a more normal phenotype [27]. Various protease inhibitors with diverse mechanisms of enzyme inhibition have been shown to modulate the characteristics of transformed cultures to approximate the restoration of a normal, non-malignant phenotype. Malignantly transformed cultures treated with inhibitors of proteolytic enzymes display: reduced saturation and growth rate; normal flattened morphology; decreased agglutinability of lectins; decreassed glucose transport rate; and enhanced cell adherence to culture dishes [reviewed in 27].

It has been demonstrated that protease inhibitors interfere with chemical transformation in C3H/10T$\frac{1}{2}$ cells [28]. In addition, protease inhibitors can suppress radiation transformation *in vitro* [29].

In summary, these studies suggested, in an indirect manner, that proteases have dramatic effects on cellular behavior relative to malignant transformation.

4.2. Enhanced protease production by transformed cells in culture

It was reported that elevated glycosidase levels followed malignant transformation by DNA tumor viruses [30], and it was demonstrated that both trypsin-like and cathepsin-like activities were also elevated in culture following viral transformation by oncogenic viruses.

Tumor cells, removed from tumor isolates of recent origin and grown in culture, were reported to differ from parental, uncloned cells by showing enhanced migration, and increased metastatic potential *in vivo* [31]; it is of interest that increased chymotrypsin-like esterase activity, glycosidase, and B-glucuronidase activity was observed. In separate sections below, the enhanced production of plasminogen activator and type IV collagenase from cultures of malignant cells shall be described in detail.

5. Effect of protease inhibitors on tumor-bearing animals

It has been reported that protease inhibitors suppress tumor formation when added in conjunction with a tumor promoter during the two-stage carcinogenesis test [32, 33]. Phorbol-12-myristate-13-acetate (PMA) is the active component of croton oil and is the most potent and best studied promoter of tumor formation in the two-stage carcinogenesis test system [34]. In this test system sub-optimal doses of specific carcinogens initiate latent changes in target cells of animals which progress to malignant tumors only following subsequent treatment with tumor promoting agents such as PMA.

Protease inhibitors have also reported to inhibit metastasis formation [35, 36], possibly by inhibition of thrombus formation following the arrest of circulating tumor cells [36]. It should be kept in mind, however, that not all reports support a dramatic role for protease inhibitors in suppression of oncogenesis or metastasis. For example, it has been shown that at least one protease inhibitor significantly suppresses liver tumors in males but not females following administration of the inhibitor in the diet [37]. In addition, at least one report suggested that a particular protease inhibitor can enhance rather than inhibit the growth of metastatic tumors in mice [38]. Nevertheless, the overall data appears to suggest that protease inhibitors can suppress or block tumorigenesis and/or metastasis and therefore suggests that the study of proteases and metastasis is worthwhile.

6. Plasminogen activator (PA), malignant transformation, and oncogenesis.

As discussed above enhanced protease activity has been documented in a variety of cells that are malignantly transformed. However, the majority of the enhanced protease activities were never defined with respect to their substrate specificity and enzymatic function. The well characterized plasminogen activator system and its correlation with the malignant phenotype is discussed below.

6.1. *Increased PA levels in transformed cells*

The production of a specific protease, plasminogen activator (PA) is substantially increased in cultures of cells that are malignantly transformed by either tumor viruses or chemical carcinogens [39, 40, 41]. Fibrinolytic activity associated with malignant transformation depends on the interaction of PA, an enzyme produced by transformed cells and plasminogen, a normal serum zymogen [42, 43, 44].

PA activity is found in low levels in normal, non-transformed chick embryo fibroblasts (CEF) and is not enhanced following infection with non-transforming avian leukosis viruses or a variety of cytocidal RNA or DNA viruses which do not cause malignant transformation [39]. However, PA levels are elevated 10- to 100-fold in primary cultures of cells malignantly transformed with RNA or DNA tumor viruses, primary tumor cell cultures, cells malignantly transformed by chemical carcinogens, in chemically induced tumors, and in tumor cells lines including human cell lines [27, 41].

Studies with Rous sarcoma virus (RSV), temperature sensitive for the expression of malignant transformation, have shown that PA is expressed at the temperature permissive for transformation but not at the restrictive temperature [39, 45].

6.2. *Correlation of PA with malignant transformation*

Studies with CEF infected with the mutant of RSV temperature sensitive for malignant transformation have demonstrated that enhanced PA activity is detectable before morphological sings of transformation are evident [39]. It therefore appears that PA production is an early event in malignant transformation and may play a causal role in modulating the morphological phenotype of malignant cells.

The rapid generation of plasmin through proteolytic activation of plasminogen by PA also yields proteolytic activity within the microenvironment of the malignant cell. Plasmin is a regulatory protease with the ability to alter cell surface proteins, modify cytoskeletal components, and induce cellular division [27].

PA production and plasmin generation as a consequence of zymogen activation have been correlated with a number of phenotypic traits of malignant cells including: growth in agar; tumorigenicity of viral transformants in nude mice; tumorigenicity of murine malignant melanoma cells; and the previously mentioned temperature sensitive expression of the RSV sarcomagenesis gene product [7, 27]. Furthermore, transformed cell morphology, adhesion, and migration are dependent, to a substantial extent, upon plasminogen or plasminogen activation to plasmin [27]. Several of these correlates shall be described in greater detail below.

PA production and plasminogen activation have been correlated with the disappearance of intracellular actin cables that is a correlate of anchorage independent growth and malignant potential [46]. A direct relationship between the production of PA, growth in agar, and the ability to give rise to tumors in nude mice has been reported for independently isolated clones of simian virus 40 (SV40) transformed rat embryo cells [47]. Therefore, the production of PA and the conversion of plasminogen to plasmin are well correlated with a characteristic of malignant cells, growth in agar, and with tumorigenic potential of transformed cells in nude mice.

Bromodeoxyuridine (BrdU) inhibits, in a reversible fashion, both the tumorigenicity and the PA activity of murine B559 melanoma cells [48]. Both the tumorigenic potential and PA activity of B559 cells are coordinately restored following the removal of BrdU from cell cultures.

A further correlation between tumorigenesis and PA production concerns a hormone dependent mouse tumor [49]. It has been shown that both tumor growth and PA production are under coordinate androgen dependence in the Shionogi SC-115 mammary carcinoma cell system [49]. Dihydrotestosterone, at physiological concentrations, can induce PA production from these cells whereas no enzymatic activity is detectable in the androgen-dependent cells cultured in the absence of the hormone.

An additional correlation between PA production and malignant transformation has been shown through the use of PMA. In studies linking proteases with tumorigenesis it has been shown that PMA treatment of the mouse ear induces a trypsin-like protease which is capable of activating human plasminogen [50]. It has also been demonstrated that PMA can induce PA levels by 10 fold in HeLa cells and in normal CEF [51]. PMA treatment of CEF that are already malignantly transformed by RSV synergistically causes a super expression of PA production and markedly increases the already enhanced levels of PA that is a consequence of RSV transformation alone [52].

The time course of PA induction in RSVCEF treated with the tumor promoter demonstrates that PMA increases extracellular levels of PA 3 to 4 h after PMA addition and increases cell associated levels as early as 1 h after treatment [52]. The PA induced by PMA is identical in molecular weight to the PA produced by untreated RSVCEF and, therefore, probably represents the same gene product [52]. PMA is capable of causing a rapid enhancement of PA activity, in both the cell associated and extracellular micro-milieu, of tumor promoter-treated cells [52].

The synergistic enhancement of PA in PMA treated RSVCEF, which is dependent upon protein synthesis, is accompanied by distinct cellular and colonial morphological alterations [52]. The clustered, colonial, super-transformed morphology of RSVCEF following long-term culture suggests that PMA selects for the outgrowth of highly malignant cells that secrete high levels of PA [52].

Recently, it has been observed that PMA also induces PA levels in highly metastatic murine B16 F10 cultures and BL 6 invasive variants of B16 F1 cells (R.H. Goldfarb and N.L. Opel, unpublished observations). The level of PMA induced PA in metastatic cells appears to be additive rather than synergistic. This data suggests that such metastatic cells, which already produce high levels of PA, can undergo only a modest boost to an apparent ceiling of enhanced activity. It is of interest that clustered super-transformed morphology is observed in such metastatic cell cultures even prior to PMA treatment.

6.3. *Role of PA in malignant transformation*

6.3.1. Direct Role of PA. The morphological alterations that accompany PMA treatment of RSV transformed cultures can be prevented by specific protease inhibitors [53, 54]. Various protease inhibitors, including diisopropylfluorophosphate (DFP), leupeptin, antipain, and nitrosophenylguanidobenzoate (NPGB) prevent the formation of cell clusters and colonial aggregates that characterize the super-transformed phenotype [53, 55]. On the other hand, plasmin inhibitors, including trasylol, epsilon amino caproic acid (EACA), and soybean trypsin inhibitor (SBTI) are incapable of inhibiting PMA induced colonial morhology [53, 56]. The former compounds, which interfere with PMA-mediated morphological changes, were shown to be inhibitors of PA by a direct fluorometric assay of the enzyme [53, 57]. The assay employed a synthetic fluorogenic peptide substrate, Cbz-gly-gly-arg-amino-4-methyl coumarin [57]. This substrate allows for direct determination of PA independently of the interfering potential of plasmin. Experimental observations demonstrate that a DFP sensitive protease with arginine specificity is involved in PMA-mediated morphological alterations [53], and it appears that PA itself, and not plasmin, mediates these changes. These results suggest that PA can catalytically act on an unidentified cellular substrate, that is not plasminogen, and modify cell behavior [53, 56]. Since PA is correlated with invasive aspects of tissue remodeling, it is possible that the protease may play an important role by directly acting on a cellular substrate such as a basement membrane component. The effect of PA on basement membrane components is described below.

6.3.2. Effect of PA on basement membrane degradation. During tumor invasion local and rapid dissolution of the basement membrane takes place [6], and penetration of the basement membrane by invasive tumor cells is necessary for metastasis. Enzymes produced by invasive tumor cells must have the ability to degrade both collagenous and non-collagenous components of the basement membrane [58, 59]. (Reviewed elsewhere in this volume.) PA may indirectly aid in the destruction of basement membrane. Plasmin generated through PA can activate latent collagenase and can also degrade glycoprotein components of basement membrane such as laminin and fibronectin.

6.3.3. Role of PA in induction of cellular proliferation. As discussed above the generation of plasmin through plasminogen activation enhances the protease content of the tumor cell microenvironment. Plasmin displays regulatory potential and can play a role in the induction of cellular proliferation [27]. The capacity to stimulate cellular growth is an important mechanism whereby proteolytic enzymes contribute to alterations over growth control and is a feature of many proteases such as alpha thrombin [55, 60]. It has been of general interest to determine whether PA has mitogenic potential.

It has been reported that PA mediated conversion of plasminogen, but not PA exogenously added to cultures, can initiate growth of quiescent cells [61]. In this study only low levels of impure PA were employed. Subsequently, it was reported that PA initiates DNA synthesis by enhancing serum mediated stimulation of resting cells [62].

A recent report has noted that PA-enriched culture fluids, derived from PMA-treated RSV transformed cultures, or purified urokinase, can function as mitogens for normal, avian and murine lymphocytes [63]. It is of interest that in this system plasmin was found to lack mitogenic activity for lymphocytes.

Several years ago it was observed that homogeneously purified PA, derived from PMA-treated RSVCEF cultures [7], is a potent mitogen for resting CEF when examined under well described conditions established for the assay of alpha thrombin mediated mitogenesis in CEF [60] (R.H. Goldfarb, B.M. Martin, and J.P. Quigley unpublished observations). More recently, it has been noted that pure human PA, urokinase, can function as a mitogen for resting CEF as well as for human lymphocyte sub-populations (R.H. Goldfarb, B.M. Martin, and G. Murano, unpublished observations). It therefore appears that PAs of various types can function in the induction of DNA synthesis and cellular proliferation, which may contribute to the malignant phenotype.

6.3.4. Role of PA in tumor angiogenesis. Tumor angiogenesis factors (TAF) have been implicated in the vascularization of malignant tumors [5, 64]. Tumor induced neovascularization appears to be a prerequisite for the metastatic spread of cancer since dormant tumors can grow only after new capillaries have been formed and have infiltrated into the tumor. TAF, which is released by solid tumors and transformed cells in culture, stimulates endothelial cells to proliferate towards the initiating tumor, which thereby continues to vascularize. A relationship may exist between tumor angiogenesis and tumor associated proteolysis. A factor, partially purified by trypsin sepharose affinity chromatography, inhibits tumor induced neovascularization and thereby inhibits tumor growth [64]. Therefore, TAF might cause vascularization by the induction of a tryptic protease with the capacity to induce the proliferation of endothelial cells. In this regard it is of interest that both plasmin and PA can function as mitogens and that endothelial cells can produce PA [65].

It has recently been observed that the anti-angiogenesis factor derived from cartilage and purified on trypsin-sepharose [64] has the capacity to inhibit the enzymatic activity of both pure and crude PAs (R.H. Goldfarb, and R. Langer, unpublished observations). It has also been observed that homogeneously pure human PA, urokinase, can cause angiogenesis in the rabbit cornea (R.H. Goldfarb, M. Ziche G. Murano, and L.A. Liotta, manuscript submitted for publication). When the pure PA was inhibited with DFP, the active site-blocked, inactive enzyme no longer caused angiogenesis. This data therefore demonstrates that the active site of PA is required for the induction of angiogenesis. It has recently been independently observed (M. Berman, personal communication) that human PA, urokinase, is angiogenic in the rabbit cornea [66].

It therefore appears that PA may be capable of mediating neovascularization during tumor invasion and function as a TAF which can markedly influence the course of tumor promotion and metastasis.

6.3.5. Role of PA in metastasis. Some very clear observations linked enhanced fibrinolytic activity with the metastatic spread of cancer [12, 14, 15]. More recent studies have quantitatively examined the role of PA in metastasis. Various reports have compared the PA production of B16 melanoma F1 cells relative to the more metastatic B16 F10 variant. It was reported [67] that high and approximately equivalent levels of PA are produced by both B16 F1, B16 F5, B16 F10, and B16 F13 cells. In contrast, it has been reported, more recently, that B16 F10 cells produce more fibrinolytic activity than B16 F1 cells due to differences in their PA production [68]. It has therefore been suggested [68] that a quantitative difference takes place in PA production in these two melanoma variants and may play a role in their differential potential for forming metastases. With regard to the production of PA in melanoma variants, it is of interest, as discussed above, that PMA can boost the already high PA levels found in B16 F10 cells.

The presence of human PA in chick embryos and newborn chicks has been used as a marker of metastasis of human epidermoid carcinoma (HEP-3) cells [69]. The tumor produces large amounts of human PA which can be distinguished from chick PA since each PA preferentially cleaves its homologous plasminogen [69].

Studies concerned with PA content of human colon tumors and normal mucosae [70] have demonstrated that tumor samples produced high PA levels relative to normal control samples. In addition, it was reported that a correlation exists between ratios of tumor/normal PA levels and invasiveness and metastases [70]. The demonstration of higher PA levels in tumors with a phenotype of invasiveness and metastasis supports the hypothesis that PA may play an important role in metastatic disease.

The direct effect of PA on metastatic tumor spread has been examined. Following long-term administration of urokinase to V2 carcinoma-bearing rabbits, the weight of tumors and the incidence of lymph node metastases was reported to be enhanced [71]. In addition, long-term urokinase treatment appears to promote the invasive nature of the V2 carcinoma [71]. However, it was also noted that the effect of PA, urokinase, on tumor spread varied as a function of the specific phase of metastasis formation. It appears that urokinase can promote invasiveness and tumor release into the vessels but may also interfere with lodgement of tumor cells in secondary, distant organ sites [71].

In summary, at least some reports in the literature suggest that a quantitative relationship exists between PA production and metastatic potential. Furthermore, many reports demonstrate that metastatic cells produce high levels of PA, and as of now, it is not known whether there is a minimum amount or maximum quantity of PA that is required for contribution to the metastatic process. Nevertheless, it appears that PA production may be a correlate of metastasis and play an active role in the invasive processes that contribute to metastasis.

7. Lack of correlation of PA and the malignant phenotype

It should be pointed out that cells other than malignant cells produce PA [27]. For many normal cells that produce and secrete PA, it appears that enzyme synthesis is a function of developmental, physiologic, temporal, or hormonal control [27]. The modulation of PA can be regulated by a number of molecules including hormones, products of lymphoid cells, and cyclic nucleotides. In such normal cells a relationship exists between cellular remodeling and PA production [41, 72]. For example, it has been reported that PA is responsible for extensive degradation of the graafian follicle at ovulation [73]. Another example of physiologic control over enzyme production is noted in trophoblast cells; transient production of PA by trophoblast cells shows an excellent temporal correlation with the invasiveness of these cells during embryonic implantation [74].

Increased levels of PA have been observed in normal cell cultures including kidney cells, lung cells, and activated macrophages [27, 41]. It is of interest that the normal cell types that display PA activity are often cells that display invasive properties associated with tissue remodeling and cell migration. PA production and plasminogen activation to plasmin might therefore confor a selective advantage upon the maintenance and promotion of the malignant state by contributing to tissue remodeling, migration, invasiveness, and metastasis.

With respect to malignant cells some exceptions have been noted in which a correlation between PA production and malignant transformation is not observed [27, 72]. In many cases, however, criticisms have been pointed out for reports that claimed a lack of correlation between PA production and the transformed phenotype [27, 72] including: lack of accurate quantitation; the study of cell populations with variable karyotypes; failure to investigate both cell associated and extracellular PA levels; failure to examine for simultaneous production of protease inhibitors; and the use of culture media with inappropriate hormone levels.

In summary, although some exceptions have been observed [27], by and large, an excellent correlation exists between the production of PA and the expression of the malignant phenotype.

8. PAs from cultured human cells: significance of multiple forms

It has become quite clear that PAs purified from malignant cells in culture from many species exist in multiple molecular weight forms and that not all of the forms are immunologically related.

It has been reported that cell cultures prepared from human brain tumors produce PA which is immunologically distinct from urokinase [76]. In contrast, anti-urokinase IgG inhibited PA derived from cultured human prostatic cells, ovarian carcinoma cells, WI38 cells, and SV40 transformed WI38 cells [76]. Additional reports have demonstrated that anti-urokinase IgG can inhibit human PAs from cultures of most normal adult tissues, from a 26-week-old embryo, and from tumors of ectodermal or mesenchymal origin [75]; in contrast, melanoma derived PA and melanoma-like PAs derived from breast carcinoma, glioblastoma, malignant teratoma, uterine sarcoma, and renal pelvis carcinoma, as well as some normal tissues, was not inhibitable by anti-urokinase IgG [75]. Other reports have demonstrated that antiurokinase-antisera inhibits PA of four lines of gastric tumor cells, two lines of lung cancer cells, one line of urinary bladder cancer, and one line of renal cancer, but failed to inhibit PA from one line of human lung cancer [77]. It has independently been concluded that human lung tumors contain PA immunologically identical to urokinase as the predominant PA [78] while the PA content of adjacent normal tissue is comprised of both urokinase like PA and mostly a PA that is anti-urokinase IgG resistant. It has also been reported that human colon tumors produce urokinase like PA, whereas normal colon biopsies contained both urokinase-like and non-urokinase-like PAs [70].

As of this time it is not clear as to whether immunologically and structurally distinct multiple PA gene products are produced by the same or different malignant cells or whether all forms of PA are involved in a product-precursor relationship, with large molecules serving as precursors to smaller molecular weight degradation products.

With the advent of the pure PAs described above and their antisera, it should be possible to investigate points raised above. It is hopeful that peptide mapping and amino acid analyses on each molecular form of pure PA will elucidate whether molecules are indeed structurally related. Furthermore, pure PAs and their antisera can be employed to examine the mechanism of export and processing of PA and to define the exact role of the enzyme in the initiation and promotion of malignancy, as well as tumor invasion and metastasis.

9. Type IV collagenase, the malignant phenotype, and malignancy

In recent years it has become increasingly clear that collagenases are another important class of proteases that contribute to invasion and metastasis. The reader is directed to a more extensive review of the subject (L.A. Liotta et al., Chapter 19, this volume).

10. Conclusions

It is clear from the work discussed in this chapter proteolytic enzymes are important regulatory molecules that modulate numerous parameters of tumor initiation, promotion, invasion, and metastasis. Proteases derived from tumor cells appear to have multiple effects: invasive degradation of basement membrane components; tumor angiogenesis; tumor cell proliferation; tumor cell migration; modulation of cell surface and cytoskeletal architecture; interaction with the immune response; and gene regulation. It is intriguing to speculate that tumor associated proteases may coordinately regulate the expression of these diverse processes through limited proteolysis and thereby function as pleiotropic modulators of the malignant state. It is quite likely that several of these regulatory proteases will work in sequential, cascade-like fashion, to achieve maximal effects through limited proteolysis.

It is hopeful that experiments with pure proteases and specific antisera will yield unambiguous correlations between these specific molecular and physiological function in order to better define the relationship between tumor associated proteases, tumor invasion, and metastasis.

References

1. Fidler IJ: Tumor heterogeneity and the biology of cancer invasion and metastasis. Cancer Res 38:2651–2660, 1978.
2. Fidler IJ, Hart IR: The origin of metastatic heterogeneity in tumors. Eur J Cancer 17:487–494, 1981.
3. Fidler IJ, Kripke ML: Metastatic heterogeneity of cells from the K-1735 melanoma. In: Metastatic tumor growth, Grundman E (ed). Stuttgart: Gustav Fischer Verlag, 1980, pp 71–81.
4. Fidler IJ, Gersten DM, Hart IR: The biology of cancer invasion and metastasis. Adv Cancer Res 28:149–250, 1978.
5. Folkman J: Tumor angiogenesis. Adv Cancer Res 19:331–358, 1974.
6. Liotta LA, Tryggvason K, Garbisa S, Rose PG, Murray JC: Interaction of metastatic tumor cells with basement membrane collagen. In: Metastatic tumor growth, Grundman E (ed). Stuttgart: Gustav Fischer Verlag, 1980, pp 21–30.
7. Goldfarb RH, Quigley JP: Purification of plasminogen activator from Rous sarcoma virus transformed chick embryo fibroblasts treated with the tumor promoter phorbol-12-myristate-13-acetate. Biochemistry 19:5463–5471, 1980.
8. Sträuli P: A concept of tumor invasion. In: Proteinases and tumor invasion, Sträuli P, Barrett AJ, Baici A (eds). New York: Raven Press, 1980, pp 1–15.
9. Peterson HI: Fibrinolysis and antifibrinolytic drugs in the growth and spread of tumors. Cancer Treat Rev 4:213–217, 1977.
10. Astrup T, Permin PM: Fibrinolysis in animal organism. Nature 159:681–683, 1947.
11. Tagon HJ, Palade GE: Activation of plasmin by a factor from mammalian tissue. J Clin Invest 29:317–324, 1950.
12. Tagnon HJ, Whitmore WF, Shulman NR: Fibrinolysis in metastatic cancer of the prostate. Cancer 5:9–12, 1952.
13. Clifton EE, Grossi CE: Fibrinolytic activity of human tumors as measured by the fibrin plate method. Cancer 8:1146–1154, 1955.
14. Peterson HL: Experimental studies on fibrinolysis in growth and spread of tumor. Acta Chir Scand 134 (suppl 394): 1968.
15. Peterson HL, Kjartansson I, Korsan-Bengsten K, Ruddenstam CM, Zettergrem L: Fibrinolysis in human malignant tumors. Acta Chir Scand 139:219–226, 1973.
16. Peterson HI, Larsson S, Zettergren L: Fibrinolysis in human bronchogenic carcinoma. Eur J Cancer 11:277–279, 1975.

17. Shulman NR, Tagnon HJ: Proteolytic activity determined with a substrate tagged with radioactive iodine. J Biol Chem 186:69–75, 1950.
18. Shulman NR: Studies on the inhibition of proteolytic enzymes by serum. I. The mechanism of the inhibition of trypsin, plasmin, and chymotrypsin by serum using fibrin tagged with I^{131} as a substrate. J Exp Med 95:571–591, 1952.
19. Sylvén B: The host tumor interzone and tumor invasion. In: Biological interactions in normal and neoplastic growth, Brennan MJ, Simpsom WL (eds). Boston: Little, Brown, 1962, pp 635–655.
20. Sylvén B: Some factors relating to invasiveness and destructiveness of solid malignant tumors. In: Mechanisms of invasion in cancer, Denoix P (ed). Berlin: Springer Verlag 1967, pp 47–60.
21. Sylvén B: Biochemical and enzymatic factors involved in cellular detatchment. In: Chemotherapy of cancer dissemination and metastasis, Gerattini S, Franchi G (eds). New York: Raven Press, 1973, pp 129–138.
22. Poole AR, Tiltman KJ, Recklies AD, Stoker TAM: Differences in secretion of the proteinase cathepsin B at the edges of human breast carcinoma and fibroadenomas. Nature 273:545–547, 1978.
23. Poole AR, Recklies AD, Mort JS: Secretion of proteinases from human breast tumors: excessive release from carcinomas of a thiol proteinase. In: Proteinases in tumor invasion, Straüli P (ed). New York: Raven Press, 1980, pp 81–93.
24. Sloane BF, Dunn JR, Honn KV: Lysosomal cathepsin B: correlation with metastatic potential. Science 212:1151–1153, 1981.
25. Sylvén B, Bois-Svennson I: On the chemical pathology of interstitial fluid. I. Proteolytic activties in transplanted mouse tumors. Cancer Res 25:458–468, 1965.
26. Bosmann HB: Elevated glycosidases and proteolytic enzymes in cells transformed by RNA tumor virus. Biochim Biophys Acta 264:339–343, 1972.
27. Quigley JP: Proteolytic enzymes of normal and malignant cells. In: Surfaces of normal and malignant cells, Hynes RO (ed). Chichester: John Wiley, 1979, 247–285.
28. Kuroki R, Drevon C: Inhibition of chemical transformation in C3H/10T½ cells by protease inhibitors. Cancer Res 39:2755–2761, 1979.
29. Kennedy AR, Little JB: Effects of protease inhibitors on radiation transformation *in vitro*. Cancer Res 41:2103–2108, 1981.
30. Bosmann HB, Hall TC: Enzyme activity in invasive tumors of human breast and colon. Proc Natl Acad Sci USA 71:1833–1837, 1974.
31. Varani J, Orr W, Ward P: Hydrolytic enzyme activities, migratory activity, and *in vivo* growth and metastatic potential of recent tumor isolates. Cancer Res 39:2376–2380, 1979.
32. Troll W, Klassen A, Janoff A: Tumorigenesis in mouse skin: inhibition by synthetic inhibitors of proteases. Science 169:1211–1213, 1970.
33. Hozumi M, Ogawa M, Sugimura T, Takeuchi T, Umezawa H: Inhibition of tumorigenesis in mouse skin by leupeptin, a protease inhibitor from Actinomycetes. Cancer Res 32:1725–1729, 1972.
34. Van Duuren BL: Tumor promoting agents in two-stage carcinogenesis. Prog Exp Tumor Res 11:31–68, 1969.
35. Saito D, Sawamura M, Umezawa H, Kanai Y, Furihata C, Matshshima T, Sugimura T: Inhibition of experimental blood-borne lung metastases by protease inhibitors. Cancer Res 40:2539–2542, 1980.
36. Giraldi T, Sava G, Kopitar M, Brzin J, Turk V: Neutral proteinase inhibitors and antimetastatic effects in mice. Eur J Cancer 16:449–454, 1980.
37. Hosaka S, Hirono I: Effect of leupeptin, a protease inhibitor, on the development of spontaneous tumors in strain A mice. Gann 71:913–917, 1980.
38. Turner GA, Weiss L: Analysis of aprotinin-induced enhancement of metastasis of Lewis lung tumors in mice. Cancer Res 41:2576–2580, 1981.
39. Unkeless JC, Tobia A, Ossowski L, Quigley JP, Rifkin DB, Reich E: An enzymatic function associated with transformation of fibroblasts by oncogenic viruses. I. Chick embryo fibroblast cultures transformed by avian RNA tumor viruses. J Exp Med 137:85–111, 1973.

40. Ossowski L, Unkeless JC, Tobia A, Quigley JP, Rifkin DB, Reich E: An enzymatic function associated with transformation of fibroblasts by oncogenic viruses. II. Mammalian fibroblast cultures transformed by DNA and RNA tumors viruses. J Exp Med 137:112–126, 1973.
41. Reich E: Activation of plasminogen: a widespread mechanism for generating localized extracellular proteolysis. In: Biological markers of neoplasia: basic and applied aspects, Ruddon RW (ed). New York: Elsevier North Holland, pp 491–500.
42. Unkeless JC, Danø K, Kellerman GM, Reich E: Fibrinolysis associated with oncogenic transformation. Partial purification and characterization of the cell factor, a plasminogen activator. J Biol Chem 249:4295–4305, 1974.
43. Quigley JP, Ossowski L, Reich E: Plasminogen, the serum proenzyme activated by factors from cells transformed by oncogenic viruses. J Biol Chem 249:4306–4311, 1974.
44. Goldberg AR: Increased protease levels in transformed cells: a casein overlay for the detection of plasminogen activator production. Cell 2:95–102, 1974.
45. Rifkin DB, Beal LP, Reich E: Macromolecular determinants of plasminogen activator synthesis. Cold Spring Harbor Conf Cell Prolif 2:841–847, 1975.
46. Pollack R, Rifkin DB: Actin-containing cables within anchorage dependent rat embryo cells are dissociated by plasmin and trypsin. Cell 6:495–506, 1975.
47. Pollack R, Risser R, Conlon S, Freedman V, Shin S, Rifkin DB: Production of plasminogen activator and colonial growth in semisolid medium are *in vitro* correlates of tumorigenicity in the immune-deficient nude mouse. Cold Spring Harbor Conf Cell Prolif 2:885–899, 1975.
48. Christman JK, Silagi S, Newcomb EW, Acs G, Silverstein S: Correlated suppression by 5-bromodeoxyuridine of tumorigenicity and plasminogen activator in mouse melanoma cells. Proc Natl Acad Sci USA 72:47–50, 1975.
49. Mak T, Rutledge G, Sutherland D: Androgen-dependent fibrinolytic activity in a murine mammary carcinoma (Shionogi SC-115) cells *in vitro*. Cell 7:233–226, 1976.
50. Troll W, Rossman T, Katz J, Levitz M, Sugimura T: Proteinases in tumor promotion and hormone action. Cold Spring Harbor Conf Cell Prolif 2:977–987, 1975.
51. Wigler M, Weinstein IB: Tumor promoter induces plasminogen activator. Nature 259:232–233, 1976.
52. Goldfarb RH, Quigley JP: Synergistic effect of tumor virus transformation and tumor promoter treatment on the production of plasminogen activator by chick embryo fibroblasts. Cancer Res 38:4601–4609, 1978.
53. Quigley JP, Goldfarb RH: Morphological changes induced by endogenous protease activity in cultures of phorbol ester treated RSV-transformed chick fibroblasts: evidence for direct proteolytic activity of plasminogen activator. J Cell Biol 79:73a, 1978.
54. Quigley JP: Phorbol ester-induced morphological changes in transformed chick fibroblasts: evidence for direct catalytic involvement of plasminogen activator. Cell 17:131–141, 1979.
55. Quigley JP, Martin BM, Goldfarb RH, Scheiner CJ, Muller WD: Involvement of serine proteases in growth control and malignant transformation. Cold Spring Harbor Conf Cell Prolif 6:219–238, 1979.
56. Quigley JP, Goldfarb RH, Scheiner CJ, O'Donnel-Tormey J, Yeo TK: Plasminogen activator and the membrane of transformed cells. Prog Clin Biol Res 41:773–796, 1980.
57. Zimmerman M, Quigley JP, Ashe B, Dorn C, Goldfarb RH, Troll W: Direct fluorescent assay of urokinase and plasminogen activators of normal and malignant cells: kinetics and inhibitor profiles. Proc Natl Acad Sci USA 75:750–753, 1978.
58. Goldfarb RH, Liotta LA, Garbisa S, Terranova VP: Degradation of basement membrane components: effects of plasminogen activator, plasmin, and alpha thrombin. Proc Am Assoc Cancer Res 22:59, 1981.
59. Liotta LA, Goldfarb RH, Brundage RG, Siegal GP, Terranova VP, Garbisa S: Effect of plasminogen activator (urokinase), plasmin, and thrombin on glycoprotein and collagenous components of the basement membrane. Cancer Res 41:4629–4636, 1981.

60. Martin BM, Quigley JP: Binding and internalization of ^{125}I thrombin in chick embryo fibrolasts: possible role in mitogenesis. J Cell Physiol 96:155–164, 1978.
61. Whur P, Silcox JJ, Boston JA, Williams DC: Plasminogen activator transforms the morphology of quiescent 3T3 cell monolayers and initiates growth. Br J Cancer 39:718–730, 1979.
62. Urquhart C, Whur P, Gordon M, Silcox JJ, Williams DC, Wright ED: The correlation between plasminogen activator stimulted DNA synthesis and cell morphology in 3T3 cells. Exp Cell Res 113:31–38, 1978.
63. Cohen SD, Israel E, Spiess-Meier B, Wainberg MA: Plasminogen activator is an apparent lymphocyte mitogen . J Immunol 126:1415–1420, 1981.
64. Langer R, Brem H, Falterman K, Klein M, Folkman J: Isolation of a cartilage factor that inhibits tumor neovascularization. Science 193:70–72, 1976.
65. Lostkutoff DJ, Edgington TS: Synthesis of a fibrinolytic activator and inhibitor by endothelial cells. Proc Natl Acad Sci USA 74:3903–3907, 1977.
66. Berman M, Winthrop S, Ausprunk D, Rose J, Langer R, Gage J: Plasminogen activator (urokinase) causes vascularization of the cornea. Invest Ophthalmol Visual Sci (in press).
67. Nicholson GL, Winkelhake JL, Nussey AC: an approach to studying the cellular properties associated with metastasis: some *in vitro* properties of tumor variants selected for enhanced metastasis. In: Fundamental aspects of metastasis, Weiss L (ed). New York: North Holland Pub, 1976, pp 288–292.
68. Wang BS, McLoughlin GA, Richie JP, Mannick JA: Correlation of the production of plasminogen activator with tumor metastasis in B16 mouse melanoma cell lines. Cancer Res 40:288–292, 1980.
69. Ossowski L, Reich E: Experimental model for quantitative study of metastasis. Cancer Res 40: 2300–2309, 1980.
70. Corasanti JG, Celik C, Camiolo SM, Mittelman A, Evers JC, Barbasch A, Hobika GH, Markus G: Plasminogen activator content of human colon tumors and normal mucosae: separation of enzymes and partial purification. J Natl Cancer Inst 65:345–351, 1980.
71. Kodama Y, Tanaka K: Effect of urokinase on growth and metastases of rabbit V2 carcinoma. Gann 69:9–18, 1978.
72. Rohrlich ST, Rifkin DB: Proteases and cell invasion. Ann Rep in Med Chem 14:229–239, 1979.
73. Beers WH, Strickland S, Reich E: Ovarian plasminogen activator: relationship to ovulation and hormonal regulation. Cell 6:387–394, 1975.
74. Strickland S, Reich E, Sherman M: Plasminogen activator in early embryogenesis: enzyme production by trophoblast and parietal endoderm. Cell 9:231–240, 1976.
75. Wilson EL, Becker MLB, Hoal EG, Dowdle EB: Molecular species of plasminogen activators secreted by normal and neoplastic human cells. Cancer Res 40:933–938, 1980.
76. Tucker WS, Kirsch WM, Martinez-Hernandez A, Fink LM: *In vitro* plasminogen activator activity in human brain tumors. Cancer Res 38:297–302, 1978.
77. Naito S, Sueishi K, Hattori F, Tanaka K: Immunological analysis of plasminogen activators from cultured human cancer cells. Virchow Arch A Pathol Anat Hist 387:251–257, 1980.
78. Markus G, Takita H, Camiolo SM, Corasanti JG, Evers JL, Hobika G: Content and characterization of plasminogen activators in human lung tumors and normal lung tissue. Cancer Res 40:841–848, 1980.

23. Collagenase immunolocalisation studies of human tomours

D. E. WOOLLEY

1. Introduction

Collagen represents the major structural protein of connective tissues and together with other macromolecular complexes such as proteoglycans, elastin and glycoproteins, probably provides an impenetrable physical barrier for most cells. The hypothesis that certain neoplasms and tumour cells invade normal tissues by their ability to secrete matrix-degrading or collagenolytic enzymes has been proposed by several research groups and has been the subject of recent reviews [1]. There are now many reports which describe a true neutral collagenase obtained either from cultured tumour explants or cells, or from direct extractions of various neoplasms [for review see 2, 3]. However, although many tumours have been shown to have the potential to elaborate collagenase, because of the heterogeneity of most specimens it remains uncertain which cells are responsible for enzyme production. One approach to this problem is the use of immunolocalisation techniques using a monospecific antibody to human collagenase.

We have used this technique to examine a variety of human tumours in an attempt to determine the distribution and cellular origin of this enzyme in specimens fixed within minutes of excision [2, 3, 4]. As the enzymatic and physicochemical properties of the true neutral collagenases have been summarised in recent reviews [5, 6], the purpose of this chapter is to describe both the present and potential advantages of collagenase immunolocalisation studies of various human tumours.

2. Antibody to human collagenase

Collagenase obtained from cultures of explanted rheumatoid synovium was purified to homogeneity and used to immunise sheep [7]. The antiserum was examined by various immunotechniques to establish monospecificity. These included double diffusion, crossed and rocket immunoelectrophoresis, enzyme inhibition/precipitation, and selective adsorption of antibody by the pure enzyme [2, 7, 8].

Because proteinases in tissues can exist in various forms, e.g. as active, latent or inhibitor-enzyme complexes, accurate interpretation of immunolocalisation data depends not only on the antibody's purity and specificity but also on knowledge of

L.A. Liotta and I.R. Hart (eds.), Tumor Invasion and Metastasis. ISBN-13: 978-94-009-7513-2.
© 1982 Martinus Nijhoff Publishers, The Hague/Boston/London.

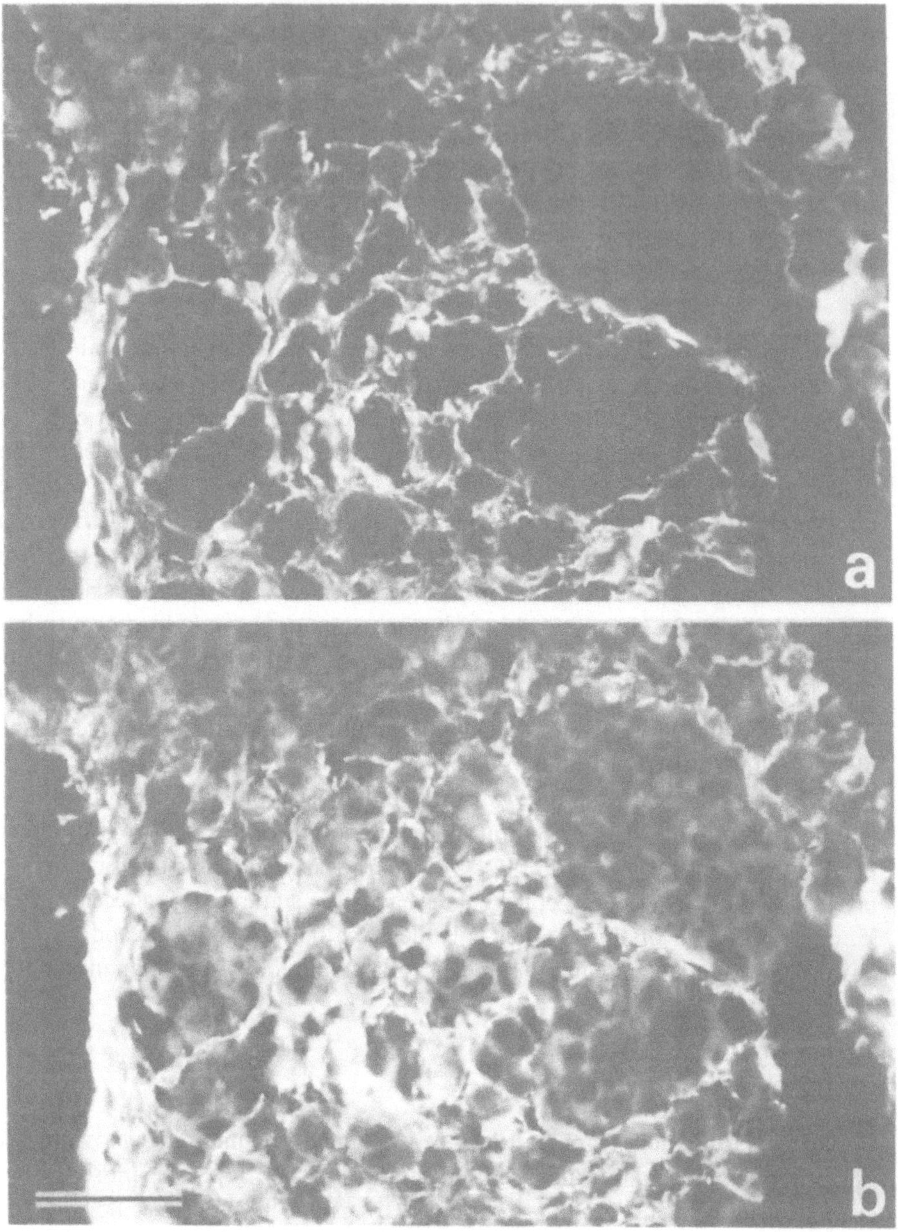

Figure 1. Immunolocalisation of collagenase in a primary melanoma from breast.
a. Frozen section showing FITC-fluorescence associated with collagenous structures which separate small nests of tumour cells. All cells appear negative for immunoreactive enzyme in this specimen.
b. Same region of tissue section shown in *a* counterstained with eriochrome black to show the distribution of cells. Bar = 25 μ.

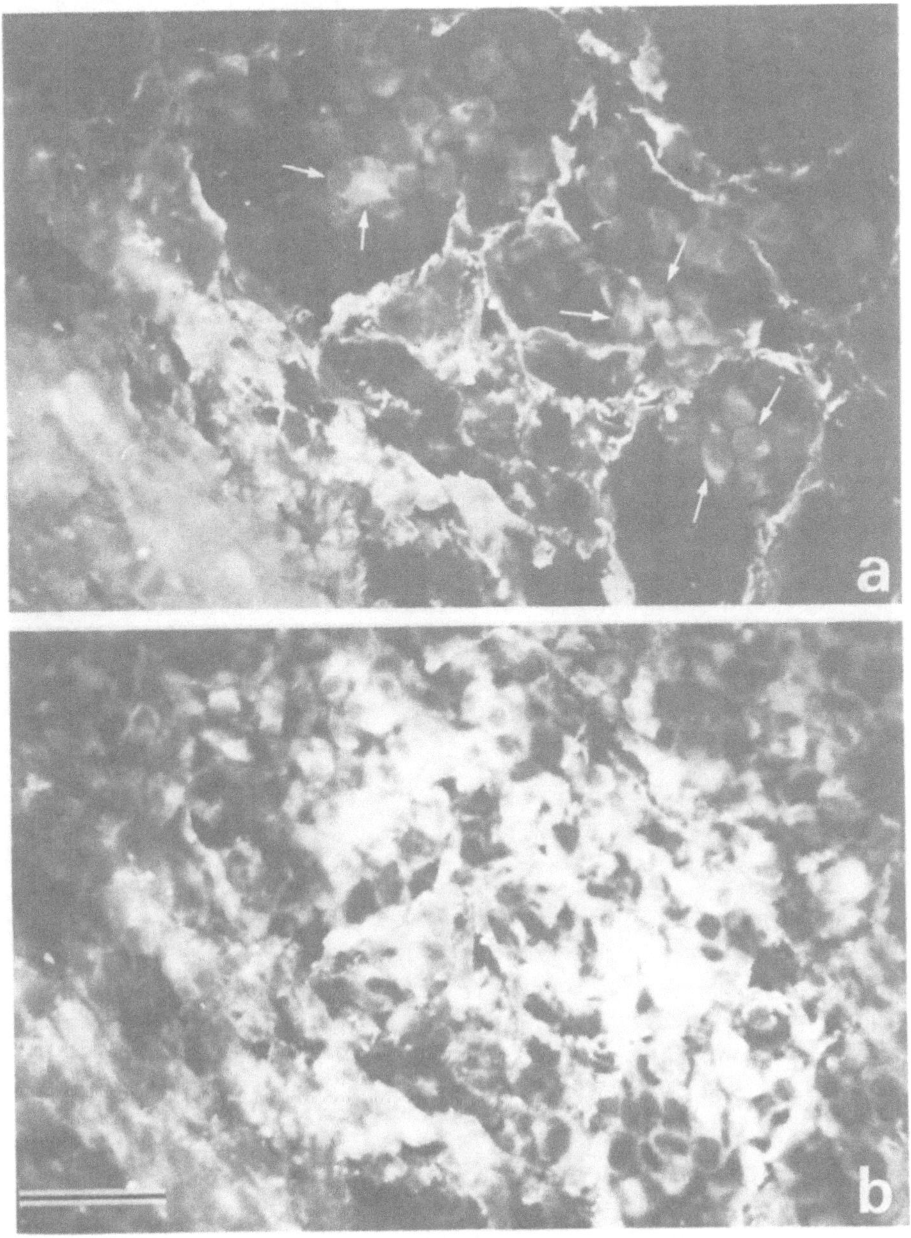

Figure 2. Immunolocalisation of collagenase in a primary melanoma from breast.

a. Immunoreactive enzyme is seen in association with connective tissue elements, especially on those bounding cells. The dense stromal tissue (bottom left) is also positive for enzyme. Whereas most cells of this specimen were negative for immunoreactive enzyme a few positive cells (arrowed) were observed in this location.

b. Same region as shown in a, counterstained with eriochrome black. Bar = 25 μ.

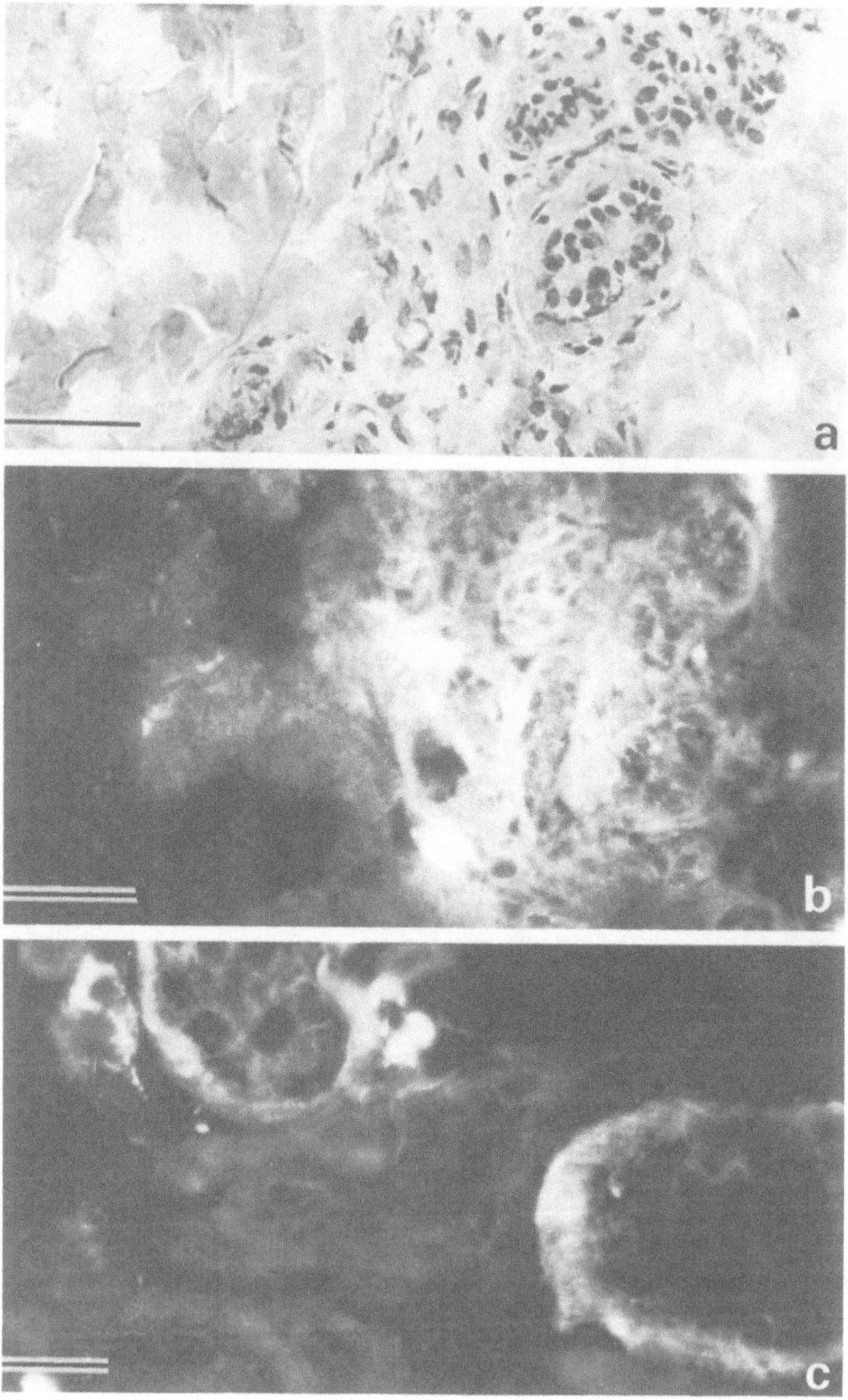
a
b
c

its cross-reactivity with all the naturally occurring forms of collagenase. Therefore, before attempting immunolocalisation studies of human tumours we first demonstrated that collagenases obtained from various neoplasms demonstrated cross-reactivity with the antibody as judged by immunodiffusion and enzyme inhibition experiments [2, 3]. We have also reported that the collagenase antibody used in our studies has no demonstrable reaction with latent collagenase preparations or serum-inhibited enzyme [2, 3] and we therefore believe that much of the immunofluorescence observed in our studies reflects active enzyme.

The collagenase antibody has been used in the indirect or sandwich immunofluorescent technique using fluorescein isothiocyanate (FITC)-labelled immunoglobulins [8]. Tumour specimens were fixed by freezing in liquid nitrogen either within minutes of excision or after 2 or 4 days in tissue culture and were stored at $-70°$ C. Cryostat sections of 6μ were exposed to antibody IgG at concentrations of 25–50μg/ml and control tissue sections were exposed to (a) non-immune sheep IgG in place of antibody; (b) immune sheep IgG previously adsorbed with pure collagenase; and (c) the FITC-conjugated antibody alone. The control sections were consistently negative for fluorescence [2, 8].

Counterstaining with eriochrome black (50:1 dilution with phosphate buffered saline [PBS] or ethidium bromide (20μg/ml in PBS) of tissue sections was used to demonstrate the presence of tumour and tissue cells. Ethidium bromide was particularly useful as it often stained tumour cells more intensely because of their high RNA content.

2.1. Immunolocalisation of collagenase in primary melanomas

Immunoreactive collagenase was detected in three out of five primary melanomas. The observations were very variable, ranging from total absence of enzyme in two specimens to regions of connective tissue which demonstrated intense fluorescence in two others. Figure 1a shows FITC-fluorescence associated with most of the collagenous tissue surrounding nests of tumour cells which are shown counter-

---

Figure 3. Immunolocalisation of collagenase in a secondary skin melanoma.
a. Photomicrograph showing a region of tumour cell infiltration of dermal tissue. Frozen section stained with Haematoxylin and cosin Bar = 25 μ.
b. Immunoreactive enzyme was demonstrated in a similar region to that shown in a and is shown in association with the cellular infiltration. Some cells within the tumour cell nests (those bounded by stromal tissue) and also those in close proximity are shown to be positive for collagenase. The surrounding dermal connective tissue is negative for enzyme. Bar = 25 μ.
c. FITC-fluorescence associated with nests of tumour cells similar to those shown in a. Note that collagenase appears associated with the stromal envelope which surrounds two nests of cells. Other nests were negative. Two cells in close proximity to a nest of tumour cells are positive for enzyme. Bar = 10 μ.

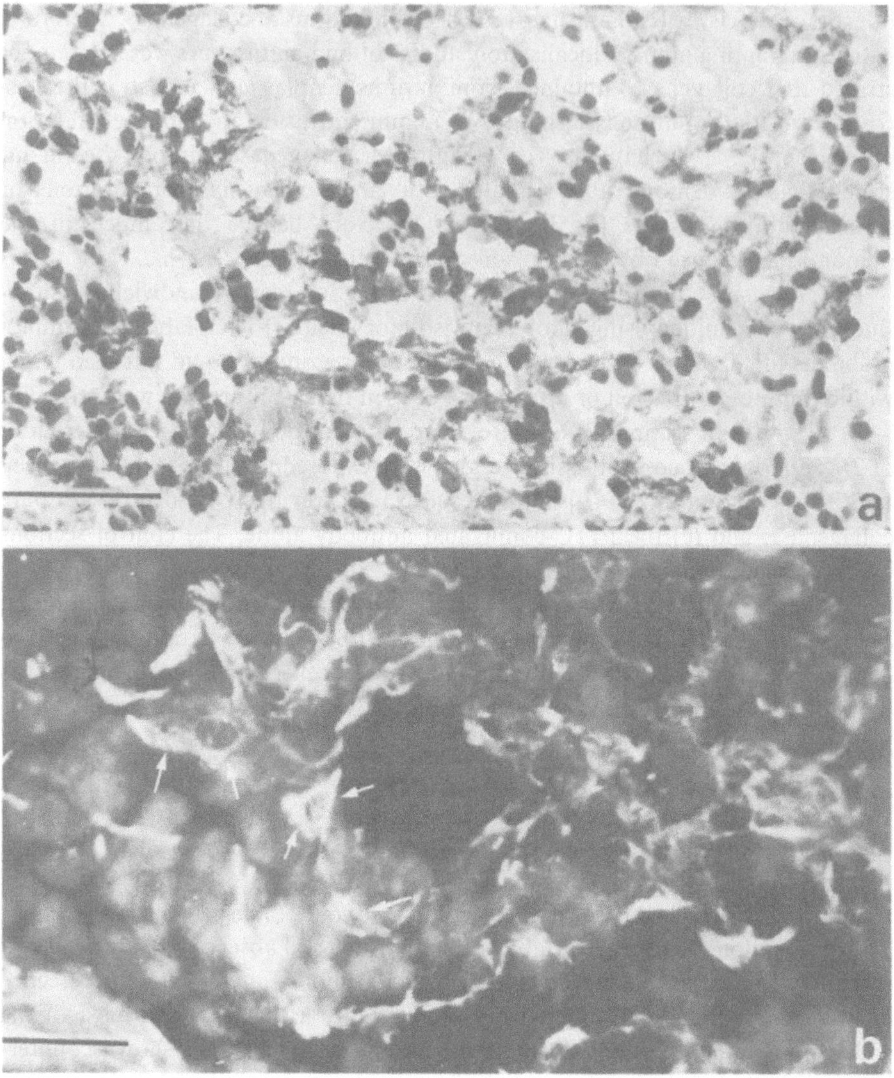

Figure 4. Immunolocalisation of Collagenase in a Secondary Skin Melanoma.

a. Frozen section of the outer margin of a melanoma fixed at time of excision showing the spread of tumour cells into dermal connective tissue with loss of collagenous structures. Haematoxylin and eosin. Bar = 25 μ.

b. FITC-fluorescence of a frozen section similar to that shown in a but at high magnification. Immunoreactive collagenase is associated with the residual collagen and three cells are positive for enzyme (arrowed). The identity of the cells is uncertain. Bar = 10 μ.

stained in Figure 1b. No FITC-fluorescence was observed with any cells of this specimen, and regions of the tissue section surrounding that shown in Figure 1 were also negative for enzyme.

Figure 2a shows immunoreactive enzyme associated with dense stromal tissue and also on thin collagenous structures which appear to separate groups of cells. In contrast to Figure 1 this primary melanoma specimen has some cells which are positive for enzyme (arrows). These make up approximately 10 percent of the cells revealed by counterstaining in Figure 2b.

Such findings suggest localised production of collagense within these primary melanomas. We have not as yet observed any tumours in which all the cells were producing enzyme; indeed, in most cases there was a striking absence of immunofluorescence. Even when alcohol fixation (which permits better intracellular access of antibody) was used in parallel with formalin fixation no significant change in FITC-fluorescence was observed for the cells.

2.2. Immunolocalisation of collagenase in secondary melanomas

Our studies on 15 metastatic human skin melanomas have recently been published [4]. When fixed within minutes of excision positive immunoreactive enzyme was detected in about 30 percent of the specimens. The observations were very variable and Figure 3 and 4 have been chosen to emphasise the variation between specimens.

Figure 3 shows infiltrations of neoplastic cells into dermal connective tissue. The nests of tumour cells are bounded by stromal tissue, but other cell types are also present. Figure 3b shows immunoreactive enzyme associated with the nests of tumour cells and also with the adjacent connective tissue. The more remote dermal tissue was negative for enzyme. Figure 3c shows FITC-fluorescence associated with the stromal tissue which surrounds the nests of tumour cells, some of which also show a weak reaction for enzyme.

Figure 4 shows an outer margin of a secondary melanoma where the dermal collagen appears to have broken down in response to a dense infiltration of tumour cells. In locations such as this, where the tumour was apparently spreading into and replacing connective tissue, we have frequently observed immunoreactive collagenase associated with the residual collagenous elements. Figure 4b illustrates this and also shows three cells which are positive for enzyme. Such observations would seem to confirm a correlation between the presence of immunoreactive collagenase and locations where collagen degradation is observed histologically.

Figure 5 shows a small region of the outer margin of a secondary subcutaneous melanoma where a small group of tumour cells have infiltrated the dermis. Other locations along the margin of this same specimen were negative for immunoreactive enzyme despite being similar histologically. Figure 5a shows immunoreactive collagenase apparently bound or associated with collagenous dermal structures. No enzyme was observed with the connective tissue matrix which is remote from the cellular infiltration, this being counterstained and shown in Figure 5b. Even within this small microenvironment it is clear that the distribution of collagenase is very variable.

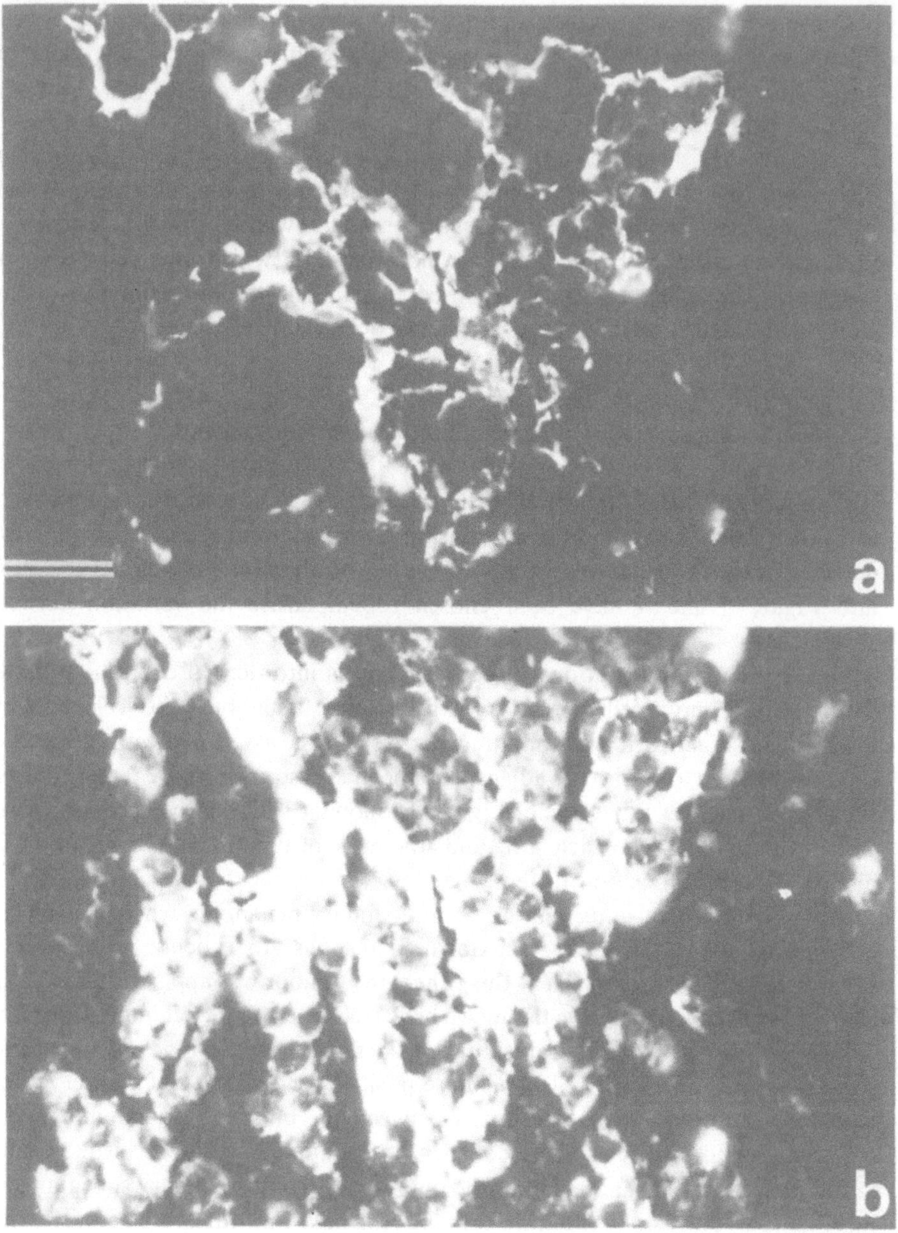

Figure 5. Immunolocalisation of collagenase at a junction of secondary melanoma with skin dermis.
a. Frozen section showing immunoreactive enzyme associated with the connective tissue structures which are in close proximity with a tumour cell infiltration of dermal tissue. Note absence of FITC-fluorescence in surrounding dermis.
b. Same region of tissue section as shown in a but counterstained with eriochrome black to show the distribution of cells. Dermal connective tissue is unstained. Bar = 10 μ.

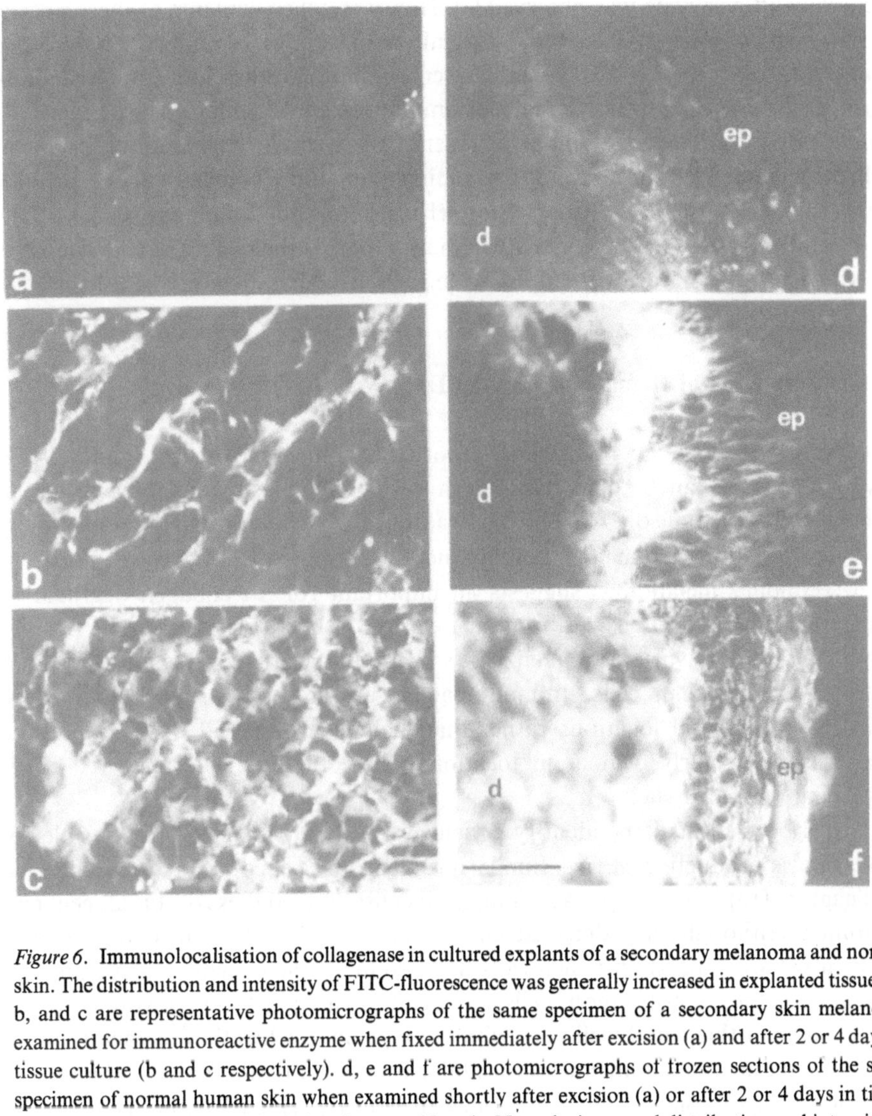

Figure 6. Immunolocalisation of collagenase in cultured explants of a secondary melanoma and normal skin. The distribution and intensity of FITC-fluorescence was generally increased in explanted tissues. a, b, and c are representative photomicrographs of the same specimen of a secondary skin melanoma examined for immunoreactive enzyme when fixed immediately after excision (a) and after 2 or 4 days in tissue culture (b and c respectively). d, e and f are photomicrographs of frozen sections of the same specimen of normal human skin when examined shortly after excision (a) or after 2 or 4 days in tissue culture (b and c respectively). d, dermis; ep, epidermis. Note the increased distribution and intensity of FITC-fluorescence of the cultured explants which suggests the accumulation or increased production of collagenase *in vitro*. Bar = 25 μ.

2.3. Immunolocalisation of collagenase in normal skin and cultured tissue explants

When ten specimens of normal skin tissue from various sites were examined for immunoreactive collagenase most were found to be devoid of enzyme when fixed at the time of excision. Occasionally single or small groups of cells were shown to be positive for enzyme, especially in the basal cell layer of the epidermis, but generally little enzyme was observed [4]. However, when explants of these normal skin specimens were subjected to tissue culture in serum-free Dulbecco's Modified Eagle's medium for 2–4 days subsequent immunolocalisation studies demonstrated an increased distribution of immunoreactive collagenase (Figure 6). Similar observations were found for most of the secondary melanoma specimens which were cultured for a similar period, including those which had been negative for enzyme at the time of excision (Figure 6). Such findings confirm the biochemical data of other workers who have reported the release of collagenase in explant cultures of various neoplasms [e.g. 9] and human skin [e.g. 10, 11].

3. Interpretation of Immunolocalisation Data

Our earlier studies [2, 3, 4] and those reported here have shown that immunoreactive collagenase can be demonstrated in various neoplasms and normal tissues when fixed at the time of excision. Whereas the majority of normal tissue specimens revealed very little enzyme the more frequent occurrence of collagenase in primary and secondary melanomas suggests an important role in collagen degradation which is often associated with tumour invasion of host tissues [12]. The positive findings were very variable and enzyme was usually restricted to connective tissue elements rather than cells. Immunoreactive enzyme was usually confined to microenvironmental locations rather than having widespread distribution, and this was particularly evident in locations where tumour cells appeared to be replacing dermal tissue.

It has been difficult to identify conclusively the types of cell responsible for collagenase production *in vivo*. Similar problems were encountered by Bauer and colleagues [13] for collagenase immunolocalisation studies of basal cell carcinomas. Although they detected enzyme associated with collagenous stromal elements it was uncertain which cells had produced the enzyme. At present it is unclear whether or not tumour cells act as collagenase producers or stimulators of host cells, but this could well vary with the type and/or location of each tumour. The general lack of significant intracellular enzyme in tissues fixed at the time of excision suggests that collagenase is not stored or packaged within cells (unlike polymorphonuclear leucocytes) but is probably synthesized and released as and when required. Our studies to date suggest that both tumour and host cells have the capacity to elaborate collagenase *in vivo*, but better histological techniques are required to examine this question in greater detail.

Tissues fixed at time of excision have usually contained a paucity of cells which reacted positively for collagenase, in contrast to tissues subjected to tissue culture for 2–4 days. The apparent increase in collagenase production in culture has previously been explained by the cells responding to the wounding effects of explantation and the absence of normal physiological restraints such as humoural and plasma factors [2]. However, it is equally possible that the increased amounts of immunoreactive enzyme observed in cultured tissue represents an accumulation of collagenase which is trapped or bound by its substrate, rather than increased production *per se*.

The general lack of immunoreactive collagenase in normal tissues and some tumours when fixed immediately after excision may have several explanations. It is possible that collagen catabolism mediated by collagenase release is not a continuous process and therefore there will be periods when little or no breakdown is occurring. As many of our observations showed enzyme associated with substrate rather than cells, this suggested that collagenase synthesis and release in many instances probably represents a short, transient phase of cell activity. Once the enzyme is released by cells it would then be subject to inhibition by extracellular inhibitors [3, 14, 15] and to subsequent elimination of the inhibited enzyme complexes either by phagocytosis or by the vascular system. Alternatively it might be argued that the antibody preparation could have poor cross-reactivity with some tumour collagenases, or that its poor ability to react with inhibited or latent forms of enzyme may account for the low incidence of positive findings in freshly fixed tissues. The latter has been discussed in detail before [6, 16]. Briefly, when cryostat sections of tissues, frozen at time of excision, were exposed to activation treatments of latent collagenase (e.g. trypsin or 4-aminophenylmercuric acetate) and subsequently examined with the FITC-immunofluorescence technique, no evidence for significant amounts of latent enzyme was found for freshly excised specimens. In contrast, frozen sections of tissue explants subjected to *in vitro* culture for 1–2 days showed an increased distribution of immunofluorescence after exposure to such activation treatments. We therefore conclude that although latent enzyme can be demonstrated in cultured tissues (after activation) we have seldom found it in tissues fixed immediately after excision.

The existence within primary tumours of specialised subpopulations of cells which have a greater potential for metastatic spread [17, 18] is of considerable interest in the light of the observations reported here. The few cells which were positive for immunoreactive collagenase were usually found at the outer growth margins of the tumours (e.g. Figures 2 and 4, ref 3). Such observations would be in agreement with the *in vitro* experiment of Liotta et al. [19] who showed that different populations of tumour cells taken from different sites of a neoplasm had different collagenolytic potentials – those from the outer margins readily solubilised basement membrane collagen in contrast to those from the central tumour mass. It therefore seems plausible that those subpopulations of tumour cells with metastatic potential might well have an enhanced capacity to produce matrix-degrading enzymes. Moreover, such cells may also have the ability to stimulate host cells such as macrophages and fibroblasts to produce proteolytic enzymes.

It seems unlikely that proteinase or collagenase production by tumour cells is sufficient in itself to account for invasion or metastatic spread. Other aggresive factors such as free locomotion, lack of response to growth restraints, high metabolic activity and changed surface properties are all likely to be important.

The full expression of malignancy might well depend on a combination of all these properties as well as the concerted action of several proteinases.

4. Future studies

Our present collagenase immunolocalisation studies of human tissues using the FITC-indirect method have produced useful information on both the frequency and distribution of this enzyme in a variety of tumours including melanomas [2, 4] and gastric adenocarcinomas [3]. However, the major problem with these studies has been the difficulty in identifying the cells responsible for collagenase production. We have therefore decided to concentrate on carefully selected specimens which demonstrate junctional regions of tumour with host tissue which suggest localised sites of invasion as judged histologically. Only with a detailed assessment of the pathology of each specimen can a good interpretation of immunolocalisation data be attempted.

All the observations reported in this chapter were obtained from frozen sections of 6 μ thickness. We have recently improved our techniques and find that plastic-embedded tissue sections of 1 μ thickness provide a much higher quality of immunohistochemical and cytochemical analysis. Together with electron microscope studies using ferritin- and peroxidase-labelled antibodies we hope that these improved techniques will provide more detailed information on the role and cellular origin of collagenase at sites of tumour invasion.

Available evidence suggests that proteinases have an important role both in tumour invasion and metastasis. Immunolocalisation techniques, using specific antibodies to other proteinases in conjunction with well-defined experimental models of tumour invasion, would appear to be the best approach for testing this hypothesis.

5. Conclusions

Our collagenase immunolocalisation studies of human melanomas may be summarised as follows:

1. In tissues frozen within minutes of excision immunoreactive collagenase has been demonstrated in both primary and secondary tumours. However, positive findings were only observed in about 30 percent of the specimens examined.
2. The immunoreactive enzyme was not widely distributed but was usually associated with connective tissue elements in microenvironmental locations. It has been difficult in identify which cells were responsible for collagenase production *in vivo*. Evidence to date suggests that both tumour and normal cells can elaborate enzyme.
3. Immunolocalisation studies of tumour explants which had been cultured in

serum-free medium for 2–4 days usually revealed intense FITC-fluorescence of the connective tissues and an increased number of positively-stained cells. Such observations suggested that most melanoma specimens had the potential to produce collagenase even though many were negative for enzyme at the time of explantation.

4. Whereas most normal tissues demonstrated insignificant amounts of immunoreactive enzyme its more frequent occurrence in both primary and secondary melanomas suggests an important role in tumour physiology. These findings support the concept that collagenase facilitates connective tissue breakdown which is commonly associated with tumour growth, invasiveness and possibly metastatic spread.

Acknowledgments

I thank Lynne Tetlow for excellent technical assistance, the surgeons and pathologists at Withington Hospital for the supply of specimens, and Professor John Evanson for his advice and constant support. This work was supported by grants from the Cancer Research Campaign.

References

1. Strauli P, Barrett AJ, Baici A (eds): Proteinases and tumor invasion, EORTC Monograph series, Vol 6. New York: Raven Press, 1980.
2. Woolley DE, Tetlow LC, Evanson JM: Collagenase immunolocalisation studies of rheumatoid and malignant tissues. In: Collagenase in normal and pathological connective tissues, Woolley DE, Evanson JM (eds). Chichester: Wileys, 1980, pp 105–125.
3. Woolley DE, Tetlow LC, Mooney CJ, Evanson JM: Human collagenase and its extracellular inhibitors in relation to tumor invasiveness. In: Proteinases and tumor invasion, Strauli P, Barrett AJ, Baici A (eds). EORTC Monograph series, Vol 6. New York: Raven Press, 1980, pp 97–115.
4. Woolley DE, Grafton CA: Collagenase immunolocalisation studies of cutaneous secondary melanomas. Br J Cancer 42:260–265, 1980.
5. Woolley DE, Evanson JM (eds); Collagenase in normal and pathological connective tissues. Chichester: Willeys, 1980.
6. Woolley DE: Human collagenases: comparative and immunolocalisation studies. In: Protein degradation in health and disease, Ciba Foundation 75, Elsevier/North Holland, 1980, pp 69–86.
7. Woolley DE, Crossley MJ, Evanson JM: Antibody to rheumatoid synovial collagenase. Eur J Biochem 69:421–428, 1976.
8. Woolley DE, Crossley MJ, Evanson JM: Collagenase at sites of cartilage erosion in the rheumatoid joint. Arthritis Rheum 20:1231–1239, 1977.
9. Dresden MH, Heilman SA, Schmidt JD: Collagenolytic enzymes in human neoplasms. Cancer Res 32:993–996, 1972.
10. Bauer EA, Eisen AZ, Jeffrey JJ: Radioimmunoassay of human collagenase. I. Specificity of the assay and quantitative determination of *in vivo* and *in vitro* human skin collagenase. J Biol Chem 247:6679–6685, 1972.
11. Woolley DE, Glanville RW, Roberts DR, Evanson JM: Purification, characterisation and inhibition of human skin collagenase. Biochem J 169:265–276, 1978.

12. Tarin D: Morphological studies on the mechanisms of carcinogenesis. In: Tissue interactions in carcinogenesis, Tarin D (ed). London: Academic Press, 1972, pp 227–290.
13. Bauer EA, Gordon JM, Reddick ME, Eisen AZ: Quantitation and immunocytochemical localisation of human skin collagenase in basal cell carcinoma. J Invest Derm 69:363–367, 1977.
14. Murphy G, Sellers A: The extracellular regulation of collagenase activity. In: Collagenase in normal and pathological connective tissues, Woolley DE, Evanson JM (eds). Chichester: Wileys, 1980, pp 65–81.
15. Baugh RJ, Schnebli HP: Role and potential therapeutic value of proteinase inhibitors in tissue destruction. In: Proteinases and tumour invasion, Strauli P, Barrett AJ, Baici A (eds). EORTC Monograph series, Vol 6. New York: Raven Press, 1980, pp 157–180.
16. Woolley DE, Brinckerhoff CE, Mainardi CL, Vater CA, Evanson JM, Harris ED, Jr: Collagenase production by rheumatoid synovial cells: morphological and immunohistochemical studies of the dendritic cell. Ann Rheum Dis 38:262–230, 1979.
17. Poste G, Fidler IJ: The pathogenesis of cancer metastasis. Nature 283:139–146, 1980.
18. Hart IR, Fidler IJ: Cancer invasion and metastasis. Quart Rev Biol 55:121–142, 1980.
19. Liotta LA, Kleinerman J, Catanzaro P, Rynbrandt D: Degradation of basement membrane collagen by murine tumor cells. J Natl Cancer Inst 58:1427–1431, 1977.

24. Host–tumor cell interactions and collagenase activity

C. BISWAS

1. Introduction

Since the discovery of the first animal collagenase in tadpole tails by Gross and Lapiere [1], enzymes with similar biochemical characteristics and substrate specificity have been demonstrated in several normal and pathological tissues [2]. It is now widely accepted that the process of collagenolysis is an important event in the remodelling or destruction of connective tissue under various physiological and pathological situations.

During the process of tumor invasion, extracellular matrix is destroyed and becomes infiltrated with tumor cells. Since collagen constitutes a major structural part of the connective tissue, several investigators have initiated studies on the role of collagenolysis in neoplastic invasion. The first direct evidence of extracellular matrix breakdown by tumor cells was provided by Birbeck and Wheatley using electron microscopy [3]. Subsequently, a number of other investigators reported the presence of increased collagenase activity associated with several human and animal tumors [4–9]. These observations supported the idea that collagenolysis is a major event in tumor invasion, but the detailed information concerning the regulation of collagenase activity and the cellular source of the enzyme in a neoplasm is still lacking.

Almost all experimental systems that have been investigated in the study of collagen degradation have used Type I collagen as a substrate. However, in an invasive, metastatic neoplasm one might expect to find an enzyme degrading Type IV collagen as well as the enzyme degrading Type I collagen. The latter may be important for tumor invasion through connective tissue matrix which most commonly contains Type I collagen; whereas the former may be important in the metastatic behaviour of the neoplasm, where the tumor cells penetrate the Type IV collagen-containing basement-membrane of blood vessel endothelial cells. In recent years, a specific enzyme degrading Type IV collagen has been reported to be associated with several metastatic tumors [10, 11]. It is not unlikely that some types of tumor might contain one type of collagenase and not the other, depending on the nature of the barriers to invasion and metastasis and the components of the cellular environment presented to the tumor cells. In addition, the requirements for tumor penetration may be met by other degradative enzymes, e.g. proteases and proteoglycanases [12, 13, 14] or macromolecular agents associated with cell

L.A. Liotta and I.R. Hart (eds.), Tumor Invasion and Metastasis. ISBN-13: 978-94-009-7513-2.
© 1982 Martinus Nijhoff Publishers, The Hague/Boston/London.

movement, e.g. hyaluronic acid [15] and chemotactic substances [16, 17].

The mechanism of tumor invasion of host tissue obviously consists of a complex series of events. Important aspects of this mechanism include interactions of host and tumor cells and participation of the host immune system. Activation of certain cell types to produce collagenase and other proteases in response to interaction with neighbouring cells, including inflammatory cells and lymphocytes, has been documented in several *in vitro* cell culture systems [18–25]. This chapter deals with the effect of such cell-cell interactions in tumors on the production of collagenase degrading Type I collagen. Events leading to production of collagenases degrading other Types of collagen are discussed in Chapter 19 by Liotta. Since the mechanisms of activation of collagenase under nonpathological conditions may also be important during tumorigenesis, these will be reviewed briefly before dealing specifically with tumor collagenase.

2. Collagenase assay

Prior to describing the relationship of collagenase to tumor invasion and the possible mechanism of its regulation, it is important to understand the methods used to measure this enzyme and to distinguish it from other proteases.

Although collagen is a major structural component of the extracellular matrix of almost all tissues, the collagens isolated from different tissues vary significantly in their amino acid and carbohydrate composition (Table 1). At least five types of collagen have now been characterized. Type I collagen has a triple helical structure, composed of two $\alpha 1$ (I) chains and one $\alpha 2$ (I) chain; it occurs in skin, bone, tendon and sclera. In certain cases collagen molecules termed Type I trimer which contain only $\alpha 1$ (I) chains have also been found, e.g. in tumors [26] and in the medium of cultured cells [27]. Type II collagen, found in cartilage and in some tissues of the eye [28] is composed of three $\alpha 1$ (II) chains. Type III collagen occurs mostly in blood vessels and skin and is commonly associated with Type I collagen

Table 1. Collagen types and sources.

Type	Composition	Tissue source
I	$[\alpha_1(I)]2\ \alpha 2$	Skin, bone, tendon
II	$[\alpha_1(II)]_3$	Cartilage, cornea, vitreous humour
III	$[\alpha_1(III)]_3$	Fetal skin, arterial wall, uterine wall
IV	$[\alpha_1(IV)]_3$*	Basement membrane
V	$[\alpha_1(V)]2\ \alpha 2\ (V)]$* (B$_2$A)	Blood vessels, smooth muscle

* The chain structures of these collagens have not yet been fully established. For example, evidence has been obtained for a second type of Type IV collagen trimer [35].

[29, 30]. Type IV is found in basement membranes and thus is a component of the structural barrier between epithelial and mesenchymal cell layers [31, 32]. Type V collagen present in skin, smooth muscle, placenta and bone [33, 34] contains two α1 (V) chains and one α2 (V) chain [for general review see 35].

Until recently only the enzyme degrading Type I collagen has been routinely investigated. However, with the increasing demand for knowledge of the mechanism of tumor metastasis and regulation of differentiation, the need to search for enzymes degrading other types of collagen has become apparent. At present, methods are available for assay of collagenase against all types of collagen, in most cases employing radioactively-labelled substrates. In this section, the enzyme assay using Type I collagen substrate will be described; others will be discussed in a separate section in this volume (Chapter 19 by Liotta).

The simplest procedure for detection of activity in a tissue is the visible lysis of a reconstituted collagen gel layered under a small living tissue explant at neutral pH and at 37° C [1]. Since serum contains a number of collagenase inhibitors it should be omitted from the system. This procedure is quite sensitive and gives a reliable indication of the presence of active collagenase in the tissue explant. The defect in this system lies in the fact that many collagenase-producing systems show collagenolytic activity only after trypsin activation, due to the presence of saturating amounts of enzyme inhibitors or of latent forms of collagenase in most tissues. Thus the absense of gel lysis does not always indicate the absence of collagenase.

The quantitative measurement of enzyme activity in culture media or tissue extracts is usually based on degradation of radioactively labelled, reconstituted collagen fibrils at neutral pH. The radioactive substrate can be prepared and purified from acetic acid-extracted guinea pig or rat skins after labelling *in vivo* by injection of ^{14}C-glycine [36] or from chick embryo calvaria incubated with ^{14}C-glycine or proline in organ culture in the presence of β-amino proprionitrile [37]. A convenient procedure for preparation of radioactive collagen is chemical acetylation of purified collagen by ^{14}C-acetic anhydride [38].

Using the labelled collagen prepared by any of the above methods the units of collagenase activity are generally measured as the micrograms of collagen digested per minute using a standard incubation protocol. The most widely used procedure involves incubation of enzyme solution subsequent to activation with protease (see section 4), with reconstituted collagen fibrils (formed by preincubation of collagen solution at 37° C) at neutral pH and measurement of the radioactivity released into the supernatant [39]. Another method involves incubation of the enzyme with a collagen solution at 27° C followed by formation of fibrils from the undigested collagen at 37° C and measurement of the soluble radioactivity remaining in solution [40]. The fall in viscosity of a reaction mixture of collagen at neutral pH and at 20–27° C is also a sensitive, useful procedure particularly for identification of characteristic reaction products by polyacrylamide gel electrophoresis [41]. Detection of the latter is of importance since animal collagenase directed towards

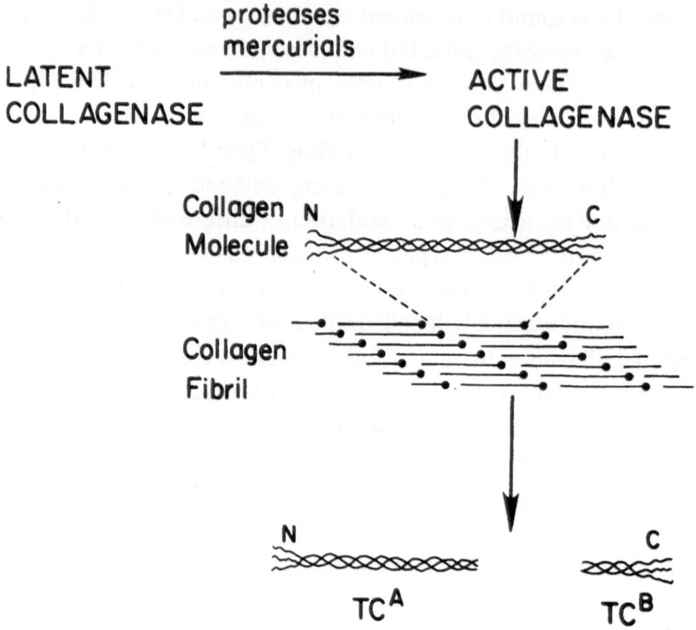

Figure 1. Schematic representation of the action of activated collagenase on collagen fibrils in the fibril lysis assay.

Type I collagen has been defined by its characteristic reaction products, TC^A and TC^B, which correspond to 75% and 25% fragments of the collagen molecule [42] (Figure 1). A relatively simple and sensitive modification of the above procedures, which allows convenient assay of a large number of samples, has been described recently [43]. This technique involves coating microwell culture plates with neutral radioactive collagen solution, polymerization to fibrils at 37° C, incubation of the dried gel film with enzyme solution and measurement of the radioactivity released into the supernatant.

Demonstration of collagenolytic activity against Type I collagen in any new biological system should include evidence for degradation of collagen by one of the above assays as well as demonstration of cleavage of peptide bonds within the helical region of the collagen molecule by characteristic polyacrylamide electrophoretic patterns or visualization of 'segment long spacing' aggregates of the products in the electron microscope [44].

3. Collagenase and tumor invasion

The degradation of extracellular matrix during tumor invasion and the involvement of collagenase in this process has been proposed by some investigators on the basis of morphologic evidence [3, 5]. These studies demonstrated disruption of connective tissue matrix associated with the presence of tumor cells. However, it is quite possible that this disruption could have been caused by neutral proteases and peptidases of neoplastic tissue origin due to their action on proteoglycan and other glycoprotein components of the extracellular matrix. Other studies have examined the levels and molecular nature of collagenase in tumors. The major conclusion from these studies has been that many invasive tumors contain large amounts of extractable Type I collagenase [8, 45–48]. In normal tissues only a low level of collagenase activity is generally detected in extracts whereas collagenase activity is almost always obtained from the media of cultured explants [2].

It should be mentioned that, until now, no clear relationship has been demonstrated between the presence of the extractable collagenase and tumor invasiveness. In our own studies we have found that rabbit V_2-carcinoma implanted in the rabbit and nude mouse contain approximately equal amounts of collagenase units even through the former is highly invasive and the latter is not. However, a difference in regulation of the enzyme activity between these two tumors was apparent in this study [49]. For example, explants taken from the rabbit produced collagenase continuously for several days of culture whereas explants from the nude mouse tumor secreted enzyme into the medium for only a short period of time. Furthermore, cycloheximide inhibited enzyme production by rabbit tumor explants and had little or no effect on that by nude mouse tumor explants. These data suggest that *de novo* synthesis of enzyme occured in the former host but not in the latter [49].

In a attempt to obtain more convincing evidence for the involvement of collagenase in tumor invasion we performed a combined morphological and biochemical study of the rabbit V_2-carcinoma implanted into the rabbit cornea [50]. This system has the following advantages: First, the highly ordered organization of the collagen fibers of the cornea allowed a better analysis of its disruption during tumorigenesis. Second, the effect of local application of medroxyprogesterone, a collagenase inhibitor [51], on tumor growth and change in corneal structure could be correlated with the level of collagenase in the tumor. Our observations indicated that, in the cornea implanted with tumor, the highly ordered collagen fibrils normally present in the extracellular space of the rabbit cornea were replaced by loose amorphous and filamentous substance (Figure 2a). In culture, corneal tumor explants produced enzyme, but in the presence of medroxyprogesterone the level of enzyme was greatly reduced. *In vivo* implantation of the hormone in the rabbit cornea containing tumors caused inhibition of tumor growth while maintaining the integrity of the connective tissue stroma [50] (Figure 2b). These data suggest strongly that tumor growth and invasion are associated with destruction of dense collagenous connective tissue.

Another approach to the demonstration of collagenase involvement in tumor growth has been to localize its distribution in tumor sections by immunohistochemical techniques. Using this approach with a variety of tumor specimens, both Bauer et al. [9] and Woolley et al. [52] observed that the enzyme was

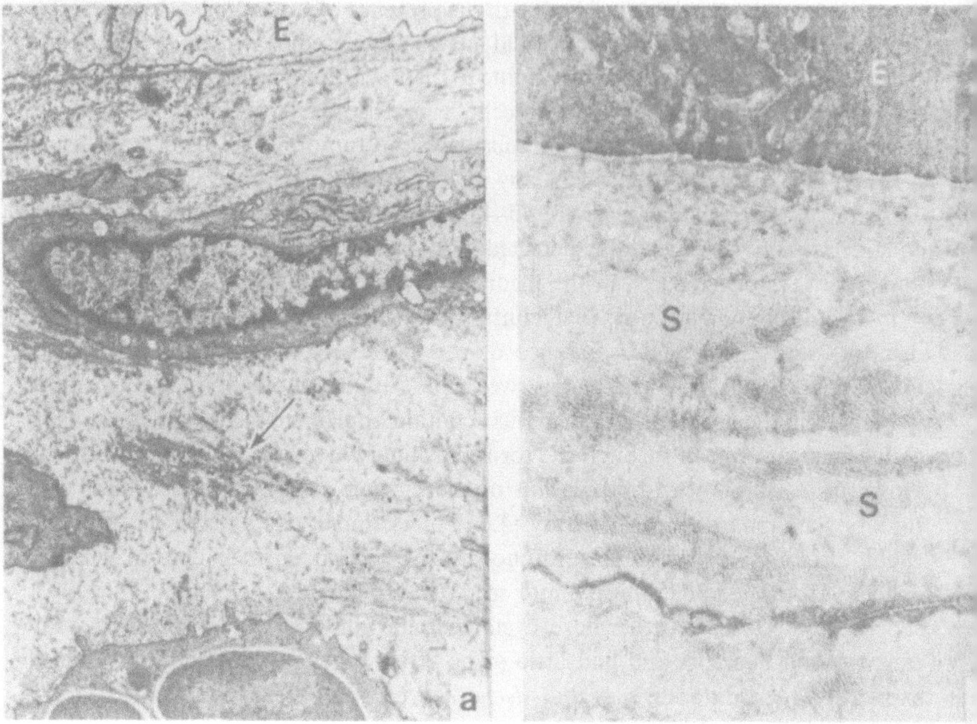

Figure 2. Electron micrographs of rabbit corneal tissue implanted with V_2-carcinoma. (a) control, showing disruption and apparent fragmentation (arrow) of normal collagenous structure of stroma near corneal epithelium (E). (x11 400) (b) Treated with medroxyprogesterone showing maintenance of ordered collagenous stroma (S). E, epithelium (x13 100). Reproduced with permission of National Academy of Sciences from [50].

associated with collagenous stroma surrounding the tumor cells but virtually no enzyme was detected inside the stroma cells. This approach is described in greater detail in Chapter 23 of this volume by Woolley.

As mentioned previously, collagenase is not the only enzyme which could conceivably be involved in extracellular matrix degradation during tumor cell invasion. For example, a synthetic substrate Pz-Pro-Leu-Gly-Pro-D-Arg (Pz = pphenyl-azo benzyl oxy carbonyl) has been used by Strauch [53] to measure the activity of a collagen peptidase in culture media of tumor tissue. The results indicate that the activity of this enzyme is higher in the invasive zone of malignant mouse carcinomas and sarcomas than the surrounding tissue zones. The collagen peptidase seemed to be specific tor cleaving native or denatured collagen only, since it did not cleave other proteins lacking the apolar Gly-Pro-n-sequence. Hence the enzyme could be of importance in a tissue undergoing massive collagenolysis by further degrading the high molecular weight collagen fragments produced by the action of collagenase. Accordingly, its presence in neoplasms provides indirect evidence of collagen degradation in tumorigenesis.

In addition to collagenase and collagen peptidase, the presence of other proteases in tumors has also been documented. Poole et al. [54] have observed large amounts of cathepsin B, a neutral proteinase, in cultures of human breast carcinomas and fibroadenomas. Neutral protease activity has also been found in extracts of Ehrlich ascites tumor cells [55]. In particular the presence of plasminogen activator has been closely correlated with malignancy. Plasminogen activator activity is elevated 10- to 100-fold in primary cultures of tumor cells as well as in tumors [56]. This enzyme may have an important role in collagen degradation since plasmin generated from plasminogen by its action catalyses the conversion of latent collagenase to active collagenase [57].

4. Regulation of collagenase activity

The possible factors and mechanisms involved in regulation of collagenase activity are rather complicated due to the existence of numerous biological and chemical substances which stimulate or inhibit enzyme activity or production. These substances can be classified into two groups: 1) those agents which activate or inhibit the enzyme directly, and 2) those agents which affect cellular production or secretion of enzyme.

4.1. Enzyme activators and inhibitors

Collagenase is often found in tissues or cell cultures as a latent or inactive form. Activation of latent enzyme by trypsin was first showed by Vaes [58] using the medium from cultured mouse bone. Since then, latent or protease-activatable forms have been described in many tissues and cells [2]. The latent enzyme can exist either as a zymogen or as an enzyme-inhibitor complex. It has been generally accepted that the zymogen is activated by limited proteolysis, whereas in the case of enzyme-inhibitor complexes, the inhibitor is released or destroyed by proteolysis. The most commonly used protease for activation of the enzyme is trypsin although plasmin is also known to be effective [57]. A physiological example is the activation of alveolar macrophage procollagenase by an endogenous protease also produced by these macrophages [59]. In addition to proteases, certain organic mercurial compounds can activate latent collagenase. These include aminophenyl mercuric acetate, 4-chloromercuric benzoate and mersalyl [60].

Collagenase activity is inhibited by EDTA, cysteine or dithiothreitol, and also by serum. α_2-Macroglobulin present in serum is a potent inhibitor of almost all proteases acting at neutral pH which contain serine, metals or thiols at their active site [61]. Woolley et al. [62] have demonstrated that serum β_1-globulin is a potent collagenase inhibitor. Whether serum contains any other type of collagenase inhibitor remains to be investigated.

In addition to the above agents a number of other inhibitors have also been isolated and partially purified from a variety of tissues and cell culture systems, e.g. from fibroblast-culture media [63], rabbit V_2-carcinoma extracts [8], embryonic chick skin culture media [64] and the cationic proteins from bovine cartilage culture media [65].

4.2. Regulation of cellular production and secretion

A number of biological and chemical substances have been shown to enhance production of collagenase by cells in culture. These include soluble factors derived from human monocytes [66], guinea pig lymphocytes [67], rabbit lymphocytes [20] and rabbit corneal epithelial cells [68]. The molecular weights of the monocyte factor and one of the factors from corneal epithelial cells were 12 000 and 19 000, respectively, as determined by gel filtration. However, their molecular nature, chemical composition and other functional aspects are not yet well enough described to conclude whether the factors from these different cellular sources are related to each other.

Proteases can stimulate the cellular release of collagenase activity in culture [69] and prostaglandins have a modulating role in collagenase production by macrophages [70, 71]. A wide range of other substances stimulate enzyme production; this list includes collagen itself [72], heparin [73]l cytochalasin B [74], endotoxin [18], phorbol myristate acetate [75], colchicine [76] and latex beads [77]. The mechanisms of activation by these agents and, specifically, whether they act via a common pathway are questions yet to be resolved.

A large number of agents are known to interfere with collagenase production by cultured cells. These include the glucocorticoids [78] and progesterone [51]. A major question is whether these agents or their physiologic analogues act via a similar mechanism. It is also important to know whether, under *in vivo* conditions, several biological agents act cooperatively to elicit a stimulatory or inhibitory effect on collagenase production or whether they act individually.

In the following section more details are given in regard to the influence of production and secretion of the above agents by one cell type on collagenase production by a second cell type.

5. Cell–cell interaction and collagenase production

This section will summarize available information on normal cell interactions in regulation of collagenase production since they may be important events in tumorigenesis. In the next section, recent studies dealing specifically with interactions between normal and tumor cells and the cellular source of collagenase within a tumor will be discussed.

5.1. Mononuclear cells and their factors

The effect of inflammatory cells on collagenase production by a variety of mesenchymal cells in culture has been studied by several investigators. Using human rheumatoid synovial cells, Dayer et al. [19] have demonstrated that these cells could be stimulated to produce collagenase by a factor released from human peripheral blood lymphocytes pretreated with concanavalin A or phytohemagglutinin. In further studies these investigators established that the cellular source of the stimulatory factor in their lymphocyte preparations was monocytes-macrophages but that the production of this factor could be modulated by T-lymphocytes [66]. The stimulatory effect of macrophages on collagenase production by both fibroblasts and synovial cells from rabbits has also been observed by Vaes et al. [23]. In this study, addition of conditioned media from macrophage culture to cultures of rabbit fibroblasts had the same effect as coculturing of both cell types together. A similar finding was made by Newsome and Gross [20] using rabbit corneal stroma cells as collagenase producers and the conditioned media from mononuclear blood cells as a source of stimulators.

The effect of macrophages on the production of collagenase and neutral protease by rabbit articular chondrocytes in culture was reported by Deshmukh-Phadke and coworkers [22]. The macrophages produced a stimulatory factor which they found to be a protein having neutral protease activity and which could be inactivated by trypsin or pronase treatment. The enhancement of degradation of the collagenous matrix of cartilage tissue in the presence of synovium tissue has been demonstrated by Fell and Jubb [79]. Their observations indicate that coculture of living cartilage with synovium tissue resulted in the degradation of both collagen and proteoglycan of the matrix. The effect was not observed when live tissue was replaced with dead tissue. Further studies by these investigators and Dingle et al. [80] identified the stimulator produced by synovium as a protein of molecular weight 20 000 which was inactivated by chymotrypsin or elastase but not by trypsin. Whether this factor is derived from macrophages or from the indigenous cells of the synovial tissue remains to be investigated.

The above studies suggest that monocytes-macrophages are the source of factors that stimulate production and secretion of collagenase by several cells and that the production of the factor may be modulated by lymphocytes. In addition to stimulating production of collagenase by other cells, macrophages themselves can be a potent source of collagenase. Significant amounts of collagenase activity have been detected in culture media of mouse peritioneal macrophages [81, 82]. Collagenase has also been demonstrated in culture media of endotoxin-activated guine pig peritoneal macrophages [18]. Wahl et al. also reported that concanavalin-A activated guinea pig lymphocytes produced substances (lymphokines) which could stimulate macrophages to secrete collagenase [67].

5.2. Epithelial cells and their factors

The influence of epithelial cells on the regulation of collagenase production by mesenchymal cells was first demonstrated by Grillo and Gross [83]. Using a wound healing system in guinea pig skin they demonstrated that the wound edge, containing both epithelium and mesenchyme, revealed a high level of enzyme activity whereas the separated epithelium and mesenchyme alone showed low activity. However, upon recombination of these cell layers the enzyme activity was restored to the same level as that of whole tissue. Recently, a cellular interaction between epithelium and stromal cells of the normal rabbit cornea which leads to stimulation of collagenase has been documented by Johnson-Muller and Gross [21]. These investigators observed that when corneal epithelial cells were cultured with stromal cells in the presence of cytochalasin B, an increased level of collagenase activity appeared in the culture medium. Epithelial cells by themselves did not produce any collagenase in the presence or in the absence of cytochalasin B whereas stromal cells occasionally produced low levels of enzyme under either condition. Furthermore, low concentrations of epithelial cells stimulated collagenase production but high concentrations inhibited collagenase production in the mixed cell cultures. Further studies have revealed that low density epithelial cells, in the presence of cytochalasin B, secrete soluble factors of molecular weights 19 000, 54 000 and 90 000 into the culture medium which stimulated collagenase production by stromal cells. High density epithelial cells on the other hand were shown to produce soluble factors, in the presence or absence of cytochalasin B, which inhibited collagenase production [68].

5.3. Other cellular agents

The studies described so far have dealt with various cellular factors of known source, monocytes-macrophages or epithelial cells, which stimulate collagenase production by mesenchymal cells. Detailed information concerning their chemical identification remains to be investigated. However, as mentioned previously (section 4.2.), the production of collagenase can be promoted by other physiological agents whose chemical and structural properties have been well characterized, notably prostaglandins, proteases and collagens. It is conceivable that these substances could be produced by one cell type but activate collagenase or stimulate its production from a second cell type.

Prostaglandins have been implicated in the regulation of collagenase production since Wahl et al. [70] observed that collagenase production by macrophages was inhibited by indomethacin, an inhibitor of prostaglandin synthesis, and could be restored by the addition of exogenous prostaglandins. However, Dayer et al. [84] reported that mononuclear cell factor stimulated the production of collagenase and prostaglandin by synovial cell but that indomethacin did not inhibit collagenase production.

Proteases are produced by a variety of cell types and could lead either to activation (section 4.1.) or to stimulation of production (section 4.2.) of collagenase from another cell type. A specific example of this phenomenon is found in bovine gingiva where fibroblast procollagenase can be activated by neutral protease derived from mast cells [85].

We have studied the effect of different types of collagen on collagenase secretion by human fibroblasts and human or rabbit synovial cells [72]. Both native and denatured forms of collagen stimulate enzyms production although their relative effect varies among the different types. In human cells the stimulatory effect of collagen was shown to be enhanced by the simultaneous presence of mononuclear cell factor. [72].

A summary of the various factors and their sources which are discussed above is given in Figure 3 [see also 86 for review].

6. Host–tumor cell interactions

In this final section two aspects of the influence of host-tumor cell interaction on collagenase activity will be discussed. These are (a) the cellular source of collagenase in tumors and (b) the effect of tumor cell-derived 'factors' on collagenase production by normal cells in culture.

6.1. Cellular source of collagenase

The cellular source of collagenase in a neoplasm could include one or more of the following:

1) Host cells may be the producers of collagenase and this event may be stimulated by the presence of tumor cells or by factor(s) released from them. 2) Tumor cells may be the producers of collagenase and they may or may not be potentiated

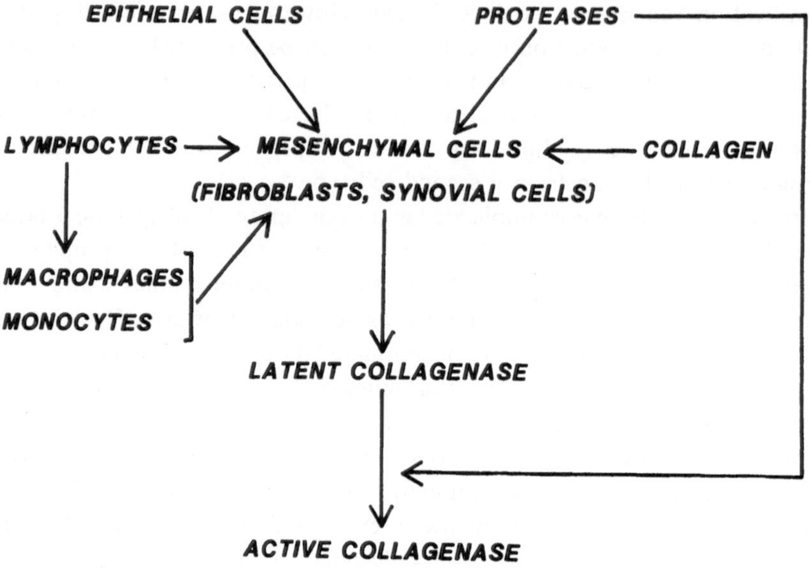

Figure 3. Factors involved in the activation and stimulation of production of collagenase by mesenchymal cells.

by factors secreted by hosts cells. 3) Host inflammatory cells may be the active collagenase producers in a neoplasm since their number increases in tumorigenesis.

Two primary experimental approaches have been used in attempts to test the above proposals. The first is by immunohistochemical localization of the enzyme in tumors which is discussed by Wolley in Chapter 23. The second is by immunological identification of enzyme extracted from a heterologous host-tumor animal model, an approach which we have used and which is described in this section. A third, indirect approach, which we have also used, has been an attempt to reproduce host-tumor cell interactions under *in vitro* culture conditions; this is discussed in the next section (6.2.).

We have employed rabbit V_2-carcinoma implanted into the nude mouse as a heterologous animal tumor model for our studies [49]. Our observations indicate that extracts from V_2-carcinoma grown in rabbit or nude mouse both contain collagenolytic activity. Since it has been reported by others [87] and confirmed by us that the collagenases from rabbit and from mouse are immunologically different we raised antibodies against rabbit enzyme and mouse enzyme for identification of the collagenase extracted from V_2-carcinoma implanted in nude mice. The species specificity of each antibody was first established in separate experiments. The partially purified enzyme from nude mouse tumor extracts was tested for its sensitivity to both antibodies separately and together. Our results indicate that enzyme present in the nude mouse tumor reacted with antibody raised against rabbit collagenase as well as with antibody raised against mouse collagenase, but that the major proportion of the nude mouse tumor enzyme reacted with the former antibody (Table 2). When both antibodies were added simultaneously to the nude mouse tumor collagenase virtually total inhibition was observed. These results indicate that the collagenase present in the neoplasm may originate from host cells as well as from tumor cells [49]. Although the type of host cells responsible for enzyme production in this study is not yet known, it seems reasonable to assume that either host fibroblasts or inflammatory cells or both could be the source. Further identification of the cell type producing collagenase needs to be explored.

6.2. *Fibroblast–tumor cell interaction in vitro*

We have studied the cellular interaction between synovial fibroblasts and tumor cells in monolayer cell culture. Since mouse cells often prove to be poor collagenase producers, we have employed rabbit synovial fibroblasts to test the possible effect of mouse tumor cells on collagenase production by the normal cells [88]. Mouse B-16 melanoma and A-10 adenocarcinoma cell lines were used as sources of tumor cells. Both cell lines are known to be tumorigenic in their respective isogenic mice, an observation which we have confirmed. When the normal cells were cocultured either with B-16 or with A-10 cells, a dramatic increase in collagenase activity in the culture media was observed. Figure 4 presents data from such an experiment where A-10 was used as the source of tumor cells. The stimulatory effect was first observed on day 6 of culture with further increase on day 8. Neither rabbit synovial cells nor tumor cells alone produced significant collagenase activity. This effect was dependent on tumor cell concentration, the optimal ratio of host cells to tumor cells being approximately 1:1 (Figure 5). Similar results were observed with B-16 melanoma cells.

Since it has been documented in other cell-cell interaction systems that soluble factors released by one cell type stimulate collagenase production by the other cell

Table 2. Sensitivity of collagenase to collagenase antibodies.

	% Inhibition of collagenase activity		
Source of	Source of enzyme		
antigen	Rabbit V_2-carcinoma	Nude mouse V_2-carcinoma	Mouse bone
Rabbit V_2-carcinoma	90	70–80	0
Mouse bone	0	30–40	80

Approximately the same number of units of collagenase from each source was incubated with each antibody and the remaining enzyme activity left in the mixture, after removal of immune complexes, was measured by enzyme assay.

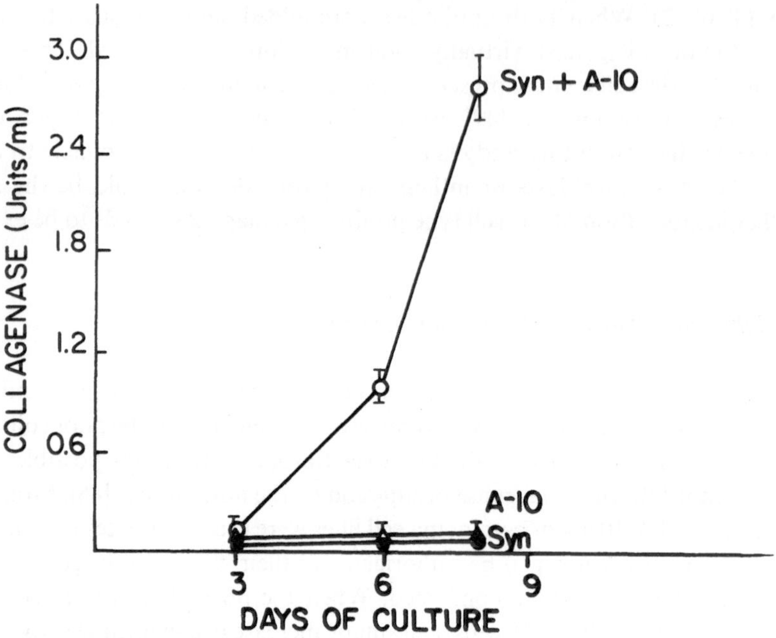

Figure 4. Cumulative collagenase production by rabbit synovial cells and A-10 adenocarcinoma cultured separately and together using 1 × 10^5 cells of each cell strain.

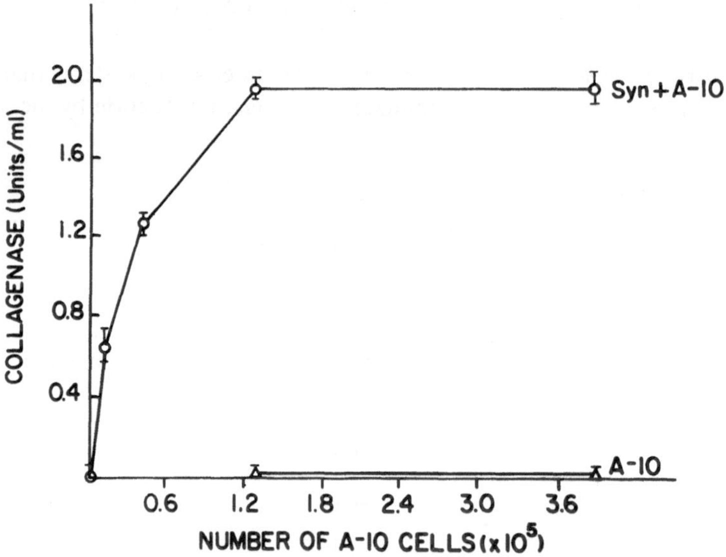

Figure 5. Effect of increasing concentration of A-10 cells on collagenase production in the presence of rabbit synovial cells (1 × 10^5 per well).

type, we explored this possibility in our study. We observed that conditioned media obtained from high density tumor cell cultures stimulated collagenase production by rabbit synovial cells (Figure 6). The effect was markedly dependent on the concentration of conditioned medium, with a maximum stimulation occurring at 40% under the conditions used. The stimulatory effect was diminished at higher concentration (Figure 6). On the contrary, addition of conditioned media from rabbit synovial cells to tumor cells did not have any effect on collagenase production. These results thus indicate that tumor cells produce soluble factor(s) which stimulate fibroblasts to produce collagenase. Since this study has been conducted in a heterologous cell culture system it is important to confirm this finding in homologous systems.

Collagenase activity has been demonstrated in the culture media of human melanoma cell lines in their early passages, but their activity diminished to a low level upon successive subculturing and cloning [89]. Interestingly, one of these cell lines regained its collagenase activity after transplantation into the nude mouse [89], suggesting thereby that interaction of tumor cells with host cells may be a prerequisite for enzyme production in this system also.

7. Summary and conclusions

Recent evidence suggests strongly that collagenase specific for Type I collagen degradation is involved in infiltration of tumor cells into and through connective tissue matrices. Collagenase production appears to involve a series of cellular and biochemical events under normal conditions and it is not unlikely that some of these events may be involved in activation or stimulation of tumor collagenase. Examples of possible sequences related to tumorigenesis are outlined below as well as in Figure 7.

The increased production of plasminogen activator by tumor cells has been discussed earlier (section 3). The plasminogen activator, a serine protease, stimulates the conversion of plasminogen to plasmin, an important event in the cascade mechanism of the clotting system. Plasmin is also an activator for the conversion of latent collagenase to active collagenase and can induce collagenase secretion by cells. The simultaneous production of collagenase and plasminogen activator by human breast carcinoma cells has been demonstrated by Paranjpe et al. [90]. Their results suggest that plasminogen activator produced by tumor cells may participate in collagenase production by these cells. Although the cells were maintained in culture for several passages the possibility of the presence of other host cells in these cultures cannot be excluded. Thus, in a mixed cell population those cells producing large amounts of plasminogen activator or other neutral proteases may cause activation of collagenase or increased production of collagenase; but the source of the collagenase could be either the tumor cells themselves or associated host cells.

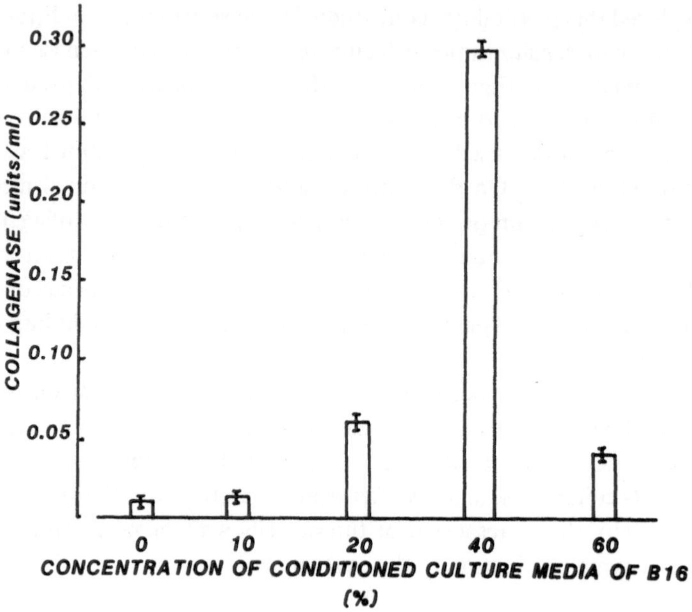

Figure 6. Effect of conditioned culture medium of B-16 cells on collagenase production by rabbit synovial cells at 3 days of culture. Media was conditioned for 3 days by 1.5×10^5 B-16 cells/ml. Synovial cells = 1×10^5.

Infiltration of macrophages at the site of a tumor lesion is known to occur in many systems [91]. Macrophages stimulated with inflammatory agents are known to secrete plasminogen activator [92] as well as collagenase [81, 82]. These cells are also capable of producing other neutral proteases which can activate latent collagenase produced by other types of cells [22] or by themselves [59]. These observations suggest that proteases from macrophages may have a direct or indirect role in stimulation of collagenolytic activity in neoplasms.

Our studies with the heterologous host-tumor model system indicate that although host cells are 'turned on' to produce collagenase, tumor cells themselves appear to be the major source of collagenase. Our *in vitro* studies with the mixed fibroblast-tumor cell culture system suggest, however, that fibroblasts can be stimulated dramatically to produce collagenase under the influence of tumor cells. A major difference between these two systems is of course the presence of other cell types and a different extracellular environment which may modulate the response and which may vary greatly from tumor to tumor and host to host. In each of these cases, however, it seems likely that factors derived from tumor cells themselves stimulate collagenase production by host fibroblasts. The relationship of these substances to the previously mentioned proteases and other cellular factors is a major question to be addressed. Figure 7 summarizes the various cellular interactions which might contribute to stimulation of collagenase activity within a tumor.

Another important consideration in studies of host-tumor cell interactions is the cellular origin of the tumor. Thus, epithelially-derived carcinomas might potentiate collagenase production by fibroblasts in a manner analogous to the epithelium-stroma interaction in wound healing [83] or in the normal rabbit cornea [21]. On the other hand, connective tissue-derived fibrosarcomas may or may not have any effect on fibroblasts but may stimulate other types of host cells, e.g. endothelial cells which may respond by producing collagenase specific for Type IV rather than Type I collagen. Furthermore, populations of fibroblasts of different tissue origin may not respond to normal or tumor cell factor(s) in the same way or to the same extent. Hence, cells from some host tissues may not respond at all to the presence of tumor cells or they may respond only in the presence of additional agents.

Thus, host-tumor cell interactions should be explored in the light of participation of other cellular agents and not only as an isolated culture system consisting of only two types of cells. Future directions of research in this area would include studies of cell-interactions in the presence of other tissue and cell factors, and their effect not only on degradation of Type I collagen but also on other types of collagen (see Liotta, Chapter 19). The information obtained from these approaches will further aid the understanding of regulation of collagen degradation in tumor invasion and metastasis.

Acknowledgement

The author thanks Dr. Jerome Gross for his support, Dr. Bryan P. Toole for his helpful criticism of the manuscript and Michelle S. Finck for assistance with the figures. The recent work included in this chapter was supported by NIH grants No. CA 19158 and AM 03564. This is publication No. 875 of the Lovett Memorial Group for the Study of Diseases Causing Deformities.

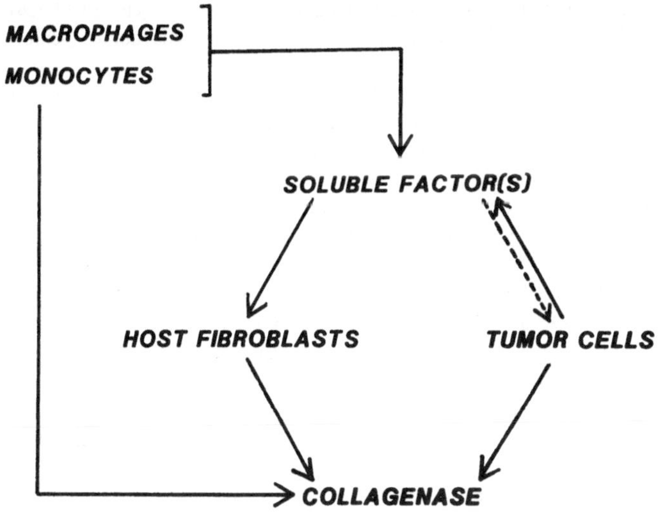

Figure 7. Possible host-tumor cell interactions leading to stimulation of collagenase production.

References

1. Gross J, Lapiere CM: Collagenolytic activity in amphibian tissues: a tissue culture assay. Proc Natl Acad Sci 48:1014–1022, 1962.
2. Gross J: Aspects of the animal collagenases. In: Biochemistry of collagen, Ramachandran GN, Reddi AH (eds). Plenum Press, 1976, pp 275–317.
3. Birbeck MSC, Wheatley DN: An electron microscopic study of the invasion of ascites tumor cells into the abdominal wall. Cancer Res 25:490–497, 1965.
4. Dresden MH, Heilman SA, Schmidt JD: Collagenolytic enzymes in human neoplasms. Cancer Res 32:993–996, 1972.
5. Hashimato K, Yamanishi Y, Dabbous MK: Electron microscopic observations of collagenolytic activity of basal cell epithelioma of the skin *in vivo* and *in vitro*. Cancer Res 32:2561–2567, 1972.
6. Hashimato K, Yamanishi Y, Maiyens E, Dabbous MK, Kanzaki T: Collagenolytic activities of squamous cell carcinoma of the skin. Cancer Res 33:2790–2801, 1973.
7. Abramson MA, Schilling RW, Huang C, Salome GR: Collagenase activity in epidermoid carcinoma of the oral cavity and larynx. Ann Otol Rhinol Laryngol 84:158–163, 1975.
8. McCroskery PA, Richards JF, Harris ED, Jr: Purification and characterization of a collagenase extracted from rabbit tumors. Biochem J 152:131–142, 1975.
9. Bauer EA, Gordon JM, Reddick ME, Eisen AZ: Quantitation and immunocytochemical localization of human skin collgenase in basal cell carcinoma. J Invest Dermatol 69:363–367, 1977.
10. Liotta LA, Abe S, Gehron-Robey P, Martin GR: Preferential digestion of basement membrane collagen by an enzyme derived from a metastatic murine tumor. Proc Natl Acad Sci USA 76:2268–2272, 1979.
11. Liotta LA, Tryggvason K, Garbisa S, Hart I, Flotz CM, Shafie S: Metastatic potential correlates with enzymatic degradation of basement membrane collagen. Nature 284:67–68, 1980.
12. Sapolsky AI, Keiser H, Howell DS, Woessner Jr JF: Metalloproteases of human articular cartilage that digest cartilage proteoglycan at neutral and acid pH. J Clin Invest 58:1030–1041, 1976.
13. Sellers A, Reynolds JJ, Meikle MC: Neutral metalloproteinases of rabbit bone. Biochem J 171: 493–496, 1978.
14. Vaes G, Eeckhout G, Lenuers-Claeyes G, Francois-Gillet CH, Druetz JE: The simultaneous release by bone explants in culture and the parallel activation of procollagenase and of a neutral proteinase that degrades cartilage proteoglycans and denatured collagens. Biochem J 172:261–264, 1978.
15. Toole BP, Biswas C, Gross J: Hyaluronate and invasiveness of the rabbit V_2-carcinoma. Proc Natl Acad Sci USA 76:6299–6303, 1979.
16. Postlehwaite AE, Snyderman R, Kang AH: The chemotactic attraction of human fibroblasts to a lymphocyte derived factor. J Exp Med 144:1188–1203, 1976.
17. Orr W, Varani J, Gonek MD, Ward PA, Mundy GR: Chemotactic responses of tumor cells to products of resorbing bone. Science 203:176–179, 1979.
18. Wahl LM, Wahl SM, Mergenhagen SE, Martin GR: Collagenase production by endotoxin activated macrophages. Proc Natl Acad Sci USA 71:3598–3601, 1974.
19. Dayer JM, Breard L, Chess L, Krane SM: Collagenase production by rheumatoid synovial cells: stimulation by a human lymphocyte factor. Science 195:181–183, 1977.
20. Newsome DA, Gross J: Regulation of corneal collagenase production: stimulation of serially passaged stromal cells by blood mononuclear cells. Cell 16:895–900, 1979.
21. Johnson-Muller B, Gross J: Regulation of corneal collagenase production: epithelial-stromal cell interactions. Proc Natl Acad Sci USA 75:4417–4427, 1978.
22. Deshmukh-Phadke K, Nada S, Lee K: Macrophage factor that induces neutral protease secretion by normal rabbit chondrocytes. Eur J Biochem 104:175–180, 1980.
23. Vaes G, Huybrechts-Godin G, Hauser P: Lymphocyte-macrophage-fibroblast cooperation in the inflammatory degradation of cartilage and connective tissue. Agent and Actions, 1980.
24. Greinder DK, Counorton KJ, David JR: Plasminogen activator production by human monocytes.

Enhancement by activated lymphocytes and lymphocyte products. J Immunol 123:2808–2813, 1980.
25. Hamilton JA, Slywka J: Stimulation of human synovial fibroblast plasminogen activator production by mononuclear cell supernatants. J Immunol 126:851–855, 1981.
26. Moro L, Smith BD: Identification of collagen αl (I) trimer and normal type I collagen in a polyoma virus-induced mouse tumor. Arch Biochem Biophys 182:33–41, 1977.
27. Mayne R, Vail M, Mayne P, Miller EJ: Changes in type of collagen synthesized as clones of chick chondrocytes grow and eventually lose division capacity. Proc Natl Acad Sci USA 73:1674–1678, 1976.
28. Linsenmayer TF, Smith GN, Hay E: Synthesis of two collagen types by embryonic chick corneal epithelium *in vitro*. Proc Natl Acad Sci USA 74:39–43, 1977.
29. Miller EJ, Epstein EH Jr, Piez KA: Identification of three genetically distinct collagens by cyanogen bromide cleavage of insoluble human skin and cartilage collagen. Biochem Biophys Res Commun 42:1024–1029, 1971.
30. Chung E, Miller EJ: Collagen polymorphism: characterization of molecules with the chain composition $\alpha_1(III)_2$ in human tissues. Science 183:1200–1201, 1974.
31. Kaefalides NA: Basement membranes: structural and biosynthetic considerations. J Invest Dermatol 65:85–92, 1975.
32. Sage H, Woodbury RG, Bornstein P: Structural studies on human type IV collagen. J Biol Chem 254:9893–9900, 1979.
33. Burgeson RE, Fouad A, Adli EL, Ilkka IK, Hollister DW: Fetal membrane collagens: identification of two new collagen alpha chains. Proc Natl Acad Sci USA 73:2579–2583, 1976.
34. Glanville RW, Rauter A, Fietzek PP: Isolation and characterization of a native placental basement membrane collagen and its component α-chains. Eur J Biochem 95:383-389, 1979.
35. Kleinman HA, Klebe RJ, Martin GR: Role of collagenous matrices in the adhesion and growth of cells. J Cell Biol 88:473–485, 1981.
36. Evanson JM, Jeffrey JJ, Krane SM: Studies on collagenase from rheumatoid synovium in tissue culture. J Clin Invest 47:2639–2651, 1968.
37. Robertson PB, Taylor RE, Fullmer HM: A reproducible quantitative collagenase radiofibril assay. Clin Chem Acta 42:43–45, 1972.
38. Gisslow Mt, McBride BC: A rapid senive collagenase assay. Anal Biochem 68:70–78, 1975.
39. Nagai Y, Lapiere CM, Gross J: Tadpole collagenase: preparation and purification. Biochemistry 5:3123–3130, 1966.
40. Sakamoto S, Goldhaber P, Glimcher MJ: A new method for the assay of tissue collagenase. Proc Soc Exp Biol Med 139:1057–1059, 1972.
41. Gross J, Nagai Y: Specific degradation of the collagen molecule by tadpole collagenolytic enzyme. Proc Natl Acad Sci USA 54:1197–1204, 1965.
42. Nagai Y, Gross J, Piez KA: Disc electrophoresis of collagen components. Ann NY Acad Sci 121:494–500, 1964.
43. Johnson-Wint B: A quantitative collagenase film assay for large number of samples. Anal Biochem 104:175–181, 1980.
44. Bruns RR, Gross J: Band pattern of the segment-long spacing form of collagen. Its use in the analysis of primary structure. Biochemistry 12:808–815, 1973.
45. Yamanishi Y, Maeyens E, Dabbous MF, Ohyama H, Hashimoto K: Collagenolytic activity in malignant melanoma: physiochemical studies. Cancer Res 33:2507–2512, 1973.
46. Dabbous MK, Roberts AN, Brinkley B: Collagenase and neutral protease activities in cultures of rabbit V_2-carcinoma. Cancer Res 37:3537–3544, 1977.
47. Steven FS, Itzhaki S: Evidence for a latent form of collagenase extracted from rabbit tumor cells. Biochim Biophys Acta 496:241–246, 1977.
48. Biswas C, Bloch KJ, Moran WP, Gross J: Collagenolytic activity of rabbit V_2-carcinoma growing at multiple sites. Biochem Biophys Res Commun 80:33–38, 1978.
49. Biswas C, Bloch KJ, Gross J: The collagenolytic activity of rabbit V_2-carcinoma implanted in

nude mouse. Submitted.

50. Gross J, Azizkhan RG, Biswas C, Bruns R, Hsieh DST, Folkman J: Inhibition of tumor growth, vascularization, and collagenolysis in the rabbit cornea by medroxyprogesterone. Proc Natl Acad Sci USA 78:1176–1180, 1981.
51. Koob TJ, Jeffrey JJ: Hormonal regulation of collagen degradation in the uterus: inhibition of collagenase expression by progesterone and cyclic AMP. Biochim Biophys Acta 354:61–70, 1974.
52. Woolley DE, Tetlow LC, Evanson JM: Collagenase immunolocalization studies of rheumatoid and malignant tissues. In: Collagenase in normal and pathological connective tissues, Woolley DE, Evanson JM (eds). New York: John Wiley, 1980, pp 105–125.
53. Strauch L: The role of collagenases in tumor invasion. In: Tissue interactions in carcinogenesis, Tarin D. (ed). New York: Academic Press, 1972, pp 399–428.
54. Poole AR, Tiltman KJ, Recklies AD, Stoker TAM: Differences in secretion of the proteinase cathepsin B at the edges of human breast carcinoma and fibroadenomas. Nature 273:545–547, 1978.
55. Steven FS, Podrazky V, Itzhaki S: The interaction of a trypsin-dependent neutral protease and its inhibitor found in tumor cells. Biochim Biophys Acta 52:170–182, 1978.
56. Quigley JP: Proteolytic enzymes of normal and malignant cells. In: Surfaces of normal and malignant cells, Hynes R.O. (ed). New York: John Wiley, 1979, pp 247–275.
57. Eeckhout Y, Vaes G: Further studies on the activation of procollagenase, the latent precursor of bone collagenase. Biochem J 166:21–31, 1977.
58. Vaes G: The release of collagenase as an inactive proenzyme by bone explants in culture. Biochem J 126:275–289, 1972.
59. Horwitz AL, Kelman JA, Crystal RG: Activation of alveolar macrophage collagenase by a neutral protease secreted by the same cell. Nature 264:772–774, 1976.
60. Harris ED Jr, Vater CA: Methodology of collagenase research: substrate preparation, enzyme activation and purification. In: Collagen in normal and pathological connective tissues, Woolley DE, Evanson JM (eds). New York: John Wiley, 1980, pp 37–63.
61. Werb Z, Burleigh MC, Barrett AJ, Starkey PM: The interaction of α_2-macroglobulin with proteinases. Biochem J 139:359–368, 1974.
62. Woolley DE, Roberts DR, Evanson JM: Small molecular weight β_1 serum proteins which specifically inhibits human collagenases. Nature 261:325–327, 1976.
63. Welgus HG, Stricklin GP, Eisen AZ, Bauer EA, Cooney RV, Jeffrey JJ: A specific inhibitor of vertebrate collagenase produced by humanskin fibroblasts. J Biol Chem 254:1938–1943, 1979.
64. Shinkai H, Kawamoto T, Hori H, Nagai Y: A complex of collagenase with low molecular weight inhibitors in the culture medium of embryonic chick skin explants. J Biochem 81:261–263, 1977.
65. Kuettner KE, Soble L, Croxen RL, Marczynski B, Hiti J, Harper E: Tumor cell collagenase and its inhibition by a cartilage-derived protease inhibitor. Science 196:653–654, 1977.
66. Dayer JM, Breard J, Chess L, Krane SM: Participation of monocyte-macrophages and lymphocytes in the production of a factor that stimulates collagenase and prostaglandin release by rheumatoid synovial cells. J Clin Invest 64:1386–1392, 1979.
67. Wahl L, Wahl SM, Mergenhagen S, Martin GE: Collagenase production by lymphokine-activated macrophages. Science 187:261–263, 1975.
68. Johnson-Wint B: Regulation of stromal cell collagenase production in the adult rabbit cornea, *in vitro* stimulation and inhibition by epithelial cell products. Proc Natl Acad Sci USA 77:5331–5335, 1980.
69. Werb Z, Aggelar J: Proteases induce secretion of collagenase and plasminogen activator by fibroblasts. Proc Natl Acad Sci USA 75:1839–1843, 1978.
70. Wahl LM, Olsen CE, Sandberg AL, Mergenhagen SE: Prostaglandin regulation of macrophage collagenase production. Proc Natl Acad Sci USA 74:4955–4958, 1977.
71. Dayer JM, Karne SM: PGE_2 modulates collagenase production by cultured adherent rheumatoid synovial cells. Clin Res 26:513A, 1978.
72. Biswas C, Dayer JM: Stimulation of collagenase production by collagen in mammalian cell culture.

Cell 18:1035–1041, 1979.

73. Sakamoto S, Sakamoto M, Goldhaber P, Glimcher P: Studies on the interaction between haparin and mouse bone collagenase. Biochim Biophys Acta 385:41–50, 1975.
74. Harris ED Jr, Reynolds JJ, Werb Z: Cytochalas in B increases collagenase production by cells *in vitro*. Nature 257:243–244, 1975.
75. Brinckerhoff CE, McMillan RM, Fahey JV, Harris Jr ED: Collagenase production by synovial fibroblasts treated with phorbol myristic acetate. Arthritis Rheum 22:1109–1115, 1979.
76. Harris Jr ED, Krane SM: Effect of colchicine on collagenase cultures of rheumatoid synovium. Arthritis Rheum 14:669–684, 1971.
77. Werb Z, Reynolds JJ: Stimulation by endocytosis of secretion of collagenase and neutral proteinase from rabbit synovial fibroblasts. J Exp Med 140:1482–1497, 1974.
78. Werb Z, Foley R, Munck A: Glucocorticoid receptors and glucocorticoid sensitive secretion of neutral proteinases in a macrophage line. J Immunol 127:115–121, 1978.
79. Fell HB, Jubb RN: The effect of synovial tissue on the breakdown of articular cartilage in organ culture. Arthritis Rheum 20:1359–1371, 1977.
80. Dingle JL, Saklatvala J, Hembry R, Tyler J, Fell HB, Jubb R: A cartilage catabolic factor from synovium. Biochem J 184:177–180, 1979.
81. Werb Z, Gordon S: Secretion of a specific collagenase by stimulated macrophages. J Exp Med 42:346–360, 1975.
82. Boxer PA, Leibovich SJ: Production of collagenase by mouse peritoneal macrophages *in vitro*. Biochim Biophys Acta 444:626–632, 1976.
83. Grillo HC, Gross J: Collagenolytic activity during mammalian wound repair. Dev Biol 15:300–317, 1967.
84. Dayer JM, Robinson DR, Krane SM: Prostaglandin production by rheumatoid synovial cells. Stimulation by a factor from human mononuclear cells. J Exp Med 145:1399–1404, 1977.
85. Birkedahl-Hansen H, Cobb CM, Taylor RE: Fullmer HM: Activation of fibroblast procollagenase by most cell proteases. Biochim Biophys Acta 438:273–286, 1976.
86. Vaes G: Cellular secretion and tissue breakdown. Cell to cell interactions in the secretion of enzymes of connective tissue breakdown collagenase and proteoglycan degrading neutral proteases. A review. Agents Actions 10:474–485, 1980.
87. Werb Z, Reynolds JJ: Rabbit collagenase. Immunological identity of the enzymes released from cells and tissues in normal and pathological conditions. Biochem J 151:665–669, 1975.
88. Biswas C, Gross J: Fibroblast-tumor cell interaction in collagenase production. Am Soc Cell Biol in Anaheim 91:163a, 1981.
89. Nayoshi T, Hashimoto K, Kanzaki T, Ohyma H: Collagenolytic activities of cultured human malignant melanoma cells. J Biochem (84)1171–1176, 1978.
90. Paranjpe M, Engel L, Young N, Liotta L: Activation of human breast carcinoma collagenase through plasminogen activator. Life Sci (26):1223–1231, 1980.
91. Thornthwaite JT, Sugarbaker EV: An examination of the macrophage response after challenge with murine, syngenic sarcoma cells. Exp Mol Pathol (33):169–184, 1980.
92. Unkeless J, Gordon S, Reich E: Secretion of plasminogen activator by stimulated macrophages. J Exp Med (139):834–850, 1974.

25. Observations on cancer metastasis in man

E. V. SUGARBAKER, D. N. WEINGRAD and J. M. ROSEMAN

1. Introduction

A malignant neoplasm is thought to arise from transformation of normal somatic cells by an oncogenic stimulus. Intrinsic to this malignant transformation is acquisition of the propensity for uncontrolled cell division which eventually creates a macroscopic primary tumor in the organ of origin.

At an as yet unpredictable size in the growth of an individual primary neoplasm, many malignancies acquire the capability of metastasis to other organs. Curtailment of human life due to malignant disease can be caused by disruption of vital physiologic functions due to unrestrained or untreatable growth at the primary tumor site. A primary astrocytoma of the brain, which is unresectable or recurrent, a primary liver hepatoma – unresectable, unresectable lung carcinoma, and other tumors can be given as examples of how the primary tumor, at the site of the initially transformed cell can cause eventual patient demise. However, despite the importance of untreatable primary cancer growth, the major cause of death in most human malignancies is due to metastasis to distant organs. About 50% of patients who develop a malignant neoplasm are currently cured by the various therapies employed. Of the 50% who die of their disease more than half succumb to metastasis, making the problem of cancer metastasis one of the most significant aspects of the biologic behavior of malignant disease in man.

The human model for metastasis, which is obviously the most relevant setting for studies of this event, cannot be manipulated as can experimental tumor systems. Thus, the experimental literature on metastasis has grown at an extremely rapid rate, particularly in the last 20–25 years. Much of the experimental data generated in these reports is of the highest scientific quality within the scope of the experimental tumor system employed. However, an infrequently printed question is: *How relevant are these experimental models to the problem of cancer metastasis in man? Is my experimental model relevant to all human cancers? If not, which aspect of the protean manifestation of cancer in man am I actually studying in this experimental model?*

One of the difficulties faced by the basic scientist in attempting to answer such poignant questions regarding model relevance, is that clinicians treating this disease have not made many attempts to provide an organized assessment of their observations on the clinical characteristics of metastasis in man. The central

L.A. Liotta and I.R. Hart (eds.), Tumor Invasion and Metastasis. ISBN-13: 978-94-009-7513-2.
© 1982 Martinus Nijhoff Publishers, The Hague/Boston/London.

objective of this chapter therefore, is to describe for the basic science oncologist, some of the aspects of biologic behavior of metastatic cancer in man. In order to accomplish this objective it will be necessary to draw upon diverse sources of clinical data in observation, not all of which were recorded with this type of analysis of clinical metastasis as its main intention.

1.1. Data bases for studies of clinical metastases

The prime objective of the oncologist in treating the patient with cancer is to eradicate the neoplastic disease and restore a normal life expectancy. However as a by-product of therapeutic intervention, many observations on the biologic behavior of cancer metastasis have been made. First, striking individual clinical observations such as spontaneous regression of metastasis [1], disease explosions [2], long delayed or dormant metastasis [3], localization of metastases at sites of trauma [4], and other observations from individual patients or small series of patients have been frequently documented in the medical literature. Such striking deviations from the central range of biologic behavior of cancer in man stimulate thought and generate hypotheses as to the mechanisms involved. The limitation is that few data points are generated so that such relatively isolated observations cannot be used to substantiate any given hypothesis and no statistical significance can be assigned. The clinician, however, is not usually apologetic about such observations, for medicine is practiced by one doctor treating one patient at a time. For a given doctor-patient interrelationship one striking observation can have considerable impact.

A second major source of information is generated by clinical-surgical pathological data evolving from careful clinical assessment of metastases which can then be correlated with an analysis of the surgical specimens excised during surgical treatment. Clinical characteristics of the primary tumor can thus be correlated with other clinical and/or pathological findings in adjacent resected lymph nodes and other organs. Autopsy data add information on the terminal phases of widespread organ cancer metastasis.

Third, treatment results from large series of patients with histologically classified and clinically staged tumors can be assessed in terms of organ site and timing of metastatic appearance after treatment. The tumor registry records initial disease characteristics and monitors the outcome during careful follow up after therapy.

Finally, the randomized prospective clinical trial has increased the quality of biologic data related to observations on metastasis by standardizing treatments, and, increasing the number of patients studied and reported.

2. Historical perspective on cancer metastasis in man

A perspective on the evolution of the cellular theory of cancer metastasis, and, the translation of this concept into surgical therapeutic procedures in the late 19th century is pertinent to the objectives of this chapter of providing a better understanding of the currently employed concepts of cancer metastasis and treatment in man.

2.1. Malignancy as a diffusing fluid

One of the first organized attempts to understand cancer dissemination was made by Galen (AD131–203). According to Galen the black bile (one of the four humors) was responsible for malignancy. Wherever it concentrated a cancer developed. In his autopsy studies he interpreted distant foci of breast cancer as pools of black bile. Only a minor modification of this theory occurred in the ensuing 1400 years. Paracelsus (1493–1541) re-interpreted Galen's black bile as representing mineral salts. Wherever such salts concentrated cancer occurred. This observation may have been related to the not infrequent findings of calcifications present in malignancy of many types. The disease was considered ubiquitous in the human host, and, the primary tumor was not distinguished from secondary deposits or metastases [5].

2.2. Historical development of the cellular theory of metastasis

In the late 18th century before the discovery of the cellular nature of all biological material (Schleiden and Schwann, 1928), some surgeons were empirically using the concept of embolic metastasis in their approaches to surgical therapy. In 1778 Guy [6] wrote in reference to breast cancer:

> '...if any of the diseased, or contaminated parts remain after the operation, even to the degree of a fibre it will reassume...a fresh disease, the same as at first.'

The cellular theory of cancer metastasis awaited the work of Johannes Peter Muller, who in 1828 established that cells were basic components of malignant diseases. In the next year Joseph Claude Recamier demonstrated the presence of secondary deposits of carcinoma of the breast in the brain of a patient. He also noted invasion of the disease into the veins at the primary site in the breast, and, he coined the term 'metastasis' to describe the secondary tumor growths [5]. Rudolph Virchow (1821–1902) expanded Muller's views and in his famous cellular pathology [7] of 1863 expounded the doctrine on this 'cellula' (all cells from a cell). Yet, paradoxically, despite his conviction of the basic cellular composition of malignant tumors, Virchow retained a humoral theory for the secondary deposits of dissemination of malignant disease:

> 'The manner in which metastatic diffusion takes place is by means of certain fluids and these possess the power of producing an infection which disposes different parts to a reproduction of a mass of the same nature as the one which originally existed.'[7]

Sir James Paget, a renowned surgeon of the same era (1814–1899) likewise maintained:

> 'We need not assume that corpuscles of pus or cancer, or any kind of germs already formed, must be thus carried for multiplication or dissemination of disease. A rudimentary liquid, an unformed cancerous blastema, mingled with blood, may be as effectual as any germs; and must almost necessarily be assumed, in the explanation of cures in which dissemination takes place ... in organs beyond.'[8]

Solid evidence was needed to refute the humoral concept of metastasis. Karl Thiersch (1822–1895) studied metastasizing epithelial tumors of the skin by serial sectioning techniques. He reasoned that the malignant epithelial cells found in lymph nodes reached this position by cellular embolism. He also stated that, although toxic fluids are released from malignant growths, it is the cancer cells themselves that produce metastases. Thiersch (1865) performed autopsy studies of a woman with carcinoma of the uterus. Metastases were present in pelvic lymph nodes, ovary and external iliac veins. Also, clusters of identical tumor cells were present in the thoracic duct. The entire pattern could be explained by the known anatomy of the circulation, further supporting the cellular theory of metastasis [5]. He also supported his conclusions with many other clinical observations. Further Langenbeck [9] showed in 1841 that cancer cells could be microscopically identified in the blood of patients dying with metastases. In 1878 Waldeyer extended Thiersch's proof by studies of metastases of gastrointestinal carcinomas tracing their origins to the epithelial primary tumors. Hoggan (1878) [19] wrote a persuasive treatise 'On Cancer and Its Relationship to Lymphatic Vessels,' which supported this concept. Von Recklinghausen (1885) [11] showed that neoplastic obstruction of lymphatics can cause re-routing and opening of collateral lymphatic channels explaining some unusual sites of metastasis. Thus in the late 19th century the cellular theory of metastasis became solidly established [5, 6, 12].

Figures 1A and 1B. Squamous cell carcinoma of the hand which metastasized to epitrochlear and axillary lymph nodes. This gentleman presented with the large squamous cell carcinoma of the ulnar aspect of the left hand. A partial hand amputation was performed sparing the thumb, index and middle finger. One year later metastases were clinically apparent in the epitrochlear lymph nodes at the level of the elbow. These underwent resection. Fourteen months after this metastasis, metastatic lymph nodes were palpable in the left axilla and he underwent a left radical axillary lymph node dissection. Since then two small recurrences have occurred in the skin of the upper arm. Currently, 5½ years after the initial picture (Figure 1A) was taken he remains free of disease locally and systemically. Such clinical observations engendered the cellular-embolic concept of cancer metastasis, and such current clinical observations remain consistent with the time-space progression of neoplastic disease in man.

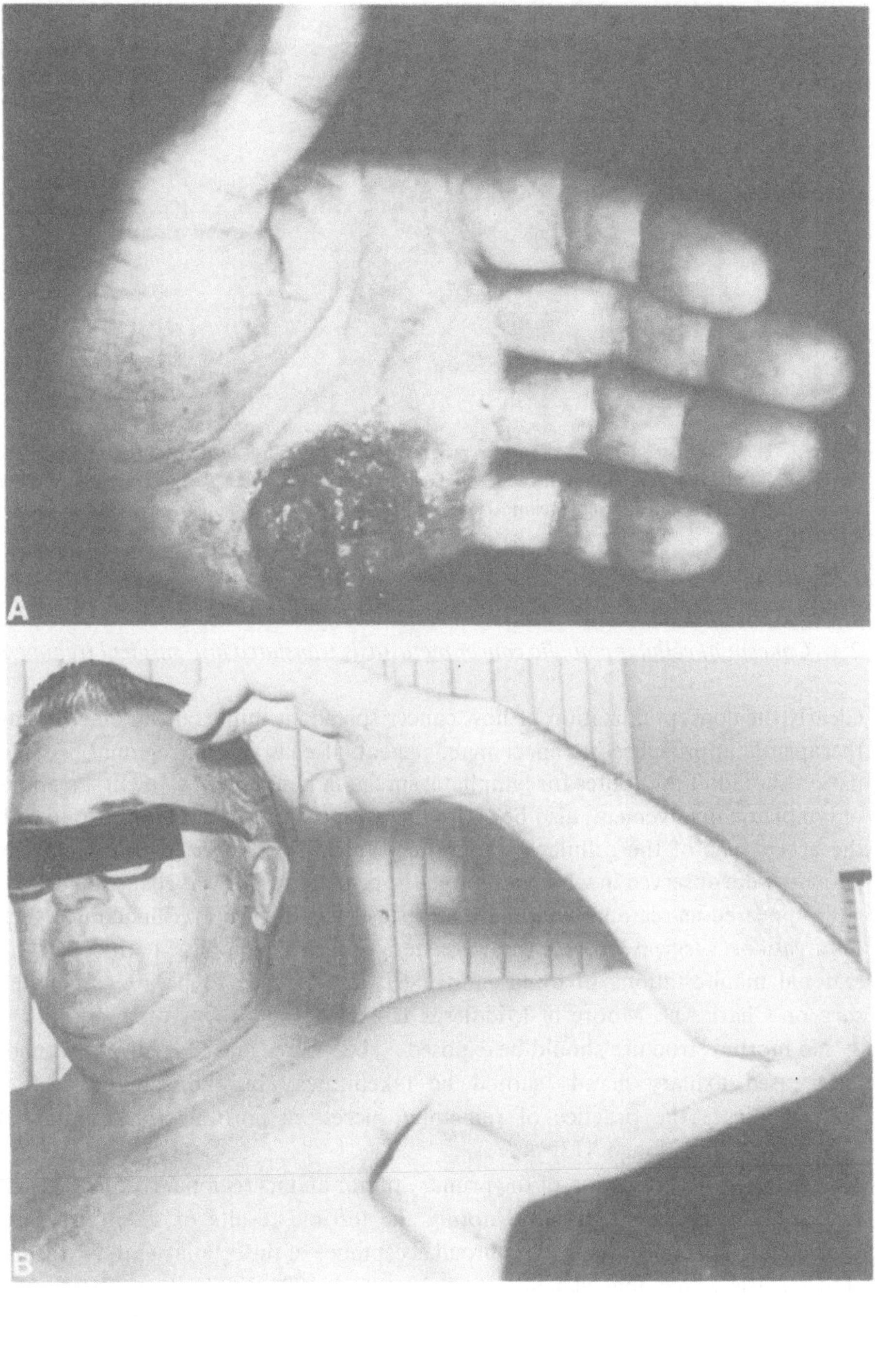
A
B

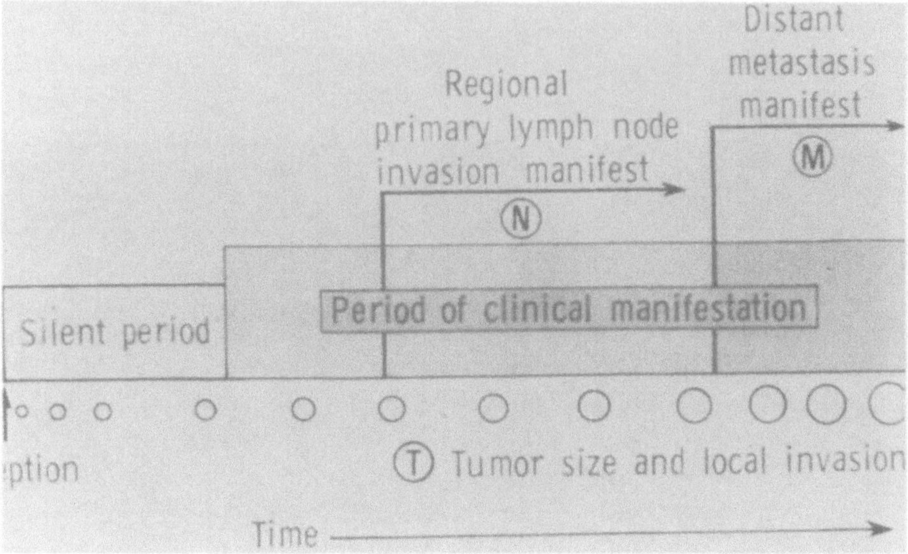

Figure 2. The time-space concept of cancer progression. Cancer surgical procedures, and also the design of radiotherapy ports utilize this concept of cancer progression. In the last decade, however, this concept has been modified in many clinical situations to include direct and early systemic or distant metastases.

2.3. Concept of cellular embolic cancer metastasis translated into surgical treatment

Clearly the conceptualization of how cancer spreads is important in determining therapeutic approaches in cancer management. If cells caused regional dissemination shouldn't the routes for lymphatic spread in lymph nodes, the first stations of lymphatic involvement, also be extirpated with the primary tumor? Along with the acceptance of the cellular-embolic mechanism for cancer metastasis, many patients were observed in whom although the primary tumor was removed, disease later appeared as regional lymphatic metastasis (see Figure 1). Pursuant to such observations surgical procedures were designed to encompass both local and regional manifestations of disease. In 1867, in reference to breast carcinoma, surgeon Charles H. Moore of Middlesex Hospital, England, wrote:

> 'No morbid structure should be exposed ... be set free and lodge in the wound. Diseased axillary glands should be taken away by the same dissection lymphatics... the practice of removing successive portions (of the tumor) should be abandoned.'[13]

The idea of *en bloc* resection of the primary tumor and its regional lymphatics was thus soundly based empirically (noting the terrible results of a limited local excision [8]) and conceptually with broad acceptance of the cellular-embolic theory of metastasis. Some final elements of proof came in 1906–1907 with publication of the classic clinico-pathological studies of malignant melanoma [14] and breast carcinoma [15] by W. Sampson Handley. These studies histologically traced the routes of metastasis through the lymphatics to regional lymph nodes in patients who had succumbed to their diseases. These clinical observations resulted in the conclusion that the regional nodes were a *filter barrier* which 'trapped' the disease, at least for a time. The necessity for surgical extirpation of regional nodes in addition to wide removal of the primary lesion was an obvious extension of logic and became widely accepted.

The time-space progression of metastasis in human malignancies as demonstrated in Figure 2 became the accepted theory.

Precise definitions of the anatomical routes for regional metastasis were provided by Sappey [16] and allowed for the design of surgical procedures which would extirpate regional lymph nodes. Between 1890 and 1908 *en bloc* procedures of radical mastectomy (Halstead) [17], in continuity node dissection for melanoma (Pringle) [18], abdominal perineal resection (Miles) [19], and radical neck dissection (Crile) [20], were designed around the cellular-embolic concept of regional cancer dissemination and immediately began to save the lives of many patients who otherwise would have succumbed to their disease. The enthusiasm of these early authors is obvious and major advances were made by these surgical applications of this concept of metastasis.

2.4. Extensions of the surgical perimeter based on cellular-embolic concept of regional cancer metastasis

When some recurrences and metastases were noted despite *en bloc* resection, a major direction in cancer therapy – from 1910 to the 1960s – was to extend the surgical perimeter to include more tissue about the primary tumor. With the well-known advances in surgical technique, blood replacement, antibiotics and intensive care over this period, super-radical extirpation became feasible. The Whipple procedure (pancreaticoduodenectomy) [21], extended radical gastrectomy [22], super radical mastectomy [23], and even hemicorporectomy were all devised within this conceptual framework and one tributes to the ingenuity and daring of surgical innovators, as well as their concern for the survival of their patients. However, this was an era of diminishing return for most patients so treated because of the problem of distant metastatic disease.

2.5. Revisions of the cellular-embolic nature of metastasis to include metastatic cancer as a systemic disease

Despite these extensions of the surgical perimeter to their absolute anatomical limits many patients still died from systemic metastasis. Surgery alone, although successful in eradicating the primary, often failed to 'trap' the disease in the regionalized state. The regional cellular theory of metastasis, which initially established this concept of *en bloc* surgical resection, had to be expanded to include the frequently systemic nature of metastatic dissemination. Experimental studies showed that shortly after vascularization of an experimental tumor, embolizing tumor cells could be identified in effluent lymphatic and/or venous drainage [24, 25, 26]. Many studies in resected human surgical specimens have demonstrated free tumor cells in the effluent veins draining the specimen of a resected breast [27] or colon specimen [28]. Likewise, circulating cancer cells have been noted in the peripheral blood of patients with 'curable' tumors and without clinically detectable distant metastases [29].

Studies of the serum and drainage from surgical wounds after completely successful resection of human malignant tumors have also demonstrated viable cancer cells. Smith [30] studied washings obtained from operative wounds in cancer patients prior to wound closure. Twenty-six percent had positive washings. Although the patients with positive washings did a little poorer then those that were negative, the positive group had in general more advanced cancers at the time of surgery. A subsequent study by this same group looked at cancer cells in operative wound catheter drainage. Six of 40 were positive and some patients did not develop positive cytology for three to five days after surgery, suggesting that these cancer cells may have seeped back into the operative wound from surgically transected lymphatics. The viability of at least some of these cells in wound catheter drainage has been documented by *in vitro* tritiated thymidine uptake experiments [31]. These observations, along with other confirmatory experimental data demonstrating the translymphnodal passage of tumor cells [32, 33, 34], have created the major current concentration on the systemic nature of most human malignancies. Not to be ignored, however, is the fact that many patients with regional lymph node metastases are still apparently cured by surgical extirpation of the primary tumor and the involved regional lymph nodes. This fact indicates at least the partial validity of this initial concept of the regional-embolic conceptualization of cancer spread. It is the concept which is still employed in most current cancer operations.

3. Observations related to regional and systemic metastasis in man

3.1. Correlation of primary tumor diameter and the probability of metastasis to regional lymph nodes in carcinoma of the breast, colon, malignant melanoma, and other malignancies

From the turn of the century most breast cancers have been treated by radical mastectomy [17]. This operative procedure gives opportunity to accurately

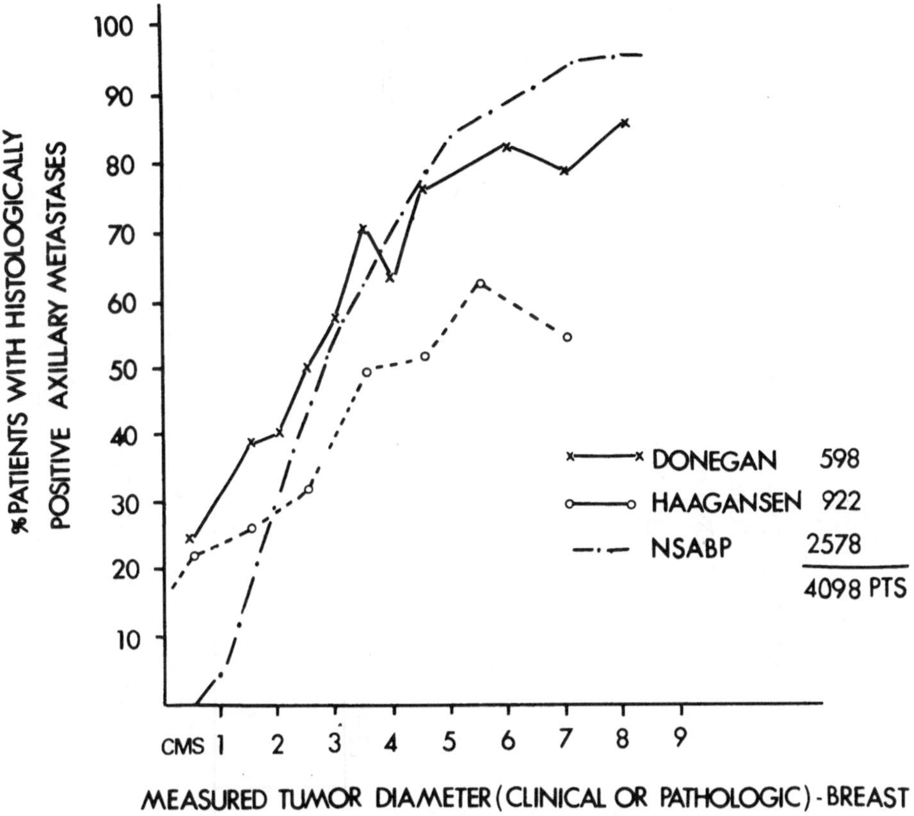

Figure 3. Correlation of the primary size of a breast malignancy with the incidence of regional axillary lymph node metastases in the surgical specimen.

measure the size of the primary tumor and to correlate the primary tumor diameter with the presence of positive metastatic lymph nodes in the simultaneously resected axilla. Haagensen [35], Spratt and Donegan [36] and Fisher et al. [37] have presented such data for a total of 4098 patients as seen in Figure 3. The striking correlation of regional axillary lymph node metastasis with the size of the primary breast cancer is readily apparent. Despite this strong association with the primary breast cancer size, however, it should be noted that between 16 and 20 percent of patients with tumors less than 1 cm in size – non-palpable – were found to have axillary metastases. As is noted in a subsequent portion of this chapter some 3–6% of patients with breast cancer present as adenocarcinoma metastatic to the axilla and no primary can be clinically detected in the breast. Conversely, even in some 15–30% of very large primary breast malignancies, in the 7–9 cm category, there is no histologic metastasis to the axilla. Thus, although size has a strong correlation with the incidence of observed metastasis, a subpopulation of breast cancers exists which metastasizes from very small lesions, or, not at all from very

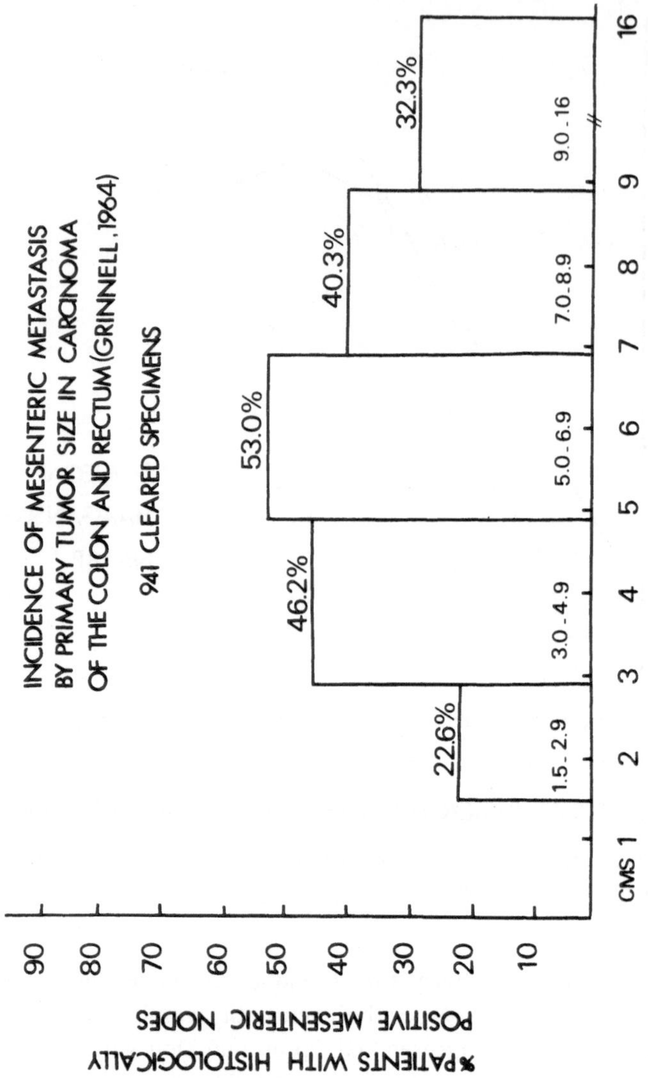

Figure 4. Incidence of mesenteric lymph node metastases correlated with the primary tumor size in colon carcinoma.

large ones. As the clinician works with an individual patient, these variations in metastatic potential interfere with precise and accurate treatment planning, and create significant controversy over individualized patient treatment decisions.

3.2. *Correlation of tumor size and metastasis in colon cancer*

Excellent data are available in the studies of Grinnell [38]. Of importance in these studies is the fact that all surgical specimens were cleared and lymph nodes were subjected to multiple histopathologic sectioning. These data (Figure 4) clearly show a size relationship of metastasis to primary colon tumor size up to the 7.0 cm diameter. Then, by virtue of the fact that patients with grossly obvious systemic metastases are not considered for surgery, only patients with better biologic variants of the disease are selected for surgical management, leading to an apparent reduction in the incidence of metastases associated with primary lesions of over 7 cm. Thus in both breast and colon carcinoma a definite size-correlation of primary tumor to the probability of lymphatic metastasis is present. Nevertheless subpopulations at either end of the size spectrum are present as were noted in breast adenocarcinoma.

It is also possible that the *time* from primary tumor residence influences the incidence of metastasis. Since patients are treated very shortly after diagnosis of malignant disease, it is not possible to accurately evaluate this possible parameter in clinical material as has been done in experimental data.

3.3. Correlation of the thickness of a primary malignant melanoma with risk of metastasis

Breslow [39] has demonstrated a similar strong correlation of melanoma thickness, as measured by an optical micrometer, with the risk of metastasis (Figures 5 and 6). As recently reviewed [40], for melanomas less than 1.5 mm in thickness the risk for a regional lymph node metastasis is only 7%. If the primary tumor thickness is greater than or equal to 1.5 mm, the risk for regional lymph node metastasis rises to 23%. Balch et al. [41], in a multifactorial analysis, showed that primary tumor thickness was one of the most important independent variables affecting risk for regional lymph node metastasis in patients with clinical stage I malignant melanoma.

Transitional carcinoma of the bladder, carcinoma of the stomach, squamous cell carcinoma of the lung, and other neoplasms also show a correlation of primary tumor size to the probability of regional lymph node metastasis and/or survival after surgical treatment. As will be discussed subsequently some malignancies of very high metastatic potential do not show any such size correlation with metastasis.

3.4. Why does primary tumor size correlate with metastasis?

As indicated by experimental models, as soon as vascularization of the initial tumor occurs, tumor cells enter the circulation. Wound washing studies [42] and studies of circulating tumor cells from surgical specimens [27, 28] or peripheral blood [29] demonstrate presence of disseminating cells even in patients who are

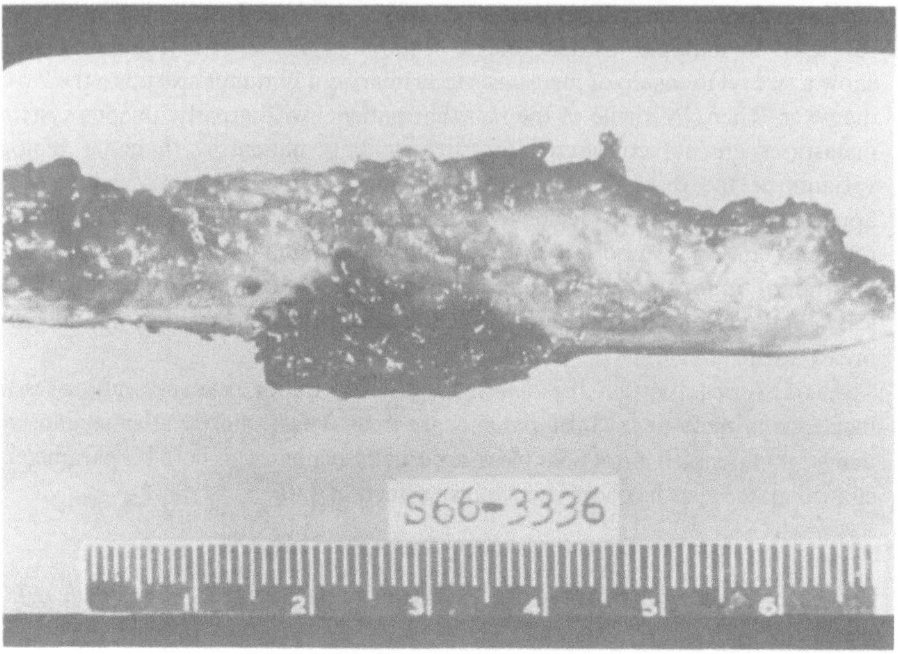

Figure 5. Cross-section of an advanced primary malignant melanoma. By taking multiple cross-sections the maximum depth of penetration (thickness as measured with an optical micronometer) can be measured and correlates directly with recurrence and/or metastasis.

cured by extirpation of the primary tumor. Why is it, then, that for most common malignancies tumor size has this important correlation with actual metastasis formation? Larger numbers of tumor cells enter the circulation from larger tumors, and thus a dose response aspect of metastasis may be partly responsible for increasing the incidence of regional and/or systemic metastasis. It is also possible that tumor cells with a greater propensity for metastasis evolve in the larger primary tumor, and, that these are the cells selected eventually for metastasis formation. The evolution of such alterations in the malignant phenotype and/or genotype could become more likely as the lesion contains more cells and more time passes. Aspects of the evolution of heterogeneity for metastasis are discussed in other portions of this book. A third possibility is that with increasing size, the host environment is eventually favorably modulated for metastasis by release of antigenic material, necrotic debris, and other cellular and/or subcellular material as is discussed in other portions of this book. The pathoetiology of this size – metastasis correlation, however, has as yet no comprehensive explanation.

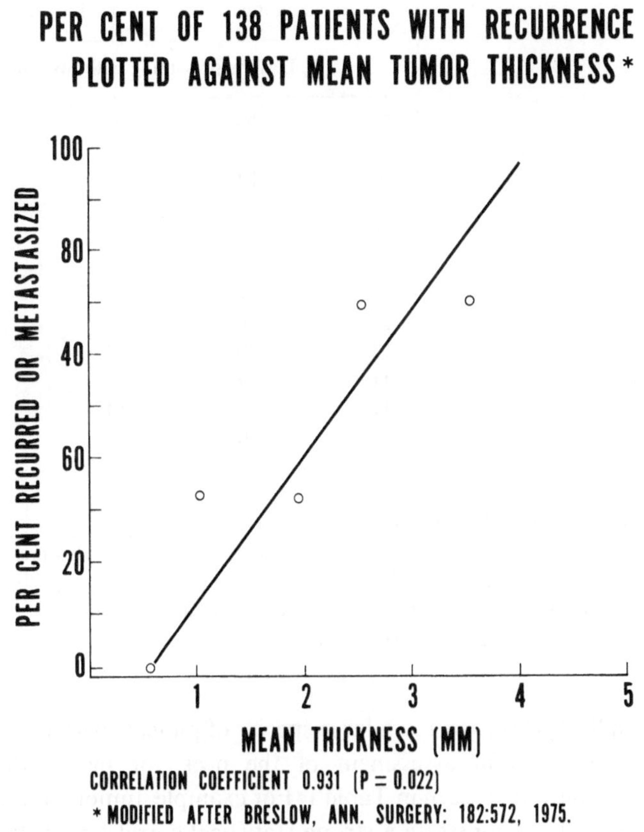

Figure 6. The correlation of recurrence with the thickness of malignant melanoma. Thickness as a measure of tumor volume and also penetration correlates well with the eventual incidence of recurrence and/or metastasis.

4. Defining metastatic potential in clinical cancer

As demonstrated, primary tumor size is statistically an important parameter of the risk for regional lymph node metastasis and eventual prognosis. Therefore, size can become a reference point in assessing metastatic potential. Let us define *metastatic potential* as the *statistical probability of metastasis in relationship to the size of the primary tumor*. To help us develop this concept let us look at a group of histologically similar squamous-cell tumors in the head and neck region. The size of the primary tumor can be accurately and directly measured by direct examination, and, the presence or absence of regional lymph node metastasis can be accurately determined by careful examination and/or biopsy of lymph nodes in the neck. This group of squamous cell carcinomas originating from multiple anatomic sites within the head and neck is known to vary widely in metastatic

Table 1. Metastatic potential of squamous cell carcinoma of head and neck by anatomical location.

	% Lesions presenting with neck metastases*			
	T_1	T_2	T_3	T_4
Nasopharynx	93	84	89	83
Base of tongue	70	71	75	84
Tonsil	70	68	70	89
Hypopharynx	63	69	79	73
Supraglottic larynx	39	41	66	59
Oropharyngeal walls	25	30	67	76
Mobile tongue	14	30	47	76
Floor of mouth	11	29	43	53
RMT-AFP	11	37	54	67
Soft palate, Uvula	8	36	65	77

Reproduced with permission from Lindberg [57].
*Those lesions presenting with the highest incidence of neck metastases also presented with more advanced neck disease (2044 cases of head and neck cancer, M.D. Anderson). T_1 = ≤ 2 cm (diameter); T_2 = >2 cm ≤ 4 cm; T_3 = >4 cm ≤ 6 cm; T_4 = >6 cm and massive tumors.
**Retromolar trigone and anterior faucial pillar.

potential. Lindberg [43] reported a large species of patients with careful (primary) staging and also careful assessment of the neck for metastatic disease. A modification of his data is seen in Table 1. For example, tumors of the tongue and floor of the mouth demonstrate a strong statistical correlation between primary tumor T-stage (measured size) and the presence of regional neck metastasis, as has already been discussed in reference to adenocarcinoma of the breast, colon, and melanoma. On the other hand, squamous cell carcinoma of the nasopharynx, tonsil, and base of the tongue shows no significant correlation between primary tumor size and the presence of neck metastasis. In these latter tumors a very high incidence of neck metastasis is present regardless of the size of the primary tumor. These cancers, including cancer of the nasopharynx, therefore, can be described as having very high metastatic potential while the metastatic potential of lesions of the tongue and floor of the mouth would be termed moderate.

4.1. Generalization of the concept of metastatic potential in human cancer

The concept of metastatic potential can provide some unification of thought about metastasis of human neoplasia, and may guide the choice of appropriate experimental models of metastasis relevant to the specific clinical cancer under study. At the high end of the spectrum of metastatic potential are the 'liquid' cancers of leukemias and many lymphomas. Diffuse organ dissemination of these

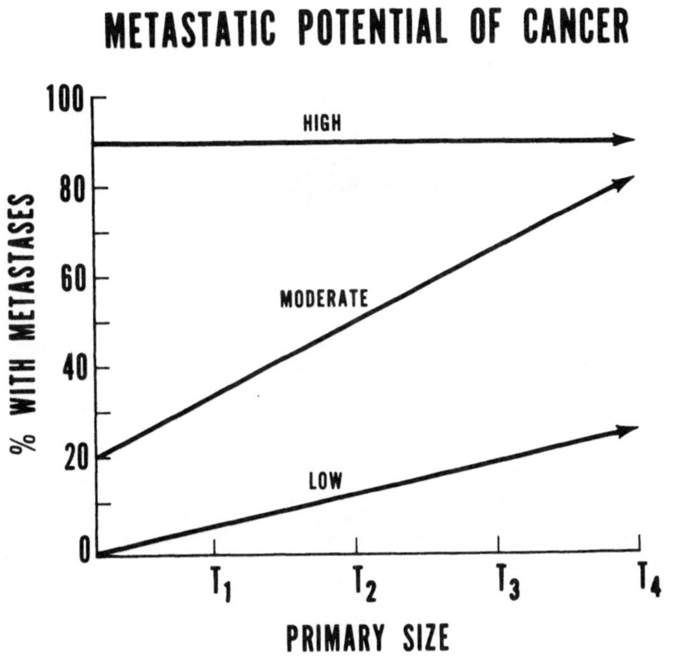

Figure 7. Metastatic potential of human cancer. One defines metastatic potential as the statistical probability of metastasis in relationship to the size of the primary tumor; most human malignancies can be broadly classified as having high, moderate, or low metastatic potential. Exceptions to this generalizing concept are noted in the text and may be very important in an individual clinical decision.

malignant diseases often takes place from inception. Small cell carcinoma of the lung, and undifferentiated carcinoma of the thyroid gland are similar lesions from which dissemination seemingly also occurs from the inception of the neoplasm (Figure 7). In the common solid epithelial tumors (breast, squamous cell carcinoma of the lung, and colon cancer), metastasis can be definitely related statistically to the size of the primary as has been discussed. Within each population of these tumors with moderate metastatic potential, however, are tumors that behave uncharacteristically and metastasize either very early, thus contribution to the problem of metastasis from an *occult* primary malignancy as subsequently is discussed, or fail to metastasize despite the primary attaining an enormous size.

At the lowest end of the spectrum of metastatic potential are the basal cell cancers, lip cancers, demoid, and ondrosarcomas which, as a rule, attain huge clinical proportions without metastasis (Figures 8, 9, 10 and 11).

One of the central problems in clinical oncology is the inability to precisely assess metastatic potential for an individual patient (as opposed to a population of patients). Thus, radical surgery may be performed and, despite the apparent success of the technique, the patient eventually may succumb to metastasis.

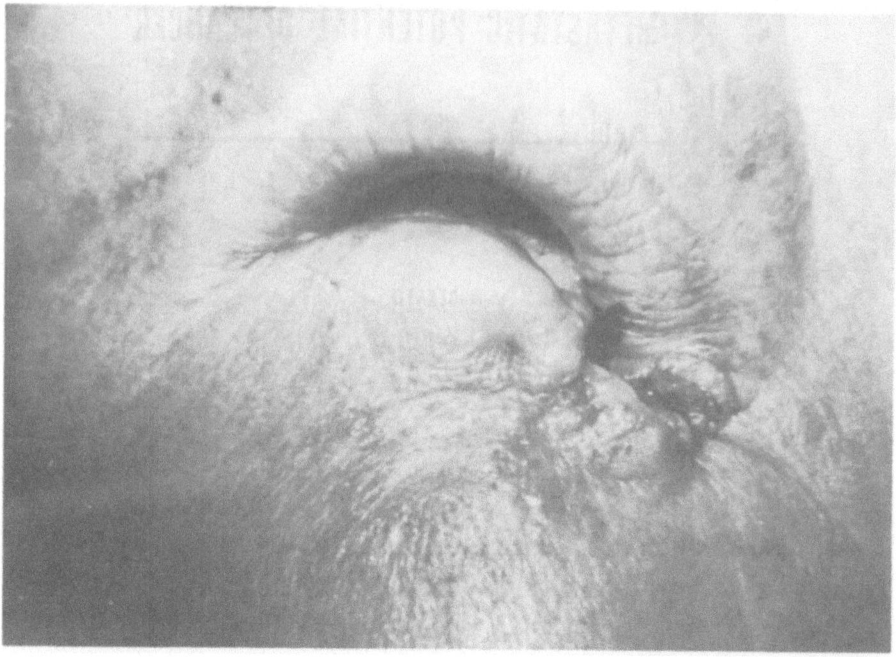

Figure 8. Large carcinoma of the lower lip with very low metastatic potential. This patients remains cured five years after an excision and reconstruction of this large invasive squamous cell carcinoma of the lip.

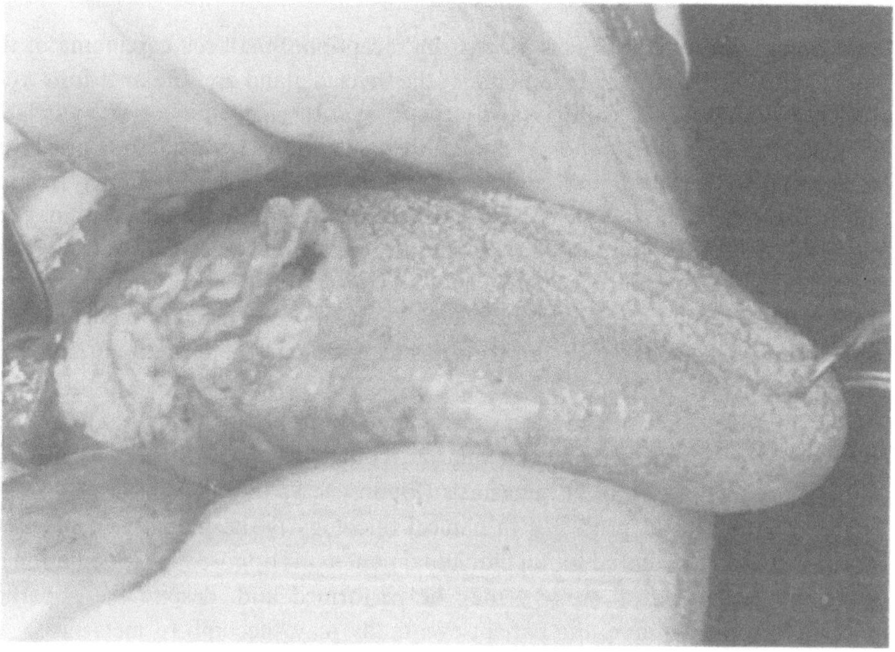

On the other hand large cancers may still carry a good prognosis encouraging aggressive therapy if somehow their low metastatic potential could be identified and characterized accurately. Of equal importance is the fact that without accurate assessment of metastatic potential, even randomized prospective clinical trials could produce spurious results. Since study design cannot include stratification for this important and unmeasured biologic variable, more patients could be included in one study arm at the expense of another, thus spuriously influencing treatment results.

Additionally, it would seem appropriate for experimental model systems of metastasis to attempt to approximate the metastatic potential of the type of human malignancy that is under study.

4.2. *Metastasis as related to the rate of primary tumor growth*

It is well known that most rapidly growing tumors prove lethal to patients or experimental animals in a short period of time, if not extirpated or treated appropriately. Burkitt's lymphoma of childhood is an example of such a lesion. The doubling times of pulmonary metastases have been measured and in a group of untreated patients reported by Spratt and Spratt [44], the shortest survival correlated, as it would be expected, with the shortest metastatic doubling time.

The questions not answered by these observations are: (1) Whether the more rapidly growing primary tumors of a given histologic type have a greater propensity for metastasis, (2) Whether they metastasize no differently from slow growing tumors of the same type, but, are associated with a shorter survival time (poor prognosis) because the rapid growth rate is also expressed by rapid growth of the metastases, or (3) a combination of both.

If indeed the primary tumor growth rate correlates with the metastatic potential of a given primary tumor, analyses of tumor cell kinetics in resected surgical specimens could help identify patients at great risk for subclinical dissemination. Also, the variability for prognosis of metastasis in any given tumor type could be reduced by considering not only the primary tumor size but also tumor cell kinetics. Preliminary studies by Temple et al. [45] indicate that flow cytometric analyses of tumor cell kinetics in primary human colon cancer add to the predictability of the Duke's staging system for metastasis and prognosis.

Figure 9. Squamous cell carcinoma of the posterior one-third of the tongue. Such squamous cell carcinomas of the posterior one-third of the tongue have a very high metastatic potential. This patient presented with palpable lymph nodes in the neck and, after radical resection of tongue along with radical neck dissection, eventually developed pulmonary metastases and expired three years after this photograph was taken.

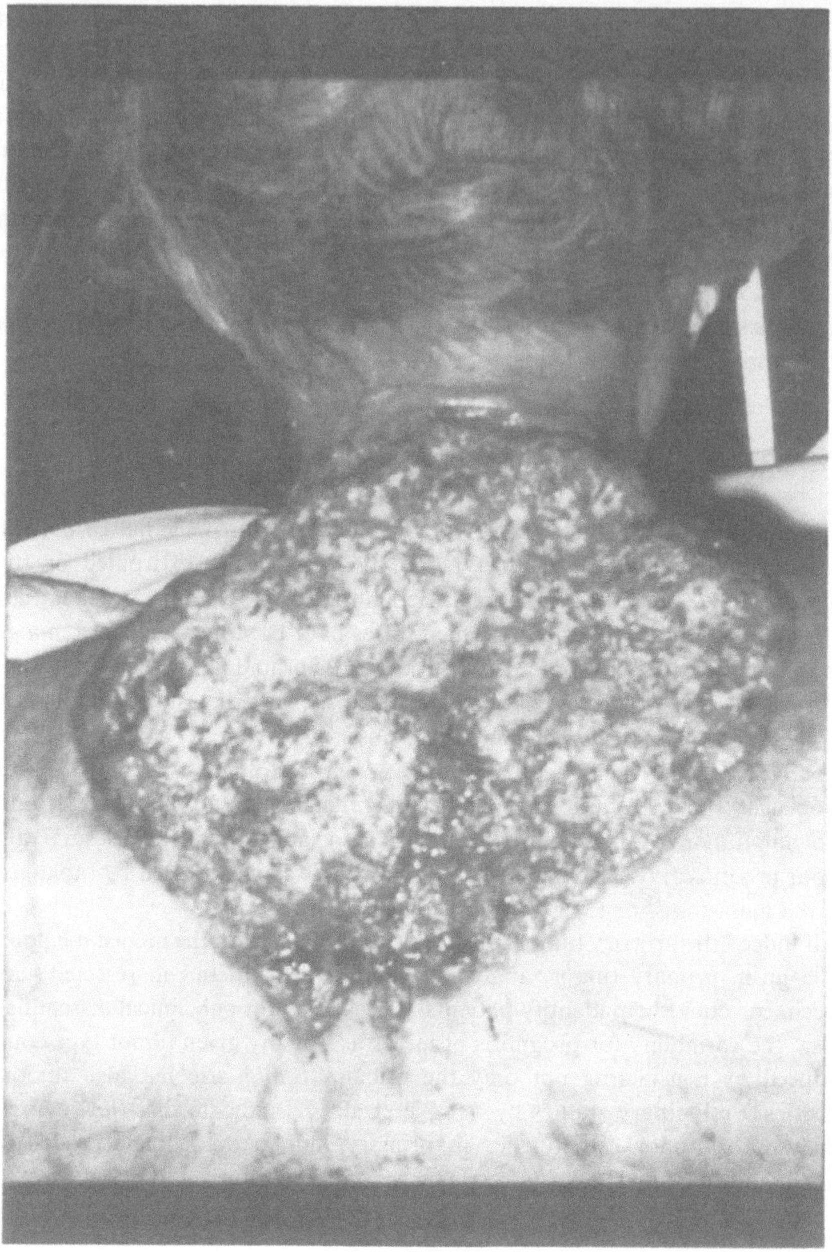

Figure 10. A massive basal cell carcinoma of the back. These lesions despite attaining massive sizes over prolonged periods of time (this patient has a ten-year history) virtually never metastasize.

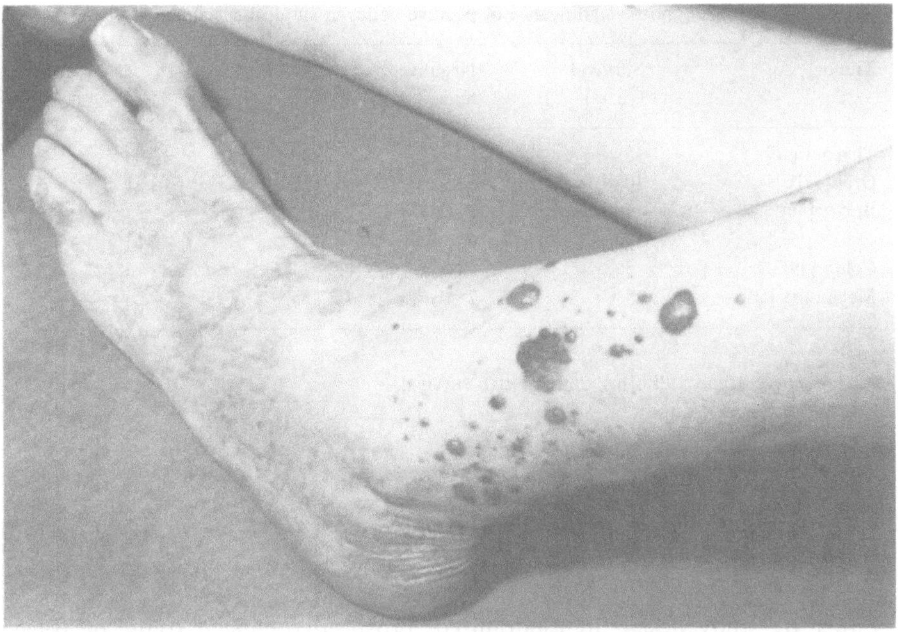

Figure 11. Malignant melanoma of the lower extremity with extensive regional intransit metastases. Despite the smaller size of primary malignant melanoma as opposed to the basal cell carcinoma noted in Figure 10, melanoma tends to metastasize more readily. The propensity for metastasis correlates with the thickness of the primary malignant melanoma as indicated in Figure 6.

4.3. Correlation of prognosis with the presence of regional lymph node metastases.

Even when all gross and microscopic regional tumor has been removed, metastasis in regional lymph nodes in a surgical specimen indicates a poorer prognosis. As indicated in Table 2 the prognosis is diminished as the number of the lymph nodes increases in colon carcinoma, breast carcinoma, and melanoma. The usual explanation for the detrimental effect of positive lymph nodes on prognosis is that when some glands are involved, the higher secondary nodes, and/or lymphatico-venous nodal collaterals, transport cells to systemic organs as occurs in experimental systems [32, 33, 34]. However, of great interest is the fact that regional lymph node metastasis from papillary carcinoma of the thyroid has absolutely no effect on prognosis with over 15 years of follow-up observation as documented in Table 2. Therefore, there is not uniformly a negative correlation of lymphatic metastasis with prognosis.

Table 2. Varying prognostic significance of positive nodes in surgical specimens.

Tumor	Survival (years)	Negative nodes	1–3 Positive	>3 Nodes
Thyroid [46]	15	89	90	92
Oral [47]*	10	57	50	31
Breast [48]	5	78	62	32
	10	65	38	13
Colon [49]	5	48	24**	6***
Melanoma [50]	5	75	55	26

*Regional recurrence; all other data refer to survival.
**Colon 1–5 nodes.
***Colon >5 nodes.

4.4. Varying growth potential of micrometastases identified in human surgical specimens

Either by study design in randomized, prospective clinical trials, or because differences of opinion exist within the medical community as to the efficacy of regional lymph node dissection, there are interesting comparisons of the incidence of occult (not clinically palpated) metastases in regional lymph nodes with the numbers of gross metastases evolving as macroscopic growths during clinical follow-up if the lymph glands are left intact. As seen in Table 3 less than 10% of occult metastases identified in papillary carcinoma of the thyroid ever grow to a clinically palpable status within a 15-year follow-up interval. Similarly, in

Table 3. Growth potential and dormancy of occult lymph node metastasis.

Histologic type	Surgical specimen positive (%)	Evolution of nodes in observed patients	Growth potential (%)
Thyroid (United States) [51]	61%	<10%	<10
Thyroid (Japan) [52]	82%		
Breast* (NSABP) [53]	40	15	37.5
Melanoma (United States) [50]	28–30%	30–35**	
Melanoma* (Europe) [54]	19.7%	24.2	~100
Squamous cell carcinoma (tongue)	23–46%	27–50%	~100

*Randomized prospective clinical trials.
**More than 5 years' observation of patients.

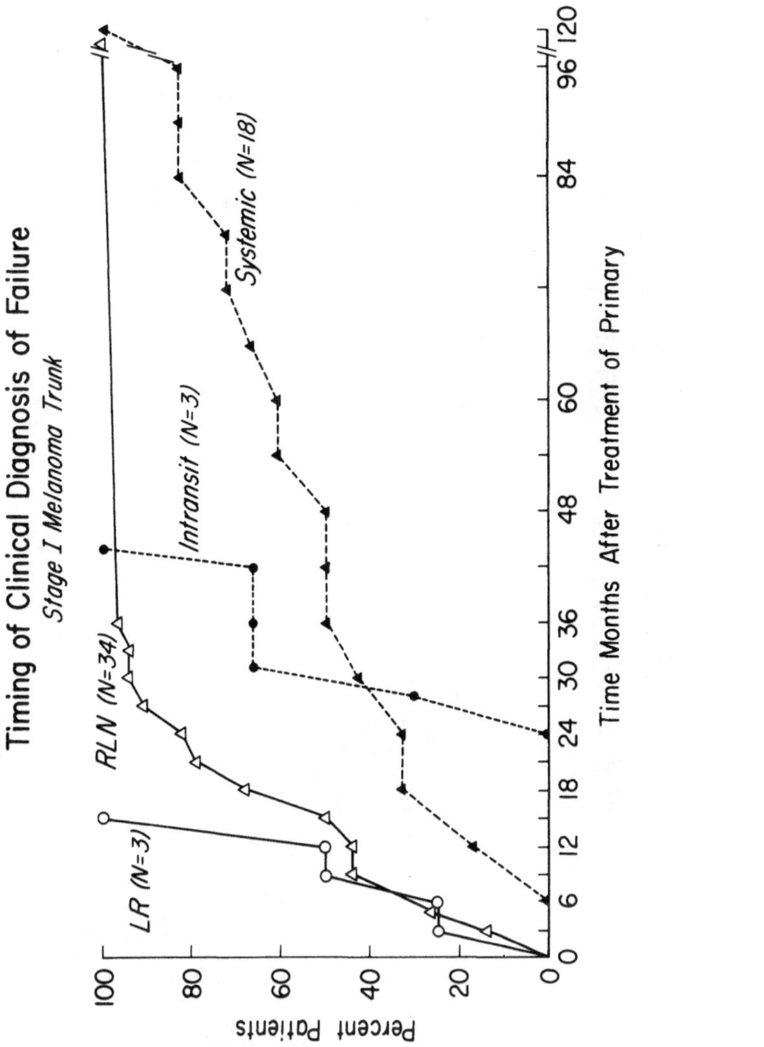

Figure 12. Time course to recurrence after excision of malignant melanoma of the trunk.

carcinoma of the breast 40% of the axillary surgical specimens were found positive for occult metastatic disease. However, in a parallel group of patients in this randomized prospective clinical trial, in which the axillary lymph nodes were not resected, only 15% grew to grossly palpable status with up to five years of observation. Thus, the growth potential of occult lymphatic metastasis in carcinoma of the breast can be approximated at 37.5%. On the other hand, in malignant melanoma and squamous cell carcinoma of the tongue, similar comparisons give an estimate of essentially 100% growth potential for occult regional metastases. Thus, even after metastasis has occurred there is significant variation in the human model as to the growth potential and/or dormancy of

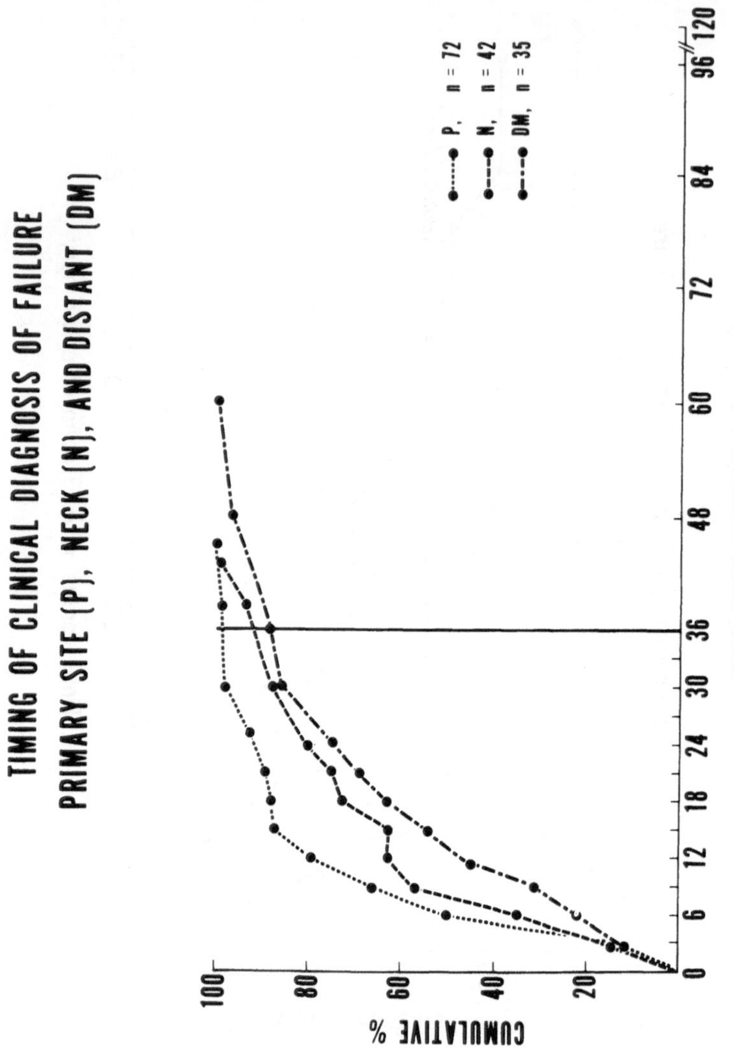

Figure 13. Time course to recurrence after definitive treatment of squamous cell carcinoma of the oropharynx.

micrometastatic regional lymphatic disease. Definitions of the conditions contributing to the dormancy of micrometastases in regional lymph nodes would be of great interest, as would the development of an appropriate experimental model for studies of this phenomenon.

4.5. Timing of appearance of metastases after surgical resection

One of the most striking differences between the appearance of metastasis in man and in experimental tumor systems is the long time interval required for the expression of metastatic disease. Experimental model systems usually evaluate times to metastasis in a few weeks or, at most, several months. In comparison, the development of metastasis in the human host is a very prolonged event, often years in length and, as noted, even dormancy of micrometastases can be demonstrated in regional lymph nodes. This prolonged residence of disseminated tumor cells intuitively adds great complexity to mechanisms of tumor-host modulation of the ability of these disseminated cells to actually succeed as a microscopic metastasis. For each histologic class of tumor, the time course to evolution of metastasis regionally, or in distant organs, follows a relatively characteristic pattern. Figures 12 and 13 compare the *sites* of *first metastasis*, after definitive treatment of primary malignant melanoma of the trunk (Figure 12) or squamous cell carcinoma of the oropharynx (Figure 13), versus the time to recurrence. For melanoma patients observed 5–10 years after treatment a broad range of time to metastasis is apparent and it is influenced by the site of metastasis. The risk for local recurrence and the evolution of positive regional lymph nodes is limited essentially to the first 24 months after treatment. However, for distant organ metastasis in melanoma, the evolution is much slower. In fact, about 50% of such metastases became clinically apparent during the 5–10 year period of observation after treatment. Examples of recurrence of malignant melanoma more than 10 years after apparent cure can be readily found (Figure 14). The course of squamous cell carcinoma of the oropharynx after definitive treatment is much less variable. More than 95% of local recurrences (primary P site failures), regional node recurrences (N) and distant metastases (DM) develop within three years. Squamous cell carcinoma of the oropharynx, therfore, tends to be much more homogeneous in terms of the development of metastatic disease.

The great variability in the clinical course of patients with malignant melanoma, breast carcinoma, thyroid carcinoma, colon cancer, and stomach cancer has fostered the concept of tumor cell dormancy [3]. The unfortunate surprise of a delayed systemic metastasis appearing 5–10 years or more after treatment, when both physician and patient have rationally and emotionally sealed the illness behind them, produces an indelible imprint in a physician's clinical experience. Therefore, this type of delayed metastasis has received a great deal of attention, and, coupled with the rare event of spontaneous regression [1] has provided great impetus to studies of host defense and contributed significantly to interest in the discipline of tumor immunology.

4.6. Early post-operative metastatic explosions and a possible inhibitory effect of the primary tumor on disseminated tumor cells

Most locally advanced human cancers are resected for apparent 'cure' after the usual systemic workup for metastasis proves negative. However, explosive

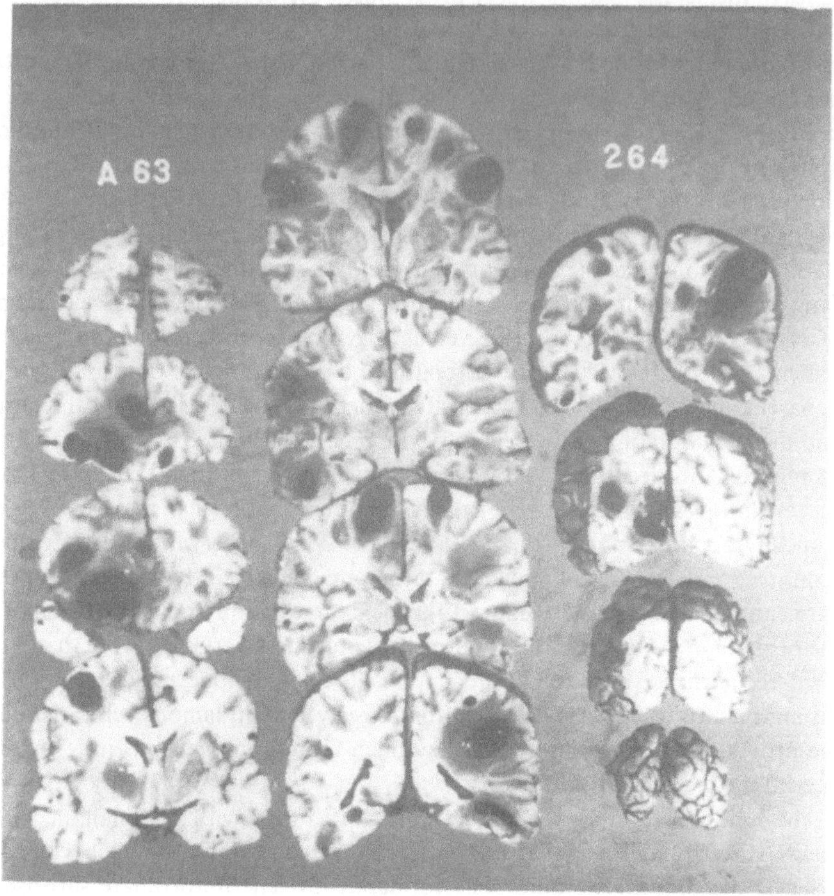

Figure 14. Dormancy of malignant melanoma. This autopsy specimen is from a patient who developed a cerebrovascular accident and expired. Fourteen years previously a melanoma had been excised from the back. These delayed metastases were the eventual cause of his demise.

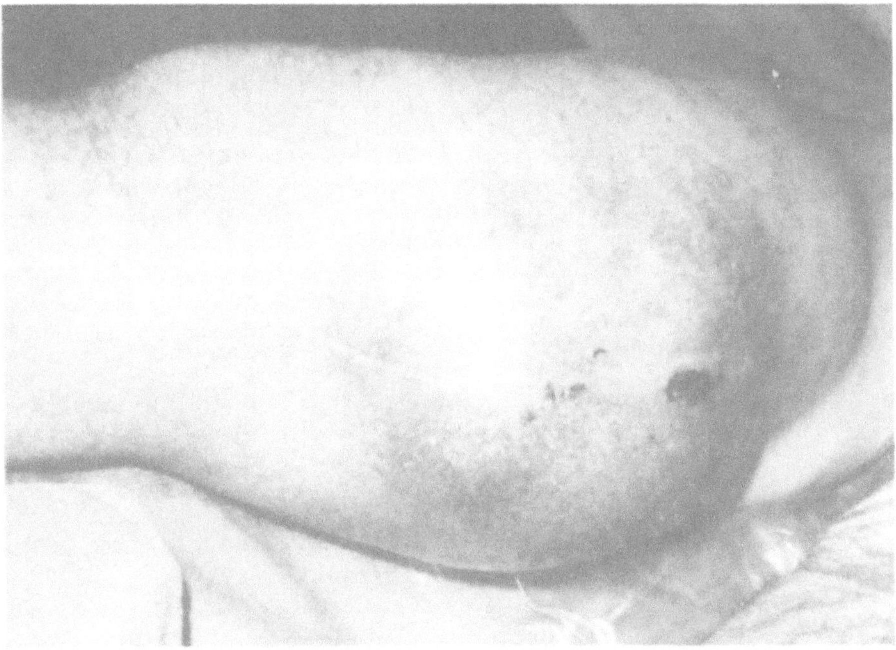

Figure 15. Large recurrent fibrosarcoma of the right thigh. For 2½ years this patient had a growth noted in the right thigh which had been partially excised on two occasions with recurrence. At this time a hip disarticulation was performed after a thorough search for metastasis. This search included full chest tomography which was negative for even small metastases in the lungs.

metastatic recurrence after resection for advanced malignancy is not an uncommon clinical observation. In other patients palliative or partial tumor resection is sometimes followed by what appears to be an accelerated development of metastatic disease. When such observations are made, questions invariably arise as to the biologic mechanisms involved. As early as 1913 Tyzzer [55] queried:

> 'In patients in which metastasis has already occurred will the growth of secondary masses be accelerated by the removal of the primary tumors ... Do ... surgical operations increase or diminish the incidence of metastasis?'

Figure 16 is a chest x-ray showing multiple pulmonary metastases that appeared four months after the resection of a large and recurrent primary extremity sarcoma (Figure 15) which had been in place for nearly two years. Immediately prior to surgery the patient had undergone full chest tomograms to exclude even small metastases. An amputation of this tumor was performed and the first post-operative chest x-ray shows multiple large pulmonary metastases. An inhibitory effect of a primary tumor on disseminated tumor cells has been demonstrated in several experimental tumor systems [2] and possible mechanisms are discussed elsewhere in this book.

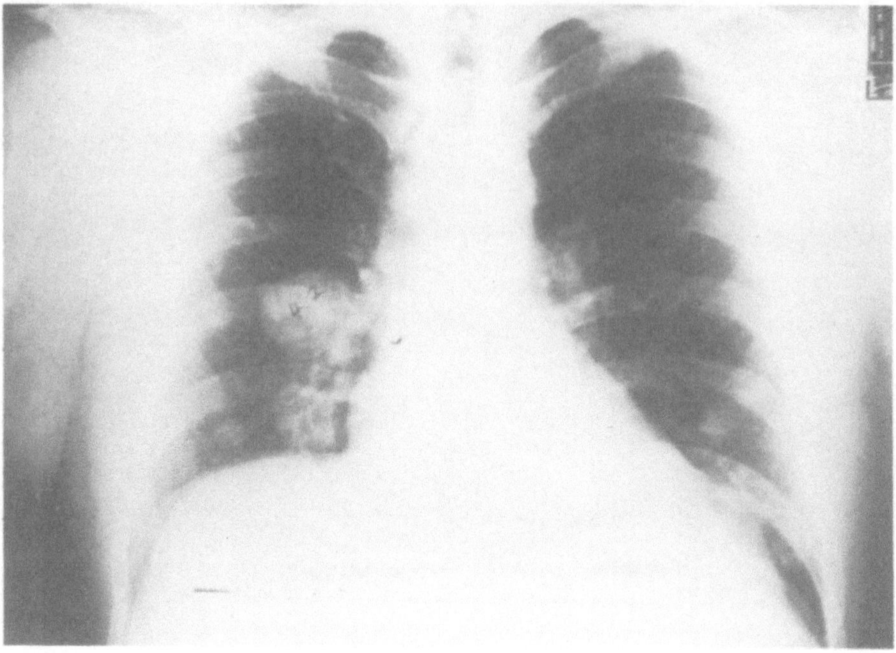

Figure 16. Multiple pulmonary metastases. This chest x-ray was obtained on the patient seen in Figure 15 four months after hip disarticulation as treatment of this sarcoma. Note that multiple pulmonary metastases are present. Such explosive appearance of metastatic disease after surgical resection has fostered the concept that the primary tumor may have an inhibitory effect on disseminated tumor cells.

4.7. Organ patterns of metastasis in human malignancies

As recently reviewed [56], two important parameters affect an observed pattern of metastases in human malignancy. The metastatic potential of the primary tumor and the stage of the malignancy at the time of the study are of importance.

Tumors of very high metastatic potential tend to involve multiple organs by the time of diagnosis and no definite pattern of organ trophism can be identified. For example, in small cell carcinoma of the lung essentially 100% of patients have multiple systemic organs involved by metastases at the time of diagnosis. A bone marrow aspirate, in fact, is positive in 50% of patients at the time of diagnosis of this malignancy, and the brain is so frequently involved that 'prophylactic' brain irradiation has become a standard part of many treatment protocols for small cell carcinoma of the lung. Similarly, multi-organ systemic metastases are usually present in undifferentiated carcinoma of the thyroid. For carcinoma of the nasopharynx – as mentioned as squamous cell carcinoma of high metastatic potential, bilateral neck metastases are usually present at the initial diagnosis and systemic metastasis is the most commonly seen amongst the squamous cell carcinomas of the head and neck.

In the moderate range of metastatic potential, the initial site of diagnosed metastasis (if indeed present at all) is most commonly determined by the anatomical relation of the regional lymphatics or draining veins of the primary tumor. For example, in squamous cell carcinomas of the head and neck classified as having moderate metastatic potential, and despite the diffuse intercommunicating collateral lymphatics, Lindberg [57] clearly demonstrated preferential or *sentinel* sites for lymph node metastasis within the neck from carcinoma of the tonsil, mobile tongue, floor of the mouth, and so on. This preference is clearly related anatomically to the site of the primary tumor and the sentinel drainage of its lymphatics. Huvos et al. [58] have shown that even within the lymphatic system of the axilla a stepwise progression of lymphatic metastasis through three defined levels is most commonly observed in patients with breast carcinoma. Similarly, for hematogenous metastasis, the first organ encountered by circulating tumor cells, for instance the lung from soft tissue and bone sarcomas, or the liver in carcinoma of the colon, becomes the dominant site for initial hematogenous metastasis.

Even though the initial pattern of metastasis in tumors with moderate metastatic potential is dominantly determined by anatomical mechanical routing of the tumor cells, there are important examples of early systemic organ metastases which are not explained by this mechanical concept. As indicated in Table 4, the fact that metastasis from hypernephroma (clear cell carcinoma of the kidney) is the most frequent metastasis seen in the thyroid gland, supports the concept of organ trophism of these tumor cells to the relatively small thyroid gland [59]. Similarly, the localization of melanoma in non-regional skin, and small bowel mucosa (Figure 17 as a frequent initial site of metastasis is peculiar and reminiscent of the embryologic dissemination of neural crest stem cells to these organs. However, ocular melanoma most frequently metastasizes to the liver [60]. The Kruckenberg tumor is the relatively frequently observed metastasis of gastrointestinal tract adenocarcinomas to the ovary [61]. And breast cancer is not infrequently attracted to the pituitary or the ovary, perhaps as an expression of the hormone trophism in estrogen receptor positive breast carcinomas. At the time of

Table 4. Early systemic metastases indicating organ trophism.

Primary site and histology	Organ of metastasis
Clear cell carcinoma (kidney) [54]	Thyroid
Cutaneous melanoma	Small bowel mucosa and non-regional subcutaneous sites
Ocular melanoma [60]	Liver
Adenocarcinomas of gastrointestinal tract [61]	Ovary (Kruckenberg tumor)
Breast	Ovary and pituitary, bone
Follicular carcinoma thyroid	Bone

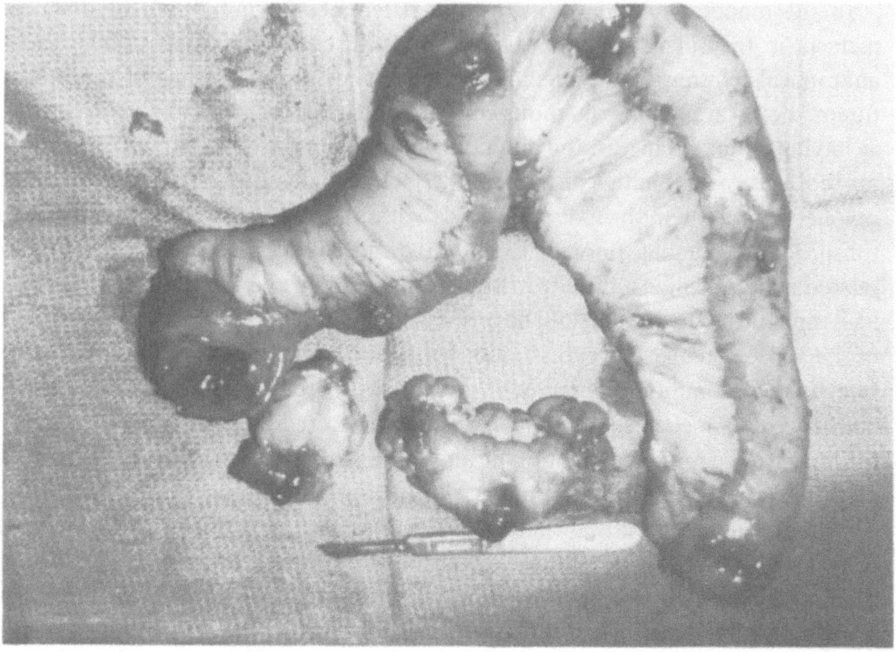

Figure 17. **Multiple metastases of malignant melanoma to the small bowel mucosa. Malignant** melanoma frequently metastasizes to the small bowel and/or other cutaneous sites. This unusual site of metastasis is considered a definitive example of organ trophism during metastasis. In a patient with a history of malignant melanoma, it is stated that the most common cause of gastrointestinal bleeding is metastatic malignant melanoma to the small bowel mucosa.

initial diagnosis the metastases listed in Table 4 are frequently solitary, further supporting organ trophism in metastasis even in the earlier stages of systemic human neoplastic dissemination.

4.8. Autopsy patterns of metastasis in man

In the terminal phases of neoplastic dissemination, particularly in patients whose primary disease has been controlled or in whom there is no disturbance with a critical organ's function by the primary tumor, full expression of a 'pattern' of metastasis should become apparent. Table 5 has been compiled from data previously published and includes a selected list of most common malignancies of humans, and analyses of metastases to most of the major internal organs [56]. This list of tumors was chosen to emphasize some of the interesting differences in patterns of metastasis observed in the different human malignancies.

Several interesting generalizations are possible from these data. The first is that the most frequent metastases in all these tumors occur in the first organ encountered by the hematogenously circulating tumor cells, emphasizing the importance of the anatomical route of venous drainage and therefore tumor cell circulation not only for early lymphatic metastasis but also, in these autopsy data, pertaining to hematogenous metastasis. However, metastases in subsequent organs from the listed primary definitely display different organ patterns of metastasis. For instance, bone, brain, adrenal, and pituitary are much more frequently involved by metastatic carcinoma of the breast, than by metastases from carcinoma of the colon. Both carcinoma of the breast and malignant melanoma originate in the peripheral soft tissues and seldom kill by virtue of large primary disease. Therefore, in patients dying of these illnesses one might expect possibly similar systemic patterns of tumor cells dissemination. The incidences of metastases in major organ sites of lung and liver are indeed quite similar. However, breast carcinoma shows a much greater affinity for bone than does melanoma. As opposed to breast carcinoma, melanoma more frequently involves the brain and has the highest reported incidence of metastasis to the spleen. All of the tumors listed show a surprising affinity for the small adrenal glands with metastases in 14–54%. Adenocarcinomas of the breast, colon, and stomach involve the ovary in a significant percentage of cases whereas primary cancer of the kidney and lung seldom produce metastases in the ovaries. The putative infrequency of metastases to the spleen, often quoted in the older literature, is not borne out by these data.

4.9. Organs that more frequently reject metastases

Thus, clinical data support an organ affinity as contributing to the pattern of

Table 5. Autopsy organ incidence of metastasis according to primary site and histology.

Autopsy organ Site of metastasis	Primary tumor (%)					
	Lung	Colon	Breast	Melanoma	Hyper nephroma	Stomach
Liver	30–50	50–60	40–61	58–70	16–27	30–40
Lung	20–40	25–40	60–80	66–80	40–65	24–33
Bone	30–50	5–10	50–85	30–49	19–40	6–11
Brain cerebrum	15–43	1	15–29	40–55	<1	5
Adrenal	17–38	14	38–54	47	20–24	21
Pituitary	1	<1	20	16	<1	<1
Ovary	1	14	15–23	10–13	<1	15
Kidney	16–23	8	12–13	31–35	—	11
Spleen	9	5	17	31	6	6

metastasis from several human malignancies. Also of interest is the fact that some organs are so infrequently the site of metastasis despite a high volume of perfusing blood. Muscle, either skeletal or cardiac, rarely becomes the site of metastasis except in metastatic melanoma [60, 62]. Similarly, the kidneys, which receive 20–25% of the cardiac output, are less commonly involved than the adrenal glands which receive proportionately much less blood and therefore many fewer tumor cells (Table 5). From experimental studies on tumor cell arrest patterns it was seen that the circulating tumor cell passes on through some resistant organs. The exact nature of such transorgan passage and/or organ resistance to metastasis is of obvious interest for future studies.

Other clinical observations demonstrate that the dominant pattern of metastasis can be altered by acute tissue trauma or inflammation [4]. Additionally, corticosteroid therapy and/or chemotherapy have been observed to alter the typical pattern of metastasis in man [56].

Knowledge of the patterns of metastasis has practical clinical value. The anatomically predicted patterns of initial lymphatic metastasis govern a careful clinical examination of regional lymph nodes, and influence the design of surgical extirpative procedures. Pre- and post-treatment diagnostic search for metastatic disease focuses on organs most likely to become the sites for metastasis for a given malignancy. For instance, lung tomograms are essential in evaluating a patient with a soft tissue sarcoma prior to surgery as this is the likely first site of metastatic disease. Bone scans are important in a patient with breast cancer, and a bone marrow biopsy is critical in a patient with small cell carcinoma of the lung. In general, the dominant sites of metastasis found in autopsy data govern the application of these organ-specific diagnostic procedures which are in search of metastatic disease. Finally, a significant number of patients present with metastases as a dominant manifestation of their disease. Knowledge of the usual patterns of metastasis for a given histologic type of occult primary tumor under such circumstances works in reverse and serves as a guide to the diagnostic search for the primary lesion as is discussed subsequently.

5. Metastases from an unknown primary tumor: an enigmatic aspect of metastasis in man

As discussed, the proposed mechanism for metastasis in that tumor cells embolize from a definable primary focus to a distant site. In clinical practice, local or systemic metastases are sometimes found as the earliest manifestation of an as yet undiagnosed or occult primary tumor. Often the primary site is not determined until well after the metastatic disease is recognized and sometimes, surprisingly, the initial focus is never identified and patients are cured by resection of the metastatic disease. In other patients who die of the malignancy the primary tumor may never be identified even after thorough autopsy evaluation. A number of possible mechanisms have been suggested for the occurrence of metastases from 'occult' or 'unknown' primary sites.

In tumors with high metastatic potential the primary tumor by virtue of its small size may be undetected. In tumors of moderate metastatic potential, such as breast carcinoma and others, occasionally regional metastases appear from clinical inapparent or undetectable primary sites. Ashikari et al. [63] have reviewed a series of female patients presenting with adenocarcinoma metastatic in the axillary lymph nodes but the breast was negative on examination and mammogram for a primary lesion. Nevertheless, mastectomies were performed and carcinomas were discovered on pathologic examination of the breast in most women and about one-third of these primary tumors were less than 1 cm in size. In ten patients no primary tumor could be found in the breast, and the survival of these patients was similar to those in which the primary tumor was eventually identified. Many patients were cured of their disease despite the fact that regional metastases had occurred. In other clinical situations the metastasis can represent an outgrowth of a metastasis which develops from a primary lesion which was iatrogenically removed or destroyed. Typically, a history may be obtained of a mole, or a colonic polyp that was removed or destroyed some time before the appearance of detectable metastases. Later a focus metastatic develops in regional lymph nodes or other organs (liver with colon polyps) and one in retrospect surmises that the initial lesion was a malignant primary tumor; sometimes this is impossible to document.

Cases of spontaneous regression in patients with melanoma have been well documented [1]. Smith and Stehlin [64] have presented arguments for this hypothesis as the usual explanation for metastases from an occult primary melanoma. An alternative, but less frequently accepted explanation, is the development of malignancy *de novo* in the distant site. Benign nevus cells [65], breast tissue [66], and thyroid tissue [67], have been documented in peripheral lymph nodes. The presumption is made that malignancy can develop by neoplastic transformation of these benign tissue rests occurring in these ectopic sites. Controversy also surrounds the development of epidermoid carcinoma in the branchiogenic cyst as the cause of an isolated focus of squamous cell carcinoma in the neck. Martin et al. [68] outlined the criteria for the diagnosis of branchiogenic carcinoma. However, recently Batsakis [69] cautioned that this diagnosis be accepted very tentatively pending the outcome of a very thorough direct search for an occult primary neoplasm in the mucosa of the head and neck area.

In the last few decades a large number of clinical reports on metastases with unknown primary have been published (Table 6). While the lung is frequently identified as a primary site, pancreas, stomach, and oropharyngeal primary malignancies are also frequently seen. The lung, liver, lymph nodes, and bone are the most common initial presenting metastatic sites when the primary is unknown. To locate the primary tumor the presenting metastatic site and histologic features are the most significant determinants. Osteen [73] has stressed the importance of

Table 6. Sites of initial metastases and eventual location of unknown primary tumor.

Author [ref]	No. cases occult primary	Site initial tumor metastasis	No. patient primary found (%)	Identified primary site (%)
Holmes & Fouts [70]	784	lymph nodes bone lung liver	98 (13)	
Nystrom et al. [71]	264	liver lung lymph nodes	125 (47)	pancreas (20) lung (18) liver (11)
Didolkar et al. [72]	254	lymph nodes lung bone	77 (30)	lung (40) pancreas (7) stomach (7)
Osteen et al. [73]	67	bone liver lymph node (neck)	38 (57)	lung (47) pancreas (16) ovary (13) colon (13)
Smith et al. [74]	53	—	15 (28)	lung (33) pharynx (27) tongue (13)

obtaining an adequate tissue sample in order to accurately identify the histology of the malignancy. Nystrom [71] has developed discriminate function values based on these factors enabling the clinician to restrict the location of the primary tumor to above or below the diaphragm accurately in 80% of patients.

In some cases the metastases might exhibit a biochemical marker that gives a clue to the site of the primary tumor. Golumb and Thomasen [75] identified estrogen receptor protein in undifferentiated carcinomas with unknown primary which suggested the origin was from breast carcinoma and also opened the therapeutic possibility of hormone manipulations. Rudnich et al. [76] report a case of gonadotropin secreting testicular tumor in a male college student that defied the detection until located as a 4 mm nodule in the testis at autopsy. In this case a hormonal marker never seen in the normal male pointed to the testis as the primary site of the tumor.

In patients presenting with metastases only in regional lymph nodes the search for the primary is based on the documented anatomical patterns of lymphatic dissemination [50]. The principle of looking towards organs in the afferent lymphatic drainage of a metastasis in patients with cervical lymph node metastases is also pertinent. Metastases in the lower neck (supraclavicular or level V) most often originate from infraclavicular sites, and those in the upper neck follow the topographic distribution of nodal metastases from known primary lesions as detailed by Lindberg [43]. Jesse et al. [77] report that when the nasopharynx is included in the radiation port for such patients with neck metastases from occult

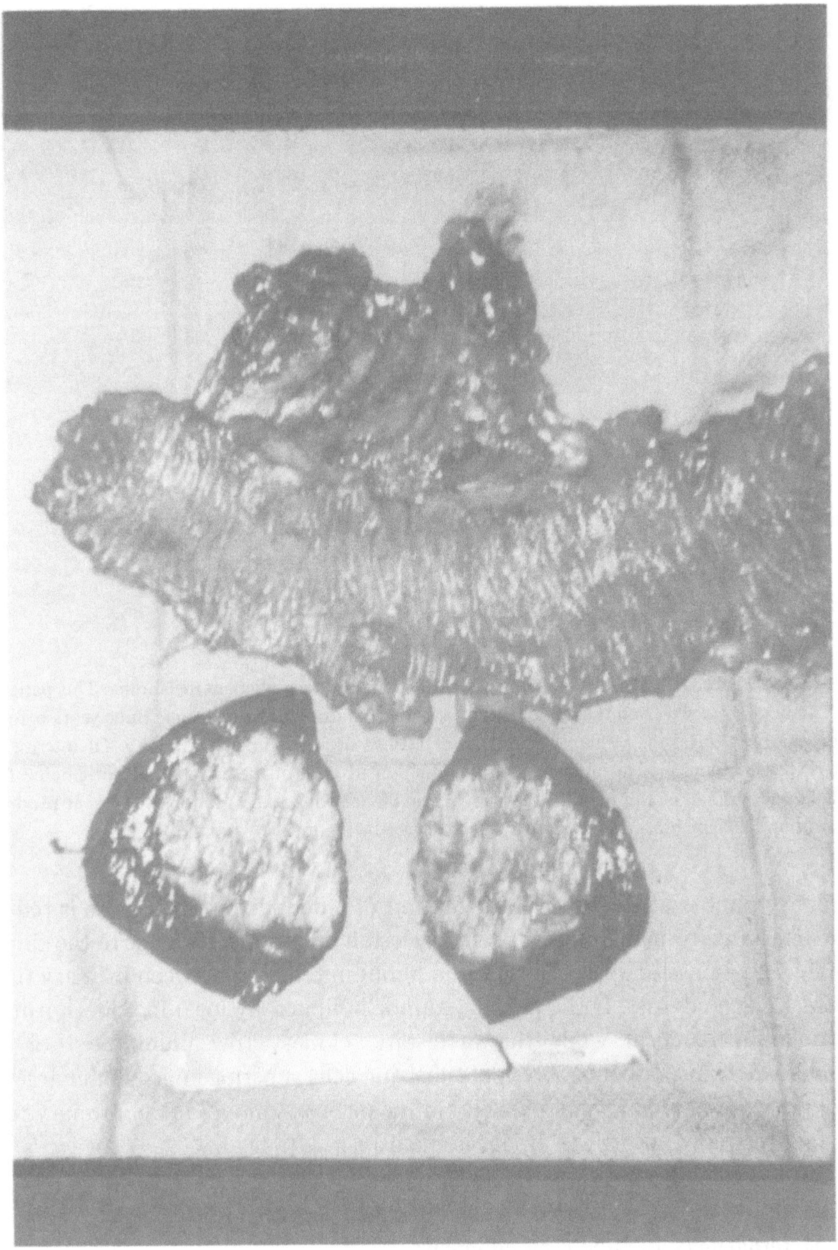

Figure 18. Possible kinetic heterogeneity in human colon carcinoma. This patient was found to have a mass in the liver and on careful seach a small carcinoma was found in the sigmoid colon. Pictured in juxtaposition to this small sigmoid carcinoma is a very large solitary liver metastasis which was simultaneously resected at the same time the colon lesion was removed. The marked size difference in the primary tumor versus the large metastases in the liver suggests possible kinetic heterogeneity in the primary human colon carcinoma, with superior growth characteristics demonstrated in the clone which grew as a liver metastasis.

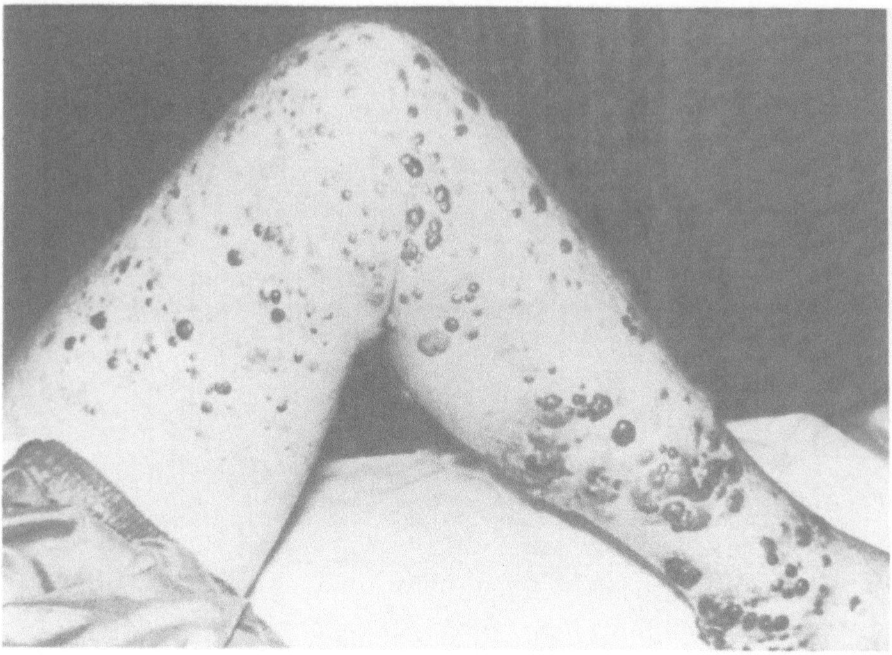

Figure 19. Heterogeneity for pigment production in metastatic malignant melanoma. This patient had a melanoma resected from the ankle, and a radical groin dissection done some three years before this photograph was taken. Miliary cutaneous metastases occurred in the extremity. Of interest is the marked heterogenity of melanin pigment production. If each of these metastases originated from a single cell or small clump of cells, they have been cloned for great variation in pigment production. Variation in pigmentation is seen to a lesser degree in Figure 11.

primary tumors, the subsequent evolution of a definable primary site is reduced.

Metastasis from an unknown primary lesion presents a challenge to the clinician and offers a possibility for speculation about interaction between primary tumor, metastases, and host. Is the primary tumor inhibited by local factors (hormonal, population kinetics) while the metastatic clones grow uninhibited or even facilitated at distant sites? Are metastasizing cells superior in growth characteristics reflecting a kinetic heterogeneity in the primary tumor? Is the primary tumor in fact restricted in growth by large metastases [2]?

6. Heterogeneity in human malignancies

Experimental tumors have been shown to be heterogeneous for many phenotypic and/or genotypic characteristics, including the propensity for metastasis [78]. In human malignancy several observable differences between primary tumors and their 'clone' metastases are consistent with this type of heterogeneity in human malignancies as well. The growth rate of metastatic tumors may vary greatly from the primary tumor. Figure 18 shows a very small primary malignant tumor of the colon and its large liver metastasis which was simultaneously resected. Such dramatic difference in size of a primary tumor and its metastasis is consistent with *kinetic heterogeneity* in human malignancy. Organ specific stimulation of tumor cell growth in the metastatic cells might also explain such an observation. Figure 19 shows extensive intransit melanoma metastasis in an extremity with a wide variation in pigment production. Some metastases are amelanotic, some partially melanotic and others show a uniformly black pigment production. If these metastases do represent clones developing from single cells (or small clumps), heterogeneity for pigment production certainly does exist in primary malignant melanoma.

Other clinical observations suggest possible antigenic heterogeneity in human malignancy. Regression zones are not uncommonly seen in primary malignant melanoma. Histologic examination of such regression zones usually reveals an area of dermal atrophy with some free melanin pigment or macrophage-contained melanin. At the inter face of such a zone with melanoma cells an intense host mononuclear cell reaction is often seen. Figure 20 shows a patient whose primary lesion was apparently completely destroyed by host reactive processes. Yet regional lymph node metastases still occurred and at the time of this photograph were about to undergo surgical extirpation. Some 3–5% of all primary malignant melanomas present with regional node metastases and an unknown primary site. As already mentioned it seems likely that host reactivity has eliminated the primary tumor in such patients, but that, the immunogenicity of the metastasizing cells is different and therefore they escape.

7. Critical clinical problems as related to metastasis in man

As has been reviewed, the process of metastasis in man is a complex, multifaceted event involving tumor characteristics, host characteristics, and a complex interrelated tumor-host modulation of this biologic event over a prolonged time course [80]. Certain practical aspects of this event, however, must be emphasized. First, as observed in man, metastases, if present, have occurred at the time diagnosis is made. Therefore therapeutic experimental models should focus on the eradication of established micrometastatic disease with emphasis on treating varying tumor burdens of 10^2–10^9 cells in each possible metastatic deposit. Secondly, the current state of the art is insufficient in its ability to accurately diagnose the presence of metastatic disease. The currently available scanning and radiographic techniques are fraught with continued considerable error. Thirdly, the risk of a given individual patient for metastasis can only be predicted with a statistical probability. Since medicine is practiced one on one, individualized treatment decisions must be made and population statistics are often found insufficient. This major deficiency in the current state of the art creates many

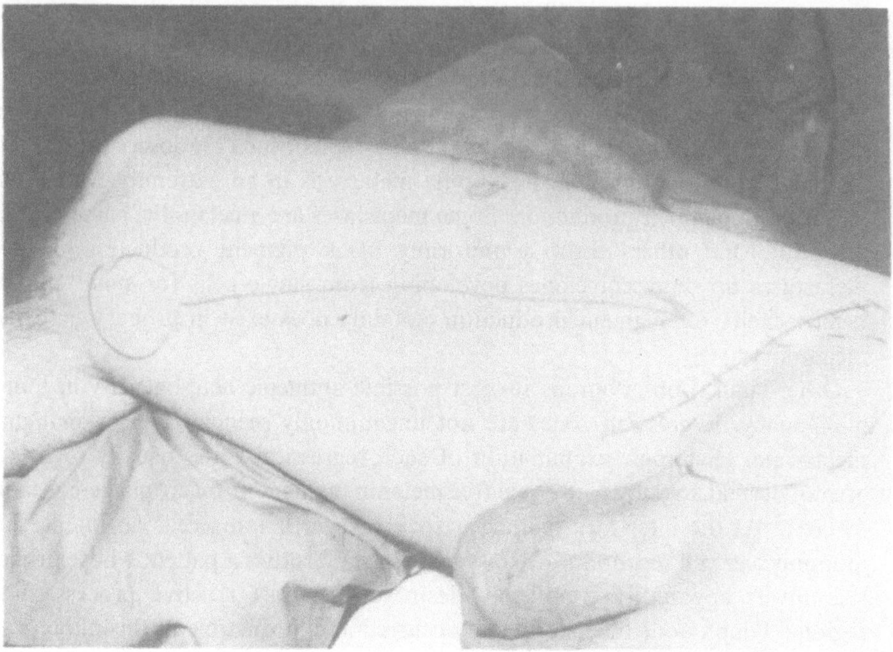

Figure 20. Heterogeneity for 'immunogenicity.' Partial regression in a primary malignant melanoma occurs in 10–15% of all primary melanomas. Sometimes this regression at the primary site is complete as occurred in the patient pictured in Figure 20. The primary site was located on the medial aspect of the right knee. However, metastases developed and at this time the patient is being prepared for a radical resection of palpable metastatic disease which is present in the groin. Total eradication of the tumor at the primary site, with simultaneous or delayed growth of regional metastases suggests that the host defenses to the primary tumor may be successful while metastatic disease escapes.

clinical dilemmas and controversies regarding appropriate treatment of individual patients. Lastly, currently available adjuvant therapy used in addition to primary tumor eradication with surgery irradiation are in general inadequate. It is hoped that continued laboratory research in models *relevant* to the clinical problem of metastases will contribute to improved therapies for this most extreme expression of the malignant cell phenotype.

References

1. Everson TC: Spontaneous regression of cancer. Ann NY Acad Sci 114:721–735, 1964.
2. Sugarbaker EV, Thornthwaite J, Ketcham AS: Inhibitory effect of a primary tumor on metastasis. In: Cancer invasion and metastasis: biologic mechanisms and therapy, Day SB, Laird WP, Myers, Stansly P, Garattini S, Lewis MG. New York: Raven Press, 1977, p 227.
3. Sugarbaker EV, Ketcham AS, Cohen AM: Studies of dormant tumor cells. Cancer 28:545, 1971.
4. DerHagopian RP, Sugarbaker EV, Ketcham AS: Inflammatory oncotaxis. JAMA 240:374–375, 1978.

5. Wilder RJ: The historical development of the concept of metastasis. J Mt Sinai Hosp 23:728, 1956.
6. Onuigbo WI: A history of the cell theory of cancer metastasis. Gesnerus 20:90, 1963.
7. Virchow R: Cellular pathology, Chance, F (trans). Philadelphia: J.B. Lippincott, 1863, p 219.
8. Paget J: Lectures on surgical pathology. London: Longman, Brown, Green and Longmans, 1863, p 580.
9. Langenbeck: On the development of cancer in the veins, and the transmission of cancer from man to the lower animals. Edinburgh Med Surg J 55:251, 1841.
10. Hoggan G: On cancer and its relationship to the lymphatic vessels. Trans Pathol Soc Lond 29:384, 1878.
11. Von Recklinghausen F: Virchows Arch Pathol Anat 100:503, 1885.
12. Onuigbo WIB: A history of hematogenous metastasis. Cancer Res 30:2821, 1970.
13. Moore H: On the influence of inadequate operations on The theory of Cancer. Roy Med Chir Soc 1:245, 1867.
14. Handley WS: The Hunterian lectures on the pathology of melanotic growths in relation to their operative treatment. Lancet 1:927, 1907.
15. Handley WS: Cancer of the breast. London: John Murray, 1906.
16. Sappey MPC: Anatomie, physiologie, pathologie des vaisseaux lymphatiques. Paris: A. DeLayaye et E. Lacrosnier, 1874.
17. Halstead WS: The results of operations for the cure of cancer of the breast performed at the Johns Hopkins Hospital from June 1889 to January 1894, Johns Hopkins Hosp Rep 4:297, 1894.
18. Pringle JH: A method of operation in cases of melanotic tumors of the skin. Edinburgh Med J 23:496, 1908.
19. Miles W: Abdominoperineal operation. Cancer 2:1812, 1908.
20. Crile G: Excision of cancer of the head and neck with special reference to plan of dissection based on 132 operations. JAMA 57:1780, 1906.
21. Whipple AO, Parson WB, Mullins CR: Treatment of carcinoma of the ampulla of Vater. Ann Surg 102:763, 1935.
22. McNeer G, Sunderland DA, McInnes G et al.: A more thorough operation for gastric cancer: anatomical basis and description of technique. Cancer 4:957, 1951.
23. Wangensteen OH, Lewis FJ, Arhelger SW: The extended or super-radical mastectomy for carcinoma of the breast. Surg Clin North Am 36:1051, 1956.
24. Gullino PM: *In vivo* release of neoplastic cells by mammary tumors. Gann 20:49, 1977.
25. Hewitt HB, Blake E: Quantitative studies of translymphoidal passage of tumour cells naturally disseminated from a nonimmunogenic murine squamous carcinoma. Br J Cancer 3:25, 1975.
26. Liotta LA, Kleinerman J, Saidel GM: Quantitative relationships of intravascular tumor cells, tumor vessels, and pulmonary metastases following tumor implantation. Cancer Res 34:997, 1974.
27. Golinger RC, Gregorio RM, Fisher ER: Tumor cells in venous blood draining mammary carcinomas. Arch Surg 112:707, 1977.
28. Griffiths JD, McKinna JA, Rowbotham HD, et al.: Carcinoma of the colon and rectum: circulating malignant cells and 5-year survival. Cancer 31:226, 1973.
29. Salsbury AJ: The significance of the circulating cancer cell. Cancer Treat Rev 2:55, 1975.
30. Smith RR, Thomas LB, Hilbers AW: Cancer cell contamination of operative wounds. Cancer 11:53–62, 1958.
31. Sako K, Marchetta FC: Radioautography of *in vitro* labeled tumor cells in postoperative wound drainage. Cancer 19:735–737, 1966.
32. Fisher B, Fisher ER: Barrier function of lymph node to tumor cells and erythrocytes. Cancer 20:1907–1919, 1967.
33. Madden RE, Gyure L: Translymphnodal passage of tumor cells. Oncology 22:281–289, 1968.
34. Hewitt HB, Blake E: Quantitative studies of translymphoidal passage of tumour cells naturally disseminated from a nonimmunogenic murine squamous carcinoma. Br J Cancer 31:25, 1975.
35. Haagensen CD: Diseases of the breast 2nd ed. Philadelphia: WB Saunders, 1971, p 401.

36. Spratt Jr, JS, Donegan WL: Cancer of the breast. In: Major problems in clinical surgery, Vol. 5, Dunphy JE (ed). Philadelphia: WB Saunders, 1967, p 63.
37. Fisher B, Montague E, Redmond C, et al.: Cancer of the breast: size of neoplasm and prognosis. Cancer 24:1071, 1969.
38. Grinnell RS: The chance of cancer and lymphatic metastasis in small colon tumors discovered on X-ray examination. Ann Surg 139:132, 1964.
39. Breslow A: Tumor thickness, level of invasion and node dissection in stage I cutaneous melanoma. Ann Surg 182:572, 1975.
40. Sugarbaker EV, Roseman JM, Weingrad DN: Malignant melanoma. In: Textbook of surgical oncology, Copeland TM (ed). J. Wiley (in press).
41. Balch CM, Soong S, Murad T, Ingalls AL, Maddox WA: A multifactorial analysis of melanoma. II. Prognostic factors of clinieal stage I disease. Surgery 86:343, 1979.
42. Arons MS, Smith RR, Myers MH: Significance of cancer cells in operative wounds. Cancer 14:1041, 1961.
43. Lindberg R: Distribution of cervical lymph node metastases from squamous cell carcinoma of the upper respiratory and digestive tracts. Cancer 29:1446–1449, 1972.
44. Spratt JS Jr, Spratt JA: The prognostic value of measuring the gross linear radial growth of pulmonary metastases and primary pulmonary cancers. J Thorac Cardiovasc Surg 71:274, 1976.
45. Temple WJ, Sugarbaker EV, Thornthwaithe JT et al.: Correlation of cell cycle analysis with Dukes staging in colon cancer patients ASCO. Abstr 22:336, 1981.
46. Cady B, Sedgwick C, Meissner WA, et al.: Changing clinical, pathologic, therapeutic, and survival patterns in differentiated thyroid carcinoma. Ann Surg 184:541, 1976.
47. Shah JT, Cendon RA, Farr HW, et al.: Carcinoma of the oral cavity. Factors affecting treatment failure at the primary site and neck. Am J Surg 132:504, 1976.
48. Fisher B, Slack N, Katrych D, Wolmark N: Ten-year follow-up results of patients with carcinoma of the breast in a co-operative clinical trial evaluating adjuvant chemotherapy. Surg Gynecol Obstet 140:528, 1975.
49. Spratt JS Jr, Spjut HJ: Prevalence and prognosis of individual clinical and pathologic variables associated with colorectal carcinoma. Cancer 20:1976, 1967.
50. Sugarbaker EV, McBride M: Melanoma of the trunk: the results of surgical excision and anatomic guidelines for predicting nodal metastasis. Surgery 80:22, 1976.
51. Frazell EL, Foote FW: Papillary thyroid carcinoma: pathological findings in cases with and without clinical evidence of node involvement. Cancer 8:1164, 1955.
52. Noguchi S, Noguchi A, Murakami N: Papillary carcinoma of the thyroid. II. Value of prophylactic lymph node dissection. Cancer 26:1061, 1970.
53. Fisher B, Montague E, Redmond C, et al.: Comparison of radical mastectomy with alternative treatments for primary breast cancer, a first report of results from a prospective randomized clinical trial. Cancer 39:2827, 1977.
54. Veronesi U, et al.: Inefficacy of immediate node dissection in Stage I melanoma of the limbs. N Engl J Med 297:627, 1977.
55. Tyzzer EE: Factors in the production and growth of tumor metastases. J Med Res 28:309, 1913.
56. Sugarbaker EV: Patterns of metastasis in human malignancies. In: Cancer biology reviews, Vol. 2, JJ Marchalonis JJ,hianna Jr, MG, Fidler IJ. New York: Marcel Dekker, 1981, pp 235–278.
57. Lindberg R: Distribution of cervical lymph node metastases from squamous cell carcinoma of the upper respiratory and digestive tracts. Cancer 29:1146, 1972.
58. Huvos AG, Hutter RVP, Berg JW: Significance of axillary macrometastases and micrometastases in mammary cancer. Ann Surg 173:44, 1971.
59. Elliott RHE, Frantz VK: Metastatic carcinoma masquerading as primary thyroid cancer: a report of authors' 14 cases. Ann Surg 151:551, 1960.
60. Patel JK, Didolkar MS, Pickren JW, Moore RH: Metastatic pattern of malignant melanoma. A study of 216 autopsy cases. Am J Surg 135:807–810, 1978.

61. McNeer G, Pack GT: Neoplasms of the stomach. Philadelphia: Lippincott, pp 435–436, 1967.
62. Moragues V: Cardiac metastasis from malignant melanoma. Am Heart J 10:579–588, 1939.
63. Ashikari R, Rosen PP, Urbau JA, Sendoo T: Breast cancer presenting as an axillary mass. Ann Surg 183:415–417, 1976.
64. Smith JL, Stehlin JS: Spontaneous regression of primary malignant melanomas with regional metastasis. Cancer 18:1379, 1965.
65. McCarthy SW, Palmer AA, Bale PA, Hirst E: Naevus cells in lymph nodes. Pathology 6:351, 1974.
66. McDivitt RW, Stewart FW, Berg JW: Tumors of the breast. In: Atlas of tumor pathology, Series 2, Fasicle 2. Washington D.C.: Armed Forces Institute of Pathology, 1968.
67. Haagensen CD, Feind CR, Herter FP, Slanetz CA, Weinberg JA: The lymphatics in cancer. Philadelphia: WB Saunders 1972, p 83.
68. Martin H, Morfit HM, Ehrlich H: The case for branchiogenic cancer (malignant melanoma). Ann Surg 132:867, 1950.
69. Batsakis JA: Tumors of the head and neck. Clinical and pathological considerations 2nd ed. Baltimore: Williams & Wilkins, 1979, p 244–245.
70. Holmes FF, Fouts TL: Metastatic cancer of unknown primary site. Cancer 26:816–820, 1970.
71. Nystrom JS, Weiner JM, Heffelfinger-Juttner J, Irwin LE, Bateman JR, Wolf RM: Metastatic and histologic presentation in unknown primary cancer. Semin Oncol 4:53–58, 1977.
72. Didolkar MS, Fanous N, Elias EG, Moore RH: Metastatic carcinomas from occult primary tumors. Ann Surg 186:625–630, 1972.
73. Osteen RT, Kopf G, Wilson RE: In pursuit of the unknown primary. Amer J Surg 135:494–498, 1978.
74. Smith PE, Krementz ET, Chapman W: Metastatic cancer without a detectable primary site. Am J Surg 1967, 113:633–637.
75. Golomb HM, Thomasen S: Estrogen receptor: Therapeutic guide in undifferentiated metastatic carcinoma in women. Arch Intern Med 135:942–945, 1975.
76. Rudnik P, Odell WD: In search of a cancer. N Engl J Med 484:405–408, 1971.
77. Jesse RH, Neff LE: Metastatic carcinoma in cervical nodes with an unknown primary lesion. Amer J Surg 112:547–553, 1966.
78. Fidler IJ, Kripke ML: Metastasis resulting from pre-existing variant cells within a malignant tumor. Science 197:893, 1977.
79. Sugarbaker EV, Cohen AM: Altered antigenicity in spontaneous pulmonary metastases from an antigenic murine sarcoma. Surgery 72:155, 1972.
80. Sugarbaker EV: Cancer metastasis: a product of tumor-host interactions. Year Book Medical Publishers, 3(7), 1979.

26. Newer methods for the diagnosis of occult metastases

P. S. DICKMAN and T. J. TRICHE

1. Introduction

It is now well accepted that the selection of appropriate therapy for both primary and metastatic malignant disease depends upon accurate histogenetic classification of the patient's tumor. This classification is, for the most part, based on histopathologic diagnosis from formalin-fixed, paraffin embedded, hematoxylin and eosin-stained sections. In recent years the application of techniques developed in research laboratories to the diagnosis of tumors has led to better understanding of the biology of many classes of malignancy and has enabled pathologists to subclassify tumors in ways that have guided the team of oncologic therapists to more refined treatment protocols, with consequent improvements in prognosis, prognostication, and treatment results. The patient who unexpectedly presents with metastatic disease, in a lymph node or the bone marrow, for example, but with no known primary, represents a special problem; for these patients, the accurate identification of primary site, or meaningful suggestion of the differential diagnosis, by the pathologist is particularly important in light of increasingly successful treatment of metastatic disease. Thus an understanding of available newer methods for the more accurate diagnosis and classification of primary and metastatic tumors will be of value to those involved in cancer research as well as to clinicians and pathologists whose daily decisions determine the therapy of cancer patients.

In the following pages we will first outline the newer methods available for better classification and diagnosis of tumors, some of which are already being used routinely in pathology laboratories. We will then discuss the application of these methods to the diagnosis of several pathologic categories of malignancy.

2. Diagnostic techniques

The key to the successful application of any of the techniques described below to tumor diagnosis is close collaboration between the clinician and the pathologist. Advance planning for tissue handling will ensure that it is at least possible to perform whatever special techniques are called for by the clinical and initial pathologic diagnosis. All of the methods to be discussed, with the exception of immunoperoxidase (IP), require initial tissue handling quite different from the routine fixation

L.A. Liotta and I.R. Hart (eds.), Tumor Invasion and Metastasis. ISBN-13: 978-94-009-7513-2.
© 1982 Martinus Nijhoff Publishers, The Hague/Boston/London.

in formaldehyde (or other light microscopic fixative) normally employed for histologic studies. Thus, electron microscopy (EM) is best performed on glutaraldehyde fixed tissue; immunofluorescence (IF) requires fresh frozen tissue; and formaldehyde fume induced fluorescence (FIF) can only be performed on rapidly dried touch preparations or frozen sections. The importance of this prospective approach to tissue handling cannot be overemphasized. It is of much greater benefit to the patient, and a much better use of the time of the clinician, pathologist, and technician, to handle and preserve tissue properly from the start, even if the special test is not performed, than to realize later that a study would be of importance to therapy but cannot be carried out, except by rebiopsying the patient, because the first, adequate tissue was all fixed in formaldehyde.

2.1. Electron microscopy

This is not a new technique, but the extensive application of ultrastructural methods to diagnostic pathology has only come about in the last decade [1–4]. There are now several textbooks [5–7] as well as a journal (*Ultrastructural Pathology*) devoted to the subject and and numerous courses are offered to diagnosticians in the methodology and application of ultrastructure to tumor diagnosis. In the past, electron microscopy suffered from being cumbersome, time-consuming, and unfamiliar to most diagnosticians. With modern microtomes and microscopes, however, and the practicability of overnight processing, ultrastructural material may be ready for examination and photography as rapidly as conventional histologic slides, thereby greatly enhancing its diagnostic value.

Electron microscopy is optimally used as an ancillary technique to enhance and expand on light microscopic diagnosis, much as a special stain is used in histopathology to further refine the diagnosis made on material stained only with hematoxylin and eosin. Nonetheless, the possible usefulness of EM should always be anticipated by fixation of small (1 mm cubed) portions of all tumors in 2.5–3% buffered glutaraldehyde soon after excision; this can always be discarded later, or embedded and stored. Buffered formaldehyde, used for routine histology, may also be used for tissue intended for ultrastructural studies, and is a good choice if glutaraldehyde is not available. Recovery of tissue from paraffin blocks or even stained slides can be performed but success is rare and proper initial fixation can avoid these frustrating situations.

Ultrastructural information should be interpreted in light of diagnostic impressions attained by light microscopy, clinical data, clinical laboratory analyses, and other, more experimental, techniques. Key features of a metastatic malignancy, such as secretion of hormones or other bioactive products, can often be confirmed by electron microscopic findings, e.g. neuroendocrine secretory granules. Structures which are inapparent or only suggested by light microscopic examination may be obvious at the fine structural level, such as myofilaments which are not organized into conventional contractile structures.

As the study of tumors has expanded to include more poorly differentiated lesions, in parallel withe clinical interest, electron microscopic study has served to identify cellular features undetectable by any other means, such as sparse structural proteins or cell-cell attachment devices, and thus contributed to the differential diagnosis of groups of tumors like soft tissue sarcomas [8, 9] and pediatric 'round-cell' tumors [10] with similar clinical presentations but widely variable outcomes. When the results of ultrastructural analyses are viewed in the context of other studies, both conventional and recently developed, its contributions to tumor diagnosis can be well appreciated.

2.2. Immunohistochemistry

The immunohistologic techniques of immunofluorescence and immunoperoxidase function as powerful tools not only in tumor classification but in many other areas of diagnostic and experimental pathology and cell biology as well [11–13]. The identification of specific intracellular, cell surface, and extracellular antigens by immunofluorescence has been a fundamental technique in experimental biology for many years. The more recent development of immunoperoxidase methodology, especially the peroxidase-antiperoxidase (PAP) technique of Sternberger [14], has added the new dimensions to tissue immunology of increased sensitivity, the opportunity for simplified examination using light instead of fluorescence microscopy, and the ability to detect antigens in formalin-fixed, paraffin embedded specimens. These methods are limited, of course, by adequacy of tissue and antigen preservation, specificity of antisera, and availability of positive and negative controls, but these limitations are more than compensated for by the power of the techniques to identify and localize numerous antigens of interest.

Specific protocols for both methods have been widely published [14–16], but the principles will be briefly outlined here. The two methods both require antisera specifically directed against the substance of interest and purified to this end or, alternatively, monoclonal antibodies prepared and selected by appropriate techniques. Thereafter, the particulars differ. In immunofluorescence, frozen sections, unfixed or fixed in acetone or alcohol, are layered with the primary antiserum in appropriate dilution, sometimes after treatment with normal serum to eliminate nonspecific adherence. Occasionally this primary antiserum has been directly coupled to the fluorescent moiety (either isothiocyanate or rhodamine), but, more commonly, a second antibody coupled to the fluorescent agent and directed against the *species* of the first (e.g. primary rabbit antigastrin, second goat anti-rabbit IgG), is used. After washing and coverslipping the slide is examined in a fluorescent microscope with appropriate incident and emission filters, and the location of the antigen is indicated by the location of bright fluorescence.

In the immunoperoxidase technique as described by Sternberger, primary antibodies to the tissue antigen are applied as in immunofluorescence. The second antibody is a bridge or link, directed against the species of the primary. A third layer, consisting of peroxidase-anti-peroxidase soluble antigen-antibody complexes, is then applied, in which the antibody in the complex is of the same species as the primary antibody and therefore also binds to the bivalent second antibody. The peroxidase activity, thus bound via the three layers to the antigen of interest, is then demonstrated using hydrogen peroxide and diaminobenzidine, resulting in a visible brown color at the site of the antigen; the color may be enhanced by exposure to osmium tetroxide.

The immunofluorescence and immunoperoxidase techniques each have specific advantages and disadvantages which affect their applications. Immunoperoxidase offers greatly increased sensitivity of antigen detection, and permits examination of formalin-fixed, paraffin embedded tissue using ordinary light microscopy. Tissue morphology is retained and antigen localization with respect to surrounding cells and structures can be seen; counterstaining with hematoxylin or other stains is possible and enables one to compare the immunoperoxidase preparation with corresponding hematoxylin adn eosin stained sections. Immunoperoxidase is superior, also, for identification of cytoplasmic antigens. With certain modifications the PAP technique can be adapted to electron microscopy, as the PAP-benzidine complexes are osmiophilic and become even more electron-dense. The major disadvantages of this technique include the toxicity of diaminobenzidine and the variable loss of antigenicity after histologic tissue processing.

Immunofluorescence, in contrast, enables the examiner to localize antigens which are labile to such fixation and processing. The technique is far superior to PAP for the localization of cell surface antigens; for example, the PAP technique is generally unrewarding in the examination of lymphocyte surface markers, while fluorescence can be used successfully. Finally, two fluorochromes are available for general use. Fluorescein and rhodamine fluoresce at different wave lengths and appear green and red, respectively. By selecting primary antisera from different animal species, the fluorescent-tagged second antisera can be differentially labeled with fluorescein and rhodamine; thus two different antigens can be identified in the same tissue section.

Recently, an improved immunohistochemical method utilizing an avidinbiotin complex has been described [17, 18]. The unparalleled affinity of biotin for avidin ($K_d > 10^{15}\ M^{-1}$) is nearly a million-fold greater than the most avid antisera and results in high sensitivity at great dilutions. This feature greatly reduces reagent volumes needed, minimizes background staining, and maximizes specificity. Experience with this variant technique is limited, but its enhanced sensitivity and decreased cost compared to conventional 2- or 3-step immunoperoxidase and immunofluorescence suggest more widespread application in the future.

It should be apparent that the choice of immunohistochemical methodology should be appropriate to the diagnostic problem at hand; otherwise the technique will be useless. When properly applied, the specificity and objectivity of the technique is unparalleled.

2.3. Immunologic surface and cytoplasmic markers

The application of the techniques of modern immunology to tumors of the organs and cells of the immune system has resulted in widespread reclassification of these tumors, the leukemias and lymphomas. Universal agreement on the optimal classification scheme does not yet exist. At the time of this writing a New International Formulation for the non-Hodgkin's lymphomas has been proposed which combines the features of many of the previous systems [19]. This classification scheme may enjoy broader support than any previous nomenclature and is also consistent with recent immunologic and histogenic data. Thus, 'histiocytic' lymphoma in the Rappaport system [20], which implied a tissue histiocyte or macrophage origin for lymphomas with a high content of transformed or 'blastic' neoplastic lymphocytes, has been replaced by the descriptive and histogenically accurate 'malignant lymphoma, large cell.'

This newer classification scheme and others already in use [21, 22] closely parallel the results of surface marker studies, unlike the older schemes. This immunologic approach to the diagnosis of lymphoma employs an ever-widening array of assays, but includes at least the following:

- Membrane bound and intracytoplasmic marker determination by immunofluorescent and immunoperoxidase methods (B cells);
- Complement receptor identification using erythrocyte-antibody-complement rosetting (B cells);
- Cytophilic antibody receptor determination by IgGEA rosettes (B cells);
- Sheep erythrocyte (E) rosette technique (T cells);
- Immunoadherence evaluation of frozen sections;
- *In vitro* phagocytosis testing for cells of monocyte-macrophage origin;
- The investigation of a variety of cytochemical markers denoting various lymphoreticular cell subsets, including: 'Non-specific' esterases, acid phosphatase, beta glucuronidase, alkaline phosphatase, and terminal deoxynucleotidyl transferase;
- Monoclonal antisera against lymphoid differentiation antigens.

Many of these techniques may be applied not only to samples from peripheral blood, bone marrow, and lymph node or tumor biopsies, but also to neoplastic cells cultured *in vitro* and frozen sections [23, 24].

2.4. Monoclonal antibody and cell sorter techniques

The past decade has witnessed the simultaneous development of hybridoma (or monoclonal) antibody techniques in parallel with the appearance of refined, commercially available fluorescence activated cell sorters. These events have made these former research tools available for diagnostic use. In conjunction with one another, they offer the ability to detect specific and immunologically defined cell populations, such as metastatic tumor cells, with a sensitivity which far exceeds that of morphologic techniques. The identification is also objective, since the cell sorter quantitatively detects fluorescence associated with the binding of fluorochrome tagged antibody to specific antigenic determinants on the tumor cell surface. It is thus possible to detect vanishingly small numbers of tumor cells in a milieu of identical-appearing normal cells with great confidence; even 0.1% metastatic neuroblastoma cells among normal marrow cells have been detected in this manner [25] (Figure 8). The early detection of tumor relapse is thought to enhance therapeutic responsiveness; cell-sorter analysis of suspected relapses or even routine monitoring of remissions may thus play an important role in improving the prognosis of patients being treated with systemic chemotherapy.

The use of cell-sorter technology in tumor cell detection is heavily dependent on the availability and use of specific antisera. Monoclonal antisera are especially valuable in this regard, since once made they are essentially inexhaustible and recognize only one antigenic determinant, as opposed to the multiple and variably cross-reacting determinants recognized by most heterologous antisera. In addition to monoclonal anti-neuroblastoma antisera [26], other diagnostically useful monoclonal antisera have recently become commercially available. A series of antisera which detects various stages of normal T cell lymphoid differentiation antigens has been used to define subtypes of human T-cell acute lymphocyte leukemia (ALL) and lymphoblastic lymphoma [27]. This is important, since the detection on these tumor cells of more mature determinants such as OKT3 appears to correlate with an improved prognosis as opposed to the presence of only the most primitive pre-T cell determinants such as OKT9. These same techniques have recently been applied to lymphoblastic lymphoma, which shares many similarities with ALL; generally similar results obtain, although the prognostic significance is yet unclear [28]. It is apparent, however, that both a normal and malignant cell population can be identified by the cell sorter in even partially involved lymph nodes. Thus, even early metastatic involvement and characterization as lymphoid versus non-lymphoid tumors may be possible with cell sorter analysis of lymph nodes suspected of harboring foci of metastatic tumor.

2.5. Formaldehyde-induced fluorescence and glyoxylic acid fluorescence

Tumors possessing characteristics of cells derived from the neural crest, termed the APUD system by Pearse [29, 30], have been of special interest to the pathologist, oncologist, and endocrinologist because of their diagnostic challenge and their neuro-endocrine secretory properties. The APUD (Amine Precursor Uptake and Decarboxylation) cells often manufacture and secrete peptide hormones, and always contain catecholamines. If tumors derived from these cells secrete hormones, there may be more than one detectable product both in the circulation and in the tumor cells. The presence of catecholamines or catechol precursors is detected by the formaldehyde fume-induced fluorescence [31, 32] and glyoxylic acid fluorescence (GAF) techniques [33]; these approaches are most useful when the more conventional methods of electron microscopy, immunofluorescence and immunoperoxidase fail to identify neurosecretory granules or specific peptide hormones.

The FIF method was developed and first described by Falck [31] and then promoted and used to great advantage by Pearse [29] to characterize the APUD system of cells and tumors. The reaction of formaldehyde and a variety of catecholamines and related compounds to form autofluorescent isoquinolone compounds is the basis of the test. Frozen sections or touch preparations from the tumor must be rapidly and thoroughly dried, then exposed to dry paraformaldehyde fumes. When examined in the fluorescent microscope, with incident illumination of 390–410 nm wave length, a bright yellow to yellow-green fluorescence is seen in cells containing catecholamines or their precursors. Rapid initial handling is essential, and positive and negative controls must be run simultaneously with the sample to avoid misinterpretation. Still, the technique is fairly simple overall and valuable for identifying APUD cells where other techniques cannot.

Because of the relatively stringent requirements of the FIF technique, the newer, more rapid, reliable and sensitive method of GAF has been proposed and implemented for diagnostic purposes [33–36], with excellent results in the study of neuroblastomas [37]. This method may be a better choice than FIF, when other diagnostic techniques fail to identify APUD characteristics, since it appears simpler to perform yet offers greater detection sensitivity when compared in parallel with FIF, as in normal neural tissues.

2.6. Collagen studies

In recent years, the elucidation and characterization of at least five major collagen types in vertebrates (as well as a host of less frequently occurring variations on these types) and improvements in the purification and specific identification of collagen and other connective tissue proteins [38] have enlarged the possibilities for biochemical analysis of not only normal tissues but also malignancies derived from collagen-producing cells [39–44]. The roles of collagenases, basement membrane collagen, cell attachment proteins, and attachment properties of tumor cells in metastasis are discussed in section III of this book and will not be further treated here. We shall instead focus on collagen production patterns of tumors *in vivo* and *in vitro* and possible applications of these findings to tumor diagnosis.

Bornstein and Sage have recently reviewed current knowledge of the various collagen types and their production patterns in a wide variety of normal vertebrate cells and tissues. At least five genetically distinct collagen types have now been described (Table 1, [45]). Each type is produced by a number of different kinds of

Table 1. Collagen types and distribution*.

Type	Tissue distribution	Molecular from
I	Bone, tendon, skin, dentin, ligament, fascia, arteries and uterus	$[\alpha 1(I)]_2\alpha 2(I)$
II	Hyaline cartilage	$[\alpha 1(II)]_3$
III	Skin, arteries and uterus	$[\alpha 1(III)]_3$
IV	Basement membranes	$[\alpha 1(IV)]_3$
V	Basement membranes and perhaps other tissues	$[\alpha 1(V)]_2\alpha 2(V)$

*Adapted from Prokop *et al.* [45]

cells, but in normal tissues the distribution of the different types is fairly characteristic. This distribution has led us and others to investigate patterns of the various collagen types in a variety of human and animal tumors [39–44]. Certain analogies between normal cells and their malignant counterparts have now become apparent. It can be seen from Table 2 that malignant tumors in many cases mimic the collagen type production patterns of their normal cellular counterparts.

While the wide range of patterns of collagen types produced by normal cells makes it dangerous to carry this analogy too far, there are some possible applications to problems in the areas to tumor diagnosis and tumor cellular histogenesis. We have recently demonstrated that tissue culture cell lines derived from primary or metastatic lesions of Ewing's sarcoma are capable of manufacturing collagen types I, III and IV simultaneously, a pattern unlike that of normal cells examined to date, and also unlike that of lymphoma, a tumor commonly confused with Ewing's sarcoma but which synthesizes *no* collagen of any type [41, 42]. This multiplicity of collagen types suggests that Ewing's sarcoma is derived from a primitive but

Table 2. Collagen type distribution in normal tissues and tumors.

Tissue	Collagen type(s)	Tumor	Collagen type(s)
Bone	I	Osteosarcoma	I
Cartilage	II	Chondrosarcoma	II
Fibrous connective tissue	I,III (80:20)	Fibrosarcoma	III
Epithelia	IV	Carcinoma Endothelioma	IV
Lymphoid	O	Lymphoma	O
Neural	O	Neuroblastoma	O
Marrow Stroma	(?)	Ewing's Sarcoma	I,III,IV

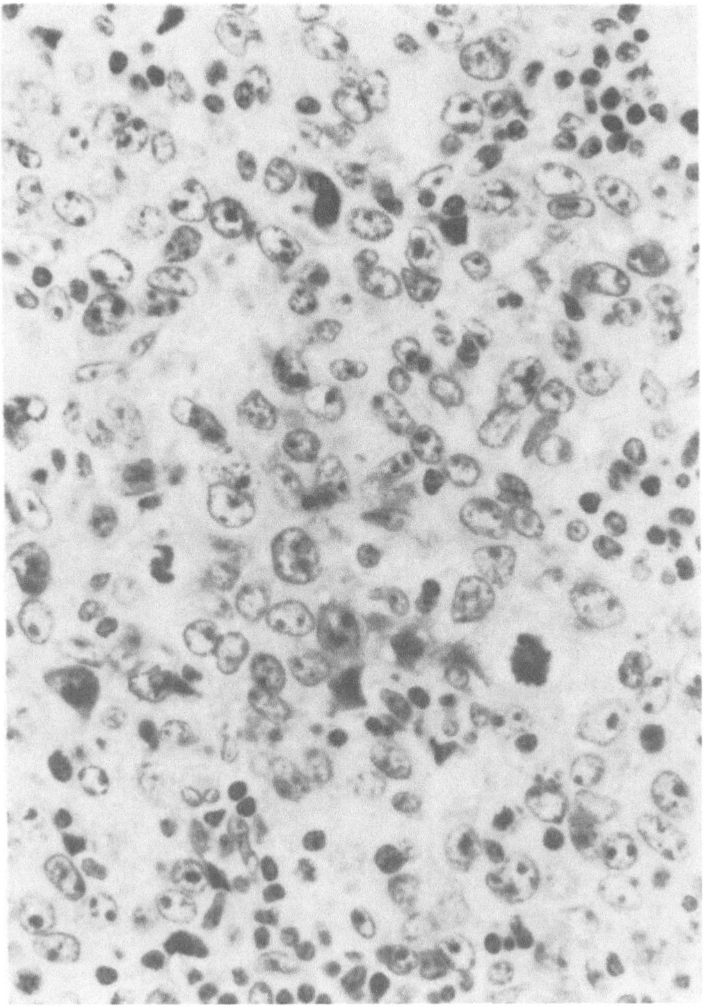

Figure 1. Metastatic tumor in axillary lymph node of 38-year-old woman with no obvious primary site. Histopathology not diagnostic. Differential diagnosis included breast carcinoma, metastatic malignant melanoma, and large cell lymphoma. (× 860).

pluripotential mesenchymal cell as yet uncommitted to fibroblastic, osteoblastic or endothelial differentiation.

The techniques used in these studies include immunofluorescence, immunoprecipitation, and polyacrylamide gel electrophoresis. The latter two methods are generally regarded as research tools; but further advance in anti-collagen antiserum production [46–51], including the possibility of monoclonal hybridoma derived sera [52, 53], may enable diagnosticians to utilize immunofluorescence or immunoperoxidase in the future to further elucidate tumor histogenesis and diagnosis. The use of anti-*pro*collagen antisera may be especially useful, since the larger collagen pre-

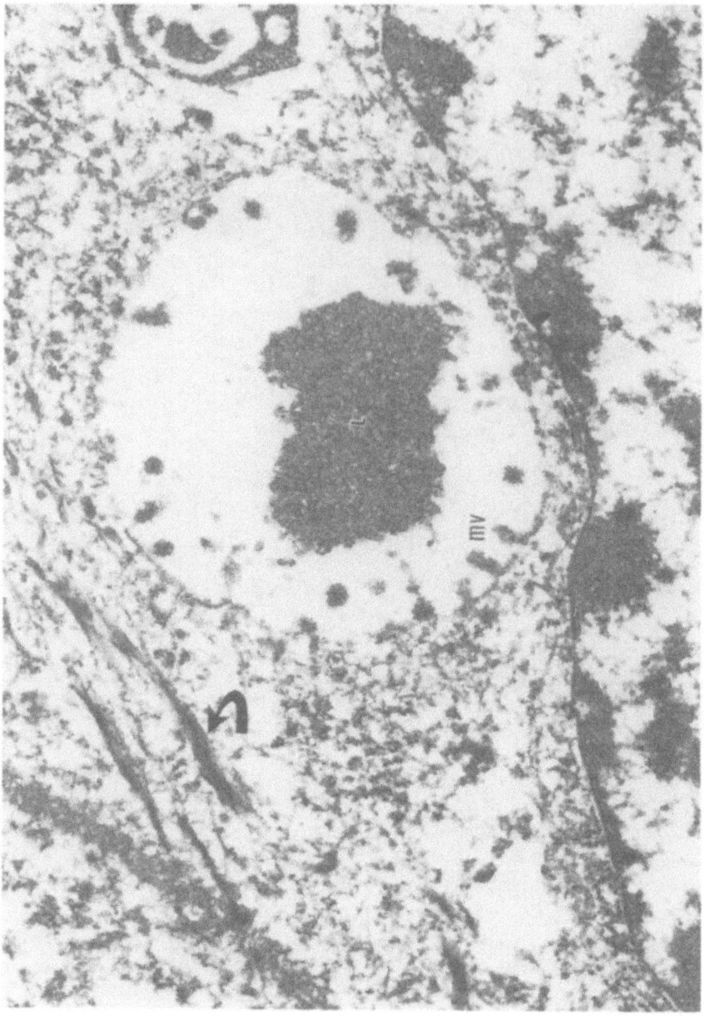

Figure 2. Diagnostic EM on tissue retrieved from paraffin block (same case as Figure 1). Ultrastructural preservation is suboptimal, but two salient diagnostic features are seen: 1) An intracytoplasmic lumen (L) with contained secretion; lumen lined by stubby microvilli (mv); 2) Coarse intermediate (10 nm) filaments (curved arrow), or tonofilaments, representing keratin. These features are never found in lymphoma or melanoma, and are routinely observed in infiltrating ductal carcinoma of the breast. (× 34 290).

cursor molecules are normally only present intracellularly and are highly antigenic, in contrast to native collagen molecules [54]. Thus, localization of collagen synthesis to morphologically detectable tumor cells and distinction from host stromal collagen would be possible. Several such antisera, specific for the C- and N-terminal non-collagenous 'pro-pieces,' in contrast to the central native collagen sequences, have been described [54–57] but are not yet widely available.

3. Applications to detection of metastases

In this section, the diagnosis of suspected metastases from a number of specific malignant neoplasms will be discussed, with emphasis on the combinations of methods (described above) which are particularly suited to the evaluation of the tumor under consideration.

3.1. Carcinomas

Identification of occult metastases as carcinomas, and differentiation from sarcomas and lymphomas, may at times, be quite difficult. A common clinical situation is that of metastatic tumor found in an enlarged cervical or axillary lymph node with no apparent primary site (Figure 1). The techniques most suitable for verifying a diagnosis of metastatic carcinoma are electron microscopy and immunohistochemistry.

Ultrastructural examination serves to identify several hallmarks of the epithelial origin of tumors, when such conventional techniques as mucin stains are negative [5, 6]. The observation of such features as desmosomes with 10 nm (keratin) tonofilaments, junctional complexes, basal lamina, and, often, intracytoplasmic lumina, generally excludes sarcomas and lymphomas from diagnostic consideration. Figure 2 illustrates such an EM finding in the case illustrated in Figure 1; the presence of an intracytoplasmic glandular lumen established the diagnosis of metastatic adenocarcinoma.

Immunohistochemical evaluation of specific epithelial protein products for the diagnosis of carcinoma is now feasible [58]. This technique has been used successfully to identify the production of basement membrane (type IV) collagen by metastatic breast carcinoma cells [59, 60] (Figure 3). More recently, the detection using immunohistochemistry of keratin production by squamous carcinoma cells and thymoma cells has been reported [13] (Figure 4). Other protein products identifiable by these methods are described in subsequent sections.

Neither of these techniques can help in distinguishing one adenocarcinoma from another, and thus several primary sites, such as breast, pancreas, and stomach, may still be under consideration once epithelial features are identified. In the case of prostate carcinoma, immunohistochemistry of a specific tissue marker is of great benefit as prostatic acid phosphatase may be detected and other sites of origin of metastatic lesions eliminated [61, 62].

3.2. APUD tumors and malignant melanoma

This group of endocrine and/or neural crest derived lesions, described earlier, have a number of features which render them susceptible to diagnosis by special tech-

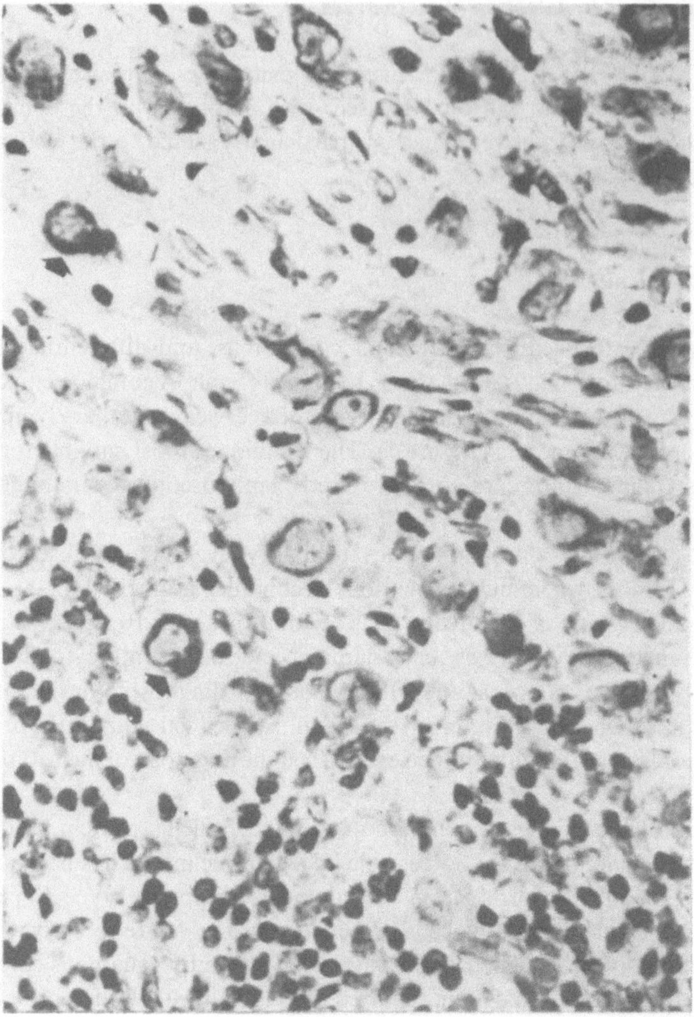

Figure 3. Immunoperoxidase staining with anti-type IV (basal lamina) collagen antibodies of routine paraffin embedded tissue sections in a case of metastatic breast carcinoma reveals intense cytoplasmic staining in tumor cells (arrows). Normal lymphocytes (small, dark cells on bottom) synthesize no collagen and thus fail to stain. Lymphoma cells and melanoma cells would likewise fail to stain. Diagnosis of metastatic carcinoma would be sustained with these results. (Approx. × 900).

niques. The applicable methods include not only ultrastructure and immunohistochemistry, but also formaldehyde-fume induced fluorescence, and enzyme histochemistry. Included among the APUD tumors is oat-cell carcinoma of the lung, an APUD tumor which presents particularly difficult diagnostic problems. Although a secretory product is not always present, these tumors may produce hormones and all the techniques described below are applicable to their identification.

The ultrastructural features of APUD tumors are quite distinctive [3, 63]. Like

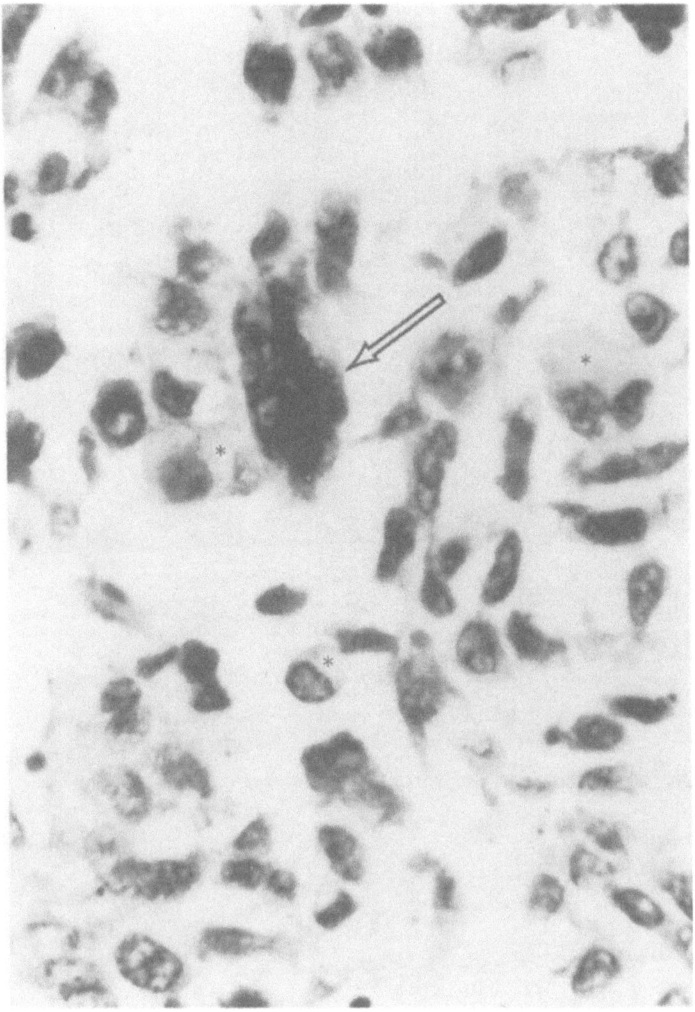

Figure 4. Immunoperoxidase staining with anti-keratin antibodies of tumor cells in poorly differentiated spindle cell carcinoma of the esophagus. Scattered giant cells are intensely reactive (arrow), indicative of keratinization. Many tumor cells are non-reactive (asterisks), but the presence of even a few reactive cells is indicative of keratinizing carcinoma. (× 1040).

their non-neoplastic counterparts, the cytoplasm usually contains varying numbers of unit membrane bound granules having cores of moderate to marked density representing the stored product, with a narrow lucent halo separating the granule from the membrane. The granules measure 100–400 nm in diameter and are usually round, though they may be oval in shape (Figure 5E-H). Granules containing glucagon (Figure 5A) usually lack the lucent halo but have an eccentric dense core, while granules containing insulin or proinsulin generally have an angular, crystal-

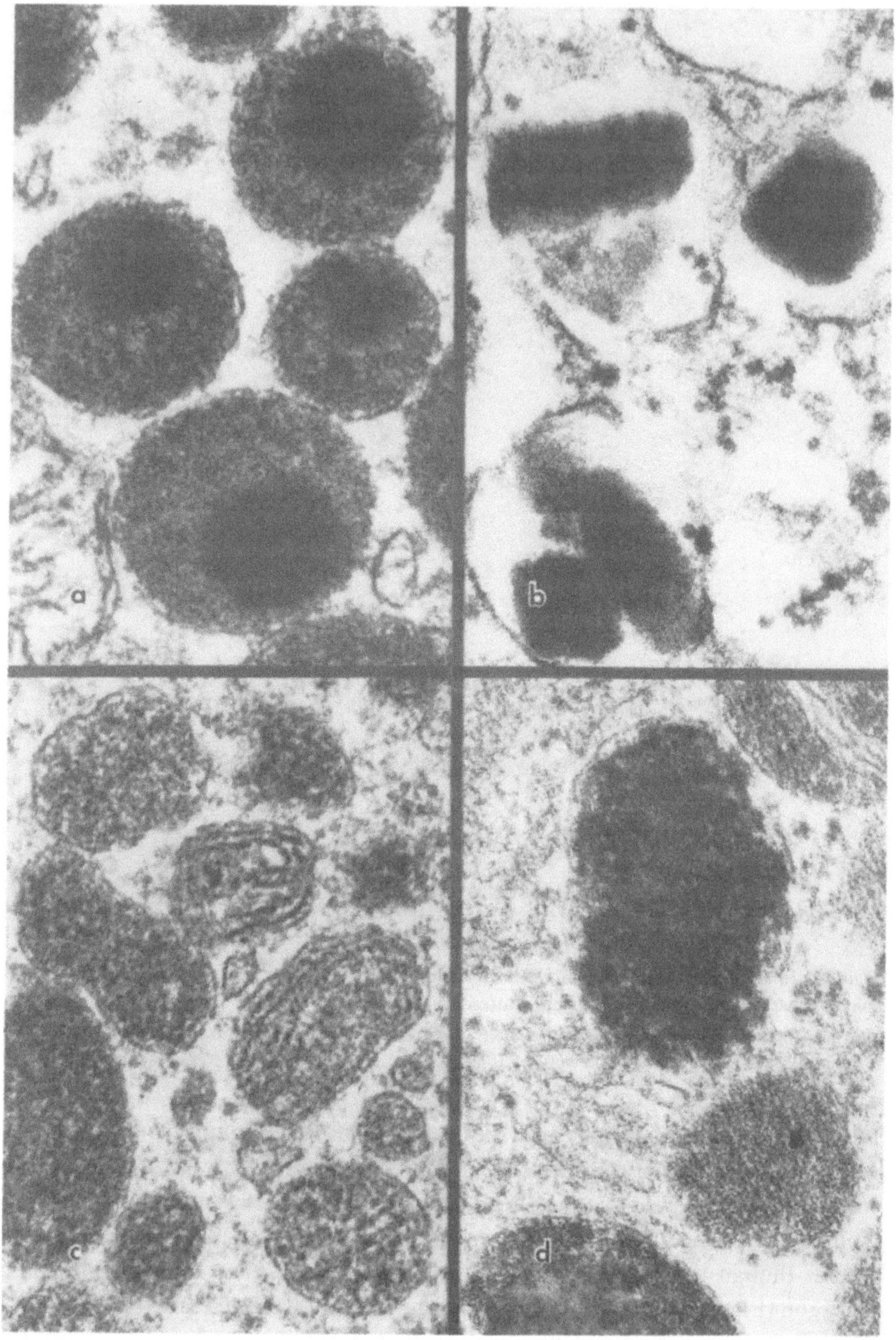
a
b
c
d

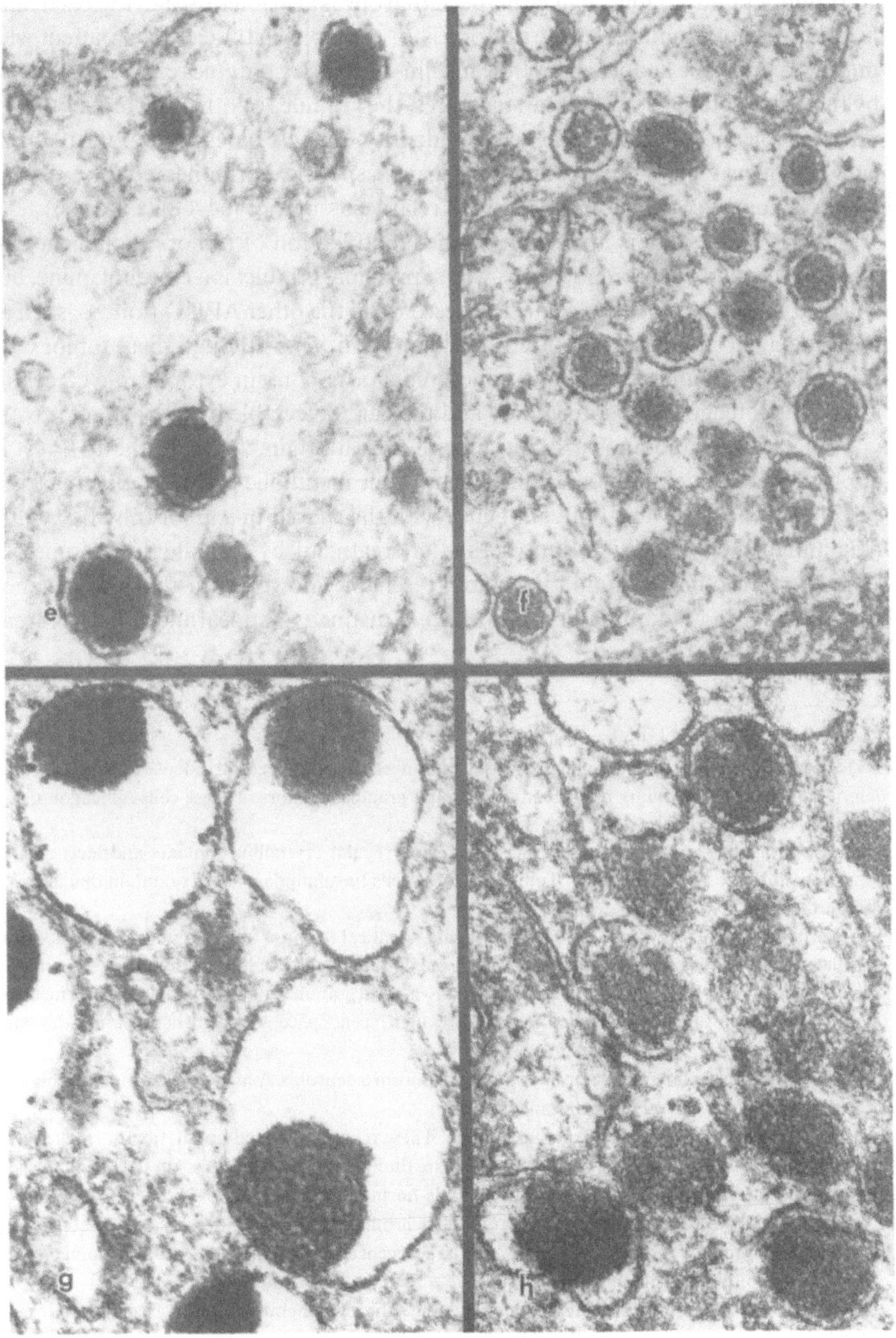
e
f
g
h

line core (Figure 5B). Granules of some cells of pheochromocytomas have eccentric cores with enlarged haloes; these may contain norepinephrine (Figure 5G).

If dense core granules are identified ultrastructurally, then the diagnosis of neural crest tumor or APUDoma can be made. Often one is also interested in the particular hormone being produced by the tumor as, for example, in the case of a patient with multiple endocrine neoplasms. While insulin-containing granules can be recognized by their characteristic crystalline structures, the granules of other hormones do not offer reliable morphologic clues to their identity. In these cases immunohistochemistry using primary antisera directed against specific hormones enables one to diagnose tumor secretion products with relative assurance [64–68] (Figure 6).

The FIF procedure is applicable to the identification of tumors such as neuroblastomas and pheochromocytomas whose principal product is a catecholamine, but will also demonstrate cytoplasmic fluorescence in the other APUD tumors, such as melanoma and small cell carcinoma of lung (Figure 7). Although these tumor cells package protein and peptide hormones, many also contain cytoplasmic catecholamines or catecholamine precursors and thus are detectable by FIF.

Malignant melanoma is also a tumor of neural origin. As such, the FIF test is applicable to its identification since melanogenic metabolic pathways diverge from catecholamine pathways but commence with the shared precursor dihydroxyphenylalanine (DOPA), which fluoresces after treatment by formaldehyde fumes or GA. Ultrastructural examination is more reliable, however, in that the melanosomes (melanin-containing granules) have a distinctive appearance when present

---

Figure 5. EM of APUD granules (all 100000 ×).

a) α cell (glucagon) granules from normal islet of Langerhans. Note eccentric dense nucleoid and less dense granular contents filling unit-membrane bound granule. Tumors of these cells (glucagonomas) often lack typical α granules.

b) β cell (insulin) granules from an islet cell. Note irregular crystalline contents and lucent space between membrane and crystalloids. Tumors of these cells (insulinomas) usually contain diagnostic β granules.

c) Early melanosomes from malignant melanoma, identical to those found in normal melanocytes. Fibrillar substructure is evident, especially in unit-membrane bound granule at center right.

d) Melanosomes from same case as in c. Mature, melanized granules contain overlying coarse melanin deposits, obscuring substructure noted in c; an irregular lucent space is evident between melanin and surrounding unit membrane.

e) Dense-core (catecholamine-containing) granules from a neuroblastoma. Note lucent halo between granule contents and surrounding unit membrane.

f) Smaller dense-core granules from gastrinoma. These represent second population of smaller granules occasionally observed in islet cell tumors, and are thought not to contain gastrin but products such as vasoactive intestinal polypeptide (VIP) in multiple-hormone secreting tumors.

g) Norepinephrine containing granules from pheochromocytoma. Eccentric position of contents is characteristic of these larger APUD granules, as is large lucent space within unit membrane; epinephrine-containing granules resemble those in e.

h) Pleomorphic dense core granules from a carcinoid. The regular granule at top resembles those in e, but many are irregular, as at lower left. This variability is typical of carcinoids.

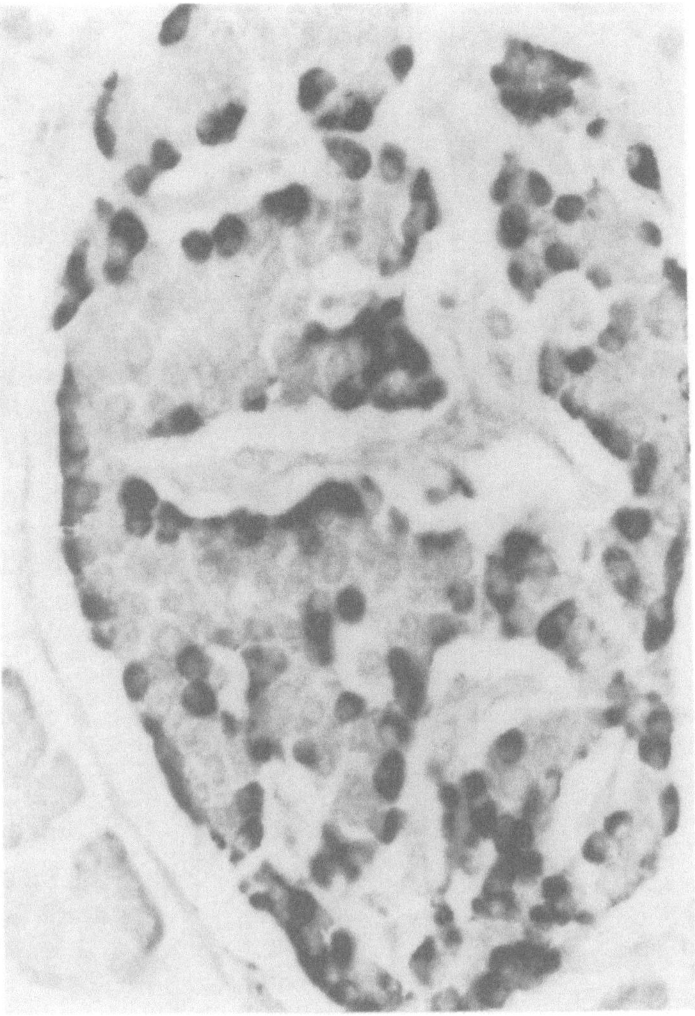

Figure 6. Immunoperoxidase preparation of normal human pancreatic islet. Note peripheral location of islet cells reactive with anti-glucagon antiserum, typical of alpha (glucagon-synthesizing) cells in endocrine pancreas. Intense reactivity of alpha cells enhanced by osmium tetroxide treatment of peroxidase reaction product. (× 680).

[6]. They are membrane bound and have a substructure composed of parallel, whorled or striated groups of membranes, often with a fingerprint pattern (Figure 5C). As the granules mature, electron-dense melanin is deposited on this membranous core, obliterating the characteristic structure (Figure 5D), but nonpigmented granule forms may usually be found to confirm the diagnosis.

Enzyme histochemistry may also be utilized to identify melanocytes and melanoma cells [69]. Melanin is formed from tyrosine and these cells contain detectable

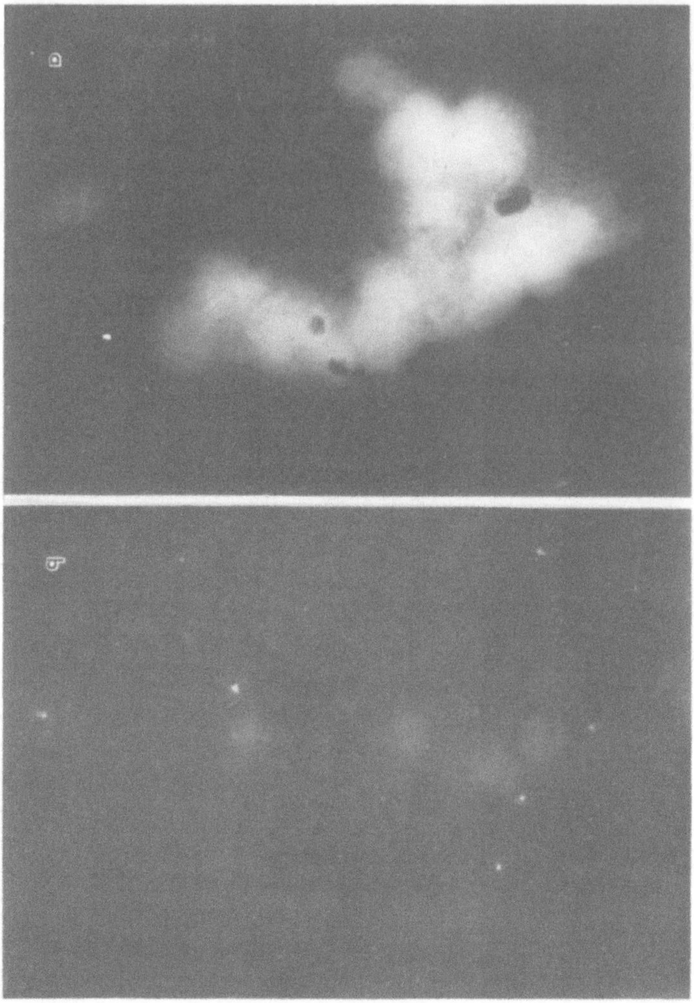

Figure 7. FIF of APUD-tumor touch preparation (A) and negative control (lymphoma) (B). Note intense cytoplasmic fluorescence in this pheochromocytoma; similar intensities observed in all APUD tumors. Negative control, which should always be included in this technique along with the unknown and positive control, is unreactive in comparison. (× 700).

tyrosinase and dihydroxyphenylalanine, both of which may be detected using suitable substrates and enzymes, as indicated above.

3.3. Neuroblastoma

This malignancy of children shows many features in common with the APUDomas.

The cells of this tumor may contain ultrastructurally identifiable dense-core granules (Figure 5E), containing catecholamines, and the FIF test demonstrates cytoplasmic fluorescence, as in Figure 7. Recently the use of the fluorescence-activated cell sorter for the identification of bone marrow metastases of neuroblastoma has been reported [26] (Figure 8). This technique is exquisitely sensitive and specific, as previously noted. An antiserum specifically directed against neuroblastoma cells is utilized to demonstrate the presence of metastatic tumor and distinguish it from normal marrow hematopoietic elements, a distinction which is often difficult to make by light microscopy and tedious to approach by ultrastructure when only small numbers of tumor cells are present. As other tumor type-specific antigens and antisera become available, the cell-sorter technique will have far more widespread application to the detection and specific diagnosis of metastatic tumors.

3.4. Rhabdomyosarcoma and soft-tissue Ewing's sarcoma

Rhabdomyosarcoma in the pediatric and young adult age groups may at times present a diagnostic challenge [10, 70]. Alveolar or embryonal rhabdomyosarcomas, with characteristic histologic patterns, recognizable myoblasts, or both, do not cause diagnostic difficulties. But many pediatric sarcomas may appear to be small round cell tumors, without obvious distinguishing features at the light microscopic level, and then the distinction among primitive rhabdomyosarcoma, Ewing's sarcoma extending to or originating in the soft tissues, neuroblastoma, and lymphoblastic lymphoma must be made. The features of neuroblastoma were discussed in previous sections, and lymphomas are dealt with below.

Ultrastructure can provide several valuable clues to the distinction between rhabdomyosarcoma and Ewing's sarcoma [70]. The identification of thick and thin filaments (15 nm and 4–6 nm) representing myosin and actin, and dense bodies representing Z-band material, firmly establish the diagnosis of rhabdomyosarcoma (Figure 9). Other helpful features include the presence of coarse collagen bundles between most tumor cells; occasionally, basement membrane material may be seen. In contrast, Ewing's sarcoma cells contain no cytoskeletal elements at all (Figure 10); thus primitive tumor cells lacking thick, myosin filaments but with abundant 6 and/or 10 nm (intermediate) filaments are unlikely to be Ewing's sarcoma and probably represent primitive rhabdomyosarcoma. Cells of Ewing's tumor also abut one another without intervening collagenous extracellular matrix (Figure 10); collagen, when present, often consists of fine, 20–30 nm fibers, further distinguishing between the lesions. Cytoplasmic glycogen, while often present in Ewing's sarcoma cells, is not of diagnostic pertinence as rhabdomyoblasts also frequently contain glycogen.

Another approach to the identification of myogenous differentiation is that of immunohistochemistry [71–74]. The immunoperoxidase technique has been successfully used to identify skeletal-muscle proteins and creatine phosphokinase

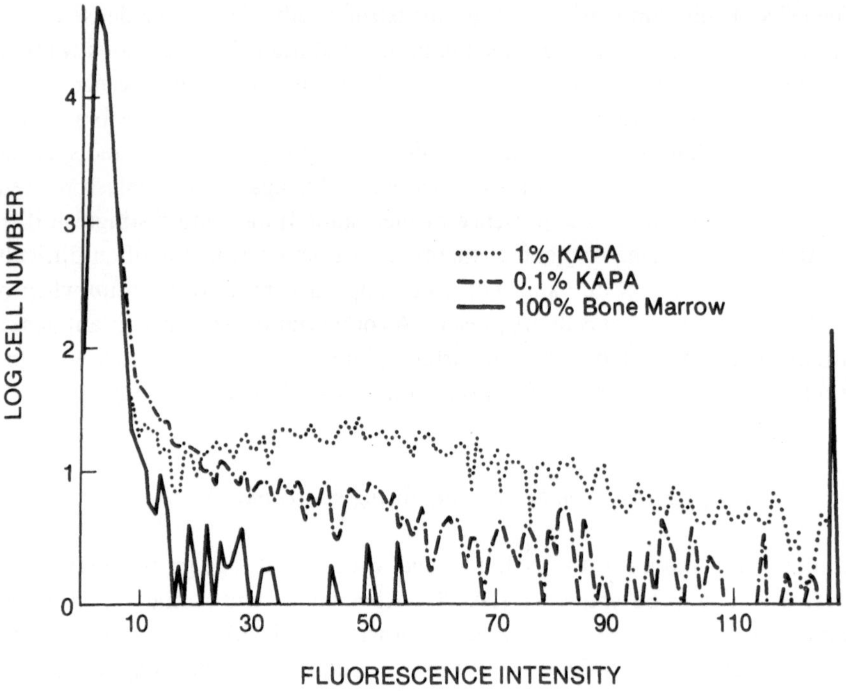

Figure 8. Fluorescence activated cell sorter graph of fluorescence versus frequency. Neuroblastoma cells stained with fluorescein-tagged monoclonal (HSAN 1) anti-neuroblastoma antiserum (broken lines) detectable above background fluorescence of normal bone marrow cells at concentrations as low as one in one thousand (0.1%). (Illustration courtesy of C.P. Reynolds and R.G. Smith.)

(MM) in cells of rhabdomyosarcomas but not in other tumors, including Ewing's sarcoma [71]. Figure 11 illustrates the detection of skeletal muscle myosin light chain in a rhabdomyosarcoma, utilizing the PAP technique.

Finally, the identification of multiple collagen types (I, III and IV) produced by tumors in short term tissue culture may, in the future, serve to identify such diagnostically difficult lesions as Ewing's sarcoma, especially as lymphomas, which are often in the differential diagnosis, do not manufacture collagen of any type [39, 41, 42].

3.5. *Lymphomas*

The identification of tumors as lymphomas and the subclassification of these lymphoid lesions has depended on the identification of surface immunoglobulin, complement or Fc receptors, sheep erythrocyte rosetting, and cytoplasmic enzymes [75]. A number of techniques may be used to detect these lymphoid markers. Immunoperoxidase or immunofluorescent studies of lymph node sections have been used with varied success [23, 24]. Better, more reliable results have been

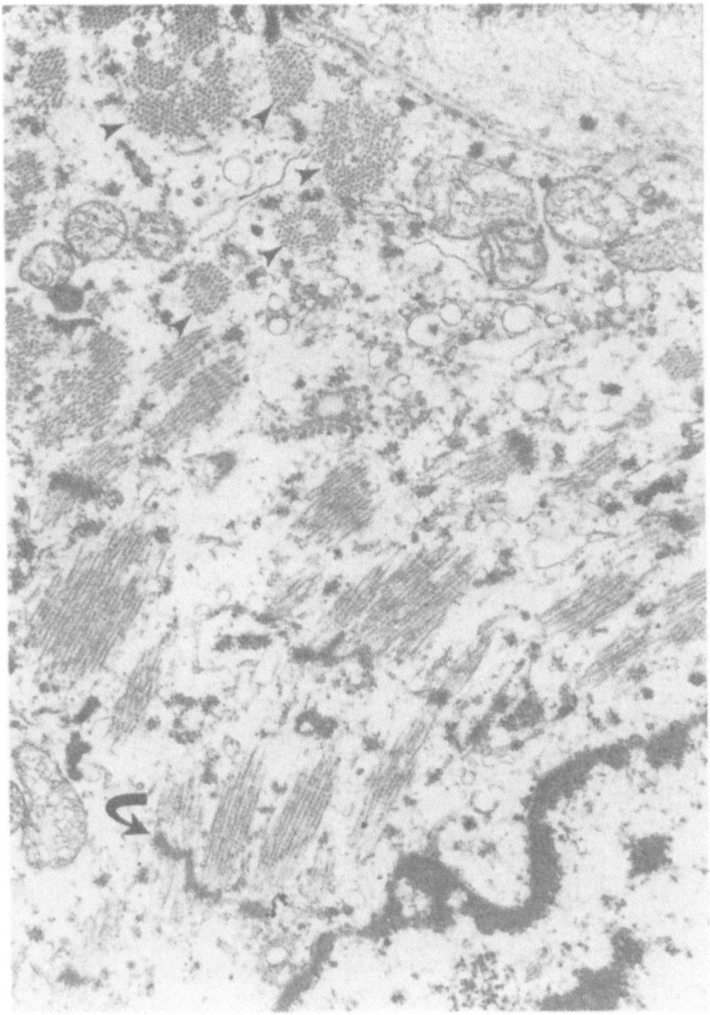

Figure 9. Electron micrograph of rhabdomyosarcoma reveals several structures specific for skeletal muscle differentiation. Z-band (curved arrow) are fragmented but numerous. Actin and myosin filaments (arrow heads) arranged in characteristic 6:1 hexagonal packing. Basal lamina, found in differentiated muscle, observed at upper right. These features are specific for skeletal muscle differentiation in this soft tissue sarcoma and are not detectable by light microscopy. (× 31570).

obtained by preparing cell suspensions from involved lymph nodes; these suspended tumor cells may then be studied, using immunofluorescence or red cell adherence techniques, in smears on glass slides [76].

More recently, monoclonal antisera and the fluorescent activated cell sorter and frozen-section studies have been applied to this classification [25, 28].

Figure 12 illustrates one example of the use of these techniques in the diagnosis

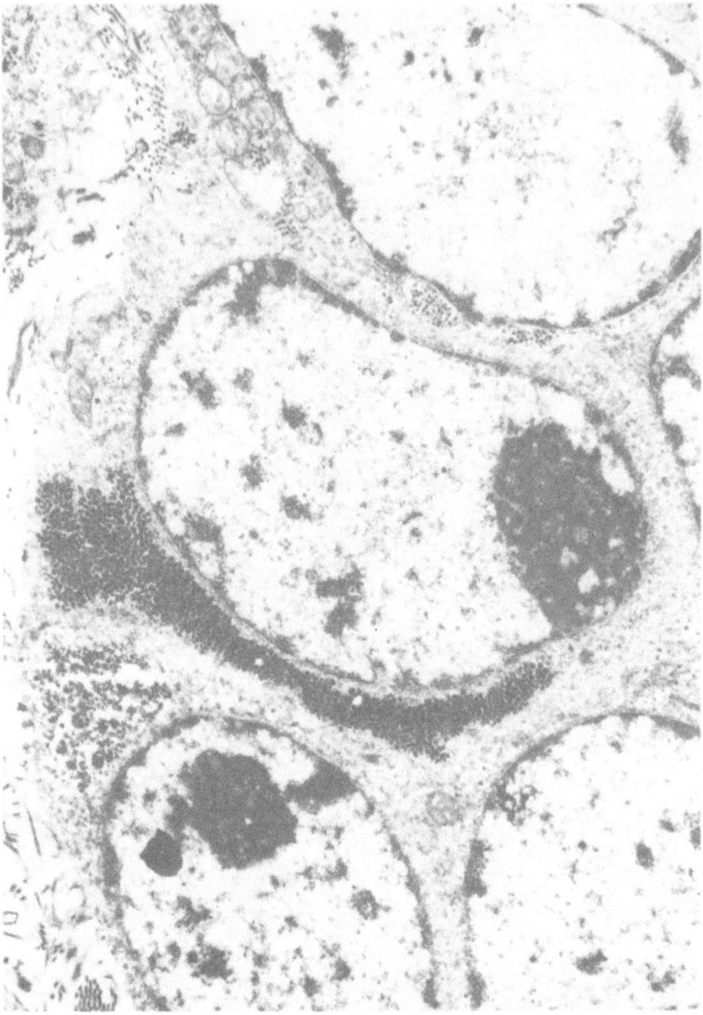

Figure 10. EM of Ewing's tumor. Tumor cells contain conspicuous amounts of cytoplasmic glycogen (black granules at left center), but lack specific differentiating features. It is readily distinguished from differentiating rhabdomyosarcoma in Figure 9 by absence of filaments. By light microscopy, the two are sometimes indistinguishable. (× 17380).

and classification of tumors. In this case, a cell suspension of tumor was smeared on a glass slide and stained with anti-terminal deoxynucleotidyl transferase (anti-TdT) antiserum. The reticular pattern of nuclear fluorescence is apparent. This positive result clearly identifies this tumor as a lymphoblastic lymphoma, since TdT-positivity is thought to be a reliable marker of this malignancy. Further subcategorization is also possible (and desirable) using the battery of immunologic techniques

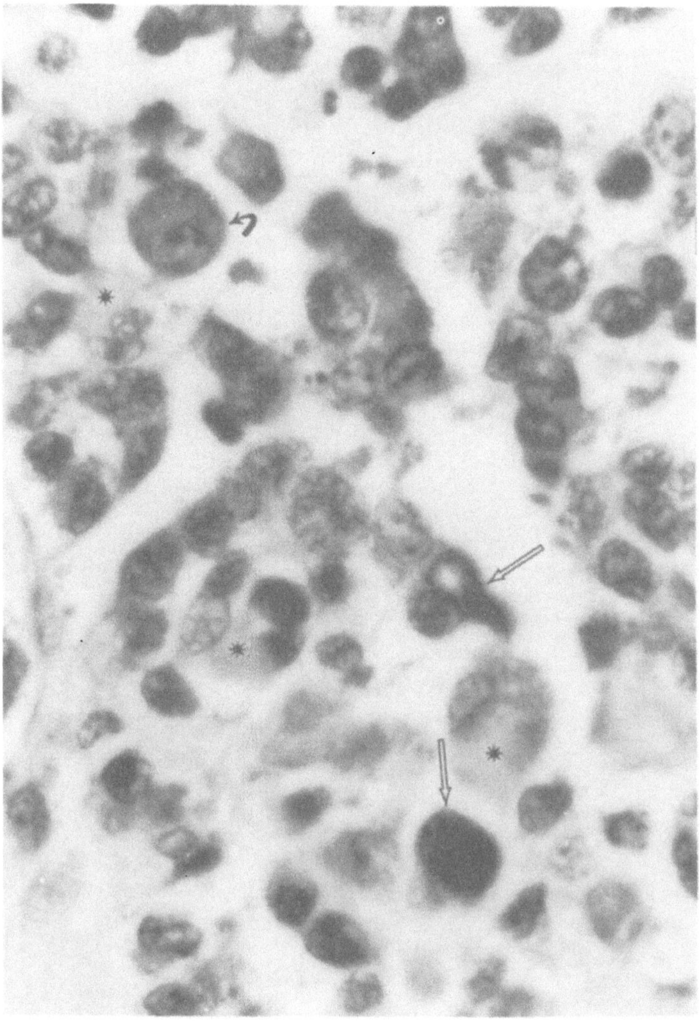

Figure 11. IP of rhabdomyosarcoma (same case as Figure 9). Note intense reactivity of some cells (open arrows), obliterating all cellular detail. Less intense reaction product is also present (curved arrow) and readily distinguishable from non-reactive cells (asterisks). Antiserum only reacts with human skeletal muscle myosin light chains. Variable tumor cell reactivity suggests that greater sampling inherent in this light microscopic preparation would detect skeletal muscle differentiation with greater sensitivity and objectivity than would electron microscopy. (× 1040).

described above. By doing so, therapeutically useful information can be obtained, since more aggressive therapy may be appropriate for the prognostically worse group of more immunologically immature lymphoblastic lymphoma.

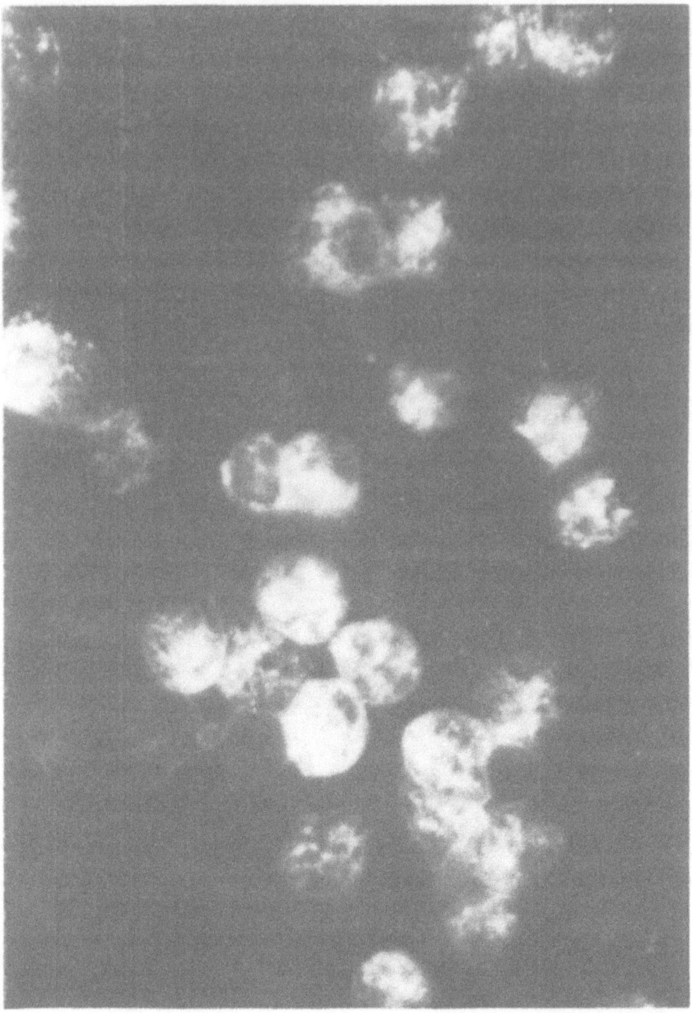

Figure 12. Immunofluorescence of lymphoblastic lymphoma treated with fluorescein-tagged anti-TdT antiserum. Bright nuclear fluorescence indicates presence of immature lymphocyte specific DNA transferase, a unique finding in lymphoblastic lymphoma, among solid lymphoid malignancies. (Approx. × 950).

4. Conclusions

It should be evident from the foregoing examples that conventional light microscopy is often an insufficient method in the detection and specific diagnosis of metastases. It is therefore important to be aware of the alternative techniques, which we have described in some detail, that are available to the clinician, pathologist, and investigator when the diagnosis of a metastatic tumor is in question. It is equally imperative to be familiar with the appropriate methods of tissue handling, which differ from fixation in formalin, so that the ancillary methods may be performed in an efficient and timely manner.

Acknowledgments

The authors would like to acknowledge the considerable help of several members of the Laboratory of Pathology, NCI, and others as indicated. We especially appreciate the opportunity to present the current work of several individuals. Dr. Lance A Liotta kindly allowed us to use his illustrations of anti-type IV collagen immunoperoxidase of metastatic breast cancer (Figure 3). Dr. Hung Chiang of this laboratory prepared the immunoperoxidase of keratin in epidermoid carcinoma (Figure 4) and skeletal muscle myosin light chains in rhabdomyosarcoma (Figure 11). Dr Ilona Linnoila provided the immunoperoxidase of glucagon in islet cells (Figure 6). Dr. Jeffrey Cossman allowed us to reproduce his immunofluorescence preparation of TdT in lymphoblastic lymphoma (Figure 12). Drs. C. Patrick Reynolds and R. Graham Smith kindly allowed us to reproduce the FACS diagram of neuroblastoma and bone marrow cells (Figure 8).

Mr. Herman Michelitch and Mr. Ralph Isenburg produced most of the illustrations for this chapter; their expert assistance is greatly acknowledged. Mrs. Sue Hostler typed the manuscript; her efforts are especially appreciated.

References

1. Sobel HJ, Marquet E: Usefulness of electron microscopy in the diagnosis of tumors. Pathol Res Pract 167:22–44, 1980.
2. Bonikos DS, Bensch KG, Kempson RL: The contribution of electron microscopy to the differential diagnosis of tumors. Beitr Pathol Bd 158:417–444, 1976.
3. Mackay B, Osborne BM: The contribution of electron microscopy to the diagnosis of tumors. Pathobiol Annu 8:359–405, 1978.
4. Gyorkey F, Min K-W, Krisko I, Gyorkey P: The usefulness of electron microscopy in the diagnosis of human tumors. Human Pathol 6:421–440, 1975.
5. Trump BF, Jones RT (eds): Diagnostic electron microscopy, Vols 1–3. New York: John Wiley, 1978–1980.
6. Ghadially FN: Ultrastructural pathology of the cell. London: Butterworths, 1975.
7. Ghadially FN: Diagnostic electron microscopy of tumours, London: Butterworths, 1980.
8. Reddick RL, Michelitch H, Triche TJ: Malignant soft tissue tumors (malignant fibrous histiocytoma, pleomorphic liposarcoma, and pleomorphic rhabdomyosarcoma): an electron microscopic study. Human Pathol 10:327–343, 1979.
9. Harris M: Differential diagnosis of spindle cell tumours by electron microscopy — personal experience and a review. Histopathol 5:81–105, 1981.
10. Triche TJ: Round cell tumors in childhood: the application of newer techniques to the differential diagnosis, chapter 11 in: Perspectives in pediatric pathology 7, Rosenberg H (ed) (in press).
11. DeLellis RA, Sternberger LA, Mann RB, Banks PM, Nakane PK: Immunoperoxidase technics in diagnostic pathology. Am J Clin Pathol 71:483–488, 1979.
12. Heyderman E: Immunoperoxidase technique in histopathology: applications, methods, and controls. J Clin Pathol 32:971–978, 1979.
13. Sieinski W, Dorsett B, Ioachim HL: Identification of prekeratin by immunofluorescence staining in the differential diagnosis of tumors. Human Pathol 12:452–457, 1981.

14. Sternberger LA: Immunocytochemistry. New York: John Wiley, 1979.
15. Taleporos P, Ornstein L: Histological methods. In: Antigen-antibody reactions *in vivo*, Methods in immunology and immunochemistry, Williams CA, Chase MW (eds). New York: Academic Press, 1976, pp 375–456.
16. Rost FWD: Fluorescence microscopy. In: Histochemistry: theoretical and applied 1: preparative and optical technology. Edinburgh: Churchill Livingstone, 1980, pp 346–378.
17. Heitzmann H, Richards FM: Use of the avidin-biotin complex for specific staining of biological membranes in electron microscopy. Proc Nat Acad Sci 71:3537–3541, 1974.
18. Hsu S-M, Raine L, Fanger H: The use of antiavidin antibody and avidin-biotin-peroxidase complex in immunoperoxidase technics. Am J Clin Pathol 75:816–821, 1981.
19. Non-Hodgkin's Lymphoma Pathologic Classification Project: National Cancer Institute sponsored study of classifications of non-Hodgkin's lymphomas: summary and description of a working formulation for clinical usage. Cancer (in press).
20. Rappaport H: Tumors of the hematopoietic system, atlas of tumor pathology, Section III – Fascicle 8, Washington: Armed Forces Institute of Pathology, 1966.
21. Berard CW, Jaffe ES, Braylan RC, Mann RB, Nanba K: Immunologic aspects and pathology of the malignant lymphomas. Cancer 42:911–921, 1978.
22. Nathwani BN: A critical analysis of the classifications of non-Hodgkin's lymphomas. Cancer 44:347–384, 1979.
23. Tubbs RR, Sheibani K, Weiss RA, Sebek BA, Deodhar SD: Tissue immunomicroscopic evaluation of monoclonality of B-cell lymphomas. Am J Clin Pathol 76:24–28, 1981.
24. Wood WG, Hood P, Rippey JH: Cell typing in lymphoproliferative disorders. Am J Surg Pathol 5:369–379, 1981.
25. Reynolds CP, Smith RG: Diagnostic and biological markers for neuroblastoma. In: Neuroblastoma: clinical and biological manifestations, Pochedly C (ed). New York: Elsevier, 1982.
26. Reynolds CP, Smith RG: Monoclonal antibody to human neuroblastoma-associated antigen. Proc Am Soc Clin Oncol 22:402, 1981.
27. Reinherz EL, Kung PC, Goldstein G, Levey RH, Schlossman SF: Discrete stages of human intrathymic differentiation: analysis of normal thymocytes and leukemia lymphoblasts of T-cell lineage. Proc Natl Acad Sci 77:1588–1592, 1980.
28. Cossman J, Chused TM, Bollum F, Jaffe ES: Diversity of immunologic phenotypes of lymphoblastic lymphoma (in preparation).
29. Pearse AGE: The cytochemistry and ultrastructure of polypeptide hormone-producing cells of the APUD series and the embryologic, physiologic, and pathologic implications of the concept. J Histochem Cytochem 17:303–313, 1960.
30. Pearse AGE: The diffuse neuroendocrine system and the APUD concept: related endocrine peptides in brain, intestine, pituitary, placenta and anura cutaneous glands. Med Biol 55:115–125, 1977.
31. Falck B: Observations on the possibilities of the cellular localization of monoamines by a fluorescence method. Acta Physiol Scand 56 (Suppl 197):6–25, 1962.
32. Falck B, Hillarp N-A, Thieme G, Torp A: Fluorescence of catechol amines and related compounds condensed with formaldehyde. J Histochem Cytochem 10:348–354, 1962.
33. Lindvall O, Bjorklund A: The glyoxylic acid fluorescence histochemical method: a detailed account of the methodology for the visualization of central catecholamine neurons. Histochemistry 39:97–127, 1974.
34. Lindvall O, Bjorklund A, Falck B, Loren I: New aspects on factors determining the sensitivity of the formaldehyde and glyoxylic acid fluorescence histochemical methods for monoamines. Histochemistry 68:169–181, 1980.
35. De la Torre JC, Surgeon JW: A methodological approach to rapid and sensitive monoamine histofluorescence using a modified glyoxylic acid technique: the SPG method. Histochemistry 49:81–93, 1976.
36. Judge DM, Dickman PS, Trapukdi S: Nonfunctioning argyrophilic tumor (APUDoma) of the

hepatic duct: simplified methods of detecting biogenic amines in tissue. Am J Clin Pathol 66:40–45, 1976.

37. Reynolds CP, German DC, Weinberg AG, Smith RG: Catecholamine fluorescence and tissue culture morphology. Am J Clin Pathol 75:275–282, 1981.
38. Bornstein P, Sage H: Structurally distinct collagen types. Ann Rev Biochem 49:957–1003, 1980.
39. Stern R, Wilczek J, Thorpe WP, Rosenberg SA, Cannon G: Procollagens as markers for the cell of origin of human bone tumors. Cancer Res 40:325–328, 1980.
40. Breitkreutz D, Diaz de Leon L, Paglia L, Gay S, Swarm RL, Stern R: Histological and biochemical studies of a transplantable rat chondrosarcoma. Cancer Res 39:5093–5100, 1979.
41. Dickman PS, Liotta LA, Triche TJ: Ewing's sarcoma: characterization in established cultures and evidence of its histogenesis. Lab Invest 42:111, 1980.
42. Triche TJ, Dickman PS, Lanzer WS, Garbisa SA, Liotta LA: Patterns of collagen type synthesis by human tumors reflect the tissue of origin. Eur J Cell Biol.22:543, 1980.
43. Alitalo K, Kurikinen M, Vaheri A, Virtanen I, Rhode H, Timpl R: Basal lamina glycoproteins are produced by neuroblastoma cells. Nature 287:465–466, 1980.
44. Lanzer WL, Liotta LA, Yee C, Azar HA, Costa JC: Synthesis of procollagen type II by a xeno-transplanted human chondroblastic osteosarcoma. Am J Pathol 104:217–226, 1981.
45. Prockop DJ, Kivirikko KI, Tuderman L, Guzman NA: The biosynthesis of collagen and its disorders. N Engl J Med 301:13–23 and 77–86, 1979.
46. Furthmayr H, Timpl R: Immunochemistry of collagens and procollagens. Int Rev Connect Tissue Res 7:61–99, 1976.
47. Hahn E, Timpl R, Miller EJ: Demonstration of a unique antigenic specificity for the collagen α 1 (II) chain from cartilaginous tissue. Immunol 28:561–568, 1975.
48. Roll FJ, Madri JA, Albert J, Furthmayr H: Codistribution of collagen types IV and AB_2 in basement membranes and mesangium of the kidney. J Cell Biol 85:597–616, 1980.
49. Timpl R, Wick G, Gay S: Antibodies to distinct types of collagens and procollagens and their application in immunohistology. J Immunol Methods 18:165–182, 1977.
50. Laurie GW, Leblond CP, Cournil I, Martin GR: Immunohistochemical evidence for the intracellular formation of basement membrane collagen (type IV) in developing tissues. J Histochem Cytochem 28:1267–1274, 1980.
51. Grimaud J-A, Druguet M, Peyrol S, Chevalier O, Herbage D, Bachawy NE: Collagen immunotyping in human liver: light and electron microscope study. J Histochem Cytochem 28:1145–1156, 1980.
52. Linsenmayer TF, Hendrix MJC, Little CD: Production and characterization of a monoclonal antibody to chicken type I collagen. Proc Natl Acad Sci 76:3703–3707, 1979.
53. Linsenmayer TF, Hendrix MJC: Monoclonal antibodies to connective tissue macromolecules: Type II collagen. Biochem Biophys Res Comm 92:440–446, 1980.
54. Cournil I, Leblond CP, Pomponio J, Hand AR, Sederlof L, Martin GR: Immunohistochemical localization of procollagens. I. Light microscopic distribution of procollagen I, III and IV antigenicity in the rat incisor tooth by the indirect peroxidase-anti-peroxidase method. J Histochem Cytochem 27:1059–1069, 1979.
55. Karim A, Cournil I, Leblond CP: Immunohistochemical localization of procollagens. II. Electron microscopic distribution of procollagen I antigenicity in the odontoblasts and predentin of rat incisor teeth by a direct method using peroxidase linked antibodies. J Histochem Cytochem 27:1070–1083, 1979.
56. Leblond CP, Wright GM: Intracellular localization of the precursors of type I collagen as shown by immunoperoxidasic and immunoradioautographic techniques. Acta Histochem Cytochem 13:23–34, 1980.
57. Garbisa S, Liotta LA, Tryggvason K, Siegal GP: Antibodies to collagenase-resistant terminal regions of pro-type IV collagen recognize whole basement membrane and 7S collagen. FEBS Lett 127:257–262, 1981.

58. Franklin WA, Ringus JC: Basement membrane antigen in Wilms' tumor. Lab Invest 44:375–380, 1981.
59. Liotta LA, Foidart JM, Gehron Robey P, Martin GR, Gullino PM: Identification of micrometastasis of breast carcinomas by presence of basement membrane collagen. Lancet 2:146–147, 1979.
60. Siegal GP, Barsky SH, Terranova VP, Liotta LA: Stages of neoplastic transformation of human breast tissue as monitored by dissolution of basement membrane components. An immunoperoxidase study. Invasion and Metastasis 1:54–70, 1981.
61. Jobsis AC, DeVries GP, Anholt RRH, Sanders GTB: Demonstration of the prostatic origin of metastases. An immunohistochemical method for formalin-fixed embedded tissue. Cancer 41:1788–1793, 1978.
62. Nadji M, Tabei SZ, Castro A, Chu TM, Morales AR: Prostatic origin of tumors. An immunohistochemical study. Am J Clin Pathol 73:735–739, 1980.
63. Pearse AGE: The APUD cell concept and its implications in pathology. Pathol Annu 9:27–42, 1974.
64. Bordi C, Ravazzola M, Baetens D, Gorden P, Unger RH, Orci L: A study of glucagonomas by light and electron microscopy and immunofluorescence. Diabetes 28:925–936, 1979.
65. DeLellis RA, Rule AH, Spiler I, Nathanson L, Tashjian AH Jr, Wolfe HJ: Calcitonin and carcinoembryonic antigen as tumor markers in medullary thyroid carcinoma. Am J Clin Pathol 70:587–594, 1978.
66. Judge DM, Demers LM, Nahrwold DL, Dickman PS, Petrokubi RJ, Trapukdi S: Vasoactive intestinal polypeptide and gastrin-producing islet cell carcinoma. Arch Pathol Lab Med 101:262–265, 1977.
67. Krejs GJ, Orci L, Conlon JM, Ravazzola M, Davis GR, Raskin P, Collins SM, McCarthy DM, Baetens D, Rubenstein A, Aldor TAM, Unger RH: Somatostatinoma syndroma. N Engl J Med 301:285–292, 1979.
68. Larsson L-I: Adrenocorticotropin-like and α-melanotropin-like peptides in a subpopulation of human gastrin cell granules: bioassay, immunoassay, and immunocytochemical evidence. Proc Natl Acad Sci 78:2990–2994, 1981.
69. Costa C, Rosai J, Philpott GW: Pigmentation of 'amelanotic' melanoma in culture. Arch Pathol 95:371–373, 1973.
70. Dickman PS, Triche TJ: Ultrastructural comparison of Ewing's sarcoma of bone with diverse pediatric soft tissue sarcomas: diagnostic criteria for soft tissue sarcoma resembling Ewing's sarcoma. Lab Invest 44:15A, 1981.
71. Tsokos M, Zweig N, Howard R, Bowling Mc, Costa JC: Immunocytochemical markers in embryonal and alveolar rhabdomyosarcoma. A diagnostic aid. Lab Invest 44:68A, 1981.
72. Sarnat HB, de Mello DE, Siddiqui SY: Diagnostic value of histochemistry in embryonal rhabdomyosarcoma. Am J Surg Pathol 3:177–183, 1979.
73. Koh S-J, Johnson WW: Antimyosin and antirhabdomyoblast sera. Their use for the diagnosis of childhood rhabdomyosarcoma. Arch Pathol Lab Med 104:118–122, 1980.
74. Mukai K, Rosai J, Hallaway BE: Localization of myoglobin in normal and neoplastic human skeletal muscle cells using an immunoperoxidase method. Am J Surg Pathol 3:373–376, 1979.
75. Mann RB, Jaffe ES, Berard CW: Malignant lymphomas – A conceptual understanding of morphologic diversity. Am J Pathol 94:105–176, 1979.
76. Jaffe ES, Braylan RC, Frank MM, Green I, Berard CW: Heterogeneity of immunologic markers and surface morphology in childhood lymphoblastic lymphoma. Blood 48:213–221, 1976.

27. Fine needle aspiration cytology of metastases

E. W. CHU and S. E. MARTIN

1. Introduction

Diagnostic cytology is the examination of cells from human organs obtained by either directly scraping the mucosal tissue or by aspirating with a fine needle. The specimen is smeared on glass slides. Under the microscope properly prepared smears show a thin layer of cells often spread out singly. After proper fixation and staining procedures, the cell membranes become transparent thus allowing the cytopathologist to scrutinize the integral parts of the nucleus and cytoplasm. Since Papanicolaou et al. [1] published a monograph on diagnostic cytology in 1943, pathologists around the world have learned the technique and applied it with great success as an adjunct to surgical pathological procedures. The clinical cytology practiced in the middle of this century consisted largely of exfoliative preparations, i.e. cells that are either exfoliated naturally into the body cavities or scraped off from the mucosal surfaces, such as in cervico-vaginal pap smears. Diagnostic cytology, as it steadily gains momentum, is no longer limited to the examination of exfoliated or scraped mucosal cells. The discipline is now encompassing all specialities of medical practice, and involving many organs which, when aspirated by a fine needle, will yield non-exfoliative types of cells for cytological examination.

2. Historical development of needle aspiration biopsy

Needle aspiration of cells for diagnosis had its beginning as early as 1900 [2] and was first applied to lymph nodes. Guthrie [3] was the first to report findings of metastatic tumor cells in a lymph node. Since then, needle aspiration has been accepted with increasing enthusiasm. In many parts of Europe and in Scandinavian countries, fine needle aspiration biopsy is employed as the main definitive diagnostic procedure for lesions of the thyroid, breast, salivary gland and soft tissue. The reader is referred to the large body of published literature in this area. Table 1 shows the areas where fine needle aspiration techniques have been commonly applied for diagnostic purposes.

L.A. Liotta and I.R. Hart (eds.), Tumor Invasion and Metastasis. ISBN-13: 978-94-009-7513-2.
© 1982 Martinus Nijhoff Publishers, The Hague/Boston/London.

Table 1. Applicable areas.

Tonsils	Prostate
Salivary gland	Testis
Thyroid gland	Lymph node
Breast	Bone
Lung	Soft tissue tumors
Kidney	

3. Clinical value and reliability

Fine needle aspiration (FNA) cytology is a refined and reliable method of detecting pathological lesions including neoplasia of both benign and malignant types. This relatively straightforward method uses simple instruments and requires minimal laboratory facilities. The diagnostic accuracy is high, approximately 90% [4]. The accuracy rating, however, is dependent upon: a) adequate aspirates for examination, b) pertinent clinical history, and c) proficiency of the examiner. When these conditions are met, the technique is very helpful in the clinic (Table 2).

For the purpose of studying metastases, fine needle aspiration smears prove to be a simple, reliable, and most rewarding method. Although FNA can often stand alone on its own merits, particularly when the previous surgical sections are available for comparison, FNA is not viewed as a replacement for the histologic biopsy but rather as an adjunct to the histologic sections. It offers an alternative method to reach a decisive diagnosis, thus aiding the clinician in his clinical management of the patient. This is particularly true in patients being treated for malignant neoplasms where the clinical objective is to detect a local tumor recurrence or to differentiate an inflammatory process from a metastasis.

Table 2. Advantages.

Fine needle aspiration	Open biopsy and/or Vim Silverman needle core biopsy
Clinic/office procedure	Operating room procedure
Painless, anesthesia not required	Anesthesia necessary
Multiple specimens in one sitting	Often not possible
No (chances of) seeding	Seeding sometimes occurs
No assistants needed	Assistants required
Diagnosis within the hour possible – saves time, may provide earlier diagnosis in malignancies	Diagnosis in five or more hours – time-consuming
Economical	Expensive

Over a three year period at the NIH Clinical Center, 178 needle aspiration specimens were submitted for diagnosis of possible metastatic lesions from various organs of the body (Table 3). Of the 178 cases, 144 cases had surgical procedures and 84 cases were lost to follow-up. There were no false positive cases reported cytologically. In one case, an aspirate from a lung nodule was reported cytologically negative because of the absence of epithelial cells and subsequent surgical excision revealed the lesion to be metastatic osteogenic sarcoma. The acceptability of a negative cytological report is contingent upon the clinician's appraisal of the patient's physical condition. A negative aspirate merely means the absence of abnormal cells. Should there be any doubt about the validity of the cytological report, be it negative or positive, either the aspiration should be repeated or an incisional biopsy should be performed.

The reliability of a cytological report is heavily dependent upon the proficiency of both the physician performing the aspiration and the cytologist interpreting the smear. A false negative report is generally the result of sampling error, i.e. missing the exact area where the metastasis is located.

Table 3. 3-year study of metastatic lesion.

	Cytology			Pathology	
Tissue	Positive for malignant cells*	Negative (benign)	Suspicious for malignancy	Malignant (biopsy)	Benign**
Lymph node	60	18	1	61	18
Lung	5	8***	2	7	8
Liver	3	4	1	3	5
Soft tissue	19	2	1	19	3
Testicle	1	3		1	3
Kidney	2	4		2	4
Bone	3	2		3	2
Vein	3	2		3	2
Total 144	96	43	5	99	45

*No false positive cases were reported cytologically.
**34 negative aspirations had no surgical follow up.
***One case was cytologically false negative.

4. Technique

The instruments required are few. One needs a pre-sterilized syringe and needle and

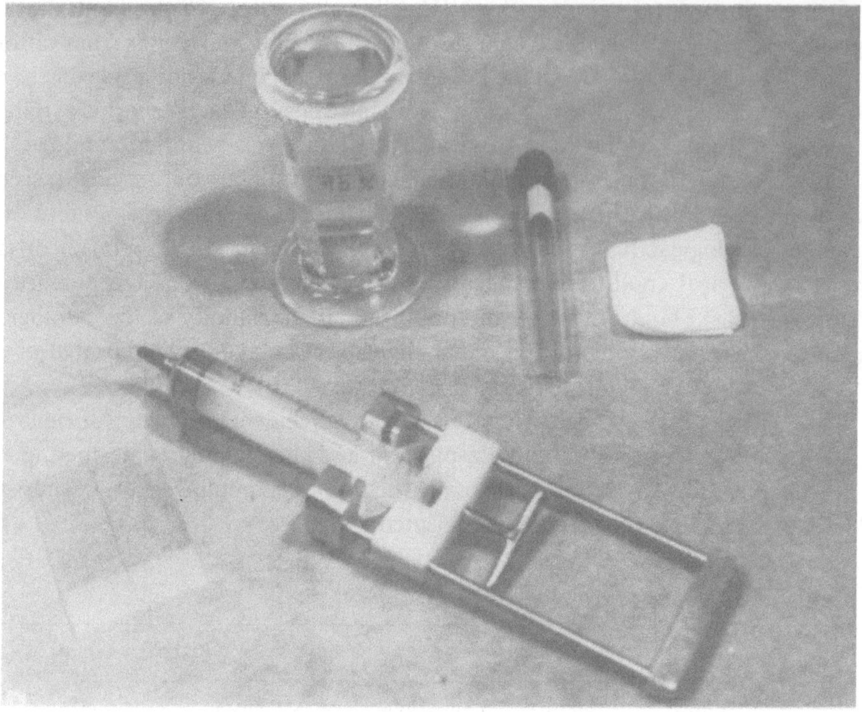

Figure 1.

a syringe holder (Figure 1). The syringe holder permits one handed operation thereby allowing the other hand to immobilize the area to be aspirated. The actual aspiration is done by using a fine gauge needle (#21 or smaller). The small caliber of the needle assures a non-traumatic puncture and also prevents admixture of blood.

4.1. Puncture

After the needle has reached the lesion, a negative pressure is created in the syringe by retracting the plunger. This manipulation allows easy aspiration of the cellular material. When a negative pressure is created, the needle is shifted slightly from area to area to insure a representative sampling (Figure 2). After completion of the aspiration, the plunger is slowly allowed to return to its normal position, releasing the excess negative pressure that is in the syringe. The needle is then withdrawn and the aspirate is placed on the glass slides in droplets.

4.2. Cytological processing

It is preferable to express one drop per slide. A smear is made by laying another slide on top of the droplet and pulling the two slides apart as in a blood smear. The smears are immediately placed into a jar of fixative; 95% ethyl alcohol is the accepted fixative in most laboratories in the U.S.A.

After the smears are made, the syringe and its attached needle are rinsed with 5 ml of isotonic saline to insure that any cells that are adherent to the syringe and needle will not be lost. The rinse is then filtered through a millipore membrane. Both the smears and the filter membrane are processed at the same time using the same fixation and staining procedures. The conventional Papanicolaou staining method is preferred by the authors.

5. Criteria for obtaining a decisive cytologic diagnosis in FNA

In order to render a decisive cytologic diagnosis on FNA biopsy material certain basic criteria must be met. First, it is absolutely critical that the clinical history be known, including any history of radiation or chemotherapy. Second, it is essential that an abundance of epithelial cells be present in the specimen. Third, provided that the foregoing criteria are met, the morphologic features of the cells indicate whether the cells are normal, reactive, or neoplastic. Fourth, the presence of non-cohesive

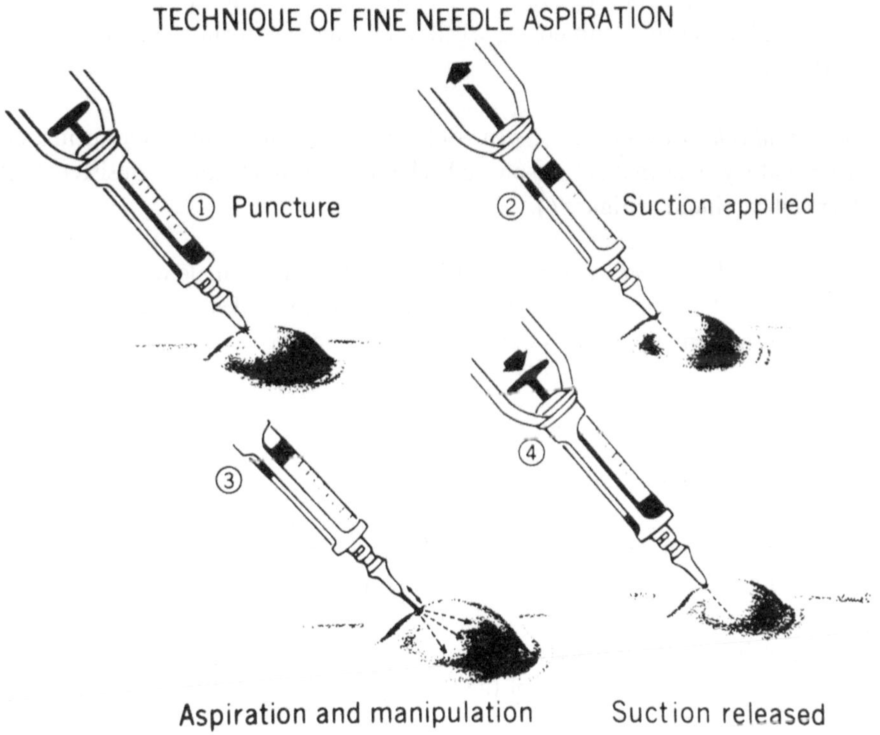

Figure 2.

atypical cells supports a diagnosis of malignancy. Finally, the presence of malignant cells alien to the location in which they are found, e.g. epithelial cells in a lymph node, is diagnostic of a metastatic process.

Sample cases

6.1. Primary lesions

6.1.1. Carcinoma of breast. During a routine examination a 48-year-old female was discovered to have a painless mass in the upper outer quadrant of her right breast. This was aspirated. The malignant cells are shown in Figure 3.

6.1.2. Squamous cell carcinoma. A 70-year-old male presented in the outpatient clinic with a 4 cm mass on his forehead. FNA was performed. The aspirates showed many malignant cells of the squamous type (Figure 4).

6.1.3. Papillary carcinoma of thyroid gland. A 29-year-old female who had undergone treatment for Hashimoto's disease for two years was found to have a 3 cm nodule in the region of the isthmus. This nodule was aspirated. The aspirates showed an abundance of non-cohesive cells and some cells forming papillary structures (Figure 5).

6.1.4. Renal cell carcinoma. A 55-year-old male was found to have a large mass in his right kidney. This mass was aspirated. The cells showed features consistent with a clear cell carcinoma (Figure 6).

6.1.5. Small cell (oat cell) carcinoma of lung. A 50-year-old male was found on x-ray to have nodules in both of his lungs. One of the nodules was aspirated. The aspirates showed many clusters of small hyperchromatic cells of the oat cell type (Figure 7).

6.2. Metastatic lesions

6.2.1. Osteogenic sarcoma – thyroid gland. A 37-year-old male, status post a left above-the-knee amputation three years previously for osteogenic sarcoma, complained of a rapidly enlarging mass in the neck. The neck mass was aspirated. The malignant cells aspirated from the thyroid gland showed features comparable to those seen in the surgical section of the tumor (Figure 8).

6.2.2. Hodgkin's disease – cervical lymph node. This 18-year-old male had been under treatment for Hodgkin's disease for the past two years. On routine follow-up examination a 1 × 1 cm nodule was found in his left neck. This was aspirated. Many classic Reed-Sternberg cells were present in the smear (Figure 9).

6.2.3. Anaplastic carcinoma – cervical lymph node. A 52-year-old female who underwent a thyroidectomy for anaplastic carcinoma two years previously noted an enlarging mass on the left side of her neck. FNA was performed. The smears showed numerous large cells with marked pleomorphism (Figure 10).

6.2.4. Renal cell carcinoma – ischium. This 50-year-old female was found on x-ray to have a lytic lesion of the right ischium. Earlier in the year, she had undergone nephrectomy for renal cell carcinoma. FNA was performed at the site of the bone lesion. The aspirates showed many abnormal cells compatible with hypernephroma (Figure 11).

6.2.5. Renal cell carcinoma – lung. This 50-year-old male had a right nephrectomy performed for renal cell carcinoma. Six months later, a chest x-ray showed a nodule in his right lung. This nodule was aspirated. Malignant cells were present in the smear (Figure 12).

6.2.6. Squamous cell carcinoma – lymph node. A 48-year-old female underwent radiation therapy for squamous cell carcinoma of the nares. A month later an enlarged submandibular nodule was discovered. This was aspirated. The aspirates showed many well-differentiated squamous cells (Figure 13).

6.2.7. Malignant melanoma – lymph node. This 22-year-old man had a malignant melanoma resected from his back in the past. He was found to have an enlarged axillary lymph node. This node was aspirated. Numerous epithelial cells showing malignant features were present (Figure 14).

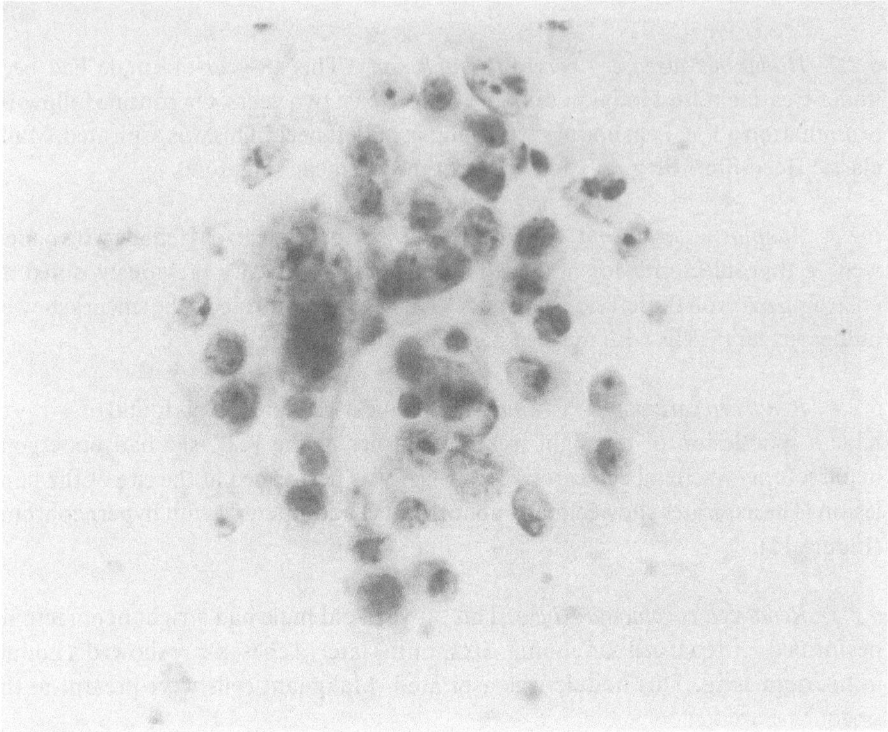

Figure 3.

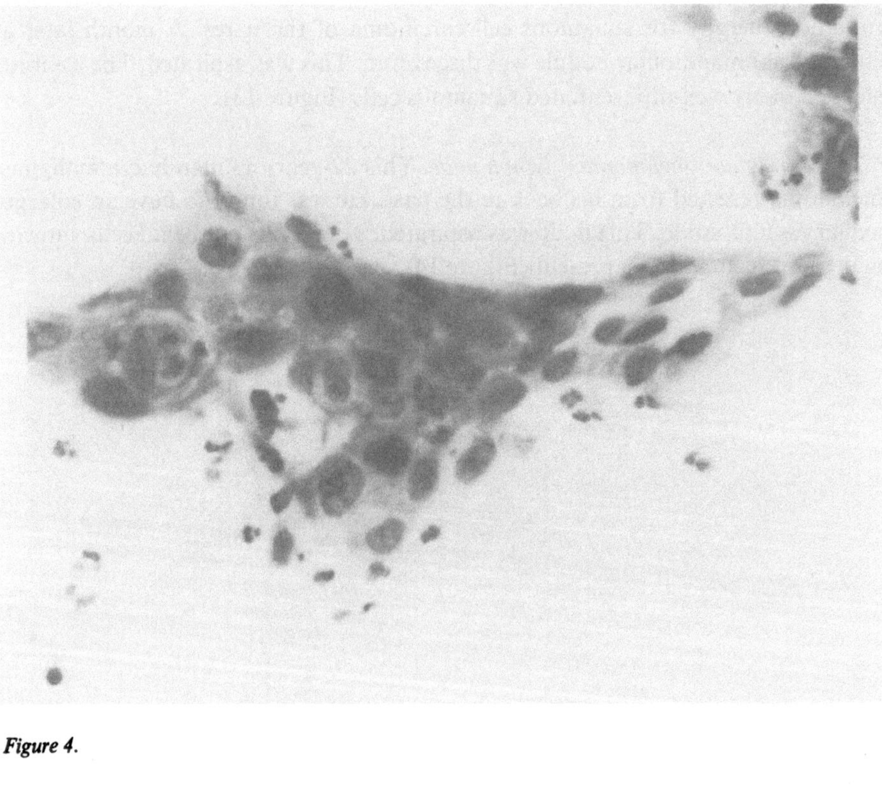

Figure 4.

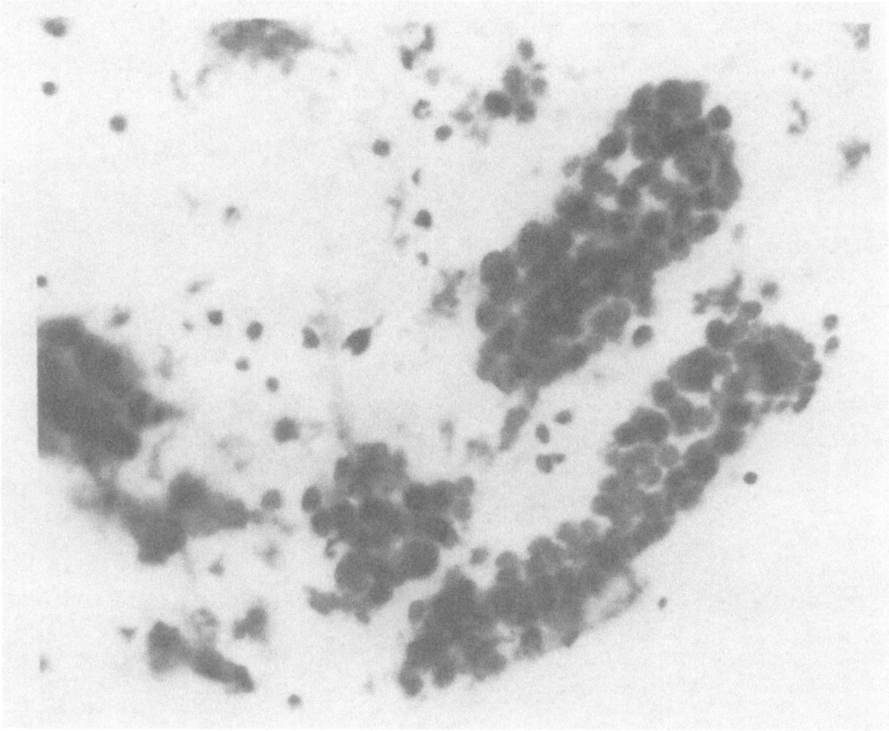

Figure 5.

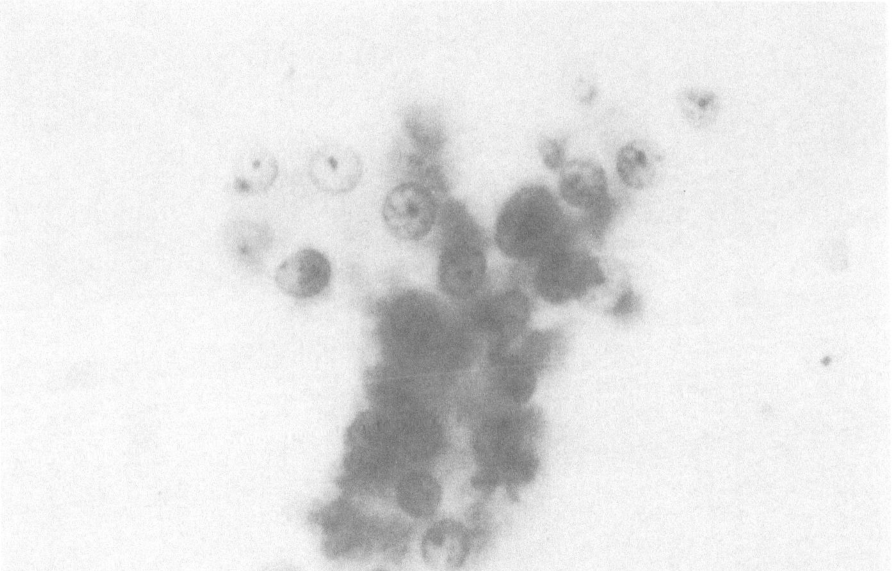

Figure 6.

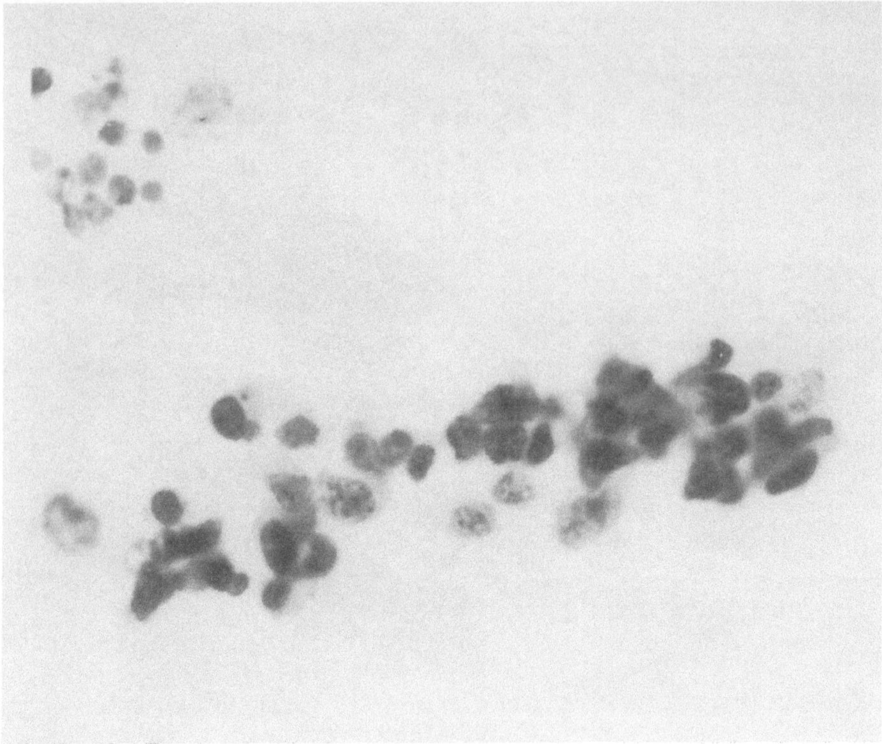

Figure 7.

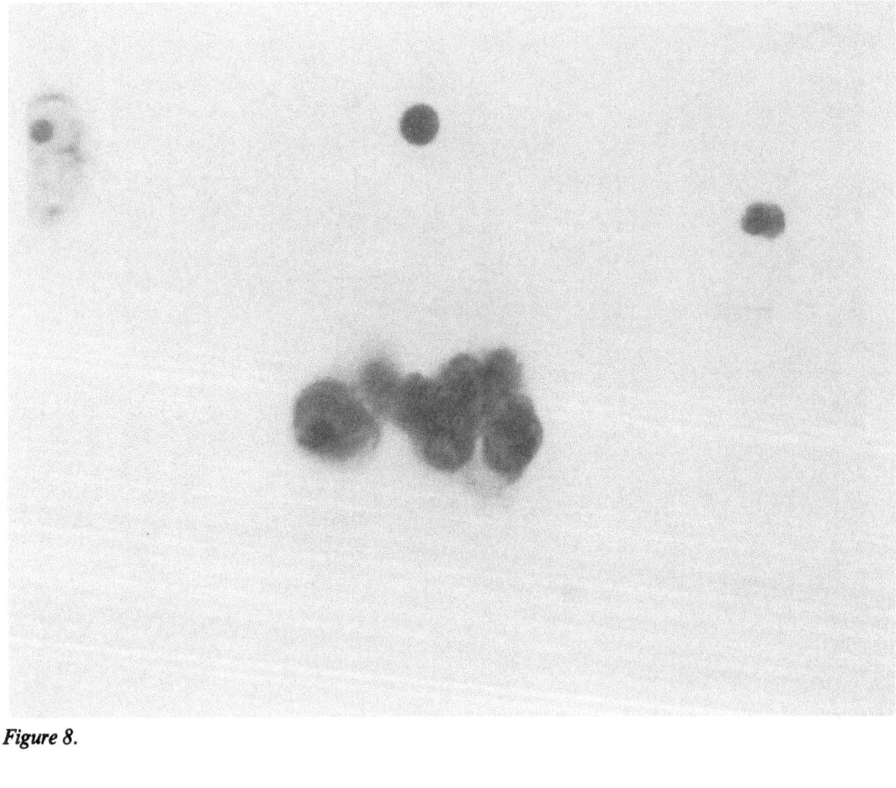

Figure 8.

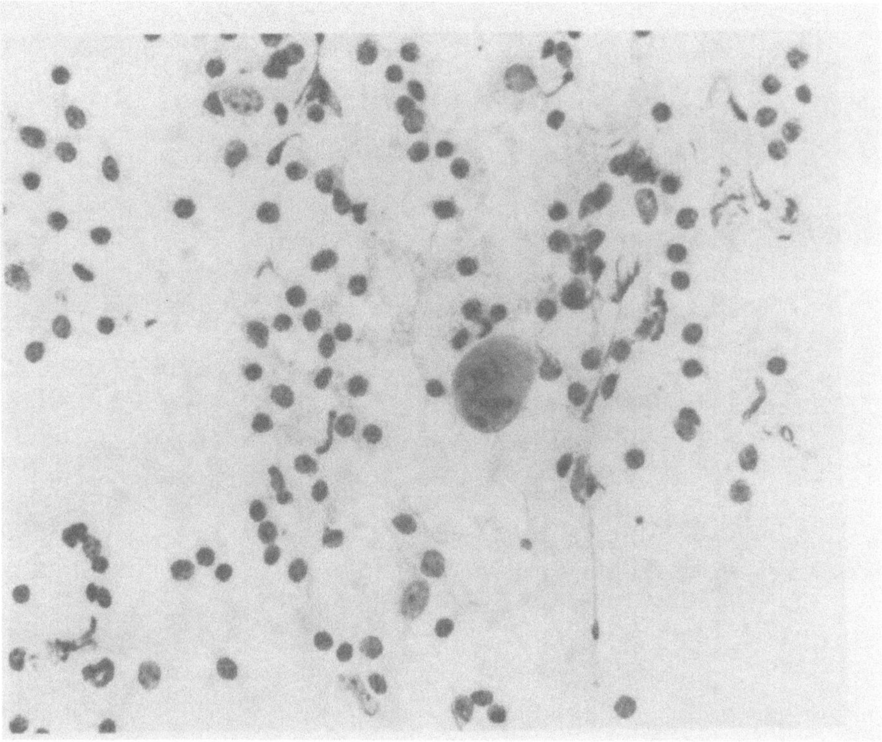

Figure 9.

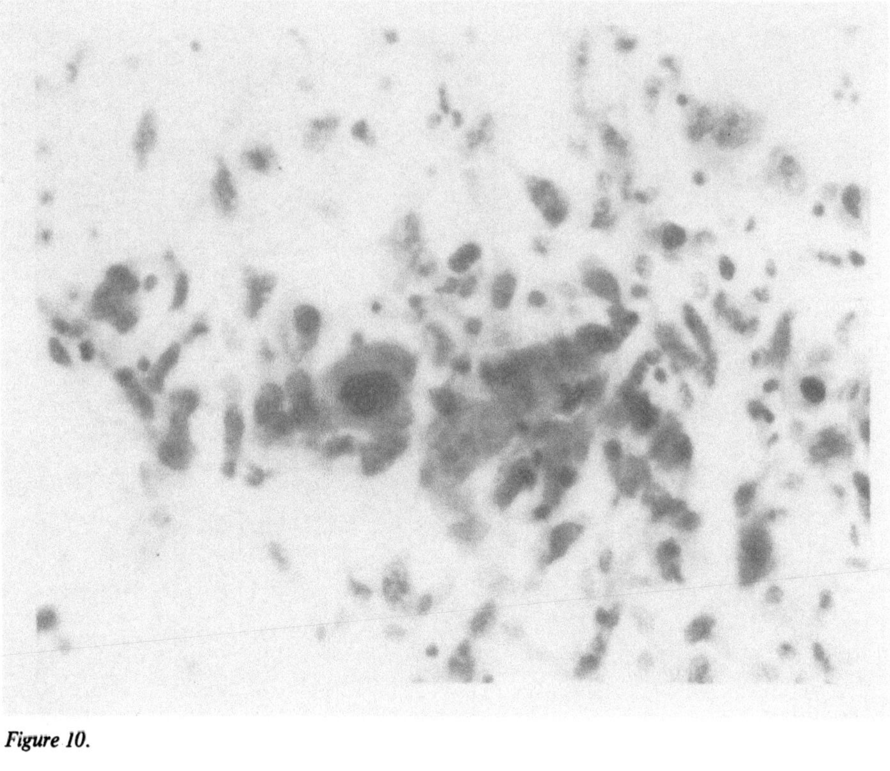

Figure 10.

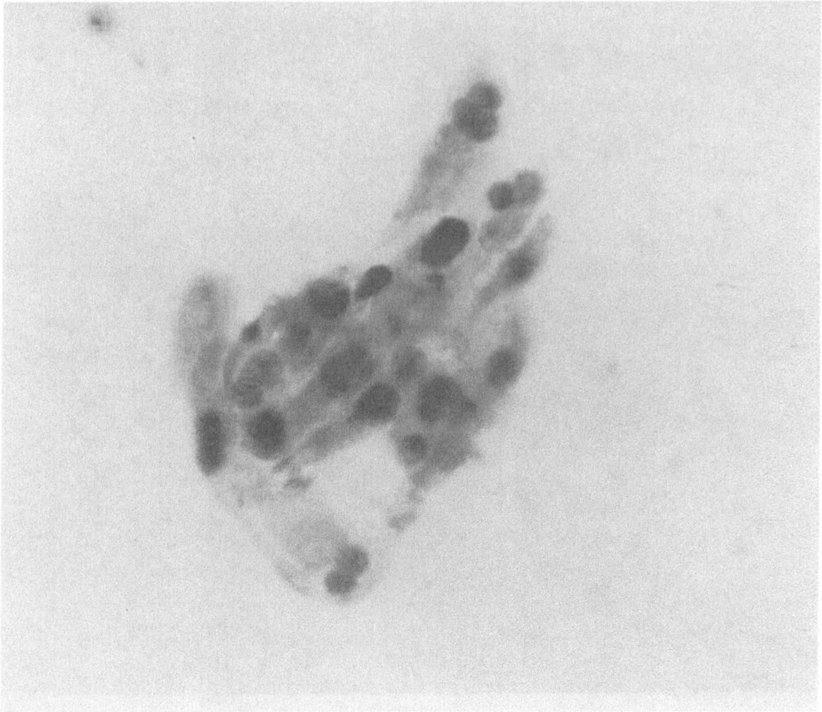

Figure 11.

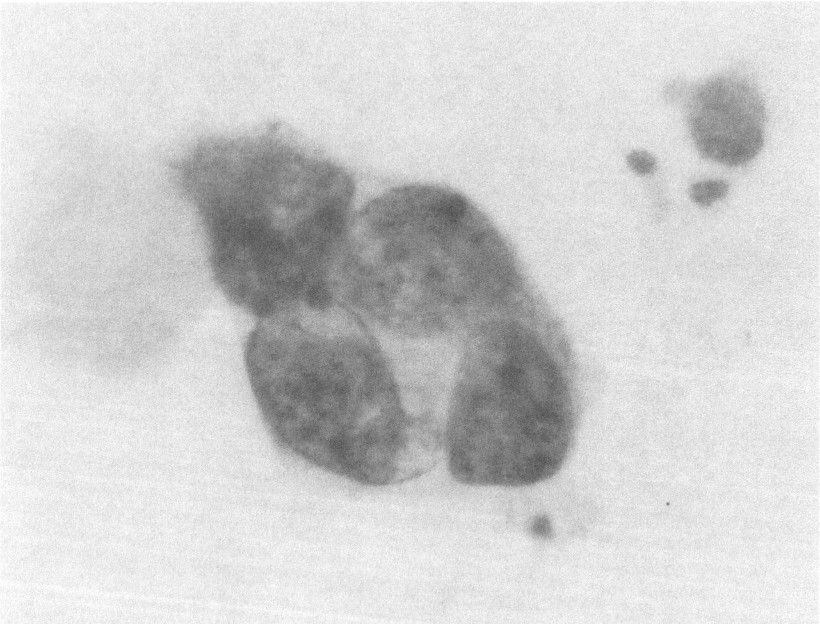

Figure 12.

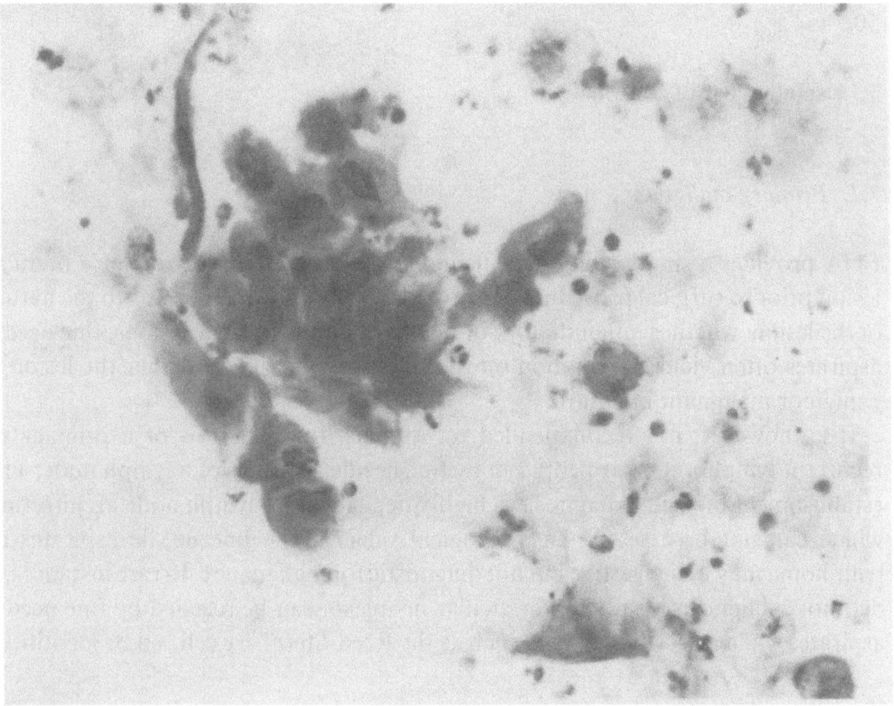

Figure 13.

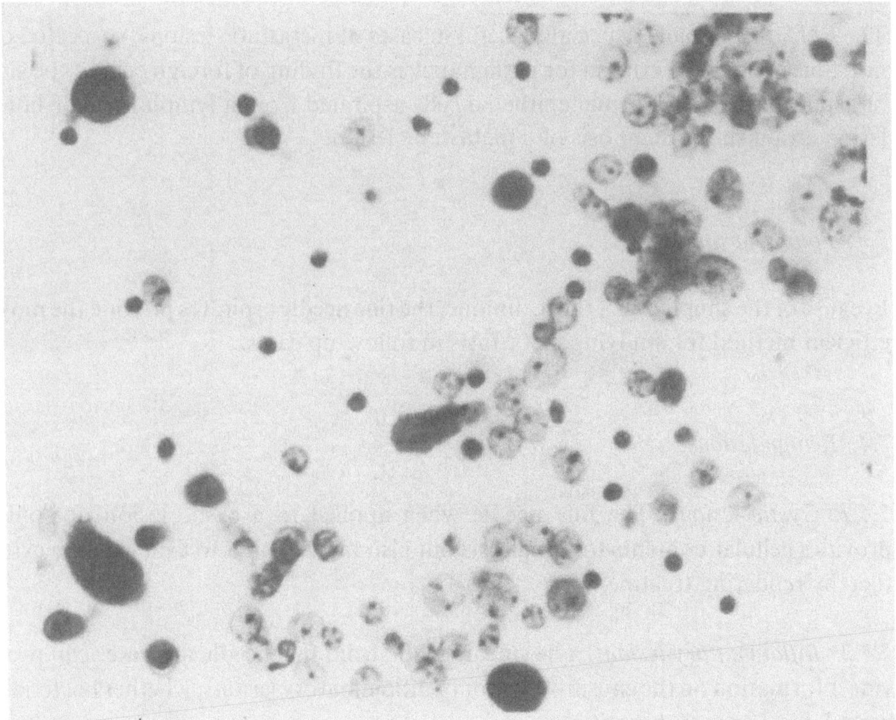

Figure 14.

7. Usefulness of FNA technique

7.1. Primary malignant lesions

FNA provides a simple and efficient method to study the aspirates of a nodular lesion prior to surgical procedures. It provides a working diagnosis as to the nature of the lesion, whether inflammatory or neoplastic. In neoplastic lesions, fine needle aspirates often yield information on the cell type as well as whether the lesion is benign or malignant in nature.

It is, however, not recommended to establish the diagnosis of a primary or recurrent lymphoreticular neoplasm by fine needle aspirates of a lymph node. The establishment of such a diagnosis is highly dependent on lymph node architecture which can not be assessed on cytological smears. The fine needle aspirates of lymphoma may be suggestive but not diagnostic for malignancy. In rare instances, a definitive diagnosis of a lymphoreticular neoplasm can be reached by fine needle aspirates when a specific cell type such as the Reed-Sternberg cell can be identified.

7.2. Metastatic lesions

The FNA technique is especially useful in cases of metastatic lesions, suspected or not. Since one of the criteria for malignancy is the finding of foreign cells at the site of aspiration, any abnormal epithelial cells aspirated from a lymph node or bone lesion establish the diagnosis of a metastatic lesion.

7.3. Follow-up studies

Because of the simplicity of the technique, the fine needle aspirates provide the most efficient method for studying metastasis in follow-up cases.

7.4. Benign lesions

7.4.1. Cystic lesions. The fine needle when applied to a cystic lesion not only provides cellular contents for diagnosis but also may be used to evacuate the cyst, thereby rendering treatment.

7.4.2. Inflammatory lesions. The smears made from fine needle aspirates can provide information on the causative factor of inflammatory lesions, whether bacterial, fungal, viral or even parasitic.

8. Potential risk factors

There is no reported case of seeding of malignant cells by a fine needle. In our ten years of experience with the FNA technique, there has been no recorded tumor seeding, hemorrhage or other complications.

9. Clinical limitations

1. FNA is of limited value in establishing the primary diagnosis of lymphoma and, likewise, in confirming recurrence and/or spread of lymphoma. 2. When chemotherapy and/or radiation therapy have already been initiated, it is not always possible to distinguish malignant changes from therapeutic effects. 3. Special cytopathology training is required to achieve proficiency in reading the cells obtained by fine needle aspiration technique.

10. Future prospects in FNA

Fine needle aspiration cytology has become a reliable diagnostic aid and is used routinely in most medical centers. It is rapid, reliable, inexpensive, and easy to perform. For these reasons, the technique, although for the most part currently practiced in referral centers, is ideally suited to primary care facilities. One of the obvious future trends in FNA is that, as the value of the technique becomes more generally appreciated, its use will become more widely disseminated throughout the medical community.

In addition to assuming an increasing role in the initial evaluation of patients, FNA will find greater use in combination with a variety of other techniques, including electron microscopy, immunology, and tissue culture. Recently, Collins and Ivarsson reported on tumor classification by electron microscopy of FNA biopsy material [5]. Using this combination of techniques, they were able to significantly increase the number of cases in which they could arrive at a preoperative diagnosis.

Perhaps the most exciting aspect of FNA and one which shows great promise for the diagnosis, classification, and, ultimately, the therapy of tumors, is the study of the cell surface using FNA biopsy material. FNA provides ready access to viable tumor cell suspensions. The cells aspirated from a tumor nodule may be placed in medium and studied immediately or maintained in culture medium for subsequent evaluation.

The recent advent of hybridoma antibody technology makes available well defined homogeneous reagents capable of specifically identifying a wide range of cell surface markers. FNA will be increasingly important in providing viable cells for precise immunological characterization of tumor cells. Questions such as the tissue origin of malignant cells, the immunological subclassification of tumors and antigenic heterogeneity within tumors should be readily addressed using monoclonal antibodies in conjunction with FNA. Further, culture of viable cells obtained from FNA may allow the study of tumor cell growth characteristics, tumor susceptibility to various cytotoxic drugs, and tumor responsiveness to growth factors. FNA may be useful in monitoring the efficiency of experimental approaches to tumor immunotherapy by providing direct information on the nature of the evoked host immune response to the tumor and in localization of parenterally administered monoclonal antibody.

In conclusion, it is safe to assume that FNA will find widespread use as a routine diagnostic procedure and as a tool to complement today's highly sophisticated biologic techniques.

References

1. Papanicolaou GN, Trant HF: Diagnosis of uterine cancer by the vaginal smear. New York: The Commonwealth Fund, 1943.
2. Menbrier P: Cancer primitif du poumon. Bull Soc Anat (Paris) 6:643–647, 1886.
3. Guthrie CG: Gland puncture as a diagnostic measure. Bull Johns Hopkins Hosp. 32:266, 1921.
4. Kline TS, Hunter SN: Needle aspiration biopsy. A critical appraisal. JAMA 239:36–39, 1978.
5. Collins VP, Ivarsson B: Tumor classification by electron microscopy of fine needle aspiration biopsy material. Acta Path Microbiol Scand Sect A. 89:103–105, 1981.

28. Applications of immunoperoxidase staining to studies of human breast disease

G. P. SIEGAL and S. H. BARSKY

1. Introduction

Beginning in the second decade and extending into the eighth, breast cancer remains the leading cause of cancer death in women in the United States [1]. More distressing still is the epidemiological evidence that, irrespective of the new therapeutic modalities, the 25-year trend in age adjusted breast cancer death rates shows no significant change [1]. In a continuing attempt to alter these dismal findings in a positive manner, pathologists and others have attempted to further recognize and subdivide breast neoplasms prior to their exhibiting highly aggressive biologic behavior. One avenue that offers some hope in this regard is the study of antigens, both host and tumor derived. Herberman, for the purposes of discussion, divides the common antigens on tumors into three major groups: i – virus induced or associated antigens, ii – fetal or carcinoembryonic antigens, and iii – tissue antigens [2]. We will subsequently discuss each of these.

Although large numbers of assays have been devised, paralleling our understanding of immunology, we will limit our discussion to immunoperoxidase (IP) techniques. By doing so, we therefore arbitrarily eliminate from our consideration some antibodies shown to have a relationship to breast disease by other techniques, for example antibodies against components of human milk fat globule [3]. Furthermore, we have, for the most part, eliminated discussing nonimmunocytochemical [e.g. 4, 5] and nonhuman [e.g. 6, 7] published reports.

2. The method

Immunoperoxidase staining of tissue sections was an outgrowth of fluorescein isothiocyanate conjugation studies allowing the histologic examination of the functional and structural status of tumors and disease processes. A number of excellent review articles [8–11] and books [12, 13] discuss the historical, theoretical, and technical aspects, to which we refer interested individuals. Although IP staining is really a group of closely related techniques (i.e. direct and indirect, conjugate and nonconjugate peroxidase methods) most recent studies use the unlabeled antibody (triple bridge) peroxidase – antiperoxidase (PAP) method, first elucidated by Sternberger and co-workers [14]. A synopsis of the technique we use [15] is as follows:

L.A. Liotta and I.R. Hart (eds.), Tumor Invasion and Metastasis. ISBN-13: 978-94-009-7513-2.
© 1982 Martinus Nijhoff Publishers, The Hague/Boston/London.

1) Warm glass slides containing fixed, paraffin embedded tissue sections
2) Deparaffinize with four changes of xylene, 2 to 4 min each
3) Absolute ethanol, 2 changes, 2 min each
4) 90%, 80%, and 70% ethanol, 1 change, 2 min each
5a) For tissue in mercury containing fixatives: 0.5% iodine in 70% ethanol for 5 min
5b) 5 min running tap water wash
5c) 5% hypo sodium thiosulfate 2 to 3 min
5d) Second 5 min water wash
6) Hydration in Tris/saline buffer (TSB) (50 mM Tris [pH 7.4], 0.85% NaCl), 2 changes, 2 min each
   This is the entry point of frozen sections
7) 1.0% H_2O_2 in absolute methanol for 20 min
8) TSB wash, 2 changes, 2 min each
9) 1.0% normal swine serum in TSB, 20 min
10) TSB wash, 2 changes, 2 min each
11) Primary antibody diluted in TSB incubated at 4° C overnight or at room temperature for 1 h in a humidified chamber
12) TSB wash, 4 changes, 2 min each
13) Secondary antisera diluted in TSB, 30 min incubation
14) TSB wash, 4 changes, 2 min each
15) PAP diluted in TSB, 30 min incubation
16) TSB wash, 4 changes, 2 min each
17) 3,3' Diaminobenzidine: H_2O_2 to develop color. Usually 2 to 8 min
18) Distilled water wash to stop reaction
19) Counterstain with Mayer's hematoxylin and lithium carbonate
20) Dehydration in ethanol cascade, rinse 2 times in xylene, permount, and cover-slip

3. The tissue

The human breast is a tubuloalveolar gland composed mainly of epithelial and myoepithelial lined ducts and alveoli, resting on a basal lamina, surrounded by prominent connective tissues, especially adipose tissue. It is subject to a whole myriad of benign and malignant neoplastic conditions [16–18]. Immunoperoxidase staining techniques as applied to the mammary gland have diagnostic as well as anatomic-physiologic usefulness and application. One can not only determine the cell type but often its *in situ* distribution, cellular products, and histogenesis. One can also observe a breast cell's ability to produce extracellular substances and its loss or gain of antigens, both inappropriate and normal. Furthermore, the production of autoantibodies and the relationship of the stroma to the cell type of interest can be monitored [10]. We will review and summarize these applications.

4. Virus and virus-related products

Antibodies have been detected in the serum of women which recognize intracytoplasmic type A particles (iAP) of mouse mammary tumor virus (MMTV) as well as type B particles. By IP techniques these antibodies bind to iAP membranes. In a study of more than 800 cases, these antibodies were found in approximately one-half of patients with proliferative mastopathy and one-third of patients with benign breast adenomas, fibroadenomas, and breast carcinomas. They were also identified in twenty-five percent of pregnant women and twelve percent of women with normal breast tissue [19]. Sera from patients and relatives of patients with breast carcinomas were tested by IP against cells of a mouse mammary tumor line. The Positive labeling observed, by immunoelectron microscopy, was localized on immature and mature type B and budding virus particles [20].

The viral component that has had the largest amount of work performed on its relationship with breast disease is a 52 000 dalton glycoprotein (GP) of MMTV. Antibodies raised against this gp 52 have been localized, by IP, on approximately 45% of human breast carcinomas but in none of 137 normal and benign breast lesions studied except for a single case of apocrine metaplasia [21–24]. In the same study, the Columbia University group found less than one percent positivity of other nonmammary carcinomas. Interestingly, of those invasive breast cancers associated with an intraductal component almost two-thirds of these cases showed positive staining, far surpassing those lesions in which only one of these conditions existed. Unfortunately there was great variability in the staining pattern and intensity and not all malignant tumor cells were positive. Although most studies found no correlation between positive staining and histologic classification or risk factors [25, 26] one study found 69 patients out of 88 with a positive family history for breast cancer had gp 52-like antigen by IP staining. [27, 28]. In a study of rapidly progressive breast carcinoma in Tunesia, 70% of patients showed positivity with antibodies against MMTV gp 52 [29]. It was also shown that these patients had enhanced immune reactivity to MMTV and tumor associated antigen. This cross reactivity between murine and human tumor antigens is now known to be due to the polypeptide component of the gp 52 [30, 31]. Edginston and Leung reported another mammary tumor glycoprotein (MTGP 20) could be localized in the cytoplasm and at the surface of human breast carcinomas but like gp 52, not in other benign tumors, hyperplasias, nor in milk secreted during lactation [32].

5. HCG and other peptide hormones

Human Chorionic Gonadotropin (HCG) has been identified in many neoplasms not associated with the placenta [33–35] and has been localized in mammary lesions in a number of studies. β chain HCG was measured by radioimmunoassay and confirmed by IP staining. In 9 of 65 malignant breast tumors it was shown to stain the cytoplasm of the tumor cells [36, 37]. In a similiar study from France, 2 out of 37 cases of adenocarcinoma of the breast were positive [38]. These low figures were offset by other studies showing about 60% of breast carcinomas were positive for HCG when antisera to αHCG was used [39, 40]. It is possible that this difference may be due to the estrogen receptor levels in these lesions since estrogen receptor negative tumors are more likely to contain β-HCG [41]. Antisera made against the α subunit of HCG has been shown to stain about 25% of breast carcinomas examined [42, 43]. Although no correlation was demonstrated between αHCG production and histology, one study found a correlation between αHCG staining in primary breast carcinomas and nodal metastases (worse prognosis) [42], although another study did not [43]. Because HCG is positive in many tumor types, it has no value as an exclusive marker for breast carcinoma [44]. In one study no tumor tissue was unequivocally negative for HCG [45].

Human growth hormone has been localized in a single case of fibroadenoma of the breast and in metastatic breast carcinoma to ovaries [46]. Luteinizing hormone-releasing factor was identified by IP in about one-half of breast carcinomas examined in a small series. Testing with antisera to LH, FSH, and TSH were all negative [47].

The pregnancy specific proteins: human placental lactogen (PL) and pregnancy specific β_1-glycoprotein (SP_1) have also been shown to be present in breast tissue [48] including 30 – 80% of malignant neoplastic cells as judged by IP [49]. One study suggests that negative staining for SP_1 and PL is an indicator for longer survival time [50]. Four other placental-specific tissue glycoproteins (PP_5, PP_{10}, PP_{11}, PP_{12}) extracted from human placentas were positive in approximately 30 – 70% of examined breast cancers [51]. One-third to one-half of other malignant tumors were also positive. PP_5 may also be produced ectopically by benign breast ductal epithelial cells [51].

6. Steroid hormones and their receptors

Normal or hyperplastic breast tissue has the ability to bind estradiol and/or progesterone. About three quarters of human breast carcinomas examined show varying degrees of binding: about one-quarter show no binding. Some tumors show 100% binding to antiestrogen antisera. With antiprogesterone antisera no tumor showed 100% positivity [52, 53]. There is an apparent correlation between the estrogen receptors in tumor cells and the percentage of cells with estradiol binding, the hormone specific staining being due to multiple classes of binding sites [52]. No correlation was seen between estrogen and/or progesterone receptors and histologic type, nodal status, amount of differentiation, endogenous peroxidase or alkaline phosphatase content of breast cancer cells [54, 55]. A second study has shown that the presence or absence of estrogen receptors in breast cancers by IP is correlated with biochemical assays for the same receptors [56]. These receptors in turn have been correlated, in multiple studies, with responsiveness of patients with breast cancer to endocrine manipulation and survival [57–60]. A single study has shown the cytologic localization of estrogen to the cytoplasmic and nuclear membranes of 35–40% of infiltrating duct adenocarcinomas [61].

In addition to estrogen and progesterone receptors there has been some work on other steroid receptors. Papamichail et al. were able to prepare antibodies to purified thymus cytoplasmic glucocorticoid receptors. By IP they were able to detect the receptor and demonstrate its specificity in a variety of normal and neoplastic cells including 100% of the breast carcinomas they examined [62, 63].

7. Oncofetal antigens

Carcinoembryonic antigen (CEA) has been localized within breast carcinoma cells [64–67]. Although CEA positivity was not appreciated in normal breast tissue, vascular endothelium, nor in tissue surrounding a nonstaining carcinoma, there was staining in normal breast ducts adjacent to positive breast carcinoma cells [64]. The same study suggested a lack of correlation between CEA presence and histologic type, lymphocyte infiltration into tumor, nodal metastases, or recurrence. Perhaps somewhat surprisingly a second study showed that patients who had CEA negative tumors (20%) had significantly higher five- (93% vs 29%) and ten- (67% vs 12%) year survival [65]. This difference was not related to stage of disease, post-operative radiotherapy treatment, or histologic type of the primary tumor. On a study of 100 cases, Shousha and Lyssiotis have shown that about two-thirds of breast carcinomas are positive. They noted a significant correlation between CEA positivity and presence of nodal metastases with CEA positivity in 90% of the primary carcinomas that eventually metastasized [66]. They also reported that 7% of dysplastic foci within acini are CEA positive but that low-grade breast malignancies (i.e. medullary and tubular carcinomas) were all CEA negative. It is apparent that the positivity of CEA (or lack of it) and its significance in breast disease is far from settled. Some authors have suggested that malignant tumors of breast are usually negative for CEA whereas benign and normal breast tissue may be positive [68–71]. Because CEA apparently cross reacts with other glycoproteins [72] the answer awaits a large scale multi-institutional cooperative study using a purified standardized antibody preparation.

To the best of our knowledge, other oncofetal antigens have not been reported to be present by IP. One study using a direct peroxidase-labeling IP technique with antibody made against the Regan isoenzyme of alkaline phosphatase (placental alkaline phosphatase) failed to demonstrate the presence of this 'carcinoplacental antigen' in a case of infiltrating duct carcinoma, metastatic to liver [73].

8. Enzymes and other proteins

In the last five years a number of papers have been published looking for the presence of isolated enzymes and other noncollagenous proteins in human neoplastic tissue including those of breast origin. In a study of the isoenzymes of creatine kinase, the β polypeptide subunit was found in normal ductal epithelium of breast, lobular *in situ*, lobular invasive, ductal and medullary adenocarcinoma [74]. A study of intracellular keratin in ductal carcinomas and cystosarcoma phyllodes was negative or weakly positive whereas the myoepithelial cells in fibroadenoma and basal or reserve cells in normal breast tissue showed intense positive staining [75]. Antibodies to keratin may be useful, the authors suggest, in studying the myoepithelial nature of breast carcinomas since the enzyme histochemical method of staining for membrane ATPase activity [76] may not be reliable [77].

Other proteins to which antibodies were prepared and tested by IP include epithelial membrane glycoprotein (EM GP-70) from mammary epithelial cells [78], α_1-acid glycoprotein purified from human breast carcinoma epithelial cells in organ culture [79, 80], colonic mucoprotein antigen [81], zinc glycinate marker antigen [82], Cap I antigen, an aqueous extract of pancreatitic cancer [83], and α1-antichymotrypsin [80]. Antisera to defatted human cream was also prepared which recognizes an epithelial membrane antigen [84]. Mason and Taylor examined the distribution of three iron binding proteins: transferin, ferritin, and lactoferrin, in breast tissue [85]. None of the antibodies made against these antigens showed exclusive staining for malignant breast tissue. Castro and his colleagues were able to identify immunoreactive insulin in six out of six cases of breast cancer examined when the tumor was shown by RIA to contain in the cytosol fraction 20 ng of insulin (or greater)/g of tissue. There was no IP staining in breast stroma, fat, normal breast, mammary dysplasia or breast cancers which produced less than 20 ng of insulin/g of tissue [86].

9. Tumor associated antibody

Building on the observation of Springer and his group [87–89] that normal human serum contains an antibody against malignant but not benign or normal breast tissue, Howard and Taylor have exploited this tumor associated antigen (TAA) in testing its ability to recognize malignant breast tumors [90–94]. This antibody, which is also known as Anti-T, has specificity against a precursor antigen of the MN blood group system. Although this IgM antitumor antibody was first thought not to stain benign lesions, more recent work has shown it to bind to breast myoepithelial cells in both benign and malignant disease [94] as well as in epithelial cells in intraductal epithelial hyperplasia [93] and florid papillomatosis [91].

10. Tissue specific markers

Human breast milk contains innumerable proteins, two of which have been studied by IP in breast disease. Casein (both total and β-casein fraction) has been localized in cases of breast cancer by Bussolati et al. [95]. Casein has also been identified within the neoplastic cells of intraductal carcinomas of the nipple and in intraepidermal cells identifiable as Paget's cells [96]. Staining was also seen in 'normal' epidermal cells of cases of Paget's disease. The possibility was raised that these may represent 'pre-Paget cells.' Casein, like the other proteins previously mentioned, is unfortunately not a tissue specific marker for breast cancer since it has been localized in cells of extramammary Paget's disease [96], other normal tissues like sweat glands of skin [97], and multiple other organ system malignancies [97]. The second 'tissue specific' mammary protein is α lactalbumin, whose presence may be linked to the presence of intact estrogen receptors [98]. Antisera to it, raised in rabbits, stained approximately 50% of primary breast carcinomas, nodal metastases, and adenosis from premenopausal women. In addition, 8% of adjacent normal breast tissue in cases of breast cancer was also stained [99]. The staining varied in intensity and distribution within breast tumors of different histology [99].

Rabbit antidenatured chicken actin has also been studied as a tissue specific marker as has human anti-actin obtained from auto-antibodies to smooth muscle in a patient with chronic hepatitis. Although both antibodies gave similiar results in fresh frozen and post fixed specimens, in fixed, paraffin-embedded tissue only the rabbit anti-actin worked, staining myoepithelial cells of breast tissue in normal, benign, dysplastic, carcinoma-*in situ*, and invasive states [100, 101]. In cases of lobular carcinoma, the distribution of myoepithelial cells (as identified by their positive staining with anti-actin) varied and at least three major patterns of staining were recognized; basket-like, nest-like, and disarranged [102]. In contradistinction to these findings, in cases of ductal CIS the myoepithelial cells either failed to stain or were widely scattered. This destruction of the myoepithelial cell layer occurred irrespective of the presence of an invasive (infiltrative) component [103]. It has been suggested that absence or gaps in the continuity of the lining myoepithelial cells in ducts may help to make the diagnosis of ductal carcinoma-*in situ* [103].

In conclusion, although certain protein products may be associated more closely with breast than other organs, it is apparent that no true tissue specific marker(s) are yet identified for the human breast.

11. Immunoglobulins and lymphocytes

Because of the frailty of surface immunoglobulins and their easy destruction during fixation and paraffin embedding, very few studies have been done with lymphocyte markers in breast disease. In one study concerned with identification of T and B lymphocytes in breast cancer (which was mostly an immunofluorescent study), of

50 consecutive breast cancer cases, T cells were found to be most consistently clustered around tumor nests. In cases of intraductal carcinoma, B cells were also identified in the surrounding lymphocyte population [104]. An interesting case report has been presented which describes in a patient with a 15-year history of a protein-losing enteropathy due to intestinal lymphangiectasia, the development of a stage IV diffuse non-Hodgkin's lymphoma of the breast. By indirect IP this tumor was shown to be of monclonal B cell origin. Both diseases were 'cured' with chemotherapy (10 + years survival) [105]. Schlom and associates prepared a monoclonal antibody to an antigen from mammary carcinoma cells using B lymphocytes from lymph nodes removed during radical mastectomies for infiltrating duct or lobular carcinoma. This IgM antibody stained about 50% of primary tumor cells and detected metastatic malignant cells in lymph nodes. It also recognized some normal mammary epithelial cells, benign tumors, and other non-breast adenocarcinomas [106]. In an IP study from Japan, lymphocytes from breast lesions were studied with anti-human T and B sera. It was found that B cells predominated in benign mammary diseases while T cells predominated in human breast carcinomas. A significant inverse correlation was also identified between intensity of T-cell infiltration and clinical stage and prognosis [107].

12. Collagens and other basement membrane proteins

As breast neoplasms pass from a stage of *in situ* to invasive carcinoma there is apparent dissolution of the basement membrane (BM) as suggested by histochemical staining and by transmission electron microscopy [108–110]. Since the BM has been demonstrated to undergo local dissolution in pathologic states [111–114], we felt it would be interesting to further study the basement membrane in different breast diseases. We did this by performing a immunoperoxidase study on a representative group of human breast lesions using antibodies prepared against two basement membrane components; type IV collagen [115, 116] and laminin, a BM noncollagenous protein [117, 118]. We determined that anti-type IV collagen and antilaminin stain continuously and intensely the BM of the breast ducts and lobules in normal, benign, and intraductal CIS (Figure 1) [15] in agreement with previous nonimmunochemical observations [119]. At sites of microinvasion, though, there was disruption of the BM with thinning and fragmentation [Figure 2]. This was demonstrated by both anti- type IV and anti- laminin staining. Furthermore, in sections of invasive adenocarcinoma and in metastatic foci, no extracellular BM-like structures (other than tiny positive linear segments) were appreciated (Figure 3). Type IV collagen and laminin appeared to accumulate, though diffusely, in the cytoplasm of the malignant cells (Figure 4) [15]. This observation confirms the previous finding of the identification of micrometastases of breast carcinomas by the presence of BM collagen [120, 121]. More recent work has suggested that type V collagen, an additional BM collagen component, has an identical staining pattern (Figure 3) [122].

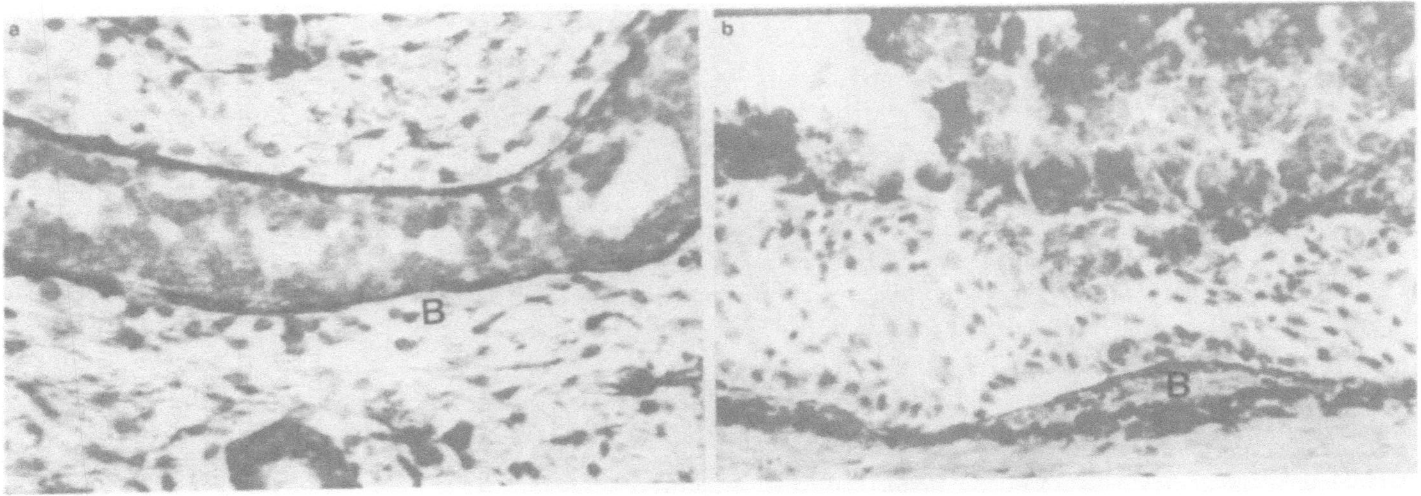

Figure 1. Ducts from both a fibroadenoma (a) and an *in situ* carcinoma (b) show intact basement membrane components as evidenced by immunoperoxidase staining utilizing antibodies to both Type IV collagen and laminin.

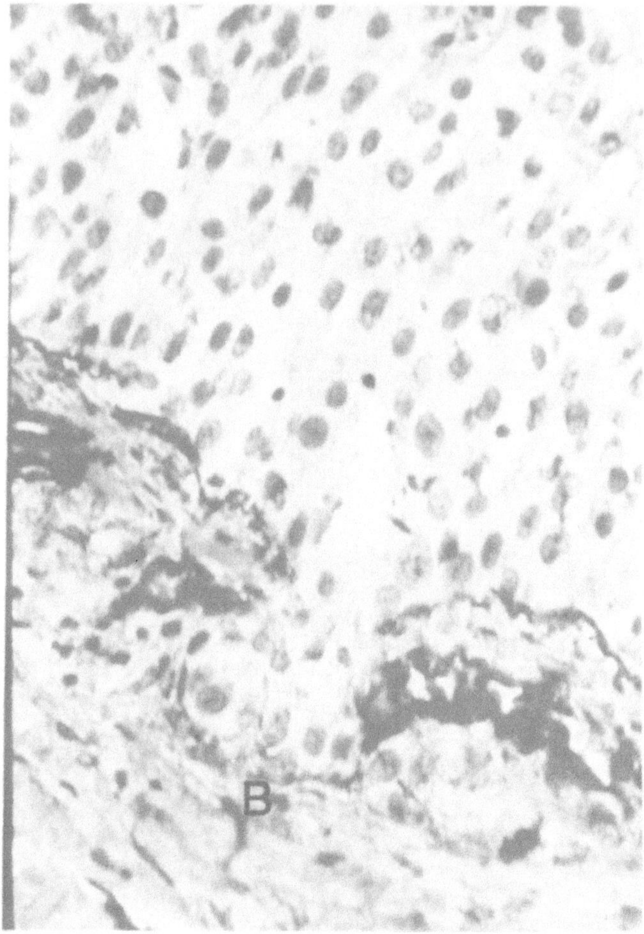

Figure 2. In contrast to Figure 1, fragmentation and disruption of the basement membrane occurs at points of tumor invasion.

The dissolution of the BM and its penetration by tumor cells is believed to occur in many tissues [123–125] including breast [121–127] and is thought to be mediated in large part by enzymatic mechanisms. In one study monospecific antibodies were made to prolyl hydroxylase, an enzyme responsible for the production of hydroxyproline, a key constituent of collagen. By indirect IP this antibody shows localization with strong avidity to the cytoplasm of malignant epithelial cells in 30 of 32 scirrhous ductal carcinomas [128]. Some preliminary observations suggest that a neutral protease which degrades type IV collagen [129] stains the stroma around invasive breast cancer cells (Siegal, Barsky, Garbisa, and Liotta, unpublished observations).

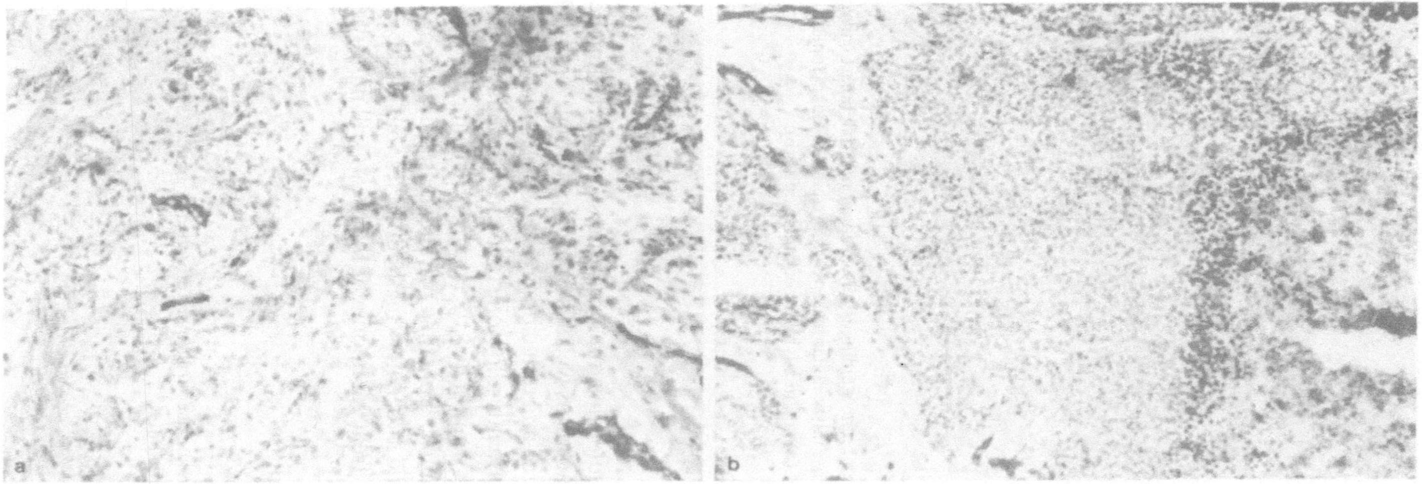

Figure 3. An invasive ductal carcinoma (a) shows no appreciable extracellular basement membrane components. The focal areas of staining represent blood vessels. Similarly a metastatic nodule in the lung (b) shows absence of staining.

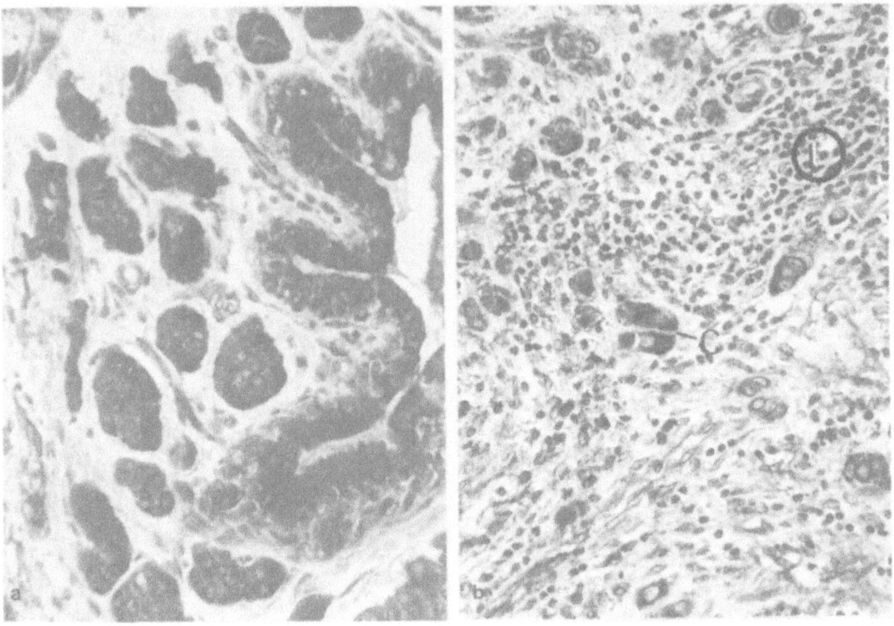

Figure 4. Although extracellular basement membrane staining is absent in all invasive breast cancers tested, the well-differentiated tumors show intense intracellular (cytoplasmic) staining. This cytoplasmic staining is observed both in the primary tumor (a) and in a lymph node metastasis (b).

13. Summary

Immunoperoxidase and other immunolocalization procedures are new techniques which already have shown their diagnostic as well as research potential. Although dozens of antibodies have been prepared and tested on breast lesions, most of these antibodies do not accurately and consistently allow one to separate benign, borderline, and frankly malignant lesions. Antibodies to basement membrane components, however, show the most promise. Hopefully, with increased use of polyclonal and monoclonal antibodies, and other new methodologies, our ability to understand, diagnose, and ultimately treat carcinoma of the breast will improve.

Acknowledgment

The authors gratefully acknowledge the support and encouragement provided by Lance A. Liotta, MD, PhD in whose laboratory this research was carried out.

References

1. Cancer facts and figures. New York: American Cancer Society, 1980.
2. Herberman RB: Immunodiagnosis of cancer in man. In: Cancer control: contemporary views on screening, diagnosis and therapy, Kessler II (ed). Baltimore: University Park Press, 1980.
3. Ceriani RL, Thompson K, Peterson JA, Abraham S: Surface differentiation antigens of human mammary epithelium cells carried on the human milk fat globule. Proc Nat Acad Sci USA 74:582–586, 1977.
4. Braunstein GD, Vaitukaitus JL, Carbone PP, Ross GT: Ectopic production of human chorionic gonadotrophin by neoplasms. Ann Inter Med 78:39–45, 1973.
5. Tormey DC, Waalkes TP, Simon RM: Biological markers in breast carcinoma. II. Clinical correlations with human chorionic gonadotrophin. Cancer 39:2391–2396, 1977.
6. Reddy S, Watkin WB: Uptake of ^{125}I-labelled human placental lactogen and placental lactogen by the tissues of normal and lactating rats. J Endocrinol 65:183–194, 1975.
7. El Etreby MF: Thyroid function in the dog and its possible relationship to mammary tumorigenesis. Pharmacol Ther 5:403–405, 1979.
8. Mesa-Tejada R, Pascal RR, Fenoglio CM: Immunoperoxidase: a sensitive immunohistochemical technique as a 'special stain' in the diagnostic pathology laboratory. Human Pathol 8:313–320, 1977.
9. Taylor CR: Immunoperoxidase techniques: practical and theoretical aspects. Pathol Lab Med 102:113–121, 1978.
10. Mukai K, Rosai J: Applications of immunoperoxidase techniques in surgical pathology. In: Progress in surgical pathology, Fenoglio CM, Wolff M (eds). New York: Masson Publishing, 1980.
11. DeLellis RA, Sternberger LA, Mann RB, Banks PM, Nakane PK: Immunoperoxidase techniques in diagnostic pathology, report of a workshop sponsored by the National Cancer Institute. Am J Clin Path 71:483–488, 1979.
12. DeLellis RA: Diagnostic immunohistochemistry. New York: Masson Publishing, 1981.
13. Sternberger LA: Immunochemistry. New York: John Wiley, 1979.
14. Sternberger LA, Hardy PH, Cuculis JJ, Meyer HG: The unlabeled antibody enzyme method of immunohistochemistry. Preparation and properties of soluble antigen-antibody complex (horseradish peroxidase–antihorseradish peroxidase) and its use in identification of spirochetes. J Histochem Cytochem 18:315–333, 1970.
15. Siegal GP, Barsky SH, Terranova VP, Liotta LA: Stages of neoplastic transformation of human breast tissue as monitored by dissolution of basement membrane components. Invasion and Metastasis 1:54–70, 1981.
16. McDivitt RW, Stewart FW, Berg JW: Tumors of the breast. Atlas of tumor pathology. Second series fascicle 2. Washington DC, AFIP, 1968.
17. Azzopardi JG: Problems in breast pathology. Major problems in pathology 11, Bennington JL (ed). Philadelphia: WB Saunders, 1979.
18. Rosai J: Ackerman's surgical pathology. St. Louis: The CV Mosby Co, 1981.
19. Muller M, Zotter S, Kemmer C: Specificity of human antibodies to intracytoplasmic type-A particles of the murine mammary tumor virus. J Natl Cancer Inst 56:295–303, 1976.
20. Hoshino M, Dmochowski L: Electron microscope study of antigens in cells of mouse mammary tumor cell lines by peroxidase-labeled antibodies in sera of mammary tumor-bearing mice and of patients with breast cancer. Cancer Res 33:2551–2561, 1973.
21. Mesa-Tejada R, Keydar I, Ramanarayanan M, Ohno T, Fenoglio C, Spiegelman S: Immunohistochemical evidence for RNA virus related components in human breast cancer. Ann Clin Lab Sci 9:202–211, 1979.
22. Mesa-Tejada R, Keydar I, Ramanarayanan M, Ohno T, Fenoglio C, Spiegelman S: Detection in human breast carcinomas of an antigen immunologically related to a group-specific antigen of mouse mammary tumor virus. Proc Natl Acad Sci USA 75:1529–1533, 1978.

23. Keydar I, Mesa-Tejada R, Ohno T, Ramanarayanan M, Spiegelman S: The detection in human breast carcinomas of an antigen immunologically related to glycoprotein (GP 52) of the mouse mammary tumor virus. Proc Am Assoc Cancer Res 19:64, 1978.
24. Branwood AM, Mesa-Tejada R, Keydar I, Ramanarayanan M, Ohno T, Fenoglio CM, Spiegelman S: Clinical-pathologic correlations in patients with breast carcinoma expressing immunohistochemically detectable mouse mammary tumor virus-related antigens. Lab Invest 40:242–243, 1979.
25. Mitchell WM, Halter SA, Schuffman SS, Hartman WH: Molecular and morphological evidence for type B retrovirus (oncornavirus) expression in human mammary carcinoma. An overview using scanning electron microscopy, immunoperoxidase staining, and transmission electron microscopy. Scan Electron Microsc 3:1–12, 1980.
26. Mesa-Tejada R, Keydar I, Ramanarayanan M, Ohno T, Fenoglio C, Spiegelman S: Immunohistochemical detection of a cross-reacting virus antigen in mouse mammary tumors and human breast carcinomas. J Histochem Cytochem 26:532–541, 1978.
27. Mesa-Tejada R, Branwood AM, Keydar I, Fenoglio CM, Spiegelman S: Increased incidence of immunohistochemically detectable mouse mammary tumor virus-related antigen in breast carcinoma tissues of patients with a family history of this disease. Proc Am Assoc Cancer Res 20:276, 1979.
28. Spiegelman S, Keydar I, Mesa-Tejada R, Ohno T, Ramanarayanan M, Nayak R, Bausch J, Fenoglio C: Possible diagnostic implications of a mammary tumor virus related protein in human breast cancer. Cancer 46(Suppl):879–892, 1980.
29. Levine PH, Mourali N, Tabbane F, Costa J, Spiegelman S, Mesa-Tejada R, Muenz LR, Bekesi JG: Immunopathologic features of rapidly progressing breast cancer (RPBC) in Tunisia. Proc Am Assoc Cancer Res 21:170, 1980.
30. Ohno T, Ramanarayanan M, Spiegelman S, Feigelson P: The human breast carcinoma antigen is immunologically related to the polypeptide of the group-specific glycoprotein of the mouse mammary tumor virus. Proc Am Assoc Cancer Res 20:277, 1979.
31. Ohno T, Mesa-Tejada R, Keydar I, Ramanarayanan M, Bausch J, Spiegelman S: Human breast carcinoma antigen is immunologically related to the polypeptide of the group-specific glycoprotein of mouse mammary tumor virus. Proc Natl Acad Sci USA 76:2460–2464, 1979.
32. Edgington TS, Leung JP: Mammary tumor glycoprotein, MTGP20: a tumor-specific marker for human breast carcinomas and candidate tumor-specific antigen. Protides Biol Fluid Proc Colloq 27:89–94, 1979.
33. Kameya T, Kuramoto H, Suzuki K, Kenjo T, Oshikiri T, Hayashi H, Itakura M: A human gastric choriocarcinoma cell line with human chorionic gonadotropin and placental alkaline phosphatase production. Cancer Res 35:2025–2032, 1975.
34. Taylor CR, Kurmann RJ, Warner NE: The potential value of immunohistologic techniques in the classification of ovarian and testicular tumors. Hum Pathol 9:417–427, 1978.
35. Buckley CH, Fox H: An immunohistochemical study of the significance of HCG secretion by large bowel adenocarcinoma. J Clin Pathol 32:368–372, 1979.
36. Castro A, Buschbaum P, Nadji M, Voigt W, Tabei S, Morales A: Ectopic human chorionic gonadotropin in breast carcinoma. Experientia 35:1392–1393, 1979.
37. Castro A, Buschbaum P, Nadji M, Voigt W, Tabei S, Morales A: Immunochemical demonstration of human chorionic gonadotropin (hCG) in tissue of breast carcinoma. Acta Endocrinol (Copenhagen) 94:511–516, 1980.
38. Bellet D, Arrang JM, Contesso G, Bohoun PV: Immunohistological and radioimmunological study of the beta subunit of the chorionic gonadotropic hormone: clinical influence. In: Clinical application of carcinoembryonic antigen. Proceedings of a symposium held in Nice (France), Oct. 7–9, 1977, Krebs BP, LaLanne CM, Schneider M (eds). Amsterdam: Excerpta Medica Int Congr Series 439:357–361, 1978.
39. Papamichail M, Tsokos G, Papapetrou P, Tsokos M, Fessas PH: Simultaneous ectopic production

of hormones by human tumors. Exerpta Med Int Ongr Series 484:321–325, 1980.
40. Nadji M, Tabei Z, Castro A, Morales AR: Immunohistochemical demonstration of human chorionic-gonadotropin in mammary-carcinoma. Cancer Treat Rep 63:1183, 1979.
41. Castro A, Nadji M, Tabei S, Voigt W, Morales A: Tissue human chorionic gonadotropin hormone (HCG-beta) in breast cancer. Cancer Treat Rep 63:1183, 1979.
42. Walker RA: Significance of alpha-subunit HCG demonstrated in breast carcinomas by the immunoperoxidase technique. J Clin Pathol 31:245–249, 1978.
43. Cove DH, Smith SCH, Walker R, Howell A: The synthesis of the glycoprotein hormone alpha subunit by human breast carcinomas. Eur J Cancer 15:693–702, 1979.
44. McManus LM, Naughton MA, Martinez-Hernandez A: Human chorionic gonadotropin in human neoplastic cells. Cancer Res 36:3476–3481, 1981.
45. Naughton MA, Merrill DA, McManus LM, Fink LM, Berman E, White MJ, Martinez-Hernandez A: Localization of the β-chain of human chorionic gonadotropin on human tumor cells and placental cells. Cancer Res 35:1887–1890, 1975.
46. Blaustein A, Kaganowicz A, Frantz A, Farkouh N: Ectopic human growth hormone in ovaries and in breast tumors. Lab Invest 40:242, 1979.
47. Seppala M, Wahlstrom T: Identification of luteinizing hormone-releasing factor and alpha subunit of glycoprotein hormones in ductal carcinoma of the mammary gland. Int J Cancer 26:267–268, 1980.
48. Horne CH, Push-Humphreys RG, Bremner RD: Practical and theoretical considerations in the detection and measurement of immunoreactive pregnancy-specific betal-glycoprotein (SP_1) in tumors. In: Carcinoembryonic proteins: chemistry, biology, clinical application. New York: Biomedical Press 1:301–311, 1979.
49. Eiermann W, Brutting G, Prechtel K: Detection of pregnancy specific proteins beta 1-(SP_1) glycoprotein and human placental lactogen in benign breast disease. In: Carcino-embryonic proteins: chemistry, biology, clinical applications, Lehmann FG (ed). New York: Biomedical Press 2:477–480, 1979.
50. Horne CH, Reid IN, Milne GD: Prognostic significance of innappropriate production of pregnancy proteins by breast cancers. Lancet 2:279–282, 1976.
51. Inaba N, Renk T, Wurster K, Rapp W, Bohn H: Ectopic synthesis of pregnancy specific beta 1-glycoprotein (SP_1) and placental specific tissue proteins (PP_5, PP_{10}, PP_{11}, PP_{12}) in nontrophoblastic malignant tumours. Possible markers in oncology. Klin Wochenschr 58:789–791, 1980.
52. Mercer WD, Lippman ME, Wahl TM, Carlson CA, Wahl DA, Lezotte D, Teague PO: The use of immunocytochemical techniques for the detection of steroid hormones in breast cancer cells. Cancer 46:2859–2868, 1980.
53. Mercer W, Wahl T, Carlson C, Teague P: Identification of estrogen and progesterone receptors in breast cancer cells by immunological techniques. Fed Proc 38:913, 1979.
54. Mercer W, Wahl T, Teague P: Identification of estrogen receptors in breast cancer cells by immunological techniques. Proc Am Assoc Cancer Res 20:332, 1979.
55. Mercer WD: The development and application of immunofluorescence and immunoperoxidase techniques for the identification of estrogen and progesterone receptors in human and rat mammary cancer. Diss Abstr Int [B] 39:4807–4808, 1979.
56. Taylor CR, Cooper CL, Kurman RJ, Goebelsmann U, Markland FS, Jr: Detection of estrogen receptor in breast and endometrial carcinoma by the immunoperoxidase technique. Cancer 47:2634–2640, 1981.
57. Jensen EV, Desombre ER, Jungblut PW: Estrogen receptors in hormone responsive tissues and tumors. In: Endogenous factors influencing host-tumor balance, Wissler RW, Dao TL, Wood S (eds). Chicago: Univ of Chicago Press, 1967.
58. McGuire W: Current status of estrogen receptors in human breast cancer. Cancer 36:638–644, 1975.
59. Cook T, George D, Shields R, Maynard P, Griffiths K: Oestrogen receptors and prognosis in early

breast cancer. Lancet 1:995–997, 1979.
60. Furmanski P, Saunders DW, Brooks SC, Rich MA and the breast cancer prognostic study clinical and pathology associates: The prognostic value of estrogen receptor determinations in patients with primary breast cancer. An update. Cancer 46:2794–2796, 1980.
61. Ghosh L, Ghosh BC, Das Gupta TK: Immunocytological localization of estrogen in human mammary carcinoma cells by horseradish-anti-horseradish peroxidase complex. J Surg Oncol 10:221–224, 1978.
62. Papamichail M, Ioanides KD, Tsawdaroglou NH, Sekeris CE: The use of specific antisera to detect glucocorticoid receptors in different cell types. Cancer Treat Rep 63:1146, 1979.
63. Papamichail M, Ioannidis C, Leventakou A, Tsawdaroglou N, Sekeris CE: The detection of glucocorticoid receptors in breast cancer by immunocytochemical and biochemical methods. Exerpta Med Int Congr Ser 484:315–320, 1980.
64. Walker RA: Demonstration of carcinoembryonic antigen in human breast carcinomas by the immunoperoxidase technique. J Clin Pathol 33:356–360, 1980.
65. Shousha S, Lyssiotis T, Godfrey VM, Scheuer PJ: Carcinoembryonic antigen in breast-cancer tissue: a useful prognostic indicator. Br Med J 1:777–779, 1979.
66. Shousha S, Lyssiotis T: Correlation of carcinoembryonic antigen in tissue sections with spread of mammary carcinoma. Histopathol 2:433–447, 1978.
67. Heyderman E, Neville M: A shorter immunoperoxidase technique for the demonstration of CEA and other cell products. J Clin Pathol 30:138–140, 1977.
68. Goldenberg DM, Sharkey RM, Primus FJ: Carcinoembryonic antigen in histopathology: immunoperoxidase staining of conventional tissue sections. J Natl Cancer Inst 57:11–22, 1976.
69. Denk H, Tappeiner G, Eckerstorfer R, Holzner JH: Carcinoembryonic antigen (CEA) in gastrointestinal and extragastrointestinal tumors and its relationship to tumor-cell differentiation. Int J Cancer 10:262–272, 1972.
70. Goldenberg DM, Primus FJ, De Land F: Tumor detection and localization with purified antibodies to carcinoembryonic antigen. In: Immunodiagnosis of Cancer, Herberman RB, McIntire KR (eds). New York: Marcel Dekker, 9 (part 1), 1979, pp 265–304.
71. Shousha S, Lyssiotis T: Granular cell myoblastoma: positive staining for carcinoembryonic antigen. J Clin Pathol 32:219–224, 1979.
72. Isaacson P, Judd MA: Immunohistochemistry of CEA: characterization of cross-reactions with other glycoproteins. Gut 18:779–785, 1977.
73. Miyayama H, Doellgast GJ, Memoli V, Gandbhir L, Fishman WH: Direct immunoperoxidase staining for Regan isoenzyme of alkaline phosphatase in human tumor tissues. Cancer Sep 38:1237–1246, 1976.
74. Wold LE, Li C-Y, Homburger HA: Localization of the B and M polypeptide subunits of creatine kinase in normal and neoplastic human tissues by an immunoperoxidase technic. Am J Clin Pathol 75:327–332, 1981.
75. Schlegel R, Banks-Schlegel S, McLeod JA, Pinkus GS: Immunoperoxidase localization of keratin in human neoplasms. A preliminary survey. Am J Pathol 101:41–50, 1980.
76. Murad TM: A proposed histochemical and electron microscopic classification of human breast cancer according to cell of origin. Cancer 27:288–299, 1971.
77. Bencosme SA, Raymond MJ, Ross RC, Mobbs B, Tsutsumi V, Ortiz H, Gonzalez R, Segura E: A histochemical and ultrastructural study of human breast carcinomas with a view to their classification by cell of origin. Exp Mol Pathol 31:236–247, 1979.
78. Imam A, Laurence DR, Neville AM: Purification, characterization and localization of a major glycoprotein from plasma membrane of human mammary epithelium. Fed Proc 39:550, 1980.
79. Tokes ZA, Gendler SJ, Srouji AH, Silverman LM, Dermer GB: The synthesis of alpha-1-acid glycoprotein by human breast adenocarcinoma. Fed Proc 39:549, 1980.
80. Tokes ZA, Gendler SJ, Silverman LM, Dermer GB: Characterization of glycoproteins synthesized by human breast surgical specimens. Proc Am Assoc Cancer Res 21:23, 1980.

81. Gold DV: Immunoperoxidase localization of colonic mucoprotein antigen in tumors. Proc Am Assoc Cancer Res 21:239, 1980.
82. O'Brien M: Comparison of immunocytochemical localization. Proc Am Assoc Cancer Res 20:401, 1979.
83. Mesa-Tejada R, Bhattacharyya J, Korat E, Fenoglio CM, Klavins JV: A widely crossreacting tumor associated antigen in carcinoma of pancreas. Fed Proc 36:1075, 1977.
84. Heyderman E, Steele K, Ormerod MG: A new antigen on the epithelial membrane: its immunoperoxidase localization in normal and neoplastic tissue. J Clin Pathol 32:35–39, 1979.
85. Mason DY, Taylor CR: Distribution of transferrin, ferritin, and lactoferrin in human tissues. J Clin Pathol 31:316–327, 1978.
86. Castro A, Ziegels-Weissman J, Buschbaum P, Voigt W, Morales A, Nadji M: Immunochemical demonstration of immunoreactive insulin in human breast cancer. Res Commun Chem Pathol Pharmacol 29:171–182, 1980.
87. Springer GF, Desai PR, Banatwala I: Blood group MN antigens and precursors in normal and malignant human breast glandular tissue. J Natl Cancer Inst 54:335–339, 1975.
88. Springer GF, Desai PR, Yang HJ, Murthy MS: Carcinoma-associated blood group MN precursor antigens against which all humans possess antibodies. Clin Immunol Immunopathol 7:426–441, 1977.
89. Springer GF, Desai PR, Murthy MS, Tegtmeye H, Scanlon EF: Human carcinoma-associated precursor antigens of the blood-group MN system and the hosts immune-responses to them. Prog Allergy 26:42–96, 1979.
90. Howard DR, Taylor CR: Immunohistological distinction of benign and malignant breast lesions utilizing antibody present in normal human sera. IRCS Med Sci Cancer 6/7:267, 1978.
91. Howard DR, Taylor CR: A method for distinguishing benign from malignant breast lesions utilizing antibody present in normal human sera. Cancer 43:2279–2287, 1979.
92. Howard DR, Taylor CR: An immunohistologic method for distinguishing benign from malignant lesion of the breast utilizing antibody present in normal human sera. Am J Clin Pathol 72:647, 1979.
93. Howard DR, Taylor CR: The significance of myoepithelial cell staining by an anti-tumor antibody in breast disease. Breast 6:10–15, 1980.
94. Howard DR, Taylor CR: An antitumor antibody in normal human serum: reaction of anti-T with breast carcinoma cells. Oncology 37:142–148, 1980.
95. Eusebi V, Betts CM, Bussolati G: Tubular carcinoma a variant of secretory breast carcinoma. Histopathol 3:407–419, 1979.
96. Bussolati G, Pich A: Mammary and extramammary Paget's disease. Am J Pathol 80:117–128, 1975.
97. Pich A, Bussolati G, Carbonara A: Immunocytochemical detection of casein and casein-like proteins in human tissues. J Histochem Cytochem 24:940–947, 1976.
98. Woods KL, Cove DH, Howell A: Predictive classification of human breast carcinomas based on lactalbumin synthesis. Lancet 2:14–16, 1977.
99. Walker RA: The demonstration of alpha lactalbumin in human breast carcinomas. J Pathol 129:37–42, 1979.
100. Bussolati G, Bonfanti S, Weber K, Osborn M: Staining of myoepithelial cells in fixed and embedded tissues by immunocytochemical techniques using antibodies to actin. Riv Istochim Norm Pathol 22:387–390, 1978.
101. Bussolati G, Alfani V, Weber K, Osborn M: Immunocytochemical detection of actin on fixed and embedded tissues: its potential use in routine pathology. J Histochem Cytochem 28:169–173, 1980.
102. Bussolati G: Actin-rich (myoepithelial) cells in lobular carcinoma *in situ* of the breast. Virchows Archiv B Cell Pathol 32:165–176, 1980.
103. Bussolati G, Botta G, Gugliotta P: Actin-rich (myoepithelial) cells in ductal carcinoma-*in-situ* of the breast. Virchows Archiv B Cell Pathol 34:251–259, 1980.

104. Schoorl R, Riviere AB, Borne AE, Feltkamp-Vroom TM: Identification of T and B lymphocytes in human breast cancer with immunohistochemical techniques. Am J Pathol 84:529–544, 1976.
105. Broder S, Callihan TR, Jaffe ES, DeVita VT, Strober W, Bartter FC, Waldmann TA: Resolution of longstanding protein-losing enteropathy in a patient with intestinal lymphangietasia after treatment for malignant lymphoma. Gastroenterology 80:166–168, 1981.
106. Schlom J, Wunderlich D, Teramoto YA: Generation of human monoclonal antibodies reactive with human mammary carcinoma cells. Proc Natl Acad Sci USA 77:6841–6845, 1980.
107. Shimokawara I, Imamura M: Identification and the significance of lymphocyte subpopulations in human breast cancer. An immunoperoxidase study with anti-human T and B cell sera. Sapporo Med J 48:453–474, 1979.
108. Ozzello L: The behavior of basement membranes in intraductal carcinoma of the breast. Am J Path 35:887–899, 1959.
109. Ozzello L, Speer FD: The mucopolysaccharides in the normal and diseased breast. Their distribution and significance. Am J Path 34:993–1009, 1958.
110. Ahmed A: Atlas of the ultrastructure of human breast diseases. London: Churchill Livingstone, 1978.
111. Babai F: Etude ultrastructural sur la pathogénie de l'invasion du muscle strié par des tumeurs transplantables. J Ultrastr Res 56:287–303, 1976.
112. Rubio CA, Biberfeld P: The basement membrane of the uterine cervix in dysplasia and squamous carcinoma: an immunofluorescent study with antibodies to basement membrane antigen. Acta Pathol Microbiol Scand A 83:744–748, 1975.
113. Birbeck MSC, Wheatley DN: An electron microscopic study of the invasion of ascites tumor cells into the abdominal wall. Cancer Res 25:490–497, 1965.
114. Wallace AC, Chew E, Jones DS: The arrest and extravasation of cancer cells in the lung. In: Pulmonary metastasis, Weiss L, Gilbert HA (eds). Boston: GK Hall, 1978, 3pp:26–42.
115. Yaoita H, Foidart JM, Katz SI: Localization of the collagenous component in skin basement membrane. J Invest Dermatol 70:191–193, 1978.
116. Garbisa S, Liotta LA, Tryggvason K, Siegal GP: Antibodies to collagenase-resistant terminal regions of pro-type IV collagen recognize whole basement membrane and 7S collagen. FEBS Lett 127:257–262, 1981.
117. Timpl R, Rhode H, Gehron-Robey P, Rennard S, Foidart JM, Martin GR: Laminin-a glycoprotein of basement membranes. J Biol Chem 254:9933–9937, 1979.
118. Terranova VP, Rohrbach DH, Martin GR: Role of laminin in the attachment of PAM 212 (epithelial) cells to basement membrane collagen. Cell 22:719–726, 1980.
119. Flotte TJ, Bell DA, Greco MA: Tubular carcinoma and sclerosing adenosis. Am J Surg Path 4:75–77, 1980.
120. Foidart JM, Liotta LA, Gehron-Robey P, Martin GR: Immunoperoxidase localization of basement membrane collagen in primary and metastatic human breast carcinoma. Fed Proc 38:1407, 1979.
121. Liotta LA, Foidart JM, Gehron-Robey P, Martin GR, Guillino PM: Identification of micrometastasis of breast carcinomas by presence of basement membrane collagen. Lancet 1:146–147, 1979.
122. Barsky SH, Siegal GP, Brundage RA, Liotta LA: Deposition of type V collagen in benign and malignant breast tissue (in preparation).
123. Liotta LA, Kleinerman J, Catanzaro P, Rynbrandt D: Degradation of basement membrane by murine tumor cells. J Natl Cancer Inst 58:1427–1431, 1977.
124. Liotta LA, Abe S, Gerhon-Robey P, Martin GR: Preferential digestion of basement membrane collagen by an enzyme derived from a metastatic murine tumor. Proc Natl Acad Sci USA 76:2268–2272, 1979.
125. Liotta LA, Lanzer WL, Garbisa S: Identification of a type V collagenolytic enzyme. Biochem Biophys Res Com 98:184–190, 1981.
126. Sadove AM, Kuettner KE: Inhibition of mammary carcinoma invasiveness with cartilage-derived

inhibitor. Surg Forum 28:499–501, 1977.
127. Poole AR, Tiltman KJ, Recklies AD, Stoker TAM: Differences in secretion of the proteinase cethepsin B at the edges of human breast carcinomas and fibroadenomas. Nature 273:545–547, 1978.
128. Al-Adnani MS, Kirrane JA, McGee JO: Inappropriate production of collagen and propyl hydroxylase by human breast cancer cells *in vivo*. Br J Cancer 31:653–660, 1975.
129. Liotta LA, Tryggvason K, Garbisa S, Gehron-Robey P, Abe S: Partial purification and characterization of a neutral protease which cleaves type IV collagen. Biochemistry 20:100–104, 1981.

INDEX